Clinical Management of the Rheumatoid Hand, Wrist, and Elbow

Kevin C. Chung
Editor

Clinical Management of the Rheumatoid Hand, Wrist, and Elbow

Springer

Editor
Kevin C. Chung, MD, MS
Comprehensive Hand Center
Section of Plastic Surgery
Department of Surgery
The University of Michigan Health System
Ann Arbor, MI, USA

Videos can also be accessed at
http://link.springer.com/book/10.1007/978-3-319-26660-2

ISBN 978-3-319-26658-9 ISBN 978-3-319-26660-2 (eBook)
DOI 10.1007/978-3-319-26660-2

Library of Congress Control Number: 2016933477

Springer Cham Heidelberg New York Dordrecht London

Printed on acid-free paper

Springer International Publishing AG Switzerland is part of Springer Science+Business Media (www.springer.com)

To Chin-yin and William for their encouragement and support in making this textbook a reality

Preface

Caring for the rheumatoid patient has been an integral part of a hand surgeon's practice. In the course of the last two decades, improvement in medical management by having innovative medications such as the biologic disease-modifying drugs has markedly decreased the rate of surgery for rheumatoid patients. These biologic medications are highly effective in decreasing synovitis and deformities that were commonly seen prior to the introduction of these medications. However, the success in applying biologics for rheumatoid arthritis does not diminish the role of surgeons in performing reconstructive procedures because some patients may be refractory to these medications, whereas others may have a delay in developing the typical deformities that invariably may still develop over time.

Rheumatoid arthritis is a worldwide disease. Many countries cannot afford the use of these highly expensive biologic medications, and surgical expertise is still needed to restore hand function. Training in the rheumatoid hand is much needed in Eastern Europe, Asia, and South America where the care of the rheumatoid hand is still in its infancy. This much anticipated textbook on the care of rheumatoid arthritis is the first of its kind, by including contributions from world experts on the care of the rheumatoid hand. All the authors and I strive to present concepts in reconstructing the rheumatoid hand, wrist, and the elbow. Additionally, we feel the care of rheumatoid arthritis patients is a collaborative effort between rheumatologists and surgeons in combating the devastating effect of this disease on our patients' quality of life. We are indebted to our rheumatology colleagues in sharing their expertise with us in this seminal textbook.

This textbook is an invaluable teaching tool for the new generation of surgeons and rheumatologists who may not have sufficient experience in evaluating and treating rheumatoid patients with these deformities that are becoming much less common in the developed world. Similarly, for those countries that still do not have the resources for intensive and costly medical treatment, understanding the pathophysiology, anatomy, and outcomes of surgical treatment is critical in the evaluation and care for the rheumatoid population. Furthermore, this textbook can be helpful to rheumatologists who should also understand surgical possibilities so that they can refer patients for surgical consultation in the early phase of the disease rather than when the deformities are so severe that options are limited.

All of the esteemed authors in this volume have made the care of rheumatoid arthritis a key component of their practices. I asked the authors to present unbiased opinions that are evidence based to share with the world the current concepts in the management of rheumatoid patients. I would very much like to acknowledge my development editor, Connie Walsh, at Springer for her dedicated stewardship of this textbook. Furthermore, I am indebted to my research assistant, Alexandra Mathews, whose guidance and care of this manuscript is unparalleled. I am grateful to my rheumatology patients who entrusted their care to me, and I am equally appreciative of my long-term rheumatology friend, Dr. David Fox, Chief of Rheumatology, University of Michigan, and his faculty who embraced me in conducting evidence-based outcomes research for the past two decades. Our friendship and collaboration is a testament of the combined effort between specialties to provide our patients with comprehensive care. This volume strives to demystify the care of the rheumatoid patient for rheumatologists and surgeons until such time when a cure is found for this disease.

Ann Arbor, MI, USA Kevin C. Chung

Contents

Contributors

Brian D. Adams, MD Department of Orthopedic Surgery, Baylor College of Medicine, Houston, TX, USA

Joshua M. Adkinson, MD Department of Surgery, Division of Plastic Surgery, Ann and Robert H. Lurie Children's Hospital of Chicago, Northwestern University Feinberg, School of Medicine, Chicago, IL, USA

Gregory Ian Bain, MBBS, FRACS, PhD Department of Orthopaedic Surgery, Flinders University, Adelaide, SA, Australia

Philippe Bellemère, MD Clinique Jeanne d'Arc, Institut de la Main Nantes Atlantique, Nantes, France

Prospero Bigazzi, MD, PhD Orthopaedics, Division of Hand Surgery and Microsurgery, Azienda Ospedaliero-Universitaria Careggi, Florence, Italy

Michel E.H. Boeckstyns, MD Clinic for Hand Surgery, Gentofte Hospital, University of Copenhagen, Hellerup, Denmark

Matthew Brown, MD The University of Michigan Medical School, Ann Arbor, MI, USA

Massimo Ceruso, MD Orthopaedics, Division of Hand Surgery and Microsurgery, Azienda Ospedaliero-Universitaria Careggi, Florence, Italy

Kevin C. Chung, MD, MS Comprehensive Hand Center, Section of Plastic Surgery, Department of Surgery, The University of Michigan Health System, Ann Arbor, MI, USA

Thomas Clifton, MBBS, BA Orthopaedics, Royal Adelaide Hospital, Adelaide, SA, Australia

John J. Costi, BEng (Mech, Hons), PhD, FIEAust Biomechanics and Implants Research Group, The Medical Device Research Institute; School of Computer Science, Engineering and Mathematics, Flinders University, Adelaide, SA, Australia

David A. Fox, MD Internal Medicine, Division of Rheumatology, University of Michigan, Ann Arbor, MI, USA

Michael C. Glanzmann, MD Orthopaedics Upper Extremities, Schulthess Clinic Zurich, Zurich, Switzerland

Daniel Herren, MD, MHA Hand Surgery, Schulthess Klinik, Zurich, Switzerland

Guillaume Herzberg, MD, PhD Orthopaedics, Herriot Lyon France, Lyon, France

Pak-cheong Ho, FHKCOS, FHKAM(Orth), FRCS(Edin) Department of Orthopaedics and Traumatology, Prince of Wales Hospital, Hong Kong, SAR, China

Hajime Ishikawa, MD, PhD Rheumatology, Niigata Rheumatic Center, Shibata, Niigata, Japan

Shepard P. Johnson, MBBS Department of Surgery, St. Joseph Mercy Ann Arbor, Ann Arbor, MI, USA

Philippe Kopylov, MD, PhD Department of Orthopedics, Central Hospital Kristianstad, Kristianstad, Sweden

Jeganath Krishnan, MBBS, FRACS, PhD Department of Orthopaedic Surgery, Flinders University, Adelaide, SA, Australia

Alberto Lluch, MD, PhD Department of Orthopaedic Surgery, Surgery of the Hand and Upper Extremity, Institut Kaplan, Barcelona, Spain

Alexandra L. Mathews, BS Section of Plastic Surgery, Department of Surgery, The University of Michigan Health System, Ann Arbor, MI, USA

Nathan T. Morrell, MD Department of Orthopaedics & Rehabilitation, University of Vermont, Burlington, VT, USA

Takeshi Ogawa, MD, PhD Department of Orthopaedic Surgery and Sports Medicine, Tsukuba University Hospital, Mito Clinical Education and Training Center, Mito, Ibaraki, Japan

Vladimir M. Ognenovski, MD Internal Medicine, Division of Rheumatology, University of Michigan, Ann Arbor, MI, USA

Alfredo Olazábal, MD Department of Orthopaedics, Hospital Aleman Buenos Aires, Buenos Aires, Argentina

Sandra Pfanner, MD Orthopaedics, Division of Hand Surgery and Microsurgery, Azienda Ospedaliero-Universitaria Careggi, Florence, Italy

Marco Rizzo, MD Department of Orthopedic Surgery, Mayo Clinic, Rochester, MN, USA

Hans-Kaspar Schwyzer, MD Orthopaedics Upper Extremities, Schulthess Clinic Zurich, Zurich, Switzerland

Erika D. Sears, MD, MS Comprehensive Hand Center, Section of Plastic Surgery, Department of Surgery, The University of Michigan Health System, Ann Arbor, MI, USA

Magnus Tägil, MD, PhD Department of Orthopedics, Lund University Hospital, Lund, Sweden

Jennifer F. Waljee, MD, MS Comprehensive Hand Center, Section of Plastic Surgery, Department of Surgery, The University of Michigan Health System, Ann Arbor, MI, USA

Arnold-Peter C. Weiss, MD Department of Orthopaedics, Brown University/ Rhode Island Hospital, Providence, RI, USA

Clara Wong Wing Yee, FRCSEd(Orth), FHKCOS, FHKAM(Orth) Department of Orthopaedics and Traumatology, Prince of Wales Hospital, Shatin, Hong Kong, SAR, China

Part I

Background Concepts

Advances in the Medical Treatment of RA: What Surgeons Need to Know

1

Daniel Herren

Introduction

Nothing has changed the face of rheumatoid arthritis (RA) as much as the medications that help to control the inflammatory aspects of the disease and reduce joint and soft tissue destruction in most patients. The biologics have also changed the pattern of disease encountered by surgeons, as reflected in the type and number of interventions now performed. Because biologics not only act locally but also have a significant impact on the patient's immune system, they affect both the surgical treatment itself and patient management before, during, and after surgery. Special precautions are needed to avoid endangering the patient. An understanding of the basic pathophysiological mechanism in RARA improves the quality of surgical indications and the management of this complex patient group. This chapter will focus on the pathogenesis of the disease, possible treatment regimens, and their effects on surgical treatment. In addition, it will address the current trends in surgical treatment imposed by the new medications.

D. Herren, MD, MHA (✉)
Hand Surgery, Schulthess Klinik,
Lengghalde 2, Zurich 8008, Switzerland
e-mail: Daniel.Herren@kws.ch

Pathophysiology of RA

RA is best characterized as an immune-mediated inflammatory disease [1]. It is the most common inflammatory arthritis and affects about 1 % of the population. The disease seems to be initiated by a complex combination of genetic predisposition and unknown extrinsic factors [2–4]. Although a genetic effect is likely, its exact influence is still unclear. Even in monozygotic twins, the range of concordance is only 15–35 %. Regarding extrinsic factors, smoking seems to be a significant risk factor for triggering the disease. Bacterial infection has often been cited as a possible cause of RA but it has never been proven to be the single driving factor.

The main tissue involved in RA is the synovial membrane in joints and around tendons. In RA, the synovial membrane is hypertrophied in all its layers, is heavily infiltrated by inflammatory cells, and shows angiogenesis. The hypertrophied synovium, also called pannus, erodes cartilage and bone to leave significant defects. The driving cytokines in this process are interleukin-1 (IL-1) and tumor necrosis factor alpha (TNFα) [5–7]. Bone destruction is mainly driven by macrophage-induced osteoclast activation. A major development in the identification and prognostic factors of RA was the detection of antibodies to cyclic citrullinated peptides (anti-CCP), which are part of the autoimmune reaction. The presence of anti-CCP is more than 98 % specific for

K.C. Chung (ed.), *Clinical Management of the Rheumatoid Hand, Wrist, and Elbow*,
DOI 10.1007/978-3-319-26660-2_1

the diagnosis of RA and generally represents a more aggressive phenotype of the disease. Although not all patients with RA develop anti-CCP, at the other extreme, these antibodies can be present up to 15 years before the first clinical symptoms. Rheumatoid factors are less specific for RA and are also found in other chronic inflammatory diseases, such as hepatitis C and tuberculosis.

The most important inflammatory mediators in RA are cytokines, including IL-1, IL-6, and TNF. These cytokines are released in the synovial membrane and are responsible for many systemic manifestations of the disease, as well as cause local destructive processes in bone and cartilage [6, 7].

There are many different pathways leading to this disease and no single disease agent that explains the pathogenesis. Interleukins, T and B cells, and macrophages interact in a complex manner to initiate and sustain the inflammatory process. This probably explains the different success rates of the various pharmaceutical agents. Even years before the clinical onset of disease, there may be raised levels of autoantibodies and cytokines in the blood.

Knowledge of the complex interactions between the different cell mediators has increased significantly over the last decade, which facilitates the development of new therapeutic approaches including biologics. The multiple immunological and inflammatory pathways that seem to be active in RA might explain the efficacy of different medications.

Medical Treatment of RA

The goal in treating RA is to gain control over the inflammatory processes in the synovial membrane and prevent joint destruction. The common principles that guide management strategies and the choice of medications have been derived from an increased understanding of the disease and from evidence provided by clinical trials and other studies. These strategies include approaches directed at achieving remission or low disease activity by more rapid and sustained control of the inflammation and by initiating disease-modifying antirheumatic drug (DMARD) therapy early in the course of disease. The fact that the inflammatory pathways may already be active some years before the disease is clinically active underlines the importance of early and aggressive control with agents that efficiently inhibit the devastating inflammatory process [8]. The anti-inflammatory potency of the different drugs can be defined in a therapeutic pyramid. The first stage of pharmacotherapy includes nonsteroidal anti-inflammatory drugs (NSAIDs) which mainly act as prostaglandin synthesis blockers. The next level consists of glucocorticosteroids, and then come the disease-modifying antirheumatic drugs. As well as having anti-inflammatory effects, corticosteroids act by an immunosuppressive mechanism in RA. The anti-inflammatory effects are seen on all cells involved in the inflammatory process and suppression of cell-mediated immunity is similarly nonspecific for the disease. Methotrexate (MTX) is the best-known and most popular DMARD. It acts as an antimetabolite in the form of a folic acid analogue. Its main effect in RA depends on the inhibition of T cells. Liver function should be monitored regularly because of its hepatotoxicity. MTX is often used in combination with corticosteroids and together with certain biologics in newer treatment regimens. There are also recent trends to use MTX in patients with severe forms of inflammatory osteoarthritis.

Sulfasalazine is another popular DMARD. It is also used in inflammatory bowel disease, including ulcerative colitis and Crohn disease. The precise reasons why sulfasalazine is effective in various forms of arthritis are not clearly understood.

Chloroquine is the third classic drug in the triad of DMARDs; it seems to be most effective in combination with MTX and possibly as triple therapy with sulfasalazine and MTX. It was originally developed as an antimalarial medication but proved to inhibit lymphocyte proliferation in RA.

Biologics, at the next level in the RA medication pyramid, were developed in the late 1990s. Their name stems from the way in which they are synthesized, as genetically engineered proteins derived from human genes [9]. Infliximab (Remicade®) [10] was the first monoclonal antibody against TNFα in clinical use. Other commonly used drugs acting in this way include etanercept (Enbrel®) and adalimumab (Humira®). TNFα inhibitors are the first-line treatment after DMARD failure. All the other biologics are not usually considered unless the therapeutic effects of anti-TNFα are not sufficient. Several targets besides TNFα are used to combat the complex inflammatory process in RA. Medication includes IL-6 blocking agents. Tocilizumab (Actemra®) is one of the most popular exponents of this class. It is often combined with MTX but can also be used as monotherapy in cases of intolerance or contraindications to MTX. Another mechanism of action is found in B-cell inhibitors such as rituximab (MabThera®). First developed as cancer therapy, it showed good effects in RA patients and also proved safe in long-term treatment. Other modes of action are found with T-cell inhibitors such as abatacept (Orencia®) and the IL-1 inhibitor anakinra (Kineret®). This last-mentioned biologic is approved only in combination with MTX. Figure 1.1 shows the different modes of action.

The newest developments are the biosimilars. These drugs are based on the different action modes of existing biologics. Because the older generation of these drugs no longer has patent protection, the biosimilars are copying the mode of action, but the biogenetical engineering is different and cheaper. With this group of pharmaceuticals, a parallel market is opened, similar to generic drugs.

Even without complete remission, most patients experience a substantial reduction in their physical disabilities, with significant pain relief 2–3 months after starting medication. The average cost of biologics is up to USD2000 per month, compared with about USD70 per month for MTX alone. In order to justify the high costs, prediction of the individual response to treatment has become a major clinical challenge in RA.

There is some evidence of biomarkers that predict the response to biopharmaceuticals [11]. Identifying and monitoring these biomarkers could enhance the efficacy of medical treatment significantly. On the other hand, the existence of these antibodies might also explain why some people are nonresponders. Knowing these patients' bioprofiles would help to choose the potentially most effective drug on an individual basis. There is also some evidence that the effects of biologics diminish with time. One of the reasons for this may be antibody production against the artificially administered antibodies.

Ideally, the goal of all of these drugs is remission of the disease, which is defined as the absence of disease activity but with the possibility of return [9, 12, 13]. The remission rate of all these biological substances is around 50 %, compared with a remission rate of around 30 % for MTX alone. Even in remission, however, it is recommended that biologics are continued at a reduced dosage instead of switching to MTX or placebo [14, 15].

There is an ongoing debate about the efficacy of the different biologics and their comparison with classic DMARDs. A recent study from China showed that traditional DMARDs were the most cost-effective in terms of improving quality of life, as measured with QALYs. There were big differences in the costs of biologics, ranging from USD26,000 to USD77,000 per QALY [16].

The adverse effects observed in RA patients treated with biologics are another concern [17, 18]. Besides the general adverse reactions, surgeons are especially interested in the discussion about possible increases in surgical site infections when immunosuppressants are administered in RA. Classic adverse reactions to MTX and even more to biologics include infections with opportunistic pathogens such as atypical fungi and mycobacteria. An increased risk of malignancies including melanoma is also suspected. Because the incidence of these adverse reactions is still low, most studies lack sufficient statistical power to provide evidence of a strong correlation. The increasing number of patients being treated with this type of medication will result in greater knowledge concerning the outcomes of long term treatment. This fact underlines the importance of collecting data from patient cohorts in large-scale studies and ideally in the form of a registry [19].

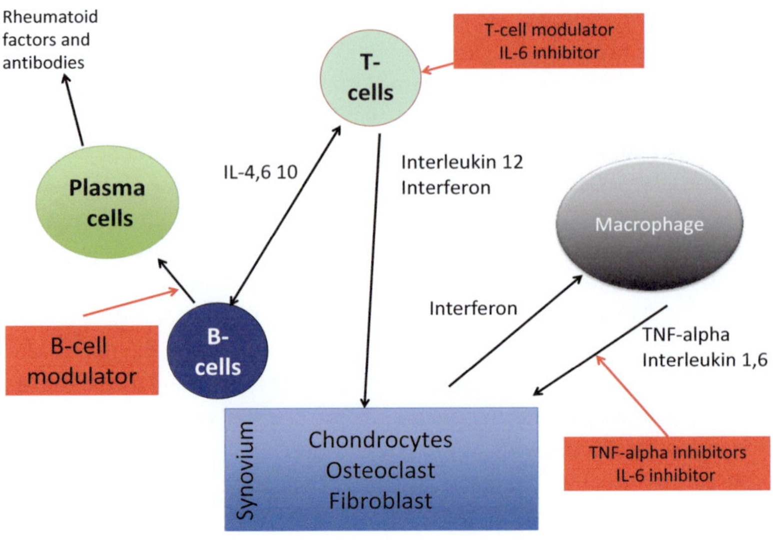

Fig. 1.1 Involved cellular elements in rheumatoid arthritis and the different drug interaction points

Risk of Infection Under Different Immunosuppressive Drugs

Although several studies and long-standing personal experience show that MTX, even in combination with corticosteroids, does not increase the risk of surgical site infections, there are major concerns about the use of biologics in a perioperative setting [20]. In their review, Polachek et al. 2012, concluded that it seems safe to use anti-TNFα and IL-6 receptor blockers during surgical interventions in RA [21]. They admitted, however, that most studies have small sample sizes, retrospective designs, and differ in the groups compared. In 2011, the Japanese orthopedic association committee on arthritis [22] published data on a large cohort of RA patients undergoing joint arthroplasty. They found a twofold risk of surgical site infection for patients on biologics, although the absolute number of infections (2.1 %) was still relatively small. In a study published by Scherrer et al. [23] analyzing 48,000 cases of degenerative arthritis orthopedic interventions versus 2500 operations in patients suffering an inflammatory rheumatic disease in one center, they showed an operation-related infection risk that was 2× higher in the inflammatory patients. The highest infection rates were in elbow (4.3 %) and foot surgery (3.4 %), whereas in the hand surgical procedures the infection rate was 0.5 %. The risk was especially high if the last dose of anti-TNFα was given less than one administration interval before surgery. In addition, patients with multiple conventional disease-modifying antirheumatic drugs had also increased rates of infections. In conclusion, the authors recommended mandatory careful planning of the discontinuation of the immunosuppressive therapy, especially in TNFα inhibitors with long administration interval. It was advised to wait at least one administration interval after the last dose before undertaking the planned orthopedic surgery. Table 1.1 shows examples of the administration times of different biologics. Figure 1.2 visualizes the time frame of drug interruption around an orthopedic procedure.

Based on these studies and personal experience, there is an informal expert consensus that interruption of the biological therapy is advisable for major surgical interventions such as joint replacement surgery, especially of larger joints [21, 22, 24–27]. There is some debate as to whether corticosteroids and/or MTX should be given in the perioperative phase in order to reduce the chances of disease flare-up. Interruption of biologics prior to surgery should be managed according to the administration time of the medication. Usually one cycle is omitted

Table 1.1 Administration interval of different biologicals according to the manufacturer

Agent	Drug	Action point	Dosage	Administration interval
Etanercept	Enbrel®	TNFα	25 mg	3.5 days
Etanercept	Enbrel®	TNFα	50 mg	7.0 days
Adalimumab	Humira®	TNFα	40 mg	14.0 days
Infliximab	Remicade®	TNFα	n.KG	56.0 days
Golimumab	Simponi®	TNFα	50 mg	30.0 days
Certolizumab pegol	Cimzia®	TNFα	200 mg	14.0 days
Certolizumab pegol	Cimzia®	TNFα	400 mg	28.0 days
Tocilizumab	Actemra®	IL-6	n.KG	28.0 days
Abatacept	Orencia®	T cell	n.KG	28.0 days

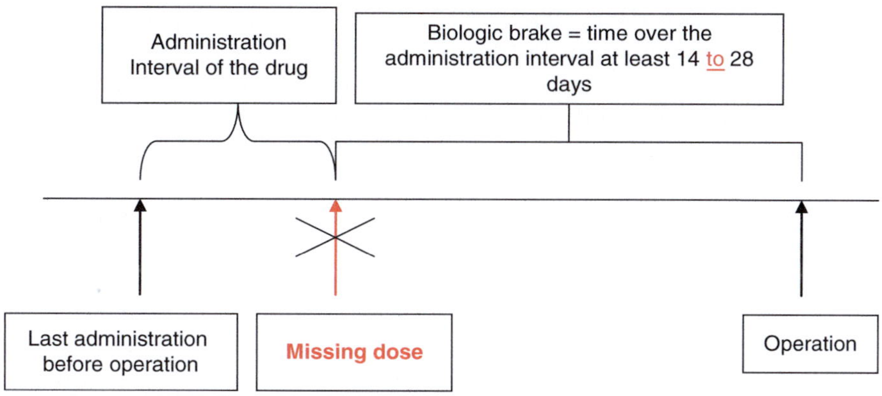

Fig. 1.2 Schematic time frame for the application of biologics around orthopedic surgical procedures

prior to surgery. According to the work of Scherrer et al. [23], another biologic break of 14–28 days is recommended to be sure the immunosuppressive action is worn out. The medication is restarted after the delay of another cycle or once wound healing is assured. However there are no precise data on this management.

Changes in Surgical Intervention Patterns Due to Improved Medical Treatment

Clinical observations indicate that the course of disease in patients with RA has become milder during the past decade. Less severe symptoms, as well as the diminishing need for orthopedic interventions, are most likely the result of the more potent drugs described previously in this chapter. There is an ongoing debate whether the type and frequency of surgical intervention have changed significantly in RA patients in recent years. Because the hand is still the main treatment target in these patients, as the hand is affected in almost 90 % of patients 10 years after the onset of disease, it can be used as an index intervention. Several studies [28, 29] have indicated a decline in the number of orthopedic interventions in RA patients over the last two decades, whereas the number of procedures in osteoarthritic patients has increased dramatically. Soft tissue procedures in RA patients in larger joints have become rare in western societies with wide access to the new treatment regimens. The number of hand and foot interventions has declined as well in the western world [29, 30]. However, there are reports of possible changes in that trend, especially in Japan. In contrast to the observations in Europe, Momohara et al. [31] found a decline in large joint replacements whereas the number of wrist and foot arthroplasties gradually increased. There are various possible explanations for this phenomenon. One possible explanation is that the new medications improve the patients' quality of life, which in turn increases their level of participation in social activities and work. These highly motivated patients place greater demands on both the functionality and the appearance of their hands and feet, so tend to seek surgical assistance more often. The appearance of the hands, as well as the feet, has a high value in societies like the Japanese, and deformities can lead to social isolation. The aesthetic aspects of these interventions should therefore not be underestimated, as shown by Chung et al. [32]. Another explanation could be the fact that fewer than 50 % of patients go into complete remission. Residual synovitis of one or more joints or tendons in the hands and/or the feet can often be observed in the remaining individuals. This leads to a further clinical observation in patients being treated with biologics: ongoing destruction of the joints, especially the wrist, has been noted in a number of patients. Despite good pain relief, the process seems to continue and can cause remarkable destruction. This process could, in fact, be called "silent destruction." Regular clinical and radiographic monitoring is therefore advisable, even in patients showing a good pain response [33].

Not only has the number of surgical interventions changed since the introduction of the new medications but also the type of procedure. Previously common procedures such as wrist fusion and metacarpophalangeal arthroplasties have become rare nowadays, whereas other surgical interventions, including wrist arthroplasties and PIP replacements, are now seen more often in RA patients. Motomiya et al. 2013 reported differences in the clinical and radiographic appearance of patients treated successfully with biologics [34]. The radiographs started to look more like those of people with osteoarthritis than those of patients with chronic inflammatory disease. On the one hand, this has changed the indications for certain interventions because good medication has the potential to improve surgical results in the long term. In particular, interventions such as partial wrist fusion rely on stable inflammatory conditions in order to maximize the results and guarantee the best possible long-term effects. Interventions such as wrist arthroplasty have therefore regained their popularity, not only with the development of new implants but also because less aggressive bone destruction allows better fixation of such devices.

It seems that soft tissue reactions to the new medications are unevenly distributed among the different anatomical areas. It is not uncommon for only certain anatomical regions to show residual synovitis, whereas other regions are in long-term remission. Why this pattern is seen more often in patients on biologics is still not clear. One possible explanation might again be the fact that different cell mediators are involved in the inflammatory processes and they may not be distributed evenly [35]. Together with possible intrinsic or extrinsic mechanical factors, there may be differences in the synovial inflammatory processes. This is all speculation and further studies still need to be performed, especially in the group of nonresponders, in order to explain this observation.

It is questionable how these trends will develop in the future. It may be that increasing numbers of patients who develop antibodies against one or more of these medications will once again necessitate more surgical interventions. And a possible increase in adverse reactions to the biologics, including neoplasia, may also mean that more patients will need to stop previously successful medical treatment. On the other hand, an increased understanding of the pathophysiological mechanisms and ongoing innovative research supported by large financial resources may broaden the spectrum of medical treatment options.

Summary

The objective of this chapter was to provide a brief overview of the new pharmacological treatment options for RA patients and indicate the different sites of action. Differences in disease pattern since the introduction of these new medications were discussed, as well as the numbers of responders and nonresponders, costs, and long-term effects. The possible adverse reactions to the modern medication of RA were highlighted, together with the consequences for surgical treatment. In addition, the goal was to increase awareness of the possible adverse reactions to biologics in surgical treatment.

The main points can be summarized as follows:

- Owing to modern treatment regimens, the number of surgical procedures has declined in most countries; however, there is a trend toward recurrence of the disease after 4–5 years of anti-TNFα treatment, possibly because of antibody formation to the medications.
- The pattern of RA patients being treated surgically has changed: these patients now either have isolated residual synovial inflammatory processes or are nonresponders with a more severe pattern of disease showing gross destruction.
- Methotrexate and corticosteroid medication can or even should be continued during surgical procedures.
- Whether anti-TNFα medication should be discontinued during surgical intervention is still open to debate, as no clear evidence of a higher risk of infection can be found in the literature. If infection should occur, however, its course might be more severe.
- If anti-TNFα medication is discontinued, the administration interval of the particular biologic must be taken into consideration, as there are substantial differences between products.
- There is a subset of patients with a disease pattern resembling degenerative arthritis with a mild inflammatory reaction; these patients can be treated according to the surgical principles for degenerative arthritis.

References

1. Aletaha D, Neogi T, Silman AJ, Funovits J, Felson DT, Bingham 3rd CO, Birnbaum NS, Burmester GR, Bykerk VP, Cohen MD, Combe B, Costenbader KH, Dougados M, Emery P, Ferraccioli G, Hazes JM, Hobbs K, Huizinga TW, Kavanaugh A, Kay J, Kvien TK, Laing T, Mease P, Menard HA, Moreland LW, Naden RL, Pincus T, Smolen JS, Stanislawska-Biernat E, Symmons D, Tak PP, Upchurch KS, Vencovsky J, Wolfe F, Hawker G. 2010 rheumatoid arthritis classification criteria: an American College of Rheumatology/European League Against Rheumatism collaborative initiative. Ann Rheum Dis. 2010;69(9):1580–8. doi:10.1136/ard.2010.138461.
2. Entezami P, Fox DA, Clapham PJ, Chung KC. Historical perspective on the etiology of rheumatoid arthritis. Hand Clin. 2011;27(1):1–10. doi:10.1016/j.hcl.2010.09.006.
3. Klein K, Gay S. Epigenetic modifications in rheumatoid arthritis, a review. Curr Opin Pharmacol. 2013;13(3):420–5. doi:10.1016/j.coph.2013.01.007.
4. Smolen JS, Aletaha D, Redlich K. The pathogenesis of rheumatoid arthritis: new insights from old clinical data? Nat Rev Rheumatol. 2012;8(4):235–43. doi:10.1038/nrrheum.2012.23.
5. Bluml S, Redlich K, Smolen JS. Mechanisms of tissue damage in arthritis. Semin Immunopathol. 2014; 36(5):531–40. doi:10.1007/s00281-014-0442-8.
6. Redlich K, Smolen JS. Inflammatory bone loss: pathogenesis and therapeutic intervention. Nat Rev Drug Discov. 2012;11(3):234–50. doi:10.1038/nrd3669.
7. Rengel Y, Ospelt C, Gay S. Proteinases in the joint: clinical relevance of proteinases in joint destruction. Arthritis Res Ther. 2007;9(5):221. doi:10.1186/ar2304.
8. Nam JL, Winthrop KL, van Vollenhoven RF, Pavelka K, Valesini G, Hensor EM, Worthy G, Landewe R, Smolen JS, Emery P, Buch MH. Current evidence for the management of rheumatoid arthritis with biological disease-modifying antirheumatic drugs: a systematic literature review informing the EULAR recommendations for the management of RA. Ann Rheum Dis. 2010;69(6):976–86. doi:10.1136/ard.2009.126573.
9. Nam JL, Ramiro S, Gaujoux-Viala C, Takase K, Leon-Garcia M, Emery P, Gossec L, Landewe R, Smolen JS, Buch MH. Efficacy of biological disease-modifying antirheumatic drugs: a systematic literature review informing the 2013 update of the EULAR recommendations for the management of rheumatoid arthritis. Ann Rheum Dis. 2014;73(3):516–28. doi:10.1136/annrheumdis-2013-204577.
10. Smolen JS. Ten years of infliximab: insights from clinical trials in rheumatoid arthritis. Eur J Pharmacol. 2009;623 Suppl 1:S5–9. doi:10.1016/j.ejphar.2009.10.026.
11. Simsek I. Predictors of response to TNF inhibitors in rheumatoid arthritis – do we have new tools for personalized medicine? Bull NYU Hosp Jt Dis. 2012;70(3):187–90.
12. Radner H, Smolen JS, Aletaha D. Remission in rheumatoid arthritis: benefit over low disease activity in patient-reported outcomes and costs. Arthritis Res Ther. 2014;16(1):R56. doi:10.1186/ar4491.

13. Smolen JS, Aletaha D. The assessment of disease activity in rheumatoid arthritis. Clin Exp Rheumatol. 2010;28(3 Suppl 59):S18–27.
14. Schoels M, Knevel R, Aletaha D, Bijlsma JW, Breedveld FC, Boumpas DT, Burmester G, Combe B, Cutolo M, Dougados M, Emery P, van der Heijde D, Huizinga TW, Kalden J, Keystone EC, Kvien TK, Martin-Mola E, Montecucco C, de Wit M, Smolen JS. Evidence for treating rheumatoid arthritis to target: results of a systematic literature search. Ann Rheum Dis. 2010;69(4):638–43. doi:10.1136/ard.2009.123976.
15. Smolen JS, Aletaha D, Bijlsma JW, Breedveld FC, Boumpas D, Burmester G, Combe B, Cutolo M, de Wit M, Dougados M, Emery P, Gibofsky A, Gomez-Reino JJ, Haraoui B, Kalden J, Keystone EC, Kvien TK, McInnes I, Martin-Mola E, Montecucco C, Schoels M, van der Heijde D. Treating rheumatoid arthritis to target: recommendations of an international task force. Ann Rheum Dis. 2010;69(4):631–7. doi:10.1136/ard.2009.123919.
16. Wu B, Song Y, Leng L, Bucala R, Lu LJ. Treatment of moderate rheumatoid arthritis with different strategies in a health resource-limited setting: a cost-effectiveness analysis in the era of biosimilars. Clin Exp Rheumatol. 2014: 20–6.
17. Genovese MC, Rubbert-Roth A, Smolen JS, Kremer J, Khraishi M, Gomez-Reino J, Sebba A, Pilson R, Williams S, Van Vollenhoven R. Longterm safety and efficacy of tocilizumab in patients with rheumatoid arthritis: a cumulative analysis of up to 4.6 years of exposure. J Rheumatol. 2013;40(6):768–80. doi:10.3899/jrheum.120687.
18. Ramiro S, Gaujoux-Viala C, Nam JL, Smolen JS, Buch M, Gossec L, van der Heijde D, Winthrop K, Landewe R. Safety of synthetic and biological DMARDs: a systematic literature review informing the 2013 update of the EULAR recommendations for management of rheumatoid arthritis. Ann Rheum Dis. 2014;73(3):529–35. doi:10.1136/annrheumdis-2013-204575.
19. Smolen JS, Landewe R, Breedveld FC, Buch M, Burmester G, Dougados M, Emery P, Gaujoux-Viala C, Gossec L, Nam J, Ramiro S, Winthrop K, de Wit M, Aletaha D, Betteridge N, Bijlsma JW, Boers M, Buttgereit F, Combe B, Cutolo M, Damjanov N, Hazes JM, Kouloumas M, Kvien TK, Mariette X, Pavelka K, van Riel PL, Rubbert-Roth A, Scholte-Voshaar M, Scott DL, Sokka-Isler T, Wong JB, van der Heijde D. EULAR recommendations for the management of rheumatoid arthritis with synthetic and biological disease-modifying antirheumatic drugs: 2013 update. Ann Rheum Dis. 2014;73(3):492–509. doi:10.1136/annrheumdis-2013-204573.
20. Barnard AR, Regan M, Burke FD, Chung KC, Wilgis EF. Wound healing with medications for rheumatoid arthritis in hand surgery. ISRN Rheumatol. 2012;2012:251962. doi:10.5402/2012/251962.
21. Polachek A, Caspi D, Elkayam O. The perioperative use of biologic agents in patients with rheumatoid arthritis. Autoimmun Rev. 2012;12(2):164–8. doi:10.1016/j.autrev.2012.04.001.
22. Suzuki M, Nishida K, Soen S, Oda H, Inoue H, Kaneko A, Takagishi K, Tanaka T, Matsubara T, Mitsugi N, Mochida Y, Momohara S, Mori T, Suguro T. Risk of postoperative complications in rheumatoid arthritis relevant to treatment with biologic agents: a report from the Committee on Arthritis of the Japanese Orthopaedic Association. J Orthop Sci. 2011; 16(6):778–84. doi:10.1007/s00776-011-0142-3.
23. Scherrer CB, Mannion AF, Kyburz D, Vogt M, Kramers-de Quervain IA. Infection risk after orthopedic surgery in patients with inflammatory rheumatic diseases treated with immunosuppressive drugs. Arthritis Care Res (Hoboken). 2013;65(12):2032–40. doi:10.1002/acr.22077.
24. Kawakami K, Ikari K, Kawamura K, Tsukahara S, Iwamoto T, Yano K, Sakuma Y, Tokita A, Momohara S. Complications and features after joint surgery in rheumatoid arthritis patients treated with tumour necrosis factor-alpha blockers: perioperative interruption of tumour necrosis factor-alpha blockers decreases complications? Rheumatology (Oxford). 2010;49(2): 341–7. doi:10.1093/rheumatology/kep376.
25. Keith MP. Perspectives on rheumatoid arthritis for the orthopedic surgeon: overview of non-tumor necrosis factor biologic drugs and perioperative management. Am J Orthop (Belle Mead NJ). 2011;40(12): E272–5.
26. Momohara S, Kawakami K, Iwamoto T, Yano K, Sakuma Y, Hiroshima R, Imamura H, Masuda I, Tokita A, Ikari K. Prosthetic joint infection after total hip or knee arthroplasty in rheumatoid arthritis patients treated with nonbiologic and biologic disease-modifying antirheumatic drugs. Mod Rheumatol. 2011;21(5):469–75. doi:10.1007/s10165-011-0423-x.
27. Pieringer H, Stuby U, Biesenbach G. Patients with rheumatoid arthritis undergoing surgery: how should we deal with antirheumatic treatment? Semin Arthritis Rheum. 2007;36(5):278–86. doi:10.1016/j.semarthrit.2006.10.003.
28. da Silva E, Doran MF, Crowson CS, O'Fallon WM, Matteson EL. Declining use of orthopedic surgery in patients with rheumatoid arthritis? Results of a long-term, population-based assessment. Arthritis Rheum. 2003;49(2):216–20. doi:10.1002/art.10998.
29. Kolling C, Herren DB, Simmen BR, Goldhahn J. Changes in surgical intervention patterns in rheumatoid arthritis over 10 years in one centre. Ann Rheum Dis. 2009;68(8):1372–3. doi:10.1136/ard.2008.100800.

30. Nikiphorou E, Carpenter L, Morris S, Macgregor AJ, Dixey J, Kiely P, James DW, Walsh DA, Norton S, Young A. Hand and foot surgery rates in rheumatoid arthritis have declined from 1986 to 2011, but large-joint replacement rates remain unchanged: results from two UK inception cohorts. Arthritis Rheumatol. 2014;66(5):1081–9. doi:10.1002/art.38344.
31. Momohara S, Inoue E, Ikari K, Ochi K, Ishida O, Yano K, Sakuma Y, Yoshida S, Koyama T, Koenuma N, Taniguchi A, Yamanaka H. Recent trends in orthopedic surgery aiming to improve quality of life for those with rheumatoid arthritis: data from a large observational cohort. J Rheumatol. 2014;41(5):862–6. doi:10.3899/jrheum.131018.
32. Waljee JF, Chung KC. Objective functional outcomes and patient satisfaction after silicone metacarpophalangeal arthroplasty for rheumatoid arthritis. J Hand Surg [Am]. 2012;37(1):47–54. doi:10.1016/j.jhsa.2011.09.042.
33. Chung KC, Nellans KW, Burns PB, Wilgis EF, Burke FD, Fox DA, Kim HM. Patient expectations and long-term outcomes in rheumatoid arthritis patients: results from the SARA (Silicone Arthroplasty in Rheumatoid Arthritis) study. Clin Rheumatol. 2014. doi:10.1007/s10067-014-2775-z.
34. Motomiya M, Iwasaki N, Minami A, Matsui Y, Urita A, Funakoshi T. Clinical and radiological results of radiolunate arthrodesis for rheumatoid arthritis: 22 wrists followed for an average of 7 years. J Hand Surg [Am]. 2013;38(8):1484–91. doi:10.1016/j.jhsa.2013.05.007.
35. Gerlag DM, Raza K, van Baarsen LG, Brouwer E, Buckley CD, Burmester GR, Gabay C, Catrina AI, Cope AP, Cornelis F, Dahlqvist SR, Emery P, Eyre S, Finckh A, Gay S, Hazes JM, van der Helm-van Mil A, Huizinga TW, Klareskog L, Kvien TK, Lewis C, Machold KP, Ronnelid J, van Schaardenburg D, Schett G, Smolen JS, Thomas S, Worthington J, Tak PP. EULAR recommendations for terminology and research in individuals at risk of rheumatoid arthritis: report from the study group for risk factors for rheumatoid arthritis. Ann Rheum Dis. 2012;71(5):638–41.doi:10.1136/annrheumdis-2011-200990.

Etiology of Rheumatoid Arthritis: A Historical and Evidence-Based Perspective

2

David A. Fox

Introduction

Rheumatoid arthritis (RA) is a chronic, inflammatory, and destructive polyarthritis with numerous autoimmune features and the potential for extra-articular and systemic complications. Its etiology is still unknown but much progress has occurred in defining important mechanistic components of RA, leading to significant advances in its treatment. RA is a multifactorial and multistage disease, beginning with preclinical autoimmunity that arises in a genetically predisposed individual who encounters one or more environmental triggers, progressing to the clinical appearance of inflammation in joints and sometimes in other organs, and leading (if effective treatment is unavailable) to destruction of the articular cartilage and adjacent bone. This chapter will consider historical, epidemiologic, genetic, environmental, autoimmune, and inflammatory aspects of the development and progression of RA.

D.A. Fox, MD (✉)
Internal Medicine, Division of Rheumatology, University of Michigan, 300 North Ingalls St., Suite 7C27, Ann Arbor, MI 48109-5422, USA
e-mail: dfox@med.umich.edu

Epidemiology and Historical Aspects of RA

In a Caucasian population sample in the United States, the incidence and prevalence of RA have fluctuated over the past five decades [1]. As of 2005, the incidence per year per 100,000 of population was 27.7 in men and 53.1 in women, with an overall prevalence of 0.72 %. The incidence of RA rises in frequency from early adulthood into the seventh decade, before declining in the eighth decade and beyond [1]. In this context, and in view of the lifelong persistence of RA in most affected individuals, the lifetime risk of developing RA is strikingly high: 3.64 % in women and 1.68 % in men [2].

Individuals with RA have an approximately 50 % increase in premature mortality (after adjustment for comorbidities and risk factors such as smoking), which equates to a reduction in life expectancy of 3–10 years [3]. Multiple factors appear to contribute to this "mortality gap" versus the general population, with accelerated cardiovascular disease identified as the most significant component [4].

The historical epidemiology of RA is intriguing and, if accurately understood, could provide clues to etiology [5]. Recognizable descriptions of RA in the medical literature are recent, beginning about 200 years ago, but some earlier European paintings show what appear to be RA-like deformities. A few skeletal remains from

K.C. Chung (ed.), *Clinical Management of the Rheumatoid Hand, Wrist, and Elbow*,
DOI 10.1007/978-3-319-26660-2_2

both the New World and the Old World, dated to points in time over the past four millennia, have shown damage interpreted as potentially due to RA (reviewed in [5]). RA may have been present in ancient times but was likely rarer than at present. If this assessment is correct, it may indicate changes in the presence of environmental triggers and/or genetic changes in the human population over time that have increased propensity to RA.

Genetics of RA

The importance of inherited risk alleles in the pathogenesis of RA is highlighted by increased concordance for RA in monozygotic compared to dizygotic twins and by the familial clustering of RA. The most important region of the human genome in RA susceptibility is the major histocompatibility complex (MHC), which encodes for genes that are essential to immune responses, notably the HLA-A, HLA-B, HLA-C, and HLA-D proteins. These structures are expressed on the surface of antigen-presenting cells and are required for recognition of peptide antigens by T lymphocytes, leading to initiation of immune responses. The RA-associated MHC allele was initially identified as HLA-DR4 [6] and later localized to a five-amino-acid sequence from residues 70–74 of the beta chain of subtypes of HLA-DR4 and selected other DR alleles, termed the "shared epitope," which is located within the MHC peptide-binding cleft [7]. More recently polymorphisms that govern additional amino acid variations in HLA-DR that are located outside the shared epitope have also been strongly associated with susceptibility to RA [8, 9]. The mechanism for MHC predisposition to RA remains to be established—while presentation of a pathogenic autoantigen by RA-associated alleles is an attractive theory, other possibilities exist, for example, unique pro-inflammatory properties of the shared epitope itself [10].

Genome-wide association studies have identified more than 100 other loci that affect susceptibility to RA, each of which has a modest effect [8, 11]. The specific genes associated with these loci mostly function in cells that mediate immune responses, such as lymphocytes and antigen-presenting cells, reinforcing the concept that RA is an autoimmune disease (Table 2.1). The known loci associated with RA, both MHC and non-MHC, are more strongly linked to seropositive RA, i.e., RA in which either rheumatoid factor (RF) or antibodies to citrulline-containing proteins (ACPA) are present. The most influential RA-associated non-MHC gene is PTPN22, which encodes a tyrosine phosphatase that is expressed in lymphocytes, regulates signaling through the T cell receptor for antigen, and influences lymphocyte development [12].

Table 2.1 Examples of RA-associated genes

Gene	Function
HLA-DR (shared epitope)	Antigen presentation, lymphocyte activation
PTPN 22 (protein-tyrosine phosphatase non-receptor type 22)	Regulation of T cell receptor signaling
PADI4 (peptidyl arginine deiminase 4)	Posttranslational conversion of arginine to citrulline
CCR6 (chemokine receptor 6)	Attraction of Th17 cells to sites of inflammation
STAT4 (signal transducer and activator of transcription 4)	Signaling downstream of cytokine receptors

Epigenetic mechanisms control gene expression in a potentially heritable manner and include DNA methylation, histone modifications such as acetylation, and microRNA control of posttranscriptional stages of gene expression. Understanding of the role of epigenetics in RA is still in its infancy, but such mechanisms are likely to be of great importance, especially in the connection of environmental triggers to changes in gene expression [8, 13]. Epigenetic changes often occur distinctly in specific cell types, such as lymphocytes or synovial fibroblasts [13, 14], increasing the complexity of analysis in a disease such as RA that involves multiple cell populations.

Environmental Triggers of RA

Smoking is the best-established environmental risk factor for RA and is receiving attention as a potential trigger for the development of RA-associated autoimmunity. Although the association of smoking with RA was suspected 25 years ago [15], this link has become much better established within the past decade [16, 17], with smoking shown to increase the risk for seropositive RA by more than twofold. Smoking synergizes with the presence and gene dosage of the MHC shared epitope allele to greatly increase the risk of developing RA [18]. Preliminary evidence suggests that cigarette smoking can induce expression in the lungs of the enzymes responsible for citrullination of various proteins, thus creating antigen targets of autoantibodies that are tightly associated with RA [18, 19]. Smoking is also associated with resistance to successful treatment of RA and more rapid disease progression [20]. Thus, smoking cessation should be viewed as part of both prevention and treatment of RA.

Infection has long been viewed as a potential trigger of RA, even though direct infection of RA joints has not been demonstrated (reviewed in [21]). A variety of bacterial and viral pathogens have been implicated, but not definitively [21]. Recently attention has refocused on the clinical association of RA and periodontal disease [22, 23]. *Porphyromonas gingivalis* (*Pg*) is a gram-negative bacterium that is strongly linked to periodontal disease. Uniquely among bacteria, it possesses the enzymatic machinery to generate citrullinated proteins, and such RA autoantigens are indeed detected in the gingival tissue of subjects with periodontitis [22, 23]. Smoking and periodontal disease are also positively associated [23].

Investigation of the microbiome is a new area of inquiry in RA and other autoimmune diseases, and is a complex task in view of the multiple microbiomes present on the skin and in the respiratory and gastrointestinal tracts and the multiple influences that can skew the composition of each microbiome. One report identified a higher level of *Prevotella copri* in feces of patients with new onset RA. This RA group was seropositive for RF and/or ACPA, and expansion of *Prevotella* was more pronounced in the subset that lacked the MHC shared epitope compared with those who were shared epitope positive [24]. This finding will require confirmation and further exploration of implications for the pathogenesis of RA.

Stages of RA

RA-associated autoimmunity precedes clinical onset of RA, and joint inflammation precedes damage to the cartilage and bone. The sequence of systemic and articular events in RA can be conceptualized as discrete stages of RA. Holmdahl et al. have delineated these stages as autoimmune priming, tissue attack, and chronic inflammation [25]. The hallmark of autoimmune priming is the appearance of RA-associated autoantibodies, especially RF and/or ACPA.

Rheumatoid factors (RFs) are antibodies that recognize a domain of the IgG Fc portion as their target antigen. Recognized since the 1950s as present in about 70 % of patients with RA, RF is however highly nonspecific and is found in many other immune-mediated and infectious conditions as well as in some apparently healthy older individuals. The presence and titer of RF correlate positively with disease severity and extra-articular manifestations, and RF has plausible roles in the pathogenesis of RA synovitis (reviewed in [21]).

ACPA recognize proteins that have undergone posttranslational conversion of arginine to citrulline at one or more arginine residues [26], a reaction that is catalyzed by peptidyl arginine deiminase (PAD). ACPA are much more specific for RA than in RF and are thus useful diagnostically [27]. The presence and titer of ACPA also predict disease severity, including the degree of joint destruction [28]. Both RF and ACPA can appear years before the clinical onset of RA [25, 29–31]. At this stage, elevated serum biomarkers of inflammation can also be detected, including pro-inflammatory cytokines [30, 31].

The high specificity of ACPA for RA has prompted consideration of a potential role for these autoantibodies in RA etiology and pathogenesis. As mentioned previously, citrullinated antigens can be formed in the lung and oral cavity as a result of cigarette smoking or by *P. gingivalis*, respectively, environmental triggers that are epidemiologically associated with risk of RA. Thus, local extra-articular inflammatory processes could create immunogens for development

Table 2.2 Key elements in the pathogenesis of RA synovitis and tissue damage

Autoantibodies	RF, ACPA
T cells	Th17 (?Th1)
Cytokines	TNF, IL-6, IL-1, IL-17
Synovial fibroblasts	Cartilage damage, interactions with lymphocytes
Osteoclasts	Bone destruction
Endothelial cells	Angiogenesis

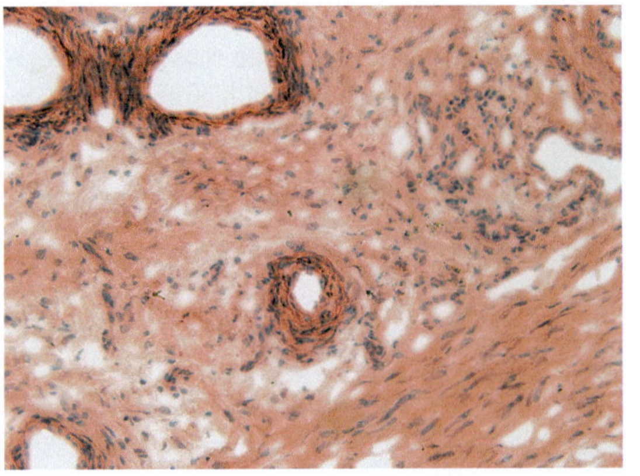

Fig. 2.1 Photomicrograph (20×) of chronic rheumatoid synovitis. Note the synovial fibroblast hyperplasia (lower right), extensive arterial and venous vascularity, and inflammatory cell infiltrate

of RA-associated autoantibodies, capable of recognizing citrullinated proteins in the joint at a later stage of disease [32].

The second stage of RA is the appearance of clinical arthritis due to a level of joint inflammation that is sufficient to generate clinical symptoms and signs. The specific trigger or triggers that localize the systemic autoimmune process to the joint are unknown and could be heterogeneous, including local trauma, transient infection of the joint itself, systemic infection that alters permeability of the synovial microcirculation, noninfectious tissue damage that generates ligands of innate immune receptors, and increase in the magnitude and affinity of autoreactive B and T lymphocyte responses that react against articular antigens. A curious feature of RA is the tendency toward symmetry of joint involvement. This mapping of the disease, which differs from other forms of inflammatory and degenerative arthritis, can be interpreted to implicate pathogenic events in the local mesenchymal cells [synovial fibroblasts (FLS), also known as type B synoviocytes] in the control of disease onset in specific joints in RA.

Synovitis is the hallmark of clinical RA (Table 2.2), and a detailed molecular understanding of this process has led to remarkable advances in the treatment of RA with both biologic and non-biologic pharmaceutical agents. The three most abundant cell populations in RA synovium are type A synoviocytes (of monocyte-macrophage lineage), FLS, and T cells. Other important participants include dendritic cells (potent antigen-presenting cells), B lymphocytes, plasma cells, endothelial cells, mast cells, neutrophils (primarily in synovial fluid rather than synovial tissue), and osteoclasts. Normal synovium is not known to be a location for initiation or propagation of immune responses, but in RA the synovium assumes characteristics of a tertiary lymphoid organ. The massive infiltration of leukocytes in RA synovium is accompanied by (and likely causes) marked hypertrophy of the synovial lining layer (Fig. 2.1). Numerous cytokines and other inflammatory mediators are produced in RA synovium as an outcome of the complex interactions between the various cellular constituents [33]. These interactions are both cognate (resulting from direct cell-cell contact mediated by various receptor-ligand pairings) and paracrine (due to local release of soluble pro-inflammatory mediators). Angiogenesis is a critical process in supporting synovial expansion and inflammation in RA, by providing avenues for the ingress of inflammatory cells and the nutrients to sustain them.

The third stage of RA is chronic inflammation that is destructive of cartilage, bone, and other structures including tendons and ligaments, leading to deformities that may require surgical intervention. Cartilage is directly invaded by chronically inflamed synovial tissue termed pannus, with a key role for FLS. Although FLS can secrete a variety of proteases and other mediators that may contribute to tissue damage in RA, a critical role has emerged for the membrane-anchored matrix metalloproteinase on the FLS surface known as MMP-14 or MT1-MMP in the invasion and destruction of collagenous structures [34]. Bone is eroded in RA through the activation of osteoclasts in the adjacent bone and through differentiation of monocyte precursors into osteoclasts in the inflamed synovial tissue, processes that are cytokine driven [35].

The distinctions between these three stages become blurred when one examines underlying mechanisms. Thus, ACPA can bind directly to citrullinated structures on the surface of osteoclasts, leading to osteoclast activation that would promote bone erosion. Sensitive imaging techniques confirm that joint damage can occur very early in clinically diagnosed RA and that osteopenia is present at the time of diagnosis in ACPA-positive patients [35]. The concept that joint destruction begins as soon as (or even before) recognizable synovitis is present reinforces the necessity for early diagnosis and aggressive treatment to minimize cartilage loss, bone erosion, soft tissue disruption, deformity, and consequent functional disability.

Cytokines and T Cells in RA

An essential role for pro-inflammatory cytokines is well established in RA, and RA has become the prototypic autoimmune disease in which cytokine blockade by biologic agents has revolutionized disease management. Of the nine biologics approved in the United States for use in RA, seven neutralize key cytokines in RA synovium—tumor necrosis factor (TNF), interleukin-1 (IL-1), or interleukin-6 (IL-6). (Of the other two biologics approved for RA, one impairs T cell activation and one depletes B lymphocytes.) Moreover, other agents that are effective in RA, such as a Janus kinase inhibitor, act primarily by blocking signaling downstream of cytokine receptor activation [36]. Cytokines appear to be important at all stages of RA, although it is possible that shifts in cytokine networks occur as RA evolves.

The search for additional cytokine targets in RA has focused in part on the cytokines secreted by differentiated effector cell subsets of CD4+ T lymphocytes. T cells have long been viewed as central to the pathogenesis of RA (reviewed in [21]). T cells in the joint respond to various local tissue antigens and interact with FLS in ways that can promote activation of both cell types [33]. Activated subsets of CD4+ cells can be defined by their cytokine products: Th1 cells secrete interferon-gamma, Th2 cells secrete interleukin 4, and Th17 cells secrete various isoforms of interleukin 17. Though Th2 cells are critical for allergic diseases, many autoimmune conditions, including RA, appeared to be driven by Th17 cells, Th1 cells, or by cells that overlap the Th1/Th17 subsets [37]. Manipulation of the function of these cells and neutralization of their secreted cytokines are current areas of clinical investigation that may shed further light on disease pathogenesis.

Future Directions

Although the cause, cure, and prevention of RA are not yet known, significant and accelerating progress has been achieved toward each of these goals. Plausible models for the development of RA that integrate genetic predisposition, environmental triggers, autoimmunity, synovial inflammation, and tissue damage have been proposed [29–32, 38]. At the same time, the notion of molecular heterogeneity of RA is gaining traction, based on distinct patterns of synovial gene expression that can predict clinical response or lack of response to various biologics and ultimately guide individualized treatment approaches [39]. Perhaps most exciting, the improving ability to define risk for RA before onset of disease is laying the groundwork for clinical trials of RA prevention [40, 41].

References

1. Myasoedova E, Crowson CS, Kremers HM, Therneau TM, Gabriel SE. Is the incidence of rheumatoid arthritis rising?: results from Olmsted County, Minnesota, 1955–2007. Arthritis Rheum. 2010;62(6):1576–82. Pubmed Central PMCID: 2929692.
2. Crowson CS, Matteson EL, Myasoedova E, Michet CJ, Ernste FC, Warrington KJ, et al. The lifetime risk

of adult-onset rheumatoid arthritis and other inflammatory autoimmune rheumatic diseases. Arthritis Rheum. 2011;63(3):633–9. Pubmed Central PMCID: 3078757.
3. Myasoedova E, Davis 3rd JM, Crowson CS, Gabriel SE. Epidemiology of rheumatoid arthritis: rheumatoid arthritis and mortality. Curr Rheumatol Rep. 2010;12(5):379–85.
4. Crowson CS, Liao KP, Davis 3rd JM, Solomon DH, Matteson EL, Knutson KL, et al. Rheumatoid arthritis and cardiovascular disease. Am Heart J. 2013;166(4):622–8.e621. Pubmed Central PMCID: 3890244.
5. Entezami P, Fox DA, Clapham PJ, Chung KC. Historical perspective on the etiology of rheumatoid arthritis. Hand Clin. 2011;27(1):1–10. Pubmed Central PMCID: 3119866.
6. Stastny P. Association of the B-cell alloantigen DRw4 with rheumatoid arthritis. N Engl J Med. 1978; 298(16):869–71.
7. Gregersen PK, Silver J, Winchester RJ. The shared epitope hypothesis. An approach to understanding the molecular genetics of susceptibility to rheumatoid arthritis. Arthritis Rheum. 1987;30(11):1205–13.
8. Viatte S, Plant D, Raychaudhuri S. Genetics and epigenetics of rheumatoid arthritis. Nat Rev Rheumatol. 2013;9(3):141–53. Pubmed Central PMCID: 3694322.
9. Okada Y, Kim K, Han B, Pillai NE, Ong RT, Saw WY, et al. Risk for ACPA-positive rheumatoid arthritis is driven by shared HLA amino acid polymorphisms in Asian and European populations. Hum Mol Genet. 2014;23(25):6916–26. Pubmed Central PMCID: 4245039.
10. Ling S, Cline EN, Haug TS, Fox DA, Holoshitz J. Citrullinated calreticulin potentiates rheumatoid arthritis shared epitope signaling. Arthritis Rheum. 2013;65(3):618–26. Pubmed Central PMCID: 3582785.
11. Kochi Y, Suzuki A, Yamamoto K. Genetic basis of rheumatoid arthritis: a current review. Biochem Biophys Res Commun. 2014;452(2):254–62.
12. Stanford SM, Bottini N. PTPN22: the archetypal non-HLA autoimmunity gene. Nat Rev Rheumatol. 2014;10(10):602–11.
13. Klein K, Gay S. Epigenetics in rheumatoid arthritis. Curr Opin Rheumatol. 2015;27(1):76–82.
14. Nakano K, Whitaker JW, Boyle DL, Wang W, Firestein GS. DNA methylome signature in rheumatoid arthritis. Ann Rheum Dis. 2013;72(1):110–7. Pubmed Central PMCID: 3549371.
15. Hernandez Avila M, Liang MH, Willett WC, Stampfer MJ, Colditz GA, Rosner B, et al. Reproductive factors, smoking, and the risk for rheumatoid arthritis. Epidemiology. 1990;1(4):285–91.
16. Padyukov L, Silva C, Stolt P, Alfredsson L, Klareskog L. A gene-environment interaction between smoking and shared epitope genes in HLA-DR provides a high risk of seropositive rheumatoid arthritis. Arthritis Rheum. 2004;50(10):3085–92.
17. Klareskog L, Stolt P, Lundberg K, Kallberg H, Bengtsson C, Grunewald J, et al. A new model for an etiology of rheumatoid arthritis: smoking may trigger HLA-DR (shared epitope)-restricted immune reactions to autoantigens modified by citrullination. Arthritis Rheum. 2006;54(1):38–46.
18. Makrygiannakis D, Hermansson M, Ulfgren AK, Nicholas AP, Zendman AJ, Eklund A, et al. Smoking increases peptidylarginine deiminase 2 enzyme expression in human lungs and increases citrullination in BAL cells. Ann Rheum Dis. 2008;67(10): 1488–92.
19. Kilsgard O, Andersson P, Malmsten M, Nordin SL, Linge HM, Eliasson M, et al. Peptidylarginine deiminases present in the airways during tobacco smoking and inflammation can citrullinate the host defense peptide LL-37, resulting in altered activities. Am J Respir Cell Mol Biol. 2012;46(2):240–8.
20. Saevarsdottir S, Rezaei H, Geborek P, Petersson I, Ernestam S, Albertsson K, et al. Current smoking status is a strong predictor of radiographic progression in early rheumatoid arthritis: results from the SWEFOT trial. Ann Rheum Dis. 2014;4.
21. Fox DA. Etiology and pathogenesis of rheumatoid arthritis. In: Koopman WJ, Moreland LW, editors. Arthritis and allied conditions. Philadelphia: LWW; 2004. p. 1089–115.
22. Bingham 3rd CO, Moni M. Periodontal disease and rheumatoid arthritis: the evidence accumulates for complex pathobiologic interactions. Curr Opin Rheumatol. 2013;25(3):345–53.
23. Scher JU, Bretz WA, Abramson SB. Periodontal disease and subgingival microbiota as contributors for rheumatoid arthritis pathogenesis: modifiable risk factors? Curr Opin Rheumatol. 2014;26(4):424–9. Pubmed Central PMCID: 4128331.
24. Scher JU, Sczesnak A, Longman RS, Segata N, Ubeda C, Bielski C, et al. Expansion of intestinal *Prevotella copri* correlates with enhanced susceptibility to arthritis. eLife. 2013;2:e01202. Pubmed Central PMCID: 3816614.
25. Holmdahl R, Malmstrom V, Burkhardt H. Autoimmune priming, tissue attack and chronic inflammation – the three stages of rheumatoid arthritis. Eur J Immunol. 2014;44(6):1593–9.
26. Schellekens GA, de Jong BA, van den Hoogen FH, van de Putte LB, van Venrooij WJ. Citrulline is an essential constituent of antigenic determinants recognized by rheumatoid arthritis-specific autoantibodies. J Clin Invest. 1998;101(1):273–81. Pubmed Central PMCID: 508564.
27. van Jaarsveld CH, ter Borg EJ, Jacobs JW, Schellekens GA, Gmelig-Meyling FH, van Booma-Frankfort C, et al. The prognostic value of the antiperinuclear factor, anti-citrullinated peptide antibodies and rheumatoid factor in early rheumatoid arthritis. Clin Exp Rheumatol. 1999;17(6):689–97.
28. Schellekens GA, Visser H, de Jong BA, van den Hoogen FH, Hazes JM, Breedveld FC, et al. The diagnostic properties of rheumatoid arthritis antibodies

recognizing a cyclic citrullinated peptide. Arthritis Rheum. 2000;43(1):155–63.
29. Demoruelle MK, Deane KD, Holers VM. When and where does inflammation begin in rheumatoid arthritis? Curr Opin Rheumatol. 2014;26(1):64–71. Pubmed Central PMCID: 4033623.
30. Holers VM. Autoimmunity to citrullinated proteins and the initiation of rheumatoid arthritis. Curr Opin Immunol. 2013;25(6):728–35. Pubmed Central PMCID: 3895448.
31. Deane KD. Preclinical rheumatoid arthritis (autoantibodies): an updated review. Curr Rheumatol Rep. 2014;16(5):419. Pubmed Central PMCID: 4059414.
32. Klareskog L, Malmstrom V, Lundberg K, Padyukov L, Alfredsson L. Smoking, citrullination and genetic variability in the immunopathogenesis of rheumatoid arthritis. Semin Immunol. 2011;23(2):92–8.
33. Fox DA, Gizinski A, Morgan R, Lundy SK. Cell-cell interactions in rheumatoid arthritis synovium. Rheum Dis Clin North Am. 2010;36(2):311–23. Pubmed Central PMCID: 2879397.
34. Sabeh F, Fox D, Weiss SJ. Membrane-type I matrix metalloproteinase-dependent regulation of rheumatoid arthritis synoviocyte function. J Immunol. 2010;184(11):6396–406.
35. Schett G, Gravallese E. Bone erosion in rheumatoid arthritis: mechanisms, diagnosis and treatment. Nat Rev Rheumatol. 2012;8(11):656–64. Pubmed Central PMCID: 4096779.
36. Fox DA. Kinase inhibition—a new approach to the treatment of rheumatoid arthritis. N Engl J Med. 2012;367(6):565–7.
37. Sarkar S, Fox DA. Targeting IL-17 and Th17 cells in rheumatoid arthritis. Rheum Dis Clin North Am. 2010;36(2):345–66.
38. Boissier MC, Semerano L, Challal S, Saidenberg-Kermanac'h N, Falgarone G. Rheumatoid arthritis: from autoimmunity to synovitis and joint destruction. J Autoimmun. 2012;39(3):222–8.
39. Dennis Jr G, Holweg CT, Kummerfeld SK, Choy DF, Setiadi AF, Hackney JA, et al. Synovial phenotypes in rheumatoid arthritis correlate with response to biologic therapeutics. Arthritis Res Ther. 2014;16(2):R90. Pubmed Central PMCID: 4060385.
40. Karlson EW, van Schaaardenburg D, van der Helm-van Mil AH. Strategies to predict rheumatoid arthritis development in at-risk populations. Rheumatology (Oxford). 2016;55(1):6–15.
41. Hunt L, Emery P. Defining populations at risk of rheumatoid arthritis: the first steps to prevention. Nat Rev Rheumatol. 2014;10(9):521–30.

Preoperative and Postoperative Medical Management for Rheumatoid Hand Surgery

3

Vladimir M. Ognenovski

Background

In rheumatoid arthritis (RA), 58 % of patients will undergo orthopedic surgery over the course of their illness [1, 2]. Hand surgery is an integral part in the management of rheumatoid arthritis patients. Among RA patients, 70 % will develop hand dysfunction [3]. About 17 % of all orthopedic surgeries done in RA will be in the hand and wrist [1]. The goals of hand surgery are preservation of function, reduction of pain, and maintenance of quality of life. In elective procedures, the surgical outcome is significantly influenced by factors such as disease activity and disease severity, comorbidities, immunosuppression, and perioperative care, reflecting the complexity of surgery in patients with rheumatoid arthritis. A close collaborative approach among the surgeons, primary care physicians, rheumatologists, anesthesiologists, and rehabilitation specialists during the perioperative period is essential for an optimal outcome.

Once a surgical indication is established, it is critically important to address factors impacting the surgical outcome such as RA activity and severity, comorbidities (cardiovascular, diabetes), and medications used to treat RA (NSAIDs, steroids, and immunosuppressive therapy). The duration of surgery, site of surgery, and revision versus primary arthroplasty all have been associated with infection risks [4, 5]. Postoperative care, wound care, and rehabilitation have equally important impacts on the surgical outcome.

Risks Associated with RA Activity

The timing of surgery has a significant impact on the surgical outcome. Active disease generally means more intensive immunosuppressive therapy which increases the risks for infections, including in the prosthetic joint. This is an inherent risk with all agents that impair the immune system function regardless of their mode of action. However, steroids have been associated with highest overall infection rates [6].

Impaired wound healing has been a concern with corticosteroid and immunosuppressive therapy, as well as NSAIDs. In animal models, long-term use of corticosteroids [7–9] or methotrexate [10, 11] has been linked to impaired wound healing. In some RA studies, long-term corticosteroid use has been linked to impaired wound healing [12, 13], whereas other studies have not supported this observation [14, 15]. In clinical studies, methotrexate use has not been linked to impaired wound healing in RA patients [12, 14–17].

V.M. Ognenovski, MD (✉)
Internal Medicine, Division of Rheumatology, University of Michigan, 300 North Ingalls Street, Suite 7C27, Ann Arbor, MI 48109-5422, USA
e-mail: vognen@med.umich.edu

K.C. Chung (ed.), *Clinical Management of the Rheumatoid Hand, Wrist, and Elbow*,
DOI 10.1007/978-3-319-26660-2_3

Anti-TNF blockade does not appear to impair wound healing in animal studies [18–20]. Tocilizumab, an Il-6 inhibitor, has been linked to delayed wound healing in one study. NSAIDs have been implicated in impairing wound healing in animal studies [21, 22].

Taken together, in elective orthopedic procedures (even though the evidence is based on small studies, variable doses of methotrexate and steroids), preoperative efforts should be directed in stabilizing the disease activity and keeping the disease under control on the lowest effective doses. Corticosteroids impair wound healing and increase risks of infections. Therefore, the maintenance corticosteroid dose should be reduced to less than 10 mg/day, preferably 5 mg/day or its equivalent. Methotrexate is less likely to impact wound healing or increase risk of infection and may not need to be interrupted in the perioperative period, depending on the dose of methotrexate, concurrent additional risk factors for infection, and the degree of frailty of the patient. Interruption of methotrexate for less than 3 weeks does not typically lead to a flare of RA. Anti-TNF agents do not appear to impair wound healing, but they increase the risk of infection as do other biologics, and they should be withheld preoperatively. NSAIDs impair wound healing and should be stopped preoperatively.

Cervical Spine

For patients undergoing general anesthesia, attention should be paid to the cervical spine stability. C1–C2 vertebral subluxation and instability is a known complication of synovitis of the atlantoaxial articulation at the odontoid process. It has been reported in as many as 61 % of RA patients undergoing joint replacement surgery [23–27]. Chronic synovitis may lead to an erosion of the odontoid process with resultant fragmentation and risks of spinal cord injury during intubation. Patients with features of more aggressive disease (progressive/erosive disease, polyarticular, nodular RA), older age, and chronic disability are at increased risk for atlantoaxial synovitis and C1–C2 instability [25]. Likewise, RA patients with neck pain and unexplained occipital headache should be imaged to assess for C1–C2 instability, although symptoms are not very reliable indicators of cervical instability [23]. Although no consensus on optimal imaging exists, at a minimum, dynamic X-rays of the cervical spine in flexion and extension should be done. Other modalities such as dynamic MRI or CT of cervical spine may identify additional abnormalities not visualized with plain X-rays. In a situation when C1–C2 instability is suspected, flexible laryngoscopy intubation or regional block may be the preferred choices for anesthesia. Fusion of C1–C2 vertebrae stabilizes the segments. Close collaboration among the surgeon, anesthesiologist, radiologist, and the rheumatologist is essential.

Risks Associated with Extra-articular RA Manifestation

Respiratory Tract Involvement with RA

RA can affect the upper airways with laryngeal inflammation and lower airways and parenchyma in the form of interstitial lung disease (ILD). When present, both can pose potential perioperative risks.

Larynx

Laryngeal involvement in RA is estimated to be present in 13–88 % of patients [28], depending on the series reported, in the form of vocal cord edema, rheumatoid nodule, and cricoarytenoid joint (CAJ) arthritis. The vocal cord function is impaired as a result of edema and impaired mobility, rheumatoid nodules, and CAJ synovitis with loss of mobility and ankylosis. When there is bilateral CAJ involvement, the vocal cords may remain fixed in adduction, leading to a life-threatening acute airway obstruction [29].

Symptoms can vary from dysphonia to life-threatening stridor. Acute postoperative obstruction following intubation has been reported [30].

If the airway is severely affected, endotracheal intubation may be difficult, and tracheostomy may be lifesaving.

ILD in RA

ILD is part of the rheumatoid lung spectrum, which also encompasses pleuropericardial disease, rheumatoid nodules, and pulmonary artery hypertension. Its prevalence is estimated at around 10 % [31, 32]; however, autopsy studies report 35 % prevalence [33]. Clinical manifestations include exertional dyspnea and cough, and when present, they should trigger additional evaluation with a chest X-ray, pulmonary function tests (spirometry with diffusion capacity), and high-resolution chest CT (HRCT). Pulmonary infection is a major contributor to morbidity and mortality in RA patients with ILD. When general anesthesia is considered, the respiratory system should be carefully assessed, and patients at risk may require additional evaluation of their pulmonary reserve.

Assessment and Management of Comorbidities

Cardiovascular diseases in RA patients are increased in prevalence, presumably due to the inflammatory state, chronic corticosteroid use, as well as traditional risk factors. The risk for death from cardiovascular disease is also higher in RA patients compared to the general population [34–36]. The risks for myocardial infarction are similar to patients with diabetes mellitus or otherwise healthy persons who are 10 years older. Therefore, preoperative risk assessment based on American Heart Association (AHA) guidelines is prudent. Those with low-risk ability to perform four metabolic equivalents (METs) may proceed with surgery. Those patients with moderate risks for CAD and unable to complete four METs should be referred to a cardiologist for additional cardiovascular risk assessment [37–39].

Comorbidities such as diabetes, hypertension, and congestive heart failure should be optimally controlled as there may be exacerbation by higher corticosteroid doses. The function of other organs such as the kidneys, liver, and bone marrow should be evaluated as they may be affected by the disease, medications, or both.

Adrenal Insufficiency

Patients with RA commonly take corticosteroids long term. Adrenal suppression can occur as early as 12 weeks on low dose of prednisone, the equivalent of 5 mg/day [40]. Symptoms of adrenal insufficiency, hypotension and electrolyte imbalance, can occur with abrupt withdrawal or in stressful situations. High perioperative doses of steroids are often given to avoid consequences of adrenal insufficiency during surgical stress [41]. This practice of giving patients supraphysiologic doses of corticosteroids preoperatively has been questioned by several studies [42–45]. Other studies have supported the safety of giving patients their maintenance corticosteroid dose in the perioperative period in orthopedic surgery [46]. Corticotropin stress test can be used to assess the adrenal reserve preoperatively; however, it may not predict which patient will need the stress dose [43]. Taken all together, it may not be necessary to use supraphysiologic stress doses of corticosteroids in RA patients undergoing hand surgery, thus minimizing risks of postoperative infections. Table 3.1 provides an example guideline for perioperative stress dosing of corticosteroids.

Osteoporosis

Prevalence of osteoporosis in women with RA is as high as twofold [47] and worsens with disease progression, usually due to systemic inflammation, long-term use of steroids, and immobility [48]. Many patients are treated either for osteoporosis or preventively, especially when prednisone is prescribed. Treatment often consists of vitamin D and calcium supplementation, along with antiresorptive therapy, most commonly bisphosphonates. Bisphosphonates do not appear to be detrimental to arthroplasty outcome [49]

Table 3.1 Guidelines for adrenal supplementation therapy

Medical or surgical stress	
Minor Rheumatoid nodule excision Carpal tunnel release Finger joint fusion procedures Trigger finger releases Distal ulna excision	25 mg of hydrocortisone po or IV or 5 mg of methylprednisolone IV on day of procedure
Moderate Total wrist fusion or arthroplasty Mertacarpophalangeal joint implant arthroplast Tendon surgery Distal radioulnar joint reconstructionArthroplast	50–75 mg of hydrocortisone IV or 10–15 mg of methylprednisolone IV on day of procedure Taper quickly (by 50 %) over next 1–2 days to maintenance dose

Data modified from Coursin [41]

and may be beneficial in improving the arthroplasty durability [50] and in preventing osteoclast-induced osteolysis [51].

Immunosuppression

Most RA patients are exposed to immunosuppressive therapy. Immunosuppressive therapy includes chronic corticosteroid use, synthetic disease-modifying antirheumatic drugs (DMARDs), and biologic DMARD agents. Used as monotherapy or in combination therapy, immunosuppression remains a cornerstone in the management of RA.

Steroids

Corticosteroids are used by 65 % of RA patients [52]. Doses vary based on disease activity, but commonly the maintenance dose of prednisone is less than 10 mg/day or its equivalent. Rheumatologists commonly target doses of prednisone at 5 mg/day or less or its equivalent. Intra-articular corticosteroids (methylprednisolone) are frequently used at doses of 40–80 mg/cc for larger joints at intervals no less than 3 months. Some of the biologics, such as rituximab infusions, are given with intravenous methylprednisolone (up to 100 mg) to reduce the risk of infusion reaction. Risk of infection with chronic steroid use is high, and 100 % of patients treated for 3 years will develop an infection [6, 53]. In order to reduce the risk and severity of an infection, it is preferable to use prednisone or its equivalent in the lowest dose possible, commonly 5 mg/day or less. Postoperatively, in addition to infections, delayed wound healing and adrenal suppression remain a concern, as discussed above. Other more serious side effects associated with chronic corticosteroid use include atherosclerosis, diabetes, mood instability, osteoporosis, avascular necrosis of bone, hypertension, cataracts, and glaucoma, to name a few.

DMARDs

DMARDs along with steroids are the backbone of pharmacotherapy in RA. Utilization of these medications is high and 75–84 % of RA patients undergoing arthroplasty will be on DMARDs [54]. Synthetic DMARDs include methotrexate, sulfasalazine, hydroxychloroquine, leflunomide, tetracyclines, tofacitinib (a Janus kinase inhibitor), and less frequently azathioprine and cyclosporine. Biologic DMARDs are a novel category of drugs comprised of inhibitors of cytokines or their receptors, antagonists of lymphocyte activation, and agents that ablate subsets of leukocytes. Synthetic DMARDs are commonly used in combination with corticosteroids, but also in combination with other synthetic DMARDs as well as biologic DMARDs.

Hand surgeons and rheumatologists are frequently faced with the decision whether to withhold DMARDs or continue therapy without interruption in the perioperative period.

Methotrexate is the most commonly used synthetic DMARD, (followed by sulfasalazine, hydroxychloroquine, leflunomide, and less frequently azathioprine and cyclosporine.) It is also the best studied DMARD in the perioperative period.

Concerns about increased perioperative risks of infection have led to a common practice to stop methotrexate 2–4 weeks prior to surgery and resume treatment once wound has healed and there is no evidence of infection. There is very little support in the literature (orthopedic/non-orthopedic surgery) for this approach, and the limited evidence based on retrospective studies suggests very low/no risk of an infection when the drug is maintained [15, 55–58].

The majority of studies demonstrate safety of methotrexate in the perioperative period; however, much of this data come from retrospective cohort studies [15, 16, 59–61]. One prospective study showed slight increase in infections in patients taking methotrexate in the perioperative period [57].

Although most studies were retrospective and the weekly dose of methotrexate was <15 mg, clinicians should feel comfortable with continuation of methotrexate at its maintenance dose in the perioperative period. However, since many patients take doses of methotrexate >15 mg, brief interruption for 1–2 weeks before surgery should be considered.

Leflunomide has a recognized risk of infections [62]. Its impact on perioperative risks of infections was reported in two studies with opposing conclusions [63, 64]. Therefore, the current approach is to hold the medication for at least 2 weeks prior to surgery (in view of its long half-life in vivo) and resume with it once the wound is healed and there is no evidence of infection.

The impact of other DMARDs such as sulfasalazine, hydroxychloroquine, and azathioprine on wound healing and risks of perioperative infection is less well studied. Limited data suggest no increased perioperative infections [59, 65, 66], and these agents are probably safe to continue during the perioperative period, with the standard immunosuppressive therapy precautions for bone marrow and liver toxicity and monitoring of renal function.

Biologic DMARDs

The use of biologic DMARDs as therapy for RA evolved over the last 15 years. The group of biological agents used in RA comprises the TNF blockers (etanercept, infliximab, adalimumab, golimumab, and certolizumab), B cell-depleting therapy (rituximab), costimulatory molecule inhibition (abatacept), interleukin-1 receptor antagonist (anakinra), and the interleukin-6 receptor antagonist (tocilizumab). They are most effective when used in combination with methotrexate, but some are effective as monotherapy.

Anti-TNF Blockers

The risk of infections is well recognized with anti-TNF therapy [67]. Multiple studies have looked into the impact of anti-TNF therapy on the risk of infection following orthopedic surgery. Although some studies show no increased risk of wound infections in association with anti-TNF use in the perioperative period [68–73], other studies point to increased risks of prosthetic joint infections in association with anti-TNF therapy [74–76]. A systematic review and meta-analysis of 11 studies of adult RA patients undergoing elective orthopedic surgery compared 3681 RA patients with anti-TNF exposure to 4310 RA patients without anti-TNF exposure. The analysis revealed significant increase in risk of surgical site infection in association with anti-TNF exposure [77]. American College of Rheumatology guidelines recommend holding biologic therapy for at least 1 week before and after surgery with further adjustment to that time frame depending on the pharmacokinetics of the individual agent [78].

The presence of an implant significantly increases the susceptibility to infection, due to the ability of the microorganisms to evade host defenses by rapidly forming a biofilm at the bone-prosthesis interface, which increases bacterial resistance [5]. Bacterial biofilms form rapidly but are initially unstable and more susceptible to host defenses early after infection than later once the biofilm has matured. However, the early innate immune response is initiated by chemokines including Il-6 and TNFα, both targets of biologic therapy, which may contribute to the increased susceptibility to infection seen in the presence of a joint prosthesis in RA patients [79].

Anti-B Cell Therapy

Rituximab is an anti-CD20 chimeric antibody commonly given as a series of two infusions every 6 months. Patients are often premedicated with methylprednisolone to prevent infusion reaction. Based on a French registry, it has a favorable safety profile for infections [80]. Comorbidities such as cardiac, pulmonary, and extra-articular disease and hypogammaglobulinemia have been associated with higher risks for infections. In a cohort of 133 patients who underwent 140 surgeries, postoperative complications were observed in 7.4 % of orthopedic surgeries. The timing of surgery does not seem to be a factor, but correcting hypogammaglobulinemia and controlling comorbidities may be a prudent preoperative approach to minimize perioperative complications [81].

Anti-costimulatory Therapy

Abatacept downregulates T-cell activation. Numerous studies suggest low risk of infection when compared to synthetic DMARDs [82]. It is dosed either weekly subcutaneously, or monthly intravenously. A single report of a small series of RA patients suggested no increased risk of perioperative complications. Given its long half-life of 14 days, surgery should be planned 2–3 weeks after the last dose.

Anti-interleukin Therapy

Tocilizumab is an anti-IL-6 receptor antagonist given as a monthly infusion or a weekly subcutaneous injection to RA patients. One study of orthopedic surgeries reported delayed wound healing in 12.4 and a 1.9 % rate of surgical site infection [76]. A smaller study showed no postoperative infections [83]. Surgery should be planned 2 weeks after the last dose, given its long half-life.

Anakinra is an anti-IL-1 receptor antagonist dosed as a daily subcutaneous injection. Although no studies of its use in orthopedic surgeries have been reported, the data from British Society for Rheumatology Biologics Register indicated that it raises the overall risk of infections in patients with RA [84]. Given its short half-life, it should be held for 1–2 days before surgery.

Anti-JAK Therapy

Tofacitinib is a Janus kinase 3 inhibitor, a representative of a novel class of antirheumatic drugs targeting signaling molecules that control the activity of nuclear factors mediating lymphocyte regulation. Although no data exist about perioperative infections yet, there is an overall increased risk of infections associated with its use [85, 86]. Given its short half-life of 3 h, discontinuation of the drug 2 days prior to surgery is prudent.

The decision to resume with an immunosuppressive agent should be made individually, based on the wound healing process and possible postoperative complications. Generally, the drug is held until wounds heal and there is no infection. Typically this may take a week or two.

NSAIDs

NSAIDs exert their effect by inhibiting cyclooxygenase-1 and cyclooxygenase-2 (COX-1 and COX-2) activity as well as via non-cyclooxygenase-dependent mechanisms [87]. The cyclooxygenase pathway inhibition results in reduction of prostaglandin production, impairing many prostaglandin-dependent functions, including wound healing and thromboxane A-dependent platelet aggregation [88].

Nonselective COX-1- and COX-2-inhibiting NSAIDs increase the risk of perioperative bleeding by reducing thromboxane A2 production. Selective COX-2-inhibiting NSAIDs do not affect platelet function. Aspirin, which irreversibly blocks COX-1 and COX-2, should be held for a week before surgery, whereas NSAIDs, which inhibit reversibly both COX-1 and COX-2, should be held for five half-lives prior to surgery. The relationship between time of discontinuation of NSAIDs with intra- and postoperative bleeding time is not well defined. For most NSAIDs, platelet function normalizes after 3 days of discontinuation, suggesting that NSAIDs should be discontinued 3 days before surgery, with the exception of ibuprofen, which can be stopped 24 h before surgery [89].

COX-2 inhibitors, although not affecting platelet function, impair wound healing and renal function and should be held preoperatively.

Summary

RA is a progressive disease of joint inflammation with systemic and extra-articular features. The evolving understanding of its pathogenesis has led to revolutionary development of targeted therapy that is changing its course and its associated morbidity and mortality. Nonetheless, a substantial number of patients will experience progression of their disease leading to disability. Reconstructive hand surgery remains an important complimentary therapeutic option in restoring function and improving quality of life for patients with RA. Preoperative management of the disease and its comorbidities is critical in optimizing the surgical outcome. Postoperative wound and joint infections remain a serious concern and can be minimized by reducing the intensity of immunosuppression. A multidisciplinary approach involving the surgeons, rheumatologists, primary care physicians, anesthesiologists, radiologists and rehabilitation specialist is essential for a successful outcome.

References

1. Kapetanovic MC, et al. Orthopaedic surgery in patients with rheumatoid arthritis over 20 years: prevalence and predictive factors of large joint replacement. Ann Rheum Dis. 2008;67(10):1412–6.
2. Massardo L, et al. A population based assessment of the use of orthopedic surgery in patients with rheumatoid arthritis. J Rheumatol. 2002;29(1):52–6.
3. de la Mata Llord J, Palacios Carvajal J. Rheumatoid arthritis: are outcomes better with medical or surgical management? Orthopedics. 1998;21(10):1085–6.
4. Doran MF, et al. Predictors of infection in rheumatoid arthritis. Arthritis Rheum. 2002;46(9):2294–300.
5. Berbari EF, et al. Risk factors for prosthetic joint infection: case-control study. Clin Infect Dis. 1998; 27(5):1247–54.
6. Smitten AL, et al. The risk of hospitalized infection in patients with rheumatoid arthritis. J Rheumatol. 2008;35(3):387–93.
7. Waters RV, et al. Systemic corticosteroids inhibit bone healing in a rabbit ulnar osteotomy model. Acta Orthop Scand. 2000;71(3):316–21.
8. Cross SE, et al. An experimental model to investigate the dynamics of wound contraction. Br J Plast Surg. 1995;48(4):189–97.
9. Del Rio JV, et al. Chronic perioperative steroids and colonic anastomotic healing in rats. J Surg Res. 1996;66(2):138–42.
10. Cohen SC, et al. Effects of antineoplastic agents on wound healing in mice. Surgery. 1975;78(2):238–44.
11. Shamberger RC, Devereux DF, Brennan MF. The effect of chemotherapeutic agents on wound healing. Int Adv Surg Oncol. 1981;4:15–58.
12. Grennan DM, et al. Methotrexate and early postoperative complications in patients with rheumatoid arthritis undergoing elective orthopaedic surgery. Ann Rheum Dis. 2001;60(3):214–7.
13. Garner RW, Mowat AG, Hazleman BL. Post operative wound healing in patients with rheumatoid arthritis. Ann Rheum Dis. 1973;32(3):273–4.
14. Perhala RS, et al. Local infectious complications following large joint replacement in rheumatoid arthritis patients treated with methotrexate versus those not treated with methotrexate. Arthritis Rheum. 1991; 34(2):146–52.
15. Jain A, et al. Influence of steroids and methotrexate on wound complications after elective rheumatoid hand and wrist surgery. J Hand Surg [Am]. 2002;27(3): 449–55.
16. Kasdan ML, June L. Postoperative results of rheumatoid arthritis patients on methotrexate at the time of reconstructive surgery of the hand. Orthopedics. 1993;16(11):1233–5.
17. Sany J, et al. Influence of methotrexate on the frequency of postoperative infectious complications in patients with rheumatoid arthritis. J Rheumatol. 1993;20(7):1129–32.

18. Iglesias E, et al. Effect of blockade of tumor necrosis factor-alpha with etanercept on surgical wound healing in SWISS-OF1 mice. J Rheumatol. 2009;36(10): 2144–8.
19. Ashcroft GS, et al. Tumor necrosis factor-alpha (TNF-alpha) is a therapeutic target for impaired cutaneous wound healing. Wound Repair Regen. 2012;20(1): 38–49.
20. Sandberg O, et al. Etanercept does not impair healing in rat models of tendon or metaphyseal bone injury. Acta Orthop. 2012;83(3):305–10.
21. Elder CL, et al. A cyclooxygenase-2 inhibitor impairs ligament healing in the rat. Am J Sports Med. 2001; 29(6):801–5.
22. Virchenko O, et al. Parecoxib impairs early tendon repair but improves later remodeling. Am J Sports Med. 2004;32(7):1743–7.
23. Collins DN, et al. Cervical spine instability in rheumatoid patients having total hip or knee arthroplasty. Clin Orthop Relat Res. 1991;272:127–35.
24. Kwek TK, et al. The role of preoperative cervical spine X-rays in rheumatoid arthritis. Anaesth Intensive Care. 1998;26(6):636–41.
25. Neva MH, et al. High prevalence of asymptomatic cervical spine subluxation in patients with rheumatoid arthritis waiting for orthopaedic surgery. Ann Rheum Dis. 2006;65(7):884–8.
26. Zikou AK, et al. Radiological cervical spine involvement in patients with rheumatoid arthritis: a cross sectional study. J Rheumatol. 2005;32(5):801–6.
27. Boden SD, et al. Rheumatoid arthritis of the cervical spine. A long-term analysis with predictors of paralysis and recovery. J Bone Joint Surg Am. 1993; 75(9):1282–97.
28. Voulgari PV, et al. Laryngeal involvement in rheumatoid arthritis. Rheumatol Int. 2005;25(5):321–5.
29. Peters JE, et al. Three cases of rheumatoid arthritis with laryngeal stridor. Clin Rheumatol. 2011;30(5): 723–7.
30. Kolman J, Morris I. Cricoarytenoid arthritis: a cause of acute upper airway obstruction in rheumatoid arthritis. Can J Anaesth. 2002;49(7):729–32.
31. O'Dwyer DN, et al. Rheumatoid arthritis (RA) associated interstitial lung disease (ILD). Eur J Intern Med. 2013;24(7):597–603.
32. Restrepo JF, et al. Clinical and laboratory factors associated with interstitial lung disease in rheumatoid arthritis. Clin Rheumatol. 2015; 34:1529–1536
33. Suzuki A, et al. Cause of death in 81 autopsied patients with rheumatoid arthritis. J Rheumatol. 1994;21(1):33–6.
34. Lindhardsen J, et al. The risk of myocardial infarction in rheumatoid arthritis and diabetes mellitus: a Danish nationwide cohort study. Ann Rheum Dis. 2011;70(6):929–34.
35. Meune C, et al. Trends in cardiovascular mortality in patients with rheumatoid arthritis over 50 years: a systematic review and meta-analysis of cohort studies. Rheumatology (Oxford). 2009;48(10):1309–13.
36. del Rincon ID, et al. High incidence of cardiovascular events in a rheumatoid arthritis cohort not explained by traditional cardiac risk factors. Arthritis Rheum. 2001;44(12):2737–45.
37. Fleisher LA, et al. ACC/AHA 2007 guidelines on perioperative cardiovascular evaluation and care for noncardiac surgery: a report of the American College of Cardiology/American Heart Association Task Force on Practice Guidelines (Writing Committee to Revise the 2002 Guidelines on Perioperative Cardiovascular Evaluation for Noncardiac Surgery): developed in collaboration with the American Society of Echocardiography, American Society of Nuclear Cardiology, Heart Rhythm Society, Society of Cardiovascular Anesthesiologists, Society for Cardiovascular Angiography and Interventions, Society for Vascular Medicine and Biology, and Society for Vascular Surgery. Circulation. 2007; 116(17):e418–99.
38. Hlatky MA, et al. A brief self-administered questionnaire to determine functional capacity (the duke activity status index). Am J Cardiol. 1989;64(10):651–4.
39. Akkara Veetil BM, Bongartz T. Perioperative care for patients with rheumatic diseases. Nat Rev Rheumatol. 2012;8(1):32–41.
40. Kirwan JR, et al. The effect of therapeutic glucocorticoids on the adrenal response in a randomized controlled trial in patients with rheumatoid arthritis. Arthritis Rheum. 2006;54(5):1415–21.
41. Coursin DB, Wood KE. Corticosteroid supplementation for adrenal insufficiency. JAMA. 2002; 287(2):236–40.
42. Thomason JM, et al. An investigation into the need for supplementary steroids in organ transplant patients undergoing gingival surgery. A double-blind, split-mouth, cross-over study. J Clin Periodontol. 1999; 26(9):577–82.
43. Glowniak JV, Loriaux DL. A double-blind study of perioperative steroid requirements in secondary adrenal insufficiency. Surgery. 1997;121(2):123–9.
44. Bromberg JS, et al. Stress steroids are not required for patients receiving a renal allograft and undergoing operation. J Am Coll Surg. 1995;180(5):532–6.
45. Marik PE, Varon J. Requirement of perioperative stress doses of corticosteroids: a systematic review of the literature. Arch Surg. 2008;143(12):1222–6.
46. Friedman RJ, et al. Use of supplemental steroids in patients having orthopaedic operations. J Bone Joint Surg Am. 1995;77(12):1801–6.
47. Haugeberg G, et al. Bone mineral density and frequency of osteoporosis in female patients with rheumatoid arthritis: results from 394 patients in the Oslo County Rheumatoid Arthritis register. Arthritis Rheum. 2000;43(3):522–30.
48. Joffe I, Epstein S. Osteoporosis associated with rheumatoid arthritis: pathogenesis and management. Semin Arthritis Rheum. 1991;20(4):256–72.
49. Gao Y, et al. The effect of surface immobilized bisphosphonates on the fixation of hydroxyapatite-

coated titanium implants in ovariectomized rats. Biomaterials. 2009;30(9):1790–6.
50. Shanbhag AS. Use of bisphosphonates to improve the durability of total joint replacements. J Am Acad Orthop Surg. 2006;14(4):215–25.
51. Matuszewski L, et al. Effect of implanted bisphosphonate-enriched cement on the trabecular microarchitecture of bone in a rat model using micro-computed tomography. Int Orthop. 2013;37(6):1187–93.
52. Caplan L, et al. Corticosteroid use in rheumatoid arthritis: prevalence, predictors, correlates, and outcomes. J Rheumatol. 2007;34(4):696–705.
53. Dixon WG, et al. The association between systemic glucocorticoid therapy and the risk of infection in patients with rheumatoid arthritis: systematic review and meta-analyses. Arthritis Res Ther. 2011;13(4):R139.
54. Goodman SM, et al. Patients with rheumatoid arthritis are more likely to have pain and poor function after total hip replacements than patients with osteoarthritis. J Rheumatol. 2014;41(9):1774–80.
55. Maderazo EG, et al. Late infections of total joint prostheses. A review and recommendations for prevention. Clin Orthop Relat Res. 1988;229:131–42.
56. Bridges Jr SL, et al. Should methotrexate be discontinued before elective orthopedic surgery in patients with rheumatoid arthritis? J Rheumatol. 1991;18(7): 984–8.
57. Carpenter MT, et al. Postoperative joint infections in rheumatoid arthritis patients on methotrexate therapy. Orthopedics. 1996;19(3):207–10.
58. Steuer A, Keat AC. Perioperative use of methotrexate—a survey of clinical practice in the UK. Br J Rheumatol. 1997;36(9):1009–11.
59. Escalante A, Beardmore TD. Risk factors for early wound complications after orthopedic surgery for rheumatoid arthritis. J Rheumatol. 1995;22(10): 1844–51.
60. Murata K, et al. Lack of increase in postoperative complications with low-dose methotrexate therapy in patients with rheumatoid arthritis undergoing elective orthopedic surgery. Mod Rheumatol. 2006;16(1):14–9.
61. Barnard AR, et al. Wound healing with medications for rheumatoid arthritis in hand surgery. ISRN Rheumatol. 2012;2012:251962.
62. Jenks KA, et al. Leflunomide-associated infections in rheumatoid arthritis. J Rheumatol. 2007;34(11): 2201–3.
63. Fuerst M, et al. Leflunomide increases the risk of early healing complications in patients with rheumatoid arthritis undergoing elective orthopedic surgery. Rheumatol Int. 2006;26(12):1138–42.
64. Tanaka N, et al. Examination of the risk of continuous leflunomide treatment on the incidence of infectious complications after joint arthroplasty in patients with rheumatoid arthritis. J Clin Rheumatol. 2003;9(2): 115–8.
65. Bibbo C. Wound healing complications and infection following surgery for rheumatoid arthritis. Foot Ankle Clin. 2007;12(3):509–24. vii.
66. Pieringer H, et al. Patients with rheumatoid arthritis undergoing surgery: how should we deal with anti-rheumatic treatment? Semin Arthritis Rheum. 2007;36(5):278–86.
67. Bongartz T, et al. Anti-TNF antibody therapy in rheumatoid arthritis and the risk of serious infections and malignancies: systematic review and meta-analysis of rare harmful effects in randomized controlled trials. JAMA. 2006;295(19):2275–85.
68. Hirano Y, et al. Influences of anti-tumour necrosis factor agents on postoperative recovery in patients with rheumatoid arthritis. Clin Rheumatol. 2010;29(5): 495–500.
69. Ruyssen-Witrand A, et al. Complication rates of 127 surgical procedures performed in rheumatic patients receiving tumor necrosis factor alpha blockers. Clin Exp Rheumatol. 2007;25(3):430–6.
70. Talwalkar SC, et al. Tumour necrosis factor alpha antagonists and early postoperative complications in patients with inflammatory joint disease undergoing elective orthopaedic surgery. Ann Rheum Dis. 2005;64(4):650–1.
71. Johnson BK, et al. Patterns and associated risk of perioperative use of anti-tumor necrosis factor in patients with rheumatoid arthritis undergoing total knee replacement. J Rheumatol. 2013;40(5):617–23.
72. Kubota A, et al. Perioperative complications in elective surgery in patients with rheumatoid arthritis treated with biologics. Mod Rheumatol. 2012;22(6): 844–8.
73. Wendling D, et al. Surgery in patients receiving anti-tumour necrosis factor alpha treatment in rheumatoid arthritis: an observational study on 50 surgical procedures. Ann Rheum Dis. 2005;64(9):1378–9.
74. Kawakami K, et al. Complications and features after joint surgery in rheumatoid arthritis patients treated with tumour necrosis factor-alpha blockers: perioperative interruption of tumour necrosis factor-alpha blockers decreases complications? Rheumatology (Oxford). 2010;49(2):341–7.
75. Giles JT, et al. Tumor necrosis factor inhibitor therapy and risk of serious postoperative orthopedic infection in rheumatoid arthritis. Arthritis Rheum. 2006;55(2): 333–7.
76. Momohara S, et al. Prosthetic joint infection after total hip or knee arthroplasty in rheumatoid arthritis patients treated with nonbiologic and biologic disease-modifying antirheumatic drugs. Mod Rheumatol. 2011;21(5):469–75.
77. Goodman S, et al. Management of perioperative tumor necrosis alpha inhibitors in rheumatoid arthritis undergoing arthroplasty: a systematic review and meta-analysis. Arthritis Rheumatol. 2014;66(11): S1031.
78. Saag KG, et al. American College of Rheumatology 2008 recommendations for the use of nonbiologic and biologic disease-modifying antirheumatic drugs in rheumatoid arthritis. Arthritis Rheum. 2008;59(6): 762–84.

79. Zimmerli W, Moser C. Pathogenesis and treatment concepts of orthopaedic biofilm infections. FEMS Immunol Med Microbiol. 2012;65(2):158–68.
80. Gottenberg JE, et al. Risk factors for severe infections in patients with rheumatoid arthritis treated with rituximab in the autoimmunity and rituximab registry. Arthritis Rheum. 2010;62(9):2625–32.
81. Godot S, et al. Safety of surgery after rituximab therapy in 133 patients with rheumatoid arthritis: data from the autoimmunity and rituximab registry. Arthritis Care Res (Hoboken). 2013;65(11):1874–9.
82. Kremer JM, et al. Longterm safety, efficacy, and inhibition of structural damage progression over 5 years of treatment with abatacept in patients with rheumatoid arthritis in the abatacept in inadequate responders to methotrexate trial. J Rheumatol. 2014;41(6): 1077–87.
83. Hirao M, et al. Laboratory and febrile features after joint surgery in patients with rheumatoid arthritis treated with tocilizumab. Ann Rheum Dis. 2009; 68(5):654–7.
84. Galloway JB, et al. The risk of serious infections in patients receiving anakinra for rheumatoid arthritis: results from the British Society for Rheumatology Biologics Register. Rheumatology (Oxford). 2011; 50(7):1341–2.
85. Wollenhaupt J, et al. Safety and efficacy of tofacitinib, an oral janus kinase inhibitor, for the treatment of rheumatoid arthritis in open-label, long term extension studies. J Rheumatol. 2014;41(5):837–52.
86. Cohen S, et al. Analysis of infections and all-cause mortality in phase II, phase III, and long-term extension studies of tofacitinib in patients with rheumatoid arthritis. Arthritis Rheumatol. 2014;66(11): 2924–37.
87. Patrono C. Aspirin as an antiplatelet drug. N Engl J Med. 1994;330(18):1287–94.
88. Diaz-Gonzalez F, Sanchez-Madrid F. NSAIDs: learning new tricks from old drugs. Eur J Immunol. 2015;45(3):679–86.
89. Cronberg S, et al. Effect on platelet aggregation of oral administration of 10 non-steroidal analgesics to humans. Scand J Haematol. 1984;33(2):155–9.

4 Setting Priorities: The Timing and Indications for Rheumatoid Surgical Procedures

Matthew Brown and Kevin C. Chung

A World of Controversy

Rheumatoid arthritis (RA) is a prevalent, destructive, and debilitating disease [1]. It is associated with loss of work/wages, lower quality of life, and increased mortality [2–5]. A sharp dichotomy exists in the opinions of surgeons and rheumatologists regarding the effectiveness of surgery in treating rheumatoid hand deformities. Surgical management of rheumatoid arthritis has endured a large degree of skepticism because of variation in practice patterns, inadequate scientific evidence in the literature, and variability in the reported clinical success of certain procedures.

Alderman et al. surveyed members of the American Society for Surgery of the Hand and members of the American College of Rheumatology and found great differences in the opinions of the effectiveness of certain hand procedures [6]. Universally, the effectiveness of surgical procedures to improve function and provide pain relief was rated higher by the hand surgeons than the rheumatologists. Furthermore, only 12.6 % of rheumatologists believed small joint synovectomy and tenosynovectomy had any role in disease prevention or delay. Many rheumatoid procedures such as tenosynovectomy or synovectomy have an optimal window prior to tendon rupture or joint destruction, but these procedures are still seen as salvage options by many referring rheumatologists.

The marked success of anti-inflammatory and disease-modifying anti-rheumatologic drugs (DMARDs) has altered the modern hand surgeon's exposure to procedures to correct damage from RA. This is reflected in the variation of surgical practice patterns both within the USA and around the world. A review of surgical practice patterns in the USA using the Healthcare Cost and Utilization Project (HCUP) database reported variation in RA surgical procedures across the country. Furthermore, this variation did not correlate with disease prevalence, the number of surgeons, or patient demographic data [7]. Men were found to be 2.4 times more likely to undergo prophylactic procedures and women were significantly more likely to undergo advanced disease reconstructive procedures. The practice of rheumatoid hand surgery in various regions of the world has also been reviewed. In addition to patient-specific factors, societal culture, patient-physician dynamic, the

M. Brown, MD (✉)
The University of Michigan Medical School, 1500 E. Medical Center Drive, 2130 Taubman Center, SPC 5340, Ann Arbor, MI 48109, USA
e-mail: msbrown67@gmail.com

K.C. Chung, MD, MS
Comprehensive Hand Center, Section of Plastic Surgery, Department of Surgery, The University of Michigan Health System, 2130 Taubman Center, SPC 5340, 1500 E. Medical Center Drive, Ann Arbor, MI 48109-5340, USA
e-mail: kecchung@med.umich.edu

K.C. Chung (ed.), *Clinical Management of the Rheumatoid Hand, Wrist, and Elbow*,
DOI 10.1007/978-3-319-26660-2_4

health care system, and economic factors were found to impact the practice of rheumatoid surgery [8].

The complexity of factors contributing to the surgical treatment of rheumatoid patients has created discord among physicians, but there is hope that long-term outcome research may provide better evidence to guide standardized practices. Closer relationships between surgeons and rheumatologists will help to provide a multidisciplinary treatment plan aimed at increasing the quality of life for patients suffering from this disease. Regardless of timing and specific interventions provided, hand surgeons should be involved as early as possible in the evaluation of rheumatoid patients, so that surgery remains an option in the treatment plan.

Indications

Rheumatoid arthritis is a complex disease and when planning surgery, the surgeon should take into account the patient's symptoms and concerns, clinical appearance, function, and X-ray studies. The decision to proceed to surgery in a rheumatoid patient is guided by four main indications: (1) pain relief, (2) restoration of function, (3) disease prevention, and (4) improvement of aesthetic deformity.

Indications for Rheumatoid Surgery

- Pain relief
- Functional improvement
- Prevention of disease progression
- Aesthetic deformity

Pain is considered the primary indication for surgery. Other indications for rheumatoid surgery should be weighed against pain relief. However, it is important to remember that pain does not correlate with the degree of deformity. Despite significant deformity, many patients may report minimal pain and are able to function well enough to complete their daily activities. In most cases, pain in joints can be reliably treated with arthrodesis or arthroplasty [9–11].

Over 70 % of rheumatoid patients report hand and wrist dysfunction [4]. Restoration of function remains the second indication for surgery, but positive outcomes have been less reliably achieved compared to pain relief. These surgeries offer an increase in motion and dexterity, but weakness remains a significant disability for most patients [12]. Some caution should be used when considering reconstructive surgery in patients with mild deformities who report a general loss of function and have minimal pain. Many patients may not have the strength or endurance to pursue their former vocations or sports activities even with corrective surgery. Additionally, there always exists the possibility of weakening the hand even further for the sake of improving range of motion or stability. Such patients need careful counseling to fully understand their disease and modify their activities.

The third indication for surgery in a rheumatoid patient is prevention of disease progression. With the advent of DMARDs, rapid joint destruction has become less common. Still, some patients may have pain in the setting of significant synovitis, which has been unresponsive to medical care. Maximal medical management should be in place for at least 6 months prior to proceeding with surgery. Other examples of preventive procedures include resection of the distal ulna and dorsal tenosynovectomy for extensor tendon ruptures. This may help prevent or delay additional extensor tendon ruptures [13]. However, the ability of these procedures to prevent problems or slow progression has not been conclusively shown [14].

The final indication for surgery in a rheumatoid patient is to improve aesthetic appearance. Although this has less weight in the decision, it cannot be dismissed as a patient concern. The aesthetic improvements in the hand have been shown to be associated with patient satisfaction after RA surgical intervention [15]. In many cases, aesthetic improvements are a natural outcome with correction of subluxed joints and reestablishment of proper anatomic alignment.

In summary, rheumatoid surgical procedures can help to alleviate pain, provide functional improvement, prevent disease progression, and improve the appearance of the rheumatoid hand. The decision to proceed with surgery is much more complex than simply fulfilling one of the above criteria; it also involves patients' goals, anesthetic planning, perioperative medical management, and a rehabilitation plan to be in place.

Timing

Rheumatoid arthritis typically occurs between the third and sixth decades of life. Women have a higher incidence at a younger age in comparison to men, but prevalence is equal by the sixth decade of life. In most cases, the pattern of onset affects the feet, hand, and wrist joints. The metacarpophalangeal (MCP) joints, proximal interphalangeal (PIP) joints, and carpus are affected earlier and more frequently than other joints such as the hip, shoulder, and elbow [16]. These smaller joints are thought to be involved partially due to their high ratio of synovium to joint surface area [17]. Additionally, joint involvement and erosive changes may be evident in the feet, but up to 70 % of patients have erosive changes in the MCP and wrist within a few years of disease onset [18].

Medical management is important in the initial treatment of RA. Abating synovial inflammation, hypertrophy, and subsequent pannus formation will help to slow disease progression. Medical treatment should be in place for 6 months in most patients prior to surgical consideration. Despite multimodality medical treatment, certain subsets of patients are less responsive to medical therapy and experience progressive wrist pain and synovial inflammation. It is in these cases that synovectomy and tenosynovectomy play an important role in early management of the disease. Synovectomy, however, should be cautioned in patients with rapidly progressive joint destruction. Clinical evaluation should be repeated every few months in progressive or unresponsive patients to determine the correct time to intervene with more reconstructive efforts. For example, acute carpal tunnel syndrome requires surgical intervention to prevent permanent median nerve dysfunction. Proliferative dorsal tenosynovitis with a diagnosed tendon rupture is also a surgical priority. Though not emergent, correcting associated deformities may prevent further tendon rupture. Most tendon ruptures occur at the wrist and can be treated with primary tendon grafting into healthy edges of the tendon. Staged tendon repair in rheumatoid patients has less promising functional outcomes. Tendon transfer can also be considered when tendon repair is not feasible. The pattern of onset and development of clinical findings will determine when the first surgical interventions are made, and judgment regarding the type and timing of surgical procedures requires experience.

Despite medical therapy, many patients experience progression and develop joint injury and destruction. After the ligamentous structures and supportive capsule have attenuated, the lack of adequate soft tissue support makes maintenance of joint realignment and functional restoration more difficult. In many instances better results are achieved when reconstruction is performed before significant subluxation or dislocation develops and the occurrence of fixed contractures (Fig. 4.1). Patients can present to the hand surgeon at a variety of stages in their disease progression with a multitude of involved joints. If proximal disease and pain at the elbow or shoulder exist, evaluation and correction is performed prior to reconstruction of the joints of the hand.

Perioperative Considerations

Before proceeding to surgery, the entire patient must be evaluated. Rheumatoid patients are unlike any other hand surgery patients. The systemic manifestations of the disease can affect preoperative medical care, anesthetic plans, and postoperative management. A thorough work-up is critical for proper care and to avoid unfavorable outcomes.

Rheumatoid arthritis affects the axial skeleton as well as the peripheral joints. As many as 85 %

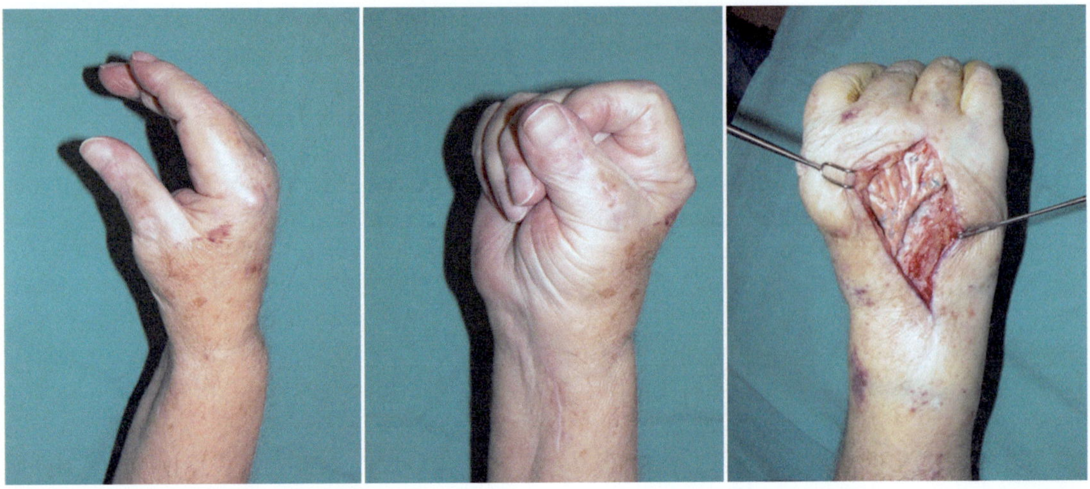

Fig. 4.1 Sixty-year-old male who previously had complex tendon reconstruction with the FDS tendon transfer. The indication for operating was his limited extension of the fingers despite therapy. He was taken to the operating room for tenolysis of the prior tendon transfer. The operation was done under local anesthesia with sedation and the release was performed until the patient was able to actively extend in the operating room. (*Left middle*) Preoperative photographs of the patient's function. (*Right*) Intraoperative photo of extensor tendon transfer with surrounding scar tissue

Table 4.1 Preoperative assessment

System	Comorbidity	Screening/interventions
Cervical spine	Alanto-axial instability/subluxation	Flexion and extension cervical spine X-rays
Airway	TMJ-decreased oral opening, vocal cord dysfunction	Anesthesia assessment, fiberoptic intubation
Respiratory	Decreased lung capacity, pulmonary fibrosis, pleural effusion	Chest X-ray pulmonary function testing
Cardiac	Coronary artery disease, impaired conduction valvular disease	EKG, possible echocardiogram or catheterization
Hematologic	Neutropenia, thrombocytopenia	Complete blood count, coagulation screen
Gastrointestinal	Decreased liver metabolism, peptic ulcer	Metabolic profile, ulcer prophylaxis

of RA patients may report neck pain, and one trial reported that as high as 12 % of patients have alanto-axial subluxation within 5 years of disease onset [19, 20]. Adequate assessment of cervical spine stability can be achieved with preoperative flexion and extension C-spine X-rays. Temporomandibular joint involvement can significantly affect mouth opening, making oral intubation techniques difficult. Additionally, nearly 80 % of RA patients may have laryngeal involvement and vocal cord dysfunction with swelling and periarytenoid inflammation [21]. In the case of cervical spine instability, fiberoptic intubation with a C-collar is recommended [22].

In addition to physical limitations, RA can affect multiple body systems, many of which can be silent. The respiratory, cardiac, renal, and gastrointestinal systems are all affected by the disease process or current treatments (Table 4.1). Studies have demonstrated a reduction in vital capacity and total lung volume in patients with RA, even in the absence of pulmonary fibrosis [23, 24]. Patients with long-standing disease or long-term use of some DMARDs are more likely to suffer from pulmonary fibrosis and pulmonary hypertension and are at increased risk for dyspnea and pleural effusion [24]. Cardiovascular disease remains one of the primary causes for mortality in rheumatoid patients. They have increased incidence of angina, myocardial infarction, heart failure, and stroke [25]. Multiple hematologic and metabolic abnormalities can also exist. Although rare, patients can suffer from Felty's syndrome (splenomegaly and neutropenia), which increases susceptibility to infection. Medications such as penicillamine and methotrexate can cause thrombocytopenia. Nonsteroidal anti-inflammatory drugs (NSAIDS) and aspirin affect platelet function, increasing bleeding risk. Methotrexate can also compromise liver function, which may affect the choice of anesthetic in surgery.

Perioperative management of rheumatologic medications must be discussed with all patients. Patients who take prednisone chronically should continue it through the perioperative period. In most instances, they also require a stress dose of steroids at the time of surgery because of a suppressed adrenal response. Various steroids can be used but dosage is usually equivalent to 100 mg IV of hydrocortisone [26]. Patients on methotrexate or other conventional DMARDs such as leflunomide, azathioprine, hydroxychloroquine, and gold should continue these during the perioperative period as well. A retrospective review of wound complications in RA surgery showed that there was no increase in wound problems for patients on steroids, methotrexate or both [27]. Patients taking biologic DMARDs, such as some of the antitumor necrosis factor (TNF) agents, are generally recommended to stop for 2–3 weeks before and after an operation because of the concern for perioperative infection, although the evidence is not clear [28, 29]. Other studies suggest that patients taking anti-TNF agents do not have an increased risk of wound complications or infection in orthopedic operations [30, 31]. This is best discussed with the patient's rheumatologist for final recommendations so that a unified plan may be established (Table 4.2).

Thorough evaluation with X-rays, electrocardiogram (EKG), basic lab work, and sometimes more cardiac testing is indicated. It is recommended that all patients have a preoperative anesthesia consultation. Although surgery is aimed at improved quality of life, in many cases surgical procedures are elective, and the risks of anesthesia, complications, and perioperative mortality should be discussed with every patient so that a well-informed decision can be made before proceeding.

Table 4.2 Perioperative medication recommendation

Corticosteroids	Continue at normal dosage, provide stress dose at time of surgery for chronic use
Methotrexate	Continue at normal preoperative dosage
Other DMARDs (gold, penicillamine, plaquenil)	Continue, discuss with rheumatologist
Biologic DMARDs	Hold for 2 weeks before and after surgery, discuss with rheumatologist

Sequence of Surgery

The main surgical procedures indicated for rheumatoid arthritis include synovectomy, tenosynovectomy, tendon surgery, arthroplasty, and arthrodesis. When a patient is evaluated early in the disease process, initial procedures such as dorsal tenosynovectomy, synovectomy, and median nerve decompression are usually considered before reconstructive surgery (Fig. 4.2). Recurrence of synovitis is expected in all patients, but the rate of recurrence is variable among patients. A multitude of reconstructive procedures exist, but the order of reconstruction can be critical.

Rheumatoid arthritis is a polyarticular disease and deformities of the proximal joints will affect the position of more distal joints. Each joint must be evaluated both individually and in context with an exam of the entire extremity. Significant involvement of one joint affects proximal, distal, and adjacent joints. For instance, if elbow flexion/movement is severely limited, correcting the flexed subluxed wrist to a position of slight extension may make it more difficult for a patient

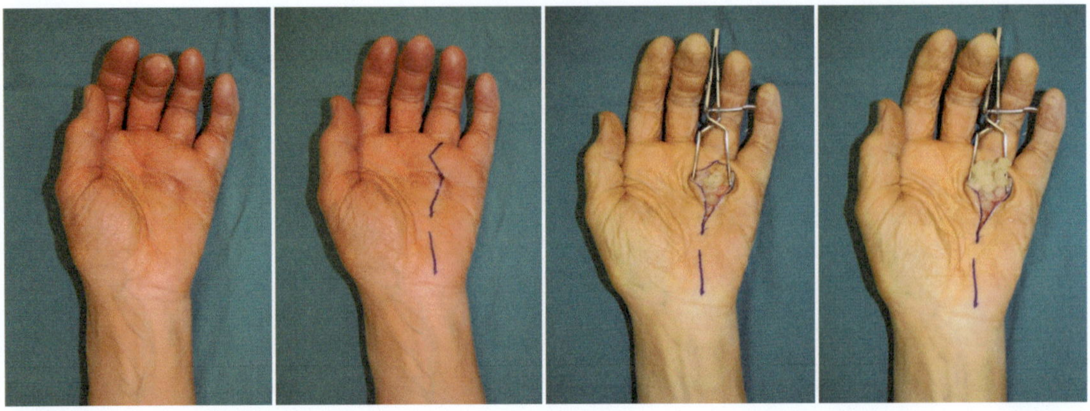

Fig. 4.2 Fifty-five-year-old female with rheumatoid who developed swelling over the palm along the flexor tendon sheath of the left index finger and presented with signs of carpal tunnel syndrome. The indications for surgery were treatment of the patient's painful mass development and presence of carpal tunnel symptoms. She had the flexor tenosynovectomy and excision of a large amount of rice bodies. After flexor tendon synovectomy, the carpal tunnel was released and synovial tissue within the carpal tunnel was excised

to get their hand to their mouth and eat. In this case, elbow range of motion should be increased first, or the wrist may be better fused in a slightly flexed position.

The carpus is affected early in the disease process, which usually begins with synovitis of the ulnar wrist, resulting in attenuation and rupture of the extensor carpi ulnaris and ligamentous attachments of the distal radioulnar joint (DRUJ). Loss of these structures leads to dorsal dislocation of the ulnar head and caput ulna syndrome. Synovitis of the volar and intercarpal ligaments causes volar and ulnar subluxation of the carpus with supination (Fig. 4.3). The intact radial wrist extensors then contribute to the radial deviation of the metacarpals at the carpometacarpal joint and compensatory ulnar drift at the metacarpal phalangeal joint. These mechanisms leading to deformity explain why correcting more proximal disease impacts the success of more distal function.

A stable wrist is necessary for a successfully reconstructed rheumatoid hand. In general, it is more physiologically and mechanically beneficial to address the wrist prior to the more distal MCP and PIP joints. For example, surgically addressing the MCP joints in a patient with significant subluxation and deviation of the wrist will have impact on functional outcome improvement at the MCP. Furthermore, some patients may find that wrist arthrodesis or arthroplasty can provide enough stability or motion so that distal surgery is not needed.

In a similar fashion, correcting MCP joint deformities before treating proximal interphalangeal (PIP) joint deformities is recommended [32]. One possible exception to this approach is a severe boutonnière deformity because a severe flexion deformity at the PIP joint compromises the result of the MP joint surgery [33]. The PIP joint can be corrected prior to or simultaneously with MCP reconstruction. Mild boutonnière deformities usually do not need to be surgically addressed because the flexed position of the fingers actually helps with grasp. Conversely, most swan-neck deformities need to be addressed to restore grasp; however, flexion at the MCP joint is unconsciously enhanced because of the need to make a fist. Therefore, theoretically an extension deformity of the PIP joint improves MCP joint arc of motion. Consequently, extension deformities at the PIP joint can usually be corrected at a later time without compromising MCP range of motion.

The decision to proceed with distal reconstructive surgery prior to addressing more proximal disease is mainly a result of patient preference. Patients without wrist pain often do not want to

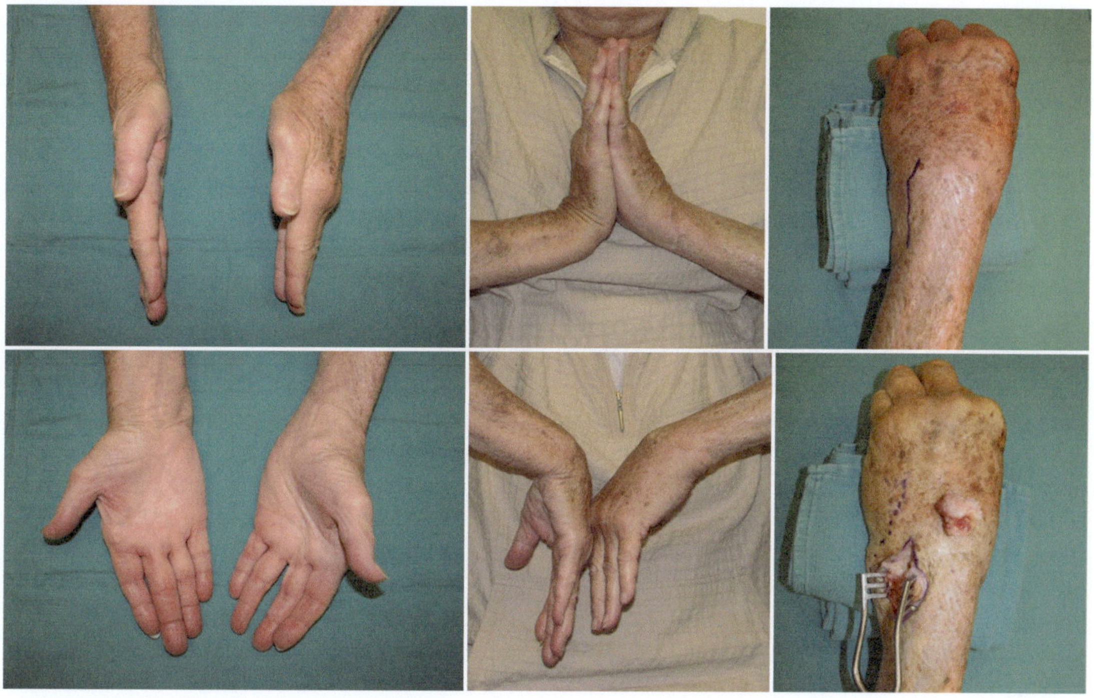

Fig. 4.3 Sixty-eight-year-old female with long-standing rheumatoid arthritis who presented with a left hand ulnar impaction syndrome due to long-term rheumatoid arthritis. The indication for surgery was the presence of significant instability of the distal radioulnar joint (DRUJ) with chronic pain and loss of function. (*Left*) The left carpus was noted to be volarly and ulnarly subluxed with prominence of the distal ulnar head dorsally. (*Center*) She had limited flexion and extension of the wrist. (*Right*) She underwent a Darrach procedure with stabilization of the distal ulna with the dorsal wrist capsule

have prophylactic correction of their wrist, which would decrease their motion. It is imperative that the patient is informed that the outcomes will not be as good when the metacarpals are deviating radially. In this circumstance, ulnar recurrence will occur faster after silicone MP arthroplasty.

Combining Procedures

The complexity of bringing a rheumatoid patient to surgery requires that efforts be made to complete as much necessary and indicated surgery in a single setting. Many procedures can be combined.

Commonly, carpal tunnel syndrome can be aggravated by any surgical procedure in the hand. Carpal tunnel release should be considered before or in conjunction with other surgical procedures on the volar aspect of the wrist. Providing median nerve decompression in many cases involves flexor tendon tenosynovectomy. Procedures that expose the flexor or extensor apparatus are easily combined with tenosynovectomy. Any large osteophytes or bony prominences can be smoothed and covered with soft tissue as well, and this surgical prophylaxis may help to delay future tendon rupture. With dorsal approaches, posterior interosseous neurectomy can also be easily added and may help with pain relief. Tenosynovectomy can also be combined with larger surgeries such as arthroplasty or arthrodesis. In some cases, occult or undiagnosed tendon injuries may be encountered during procedures. Patients should be counseled and if correction of the underlying cause of the tendon rupture is being addressed then it is reasonable to proceed with simultaneous reconstruction. The surgeon should be mindful when adding procedures to keep tourniquet time to less than 2 h if possible. Tissue swelling with longer cases may make wound closure difficult.

Outlining a Plan

Patients will seek surgery for a variety of reasons. One study examining patient preference found that younger age and female gender were significantly associated with an increased likelihood for choosing MCP joint arthroplasty surgery. Additionally patients with increased pain and decreased function as assessed by the Michigan Hand Questionnaire (MHQ) were more likely to choose arthroplasty [34]. Surgeons must be careful not to introduce their own biases into trying to understand a patient's surgical priorities. In a study analyzing men's and women's surgical priorities in rheumatoid surgery, it was found that physicians' biases conflicted with patient preferences [35]. Physicians believed that women valued aesthetics more, but patient surveys revealed that women and men were equally willing to have hand surgery, and they placed similar value on hand appearance, functional improvement, and pain relief. An in-depth preoperative discussion between the surgeon and patient can help align the preoperative goals.

With a full understanding of the indications for rheumatoid procedures, an individualized plan can be created. A treatment plan for a patient involves a stepwise approach to address the critical surgical issues first (Fig. 4.4). Patients with RA that is more progressed may proceed directly to reconstructive procedures, often combining with other procedures such as tenosynovectomy. With more aggressive operations, the surgeon should consider how the patient would provide self-care while going through rehabilitation of the operated limb. Many RA patients need assistance with ambulation using crutches or canes or may have greater difficulties necessitating use of a wheelchair. Their mobility will be further compromised during the recovery period after hand surgery. The same is true of shoulder and elbow reconstruction if indicated. These should be performed prior to hand reconstruction because it will aid the rehabilitation of the hand by eliminating more proximal problems. Patients need to be informed of limb limitations during rehabilitation after surgery so that preparations can be made to help optimize outcomes.

Additionally, almost all patients have rheumatoid disease that affects both hands. Many patients however may have preferential use of one hand and a patient should help decide which hand to operate on first. The workload of the non-operative hand will increase and this can exacerbate that hand's synovitis and pain. It may be practical to operate on the less involved hand first. This approach can prevent progressive deformity, provide improvement in a hand, and allow the patient to assess the potential for further reconstruction.

If surgery is chosen, the goal should be for patient and surgeon expectations of results to match. They must know that some deformity, especially at the metacarpophalangeal (MP) joints, is likely to recur after surgery. Good patient rapport is essential because the reconstructive process usually spans many months and often years with multiple procedures. Surgical plans and functional goals may be altered as a patient's disease progresses. Complications and risks should be discussed with each surgical procedure. For instance, although wrist arthroplasty may have higher complication rates, a patient may accept that risk for the chance of improved range of motion.

In summary, carefully listening to the patient's concerns and goals in combination with assessment of the patient's symptoms and exam findings provide the primary guidance for where the initial reconstructive process should start. From this point a sequence of surgical interventions

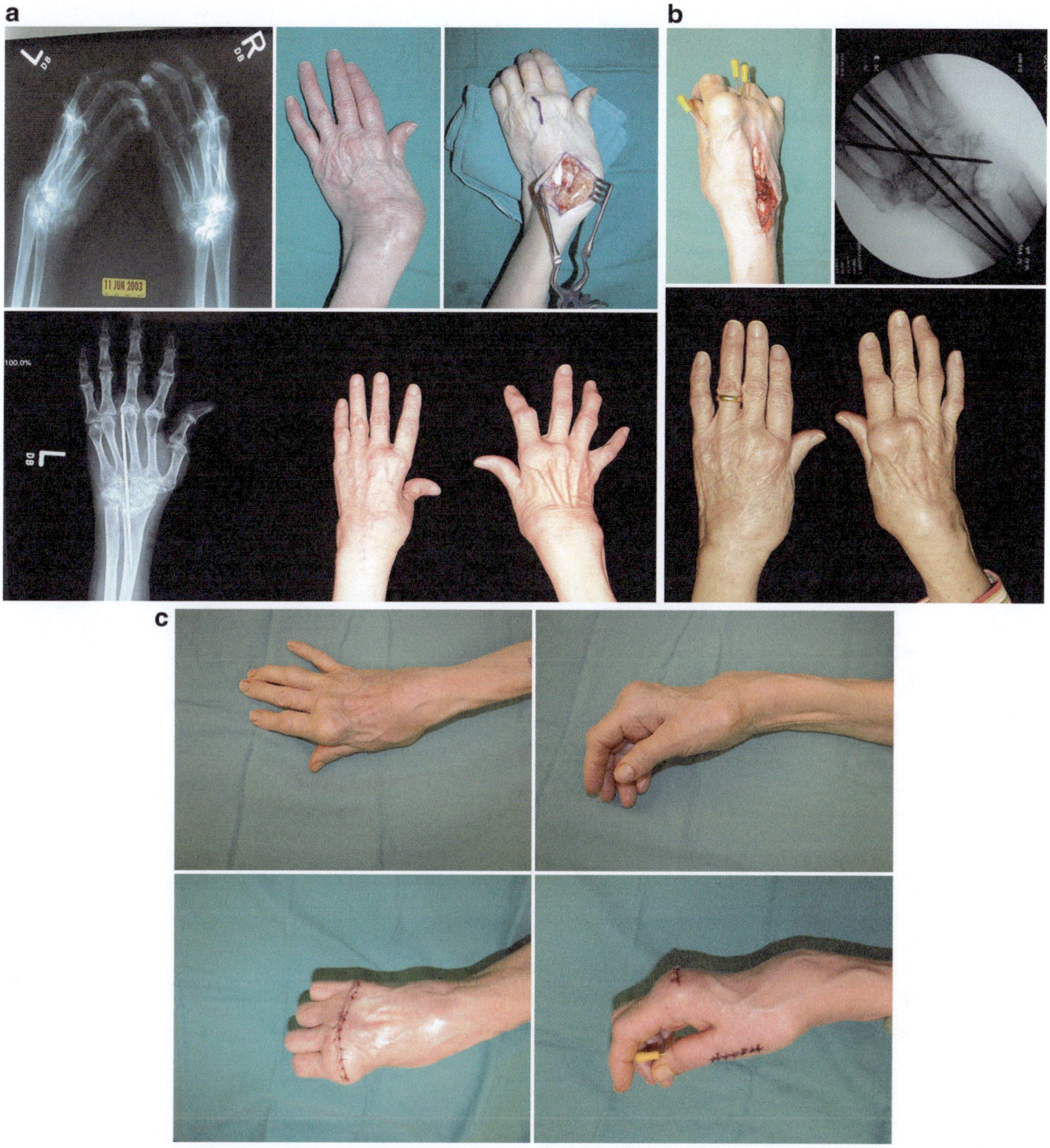

Fig. 4.4 Fifty-six-year-old female who presented with bilateral severe rheumatoid arthritis. She had pain as well as significant loss of function with bilateral caput ulna syndrome. (**a**) Her initial operation consisted of (1) left wrist fusion with a Steinmann pin; (2) extensor synovectomy of the second, third, fourth, and fifth extensor compartments and radical synovectomies; and (3) left distal ulna excision. (*Top left*) Preoperative radiographs. (*Top middle*) Left wrist preoperative. (*Top right*) Intraoperative photo demonstrating significant synovitis surrounding the extensor tendons. (*Bottom left*) Postoperative X-ray with correction of the wrist deformity. (*Bottom right*) Postoperative photos after treatment of the left wrist. The right wrist had not been treated yet. (**b**) Four years later, patient now with progressive right wrist pain because of subluxation and DRUJ instability from her ongoing RA. The right hand was treated with wrist fusion and aided by Kirschner wires, distal ulna excision, and extensor tenosynovectomy. (*Top*) Intraoperative photo and X-ray illustrating wire placement to facilitate wrist fusion. (*Bottom*) Postoperative photo. (**c**) After treatment of the wrist and recovery, the patient still had progressive MP pain and limited function because of subluxation and deviation of the right thumb. Patient went on to have fusion of the MP of the thumb and MP joint arthroplasty of the other fingers. (*Top*) Preoperative photos. (*Bottom*) Postoperative photographs

necessary to achieve final objectives can be established. Every patient presents his or her own unique challenges, but with careful planning, surgery can positively impact each patient's quality of life.

References

1. Lawrence RC, Helmick CG, Arnett FC, Deyo RA, Felson DT, Giannini EH, et al. Estimates of the prevalence of arthritis and selected musculoskeletal disorders in the United States. Arthritis Rheum. 1998; 41(5):778–99.
2. Katz PP. The impact of rheumatoid arthritis on life activities. Arthritis Care Res. 1995;8(4):272–8.
3. March L, Lapsley H. What are the costs to society and the potential benefits from the effective management of early rheumatoid arthritis? Best Pract Res Clin Rheumatol. 2001;15(1):171–85.
4. Pincus T, Callahan LF, Sale WG, Brooks AL, Payne LE, Vaughn WK. Severe functional declines, work disability, and increased mortality in seventy-five rheumatoid arthritis patients studied over nine years. Arthritis Rheum. 1984;27(8):864–72.
5. Yelin E, Meenan R, Nevitt M, Epstein W. Work disability in rheumatoid arthritis: effects of disease, social, and work factors. Ann Intern Med. 1980; 93(4):551–6.
6. Alderman AK, Chung KC, Kim HM, Fox DA, Ubel PA. Effectiveness of rheumatoid hand surgery: contrasting perceptions of hand surgeons and rheumatologists. J Hand Surg Am. 2003;28(1):3–11. discussion 2–3.
7. Alderman AK, Chung KC, Demonner S, Spilson SV, Hayward RA. The rheumatoid hand: a predictable disease with unpredictable surgical practice patterns. Arthritis Rheum. 2002;47(5):537–42.
8. Kotsis SV, Chung KC. A qualitative assessment of rheumatoid hand surgery in various regions of the world. J Hand Surg Am. 2005;30(4):649–57.
9. Chung KC, Burns PB, Kim HM, Burke FD, Wilgis EF, Fox DA. Long-term followup for rheumatoid arthritis patients in a multicenter outcomes study of silicone metacarpophalangeal joint arthroplasty. Arthritis Care Res (Hoboken). 2012;64(9):1292–300.
10. Cavaliere CM, Chung KC. A systematic review of total wrist arthroplasty compared with total wrist arthrodesis for rheumatoid arthritis. Plast Reconstr Surg. 2008;122(3):813–25.
11. Cavaliere CM, Oppenheimer AJ, Chung KC. Reconstructing the rheumatoid wrist: a utility analysis comparing total wrist fusion and total wrist arthroplasty from the perspectives of rheumatologists and hand surgeons. Hand (N Y). 2010;5(1):9–18.
12. Waljee JF, Chung KC. Objective functional outcomes and patient satisfaction after silicone metacarpophalangeal arthroplasty for rheumatoid arthritis. J Hand Surg Am. 2012;37(1):47–54.
13. Ishikawa H, Hanyu T, Tajima T. Rheumatoid wrists treated with synovectomy of the extensor tendons and the wrist joint combined with a Darrach procedure. J Hand Surg Am. 1992;17(6):1109–17.
14. Allieu Y, Lussiez B, Asencio G. Long-term results of surgical synovectomies of the rheumatoid wrist. Apropos of 60 cases. Rev Chir Orthop Reparatrice Appar Mot. 1989;75(3):172–8.
15. Goldfarb CA, Stern PJ. Metacarpophalangeal joint arthroplasty in rheumatoid arthritis. A long-term assessment. J Bone Joint Surg Am. 2003;85-A(10): 1869–78.
16. Fleming A, Benn RT, Corbett M, Wood PH. Early rheumatoid disease. II. Patterns of joint involvement. Ann Rheum Dis. 1976;35(4):361–4.
17. Mens JM. Correlation of joint involvement in rheumatoid arthritis and in ankylosing spondylitis with the synovial: cartilaginous surface ratio of various joints. Arthritis Rheum. 1987;30(3):359–60.
18. Brook A, Corbett M. Radiographic changes in early rheumatoid disease. Ann Rheum Dis. 1977;36(1):71–3.
19. Paimela L, Laasonen L, Kankaanpaa E, Leirisalo-Repo M. Progression of cervical spine changes in patients with early rheumatoid arthritis. J Rheumatol. 1997;24(7):1280–4.
20. Wasserman BR, Moskovich R, Razi AE. Rheumatoid arthritis of the cervical spine—clinical considerations. Bull NYU Hosp Jt Dis. 2011;69(2):136–48.
21. Charlin B, Brazeau-Lamontagne L, Levesque RY, Lussier A. Cricoarytenoiditis in rheumatoid arthritis: comparison of fibrolaryngoscopic and high resolution computerized tomographic findings. J Otolaryngol. 1985;14(6):381–6.
22. Malcharek MJ, Rogos B, Watzlawek S, Sorge O, Sablotzki A, Gille J, et al. Awake fiberoptic intubation and self-positioning in patients at risk of secondary cervical injury: a pilot study. J Neurosurg Anesthesiol. 2012;24(3):217–21.
23. Massey H, Darby M, Edey A. Thoracic complications of rheumatoid disease. Clin Radiol. 2013;68(3): 293–301.
24. Amital A, Shitrit D, Adir Y. The lung in rheumatoid arthritis. Presse Med. 2011;40(1 Pt 2):e31–48.
25. Jurcut C, Jurcut R, Tanasescu C. Cardiovascular risk and rheumatoid arthritis: from mechanisms of atherosclerosis to therapeutic approach. Rom J Intern Med. 2004;42(4):659–69.
26. Wakim JH, Sledge KC. Anesthetic implications for patients receiving exogenous corticosteroids. AANA J. 2006;74(2):133–9.
27. Jain A, Witbreuk M, Ball C, Nanchahal J. Influence of steroids and methotrexate on wound complications

after elective rheumatoid hand and wrist surgery. J Hand Surg Am. 2002;27(3):449–55.
28. Giles JT, Bartlett SJ, Gelber AC, Nanda S, Fontaine K, Ruffing V, et al. Tumor necrosis factor inhibitor therapy and risk of serious postoperative orthopedic infection in rheumatoid arthritis. Arthritis Rheum. 2006;55(2):333–7.
29. Bongartz T. Elective orthopedic surgery and perioperative DMARD management: many questions, fewer answers, and some opinions. J Rheumatol. 2007;34(4):653–5.
30. Hirano Y, Kojima T, Kanayama Y, Shioura T, Hayashi M, Kida D, et al. Influences of anti-tumour necrosis factor agents on postoperative recovery in patients with rheumatoid arthritis. Clin Rheumatol. 2010;29(5):495–500.
31. den Broeder AA, Creemers MC, Fransen J, de Jong E, de Rooij DJ, Wymenga A, et al. Risk factors for surgical site infections and other complications in elective surgery in patients with rheumatoid arthritis with special attention for anti-tumor necrosis factor: a large retrospective study. J Rheumatol. 2007;34(4):689–95.
32. Nalebuff EA. Metacarpophalangeal surgery in rheumatoid arthritis. Surg Clin North Am. 1969;49(4):823–32.
33. Nalebuff EA, Millender LH. Surgical treatment of the boutonniere deformity in rheumatoid arthritis. Orthop Clin North Am. 1975;6(3):753–63.
34. Chung KC, Kotsis SV, Kim HM, Burke FD, Wilgis EF. Reasons why rheumatoid arthritis patients seek surgical treatment for hand deformities. J Hand Surg Am. 2006;31(2):289–94.
35. Alderman AK, Arora AS, Kuhn L, Wei Y, Chung KC. An analysis of women's and men's surgical priorities and willingness to have rheumatoid hand surgery. J Hand Surg Am. 2006;31(9):1447–53.

5 Upper Extremity Compression Neuropathies in Rheumatoid Patients

Joshua M. Adkinson

Introduction

Rheumatoid arthritis (RA) is a chronic systemic inflammatory disease characterized by symmetric polyarthritis [1]. Extra-articular involvement occurs in approximately 10–40 % of patients with RA [2, 3]. The extra-articular manifestations most commonly affect the cardiovascular system, lungs, skin, and blood, and these have considerable prognostic implications [4, 5]. Although reported incidences vary, clinically significant neuropathy affects approximately 20 % of RA patients [5, 6]. The most commonly encountered neuropathies in patients with RA include compression, mononeuritis multiplex, distal sensory, and distal motor [5–10]. Compression neuropathies are the most common and comprise between 50 and 90 % of all neuropathy in RA patients [2]. Most studies have failed to show a relationship between compression neuropathies and gender, duration of RA, presence of other extra-articular symptoms, and serologic findings [11].

J.M. Adkinson, MD (✉)
Department of Surgery, Division of Plastic Surgery, Ann and Robert H. Lurie Children's Hospital of Chicago, Northwestern University Feinberg, School of Medicine, 225 E. Chicago Ave, Box 93, Chicago, IL 60611, USA
e-mail: joshadkinson8@gmail.com; jadkinson@luriechildrens.org

Whereas upper extremity entrapment neuropathy and RA may occur coincidentally [12], joint swelling and deformity resulting from synovitis and pannus formation frequently cause compression of adjacent structures [13]. Furthermore, evidence has shown the intrinsic effects on nerve anatomy and physiology in patients with RA. In a study by Conn et al. [14], sural nerve biopsies revealed epineurial and endoneurial arterial damage; this predisposes to axonal degeneration and neuronal demyelination [13]. Others have shown electrophysiologic and histologic evidence of nerve damage in asymptomatic RA patients [6, 7, 15]. As a result, even mild nerve compression in RA patients may lead to clinically significant neuropathy.

Diagnosis

Diagnosis of compression neuropathies in RA patients can be difficult and is often delayed. Patients frequently have coexisting joint pain, limited motion, and disuse atrophy of intrinsic muscles [13]. These examination findings complicate the assessment of neurologic impairment. Furthermore, symptoms of peripheral neuropathy in RA patients can also be caused by vasculitis and RA-related drug toxicity [12]. Nevertheless, traditional examination findings combined with electromyography and nerve conduction studies (NCS) are typically sufficient for diagnosis.

K.C. Chung (ed.), *Clinical Management of the Rheumatoid Hand, Wrist, and Elbow*,
DOI 10.1007/978-3-319-26660-2_5

As in patients without RA, compression neuropathies manifest as paresthesias, dysesthesias, and a burning sensation (these findings may be masked by arthritic pain) [16]. Provocative tests, such as the nerve percussion test (i.e., Tinel sign) [17] and the scratch collapse test [18], elicit useful diagnostic information that may localize the site of compression. A Phalen test [19] may not be possible as a result of limited wrist mobility in patients with RA. Similarly, carpal compression (i.e., Durkan test) [20] over the carpal tunnel may elicit pain from arthritis rather than the diagnostic paresthesias. In addition to the standard assessment for peripheral neuropathy, patients with RA require a full examination of the elbow, shoulder, and neck to assess for evidence of proximal nerve compression [21] or multiple sites of compression (i.e., the double-crush mechanism).

Nonsurgical Treatment of Compression Neuropathies

Conservative treatment generally involves medical optimization of the underlying inflammatory process. Whereas patients without RA suffering from mild compression neuropathy may be treated with activity modification, anti-inflammatory medications, elbow padding (for cubital tunnel syndrome), splinting, and corticosteroid injections [22–24], these modalities are rarely effective in patients with RA. As such, surgery is generally the treatment of choice, particularly in patients presenting with sensory or motor deficits [25, 26].

Carpal Tunnel Syndrome

Carpal tunnel syndrome is the most commonly diagnosed upper extremity compression neuropathy and has been estimated to affect between 6 and 69 % of patients with RA [7, 27, 28]. In fact, patients with RA are significantly more likely to develop carpal tunnel syndrome than age- and gender-matched controls [29]. Carpal tunnel syndrome in patients with RA is typically attributed to tenosynovial proliferation causing compression of the median nerve [30]. Alternatively, substantial wrist destruction with volar subluxation of the carpus can occur in severe RA and this may lead to median nerve compression [31]. Patients with carpal tunnel syndrome present with classic symptoms of pain, numbness, and paresthesias in the median nerve distribution, all of which are worse in the evening [32]. Weakness, loss of dexterity, and muscle atrophy may be noted in severe cases. The volar wrist may assume a dumb bell-shaped appearance in the setting of significant flexor synovitis due to restriction from the transverse carpal ligament [33]. Locking and triggering of the flexor tendons may be noted at the level of the carpal tunnel [34]. Magnetic resonance imaging (MRI) is a valuable adjunct in assessing the anatomic characteristics of the carpal tunnel as well as the degree of synovial proliferation [35]. Pierre-Jerome et al. [36] noted that 96 and 70 % of patients with RA undergoing a wrist MRI demonstrated synovial hypertrophy and a hyperintense signal in the median nerve.

Anatomy

The median nerve is derived from branches of the medial and lateral cords of the brachial plexus. The motor contribution is from the medial cord, whereas sensory nerve fibers are derived from the lateral cord [17]. The median nerve continues distally between the medial intermuscular septum and the brachialis before crossing the antecubital fossa under the lacertus fibrosus [37]. After coursing between the deep and superficial heads of the pronator teres, the median nerve enters the forearm deep to the fibrous arch of the flexor digitorum superficialis (FDS) muscle. The nerve then gives off the anterior interosseous nerve branch approximately 5.0–8.0 cm distal to the medial epicondyle [38, 39]. After providing motor innervation to forearm musculature, the median nerve enters the carpal tunnel at the anterior wrist along with the flexor pollicis longus, FDS, and flexor digitorum profundus (FDP) tendons. The carpal tunnel is bordered superficially by the transverse carpal ligament, radially by the scaphoid and trapezium, and ulnarly by the hamate and pisiform [24]. Distally, the median nerve gives off a recurrent motor branch to the thenar intrinsic muscles and digital sensory branches to the thumb, index, middle, and radial ring fingers [17].

Surgical Treatment

In RA patients with evidence of median nerve compression, we perform an extended open carpal tunnel release with a concomitant flexor tenosynovectomy (Fig. 5.1). Patients without evidence of tenosynovitis may also be considered for endoscopic carpal tunnel release [40], although this is not our practice. An open release allows an examination for attritional damage or rupture of the flexor tendons, which can occur because of synovial hypertrophy and invasion of tendon structures. Furthermore, the floor of the carpal tunnel may be simultaneously examined for bony prominences that are typically amenable to simple debridement with a rongeur and volar capsular flap coverage [21, 41]. In rare cases, concomitant ulnar nerve compression at the wrist from a synovial cyst [12] can be relieved by releasing Guyon's canal through the same incision.

Surgery for carpal tunnel syndrome in RA patients generally results in symptom relief. Shinoda et al. [30] reported symptom relief in all 20 hands operated on for carpal tunnel syndrome with RA using either open or endoscopic techniques. Muramatsu et al. [13] achieved good or excellent results in 13 out of 15 RA patients treated with open release and synovectomy. Conversely, Louie et al. [42] reported that patients with a carpal tunnel syndrome-confounding comorbidity, such as diabetes mellitus, polyneuropathy, rheumatoid arthritis, or osteoarthritis, had worse function and satisfaction after surgery as compared to those without a confounding morbidity at 10-year follow-up.

Cubital Tunnel Syndrome

Cubital tunnel syndrome is the second most common compression neuropathy in the upper extremity [43]. Patients with RA are at risk for compression of the ulnar nerve at the elbow from a synovial cyst within the elbow joint [44], instability or valgus deformity of the elbow [45], inflammatory swelling of the medial collateral

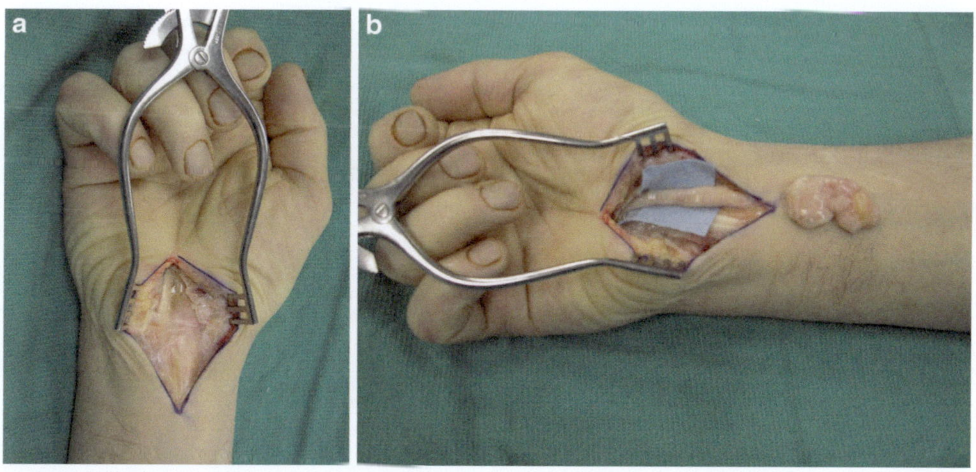

Fig. 5.1 Carpal tunnel decompression with flexor tenosynovectomy: (**a**) exposure after release of transverse carpal ligament and (**b**) median nerve isolated after tenosynovectomy and evaluation of flexor tendons for attritional damage. From Ono S, Sebastin SJ, Chung KC. Synovectomy. In: Chung KC, ed. Operative Techniques: Hand and Wrist Surgery, 2nd ed. 2012. Elsevier Saunders, Philadelphia, PA

ligament [13], or a geode (subarticular cystic lesion) of the olecranon [46]. Patients may complain of a dull ache in the medial elbow and forearm. Initial findings may include loss of vibratory and light touch sensation with subsequent progression to altered two-point discrimination, intrinsic atrophy, and clawing. With severe disease, Wartenberg and Froment signs may become evident [17, 47–50]. A Tinel sign is commonly associated with cubital tunnel syndrome and has a 98 % negative predictive value [51, 52]. Clinical evaluation is paramount in the diagnosis of cubital tunnel syndrome as electromyography (EMG) and NCS are not adequately sensitive to detect changes associated with nerve compression [17, 22, 47]. Depending upon the medical history and clinical findings, there may also be a role for plain radiographs of the neck, chest, and elbow [22] to rule out pathology including cervical disc disease (e.g., atlantoaxial subluxation), lung carcinoma, thoracic outlet obstruction, and elbow trauma or arthritis.

Anatomy

The ulnar nerve originates from the ventral rami of the C8 and T1 nerve roots and is the terminal branch of the medial cord of the brachial plexus. The nerve courses anterior to the medial intermuscular septum and passes through the arcade of Struthers 8 cm proximal to the medial epicondyle. Continuing toward the elbow, the ulnar nerve travels posterior to the septum, entering the cubital tunnel between the medial epicondyle and the olecranon. The roof of the cubital tunnel is comprised of Osborne's ligament as well as flexor carpi ulnaris (FCU) fascia. The floor of the cubital tunnel consists of the medial collateral ligament and the elbow joint capsule. The nerve then travels into the forearm between the humeral and ulnar heads of the FCU and continues in the interval between the FCU and FDP muscle bellies toward the wrist and hand [48, 53].

Surgical Treatment

Whereas a trial of nonoperative modalities is attempted in patients without RA, the fact that there are multiple case reports of attritional rupture of the ulnar nerve in neglected RA-related nerve compression [54–56] advocates for early nerve release. The amount of comparative evidence for the use of in situ cubital tunnel release is growing and all existing studies show benefit [43]; this is our procedure of choice. However, in patients with a valgus deformity of the elbow or in those having failed a previous in situ release, we recommend subcutaneous anterior ulnar nerve transposition (Fig. 5.2). One must also remember that RA patients with advanced elbow

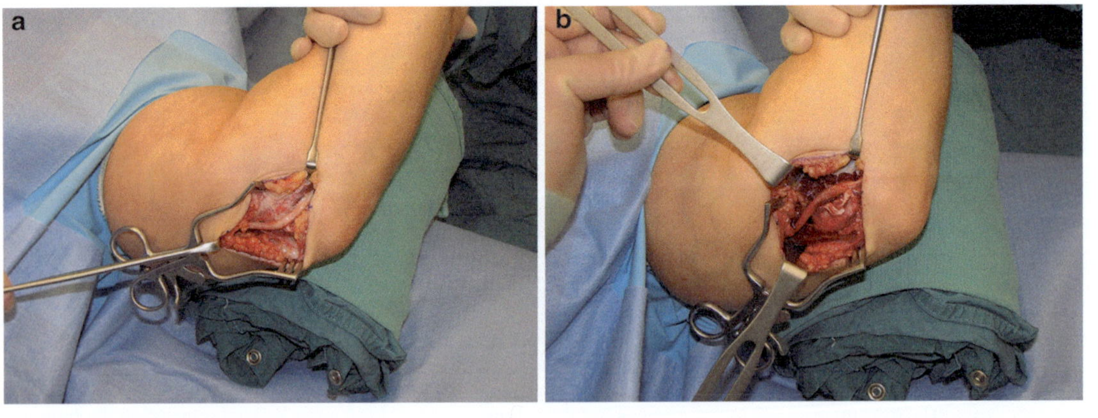

Fig. 5.2 Cubital tunnel release with ulnar nerve transposition: (**a**) decompression of ulnar nerve and (**b**) position of nerve after transposition

Table 5.1 Differential diagnosis of loss of active finger extension in RA patients

Diagnosis	Physical examination	Treatment
MCP joint dislocation	Flexed, ulnarly deviated posture of MCP joint, lack of passive extension, visible/palpable extensor tendon	MCP joint arthroplasty
Extensor tendon subluxation	Patient may keep MCP joint extended after passively extended by examiner	Extensor tendon centralization, ±MCP joint arthroplasty
Attritional tendon rupture	Loss of MCP joint extension through wrist tenodesis effect, soft tissue swelling about the wrist, possible caput ulnae syndrome	Synovectomy, tendon repair/transfer
PIN compression at the elbow	MCP joint extension through wrist tenodesis effect, radial deviation of wrist due to ECU paralysis, soft tissue swelling about the elbow	Corticosteroid injection, PIN decompression with synovectomy, tendon transfers if chronic

MCP metacarpophalangeal, *PIN* posterior interosseous nerve

arthritis may need a future total elbow arthroplasty. In these cases, transposition is recommended to position the nerve away from the anticipated future osteotomy sites [33]. Although there are case reports of good results after surgery [13, 44, 46], there are no outcome studies evaluating large groups of RA patients after cubital tunnel decompression.

Posterior Interosseous Nerve Palsy

There are multiple potential causes for the loss of active finger extension (Table 5.1). The differential diagnosis includes metacarpophalangeal (MCP) joint dislocation (most commonly), extensor tendon subluxation between the metacarpal heads, attritional tendon rupture, and posterior interosseous nerve (PIN) compression at the elbow [57]. Although the diagnosis can often be made using examination alone, a systematic evaluation is mandatory to prevent misdiagnosis and/or a delay in treatment.

PIN palsy is a rare occurrence in RA patients [58]. This uncommon finding typically results from synovial hypertrophy of the elbow leading to mechanical compression of the PIN as it passes under the supinator and arcade of Fröhse [59, 60]. RA-related anterior subluxation of the radial head has also been reported to cause compression of the PIN [61]. In addition to the loss of active finger extension, PIN compression will lead to radial wrist deviation with active wrist extension due to the loss of extensor carpi ulnaris function. Furthermore, there may be soft tissue swelling about the elbow resulting from synovitis of the radiohumeral and ulnohumeral joints [57]. Because the extensor tendons remain in continuity, MCP joint extension is possible through wrist flexion (tenodesis). Whereas attritional rupture typically affects the ring and small finger extensors first, PIN palsy leads to more profound weakness of the middle and ring fingers with less involvement of the index and small fingers [57].

Pathology about the elbow joint may be characterized with MRI [12], and EMG/NCS typically confirms the diagnosis of PIN palsy. EMG abnormalities will be found only in the muscles innervated by the PIN [58, 62]. These studies reveal scant or absent axonal regeneration and a decreased amplitude and conduction velocity. EMG/NCS are also useful to rule out a vasculitic etiology for nerve palsy. In these cases, decreased amplitudes are found, but conduction velocities are typically normal [63].

Anatomy

The radial nerve, from which the PIN originates, is a terminal branch of the posterior cord of the brachial plexus. Beginning posterior to the axillary artery, the radial nerve continues distally along the spiral groove of the humerus [17, 64]. The nerve then penetrates the lateral intermuscular septum as it courses from the posterior to the anterior compartment of the arm. The radial nerve splits into the terminal motor PIN and the radial sensory nerve approximately 6.0–10.5 cm proximal to the supinator [65, 66] prior to entering the forearm. The PIN subsequently enters the radial tunnel, which extends from the humeroradial joint to the proximal edge of the superficial head of the supinator [67]. The radial tunnel is bordered by the brachioradialis (BR), extensor carpi radialis longus (ECRL), extensor carpi radialis brevis (ECRB), biceps tendon, and brachialis. The floor of the radial tunnel is comprised of the radiocapitellar joint [68]. The nerve then passes underneath the proximal leading edge of the supinator (i.e., arcade of Fröhse) before continuing into the forearm, providing motor innervation to the extensor muscles and abductor pollicis longus [17]. It does not innervate the BR, ECRL, or anconeus muscles. Most authors agree that the arcade of Fröhse is the most common cause of PIN compression [64].

Surgical Treatment

The absence of evidence-based guidelines for treatment underscores the rarity of PIN compression in RA patients. Surgery is not the only option for treatment of PIN compression in RA patients. In fact, intra-articular corticosteroid injections may lead to symptom resolution in up to 50 % of patients [59, 69, 70]. Some authors recommend PIN decompression only in those failing medical management or with confirmation of a compressive lesion [60]. We, however, agree with the recommendation for early decompression of the PIN in RA patients [13, 26] as the results of nonoperative treatment are highly variable [26, 69] and surgery is nearly uniformly successful [51, 52, 71–73].

Decompression may be performed through an anterolateral or posterolateral approach. The anterolateral approach is commonly used for decompression [26], but the posterolateral approach is recommended if concomitant radial head excision is to be performed [70]. The anterolateral approach is advocated as it can easily be extended proximally, but it can be difficult to retract the BR radially enough to visualize the radial tunnel and distal sites of compression may be inadequately visualized. Although the posterolateral approach is limited by the inability to extend the surgical exposure more proximally, we have not found that this compromises the ability to achieve adequate nerve release; this is our preferred technique (Fig. 5.3). A 5–10 cm incision is designed extending from the lateral epicondyle distally along the posterior border of the BR. The interval between the BR and the ECRL is bluntly defined. The ECRB fascia is incised and the supinator is identified. As the plane is developed, the PIN will be found within the surrounding fat. With the nerve protected, the recurrent radial vessels of Henry are exposed, ligated, and divided. The arcade of Fröhse and the superficial head of the supinator are subsequently released. A simultaneous synovectomy is performed.

Conclusions

With ongoing advances in drug development over the past few decades, medical management of RA has substantially improved [74]. Despite this progress, patients with RA will continue to be afflicted with peripheral compression neuropathies. The unique nature of nerve compression in patients with RA requires an experienced hand surgeon with sufficient understanding of the various potential etiologies. Using the aforementioned diagnostic principles and surgical techniques, satisfactory outcomes may be achieved.

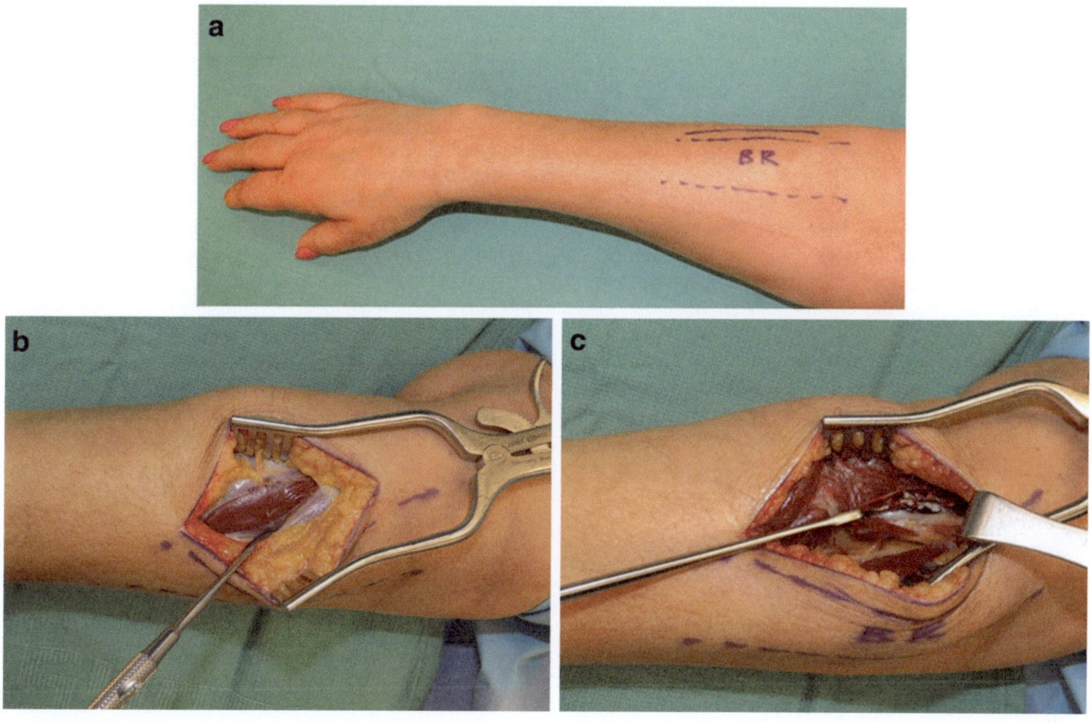

Fig. 5.3 Posterolateral approach to the posterior interosseous nerve: (**a**) skin markings, (**b**) superficial dissection through the brachioradialis/extensor carpi radialis longus interval, and (**c**) deep exposure of PIN and dorsal radial sensory branch after release of extensor carpi radialis brevis fascia

References

1. Waljee JF, Chung KC. Outcomes research in rheumatoid arthritis. Hand Clin. 2011;27(1):115–26.
2. Aneja R, Singh MB, Shankar S, et al. Prevalence of peripheral neuropathy in patients with newly diagnosed rheumatoid arthritis. Indian J Rheumatol. 2007;2(2):47–50.
3. Cimmino MA, Salvarani C, Macchioni P, et al. Extra-articular manifestations in 587 Italian patients with rheumatoid arthritis. Rheumatol Int. 2000;19(6):213–7.
4. Turesson C, Jacobsson LT. Epidemiology of extra-articular manifestations in rheumatoid arthritis. Scand J Rheumatol. 2004;33(2):65–72.
5. Agarwal V, Singh R, Wiclaf, et al. A clinical, electrophysiological, and pathological study of neuropathy in rheumatoid arthritis. Clin Rheumatol. 2008; 27(7):841–4.
6. Lanzillo B, Pappone N, Crisci CDI, et al. Subclinical peripheral nerve involvement in patients with rheumatoid arthritis. Arthritis Rheum. 1998;41(7): 1196–202.
7. Sivri A, Guler-Uysal F. The electroneurophysiological findings in rheumatoid arthritis patients. Electromyogr Clin Neurophysiol. 1999;39(7): 387–91.
8. Bharadwaj A, Haroon N. Interstitial lung disease and neuropathy as predominant extra-articular manifestation in patients with rheumatoid arthritis. Med Sci Monit. 2005;11(10):CR498–502.
9. Nadkar MY, Agarwal R, Samant RS, et al. Neuropathy in rheumatoid arthritis. J Assoc Physicians India. 2001;49:217–20.
10. Lang AH, Kalliomäki JL, Puusa A, et al. Sensory neuropathy in rheumatoid arthritis: an electroneurographic study. Scand J Rheumatol. 1981;10(2):81–4.
11. Herbison GJ, Teng C, Martin JH, et al. Carpal tunnel syndrome in rheumatoid arthritis. Am J Phys Med. 1973;52(2):68–74.
12. Vallat J-M, Rabin M, Magy L. Peripheral neuropathies in rheumatic disease—a guide to diagnosis. Nat Rev Rheumatol. 2012;8(10):599–609.
13. Muramatsu K, Tanaka H, Taguchi T. Peripheral neuropathies of the forearm and hand in rheumatoid arthritis: diagnosis and options for treatment. Rheumatol Int. 2008;28(10):951–7.
14. Conn DL, McDuffie FC, Dyck PJ. Immunopathologic study of sural nerves in rheumatoid arthritis. Arthritis Rheum. 1972;15(2):135–43.

15. Bekkelund SI, Torbergsen T, Husby G, et al. Myopathy and neuropathy in rheumatoid arthritis. A quantitative controlled electromyographic study. J Rheumatol. 1999;26(11):2348–51.
16. Sivri A, Güler-Uysal F. The electroneurophysiological evaluation of rheumatoid arthritis patients. Clin Rheumatol. 1998;17(5):416–8.
17. Mackinnon SE, Novak CB. Compression neuropathies. In: Wolfe SW, Hotchkiss RN, Pederson WC, Kozin SH, editors. Green's operative hand surgery. 6th ed. Philadelphia, PA: Elsevier; 2011. p. 977–1014.
18. Cheng CJ, Mackinnon-Patterson B, Beck JL, et al. The scratch collapse test for evaluation of carpal and cubital tunnel syndrome. J Hand Surg Am. 2008; 33(9):1518–24.
19. Phalen GS. The carpal tunnel syndrome: seventeen years' experience in diagnosis and treatment of six hundred and fifty four hands. J Bone Joint Surg Am. 1966;48(2):211–28.
20. Durkan JA. A new diagnostic test for carpal tunnel syndrome. J Bone Joint Surg Am. 1991;73(4):535–8.
21. Papp SR, Athwal GS, Pichora DR. The rheumatoid wrist. J Am Acad Orthop Surg. 2006;14(2):65–77.
22. Szabo RM, Kwak C. Natural history and conservative management of cubital tunnel syndrome. Hand Clin. 2007;23(3):311–8.
23. Celiker R, Arslan S, Inanici F. Corticosteroid injection vs. nonsteroidal antiinflammatory drug and splinting in carpal tunnel syndrome. Am J Phys Med Rehabil. 2002;81(3):182–6.
24. Bickel KD. Carpal tunnel syndrome. J Hand Surg Am. 2010;35(1):147e–52.
25. Grabois M, Puentes J, Lidsky M. Tarsal tunnel syndrome in rheumatoid arthritis. Arch Phys Med Rehabil. 1981;62(8):401–3.
26. White SH, Goodfellow JW, Mowat A. Posterior interosseous nerve palsy in rheumatoid arthritis. J Bone Joint Surg Br. 1988;70(3):468–71.
27. Geoghegan JM, Clark DI, Bainbridge LC, et al. Risk factors in carpal tunnel syndrome. J Hand Surg Br. 2004;29(4):315–20.
28. Karadag O, Kalyoncu U, Akdogan A, et al. Sonographic assessment of carpal tunnel syndrome in rheumatoid arthritis: prevalence and correlation with disease activity. Rheumatol Int. 2012;32(8):2313–9.
29. Stevens JC, Beard CM, O'Fallon WM, et al. Conditions associated with carpal tunnel syndrome. Mayo Clin Proc. 1992;67(6):541–8.
30. Shinoda J, Hashizume H, McCown C, et al. Carpal tunnel syndrome grading system in rheumatoid arthritis. J Orthop Sci. 2002;7(2):188–93.
31. Feldon P, Terrono AL. Carpal tunnel syndrome in rheumatoid arthritis. Tech Orthop. 2006;21(1): 42–7.
32. Duckworth AD, Jenkins PJ, McEachan JE. Diagnosing carpal tunnel syndrome. J Hand Surg Am. 2014; 39(7):1403–7.
33. Hayton M. Vascular and neurological considerations in rheumatoid arthritis. Int Congr Ser. 2006;1295: 34–42.
34. Clayton ML. Surgical treatment at the wrist in rheumatoid arthritis: a review of thirty-seven patients. J Bone Joint Surg Am. 1965;47:741–50.
35. Britz GW, Haynor DR, Kuntz C, et al. Carpal tunnel syndrome: correlation of magnetic resonance imaging, clinical electrodiagnostic, and intraoperative findings. Neurosurgery. 1995;37(6):1097–103.
36. Pierre-Jerome C, Bekkelund SI, Mellgren SI, et al. The rheumatoid wrist: bilateral MR analysis of the distribution of rheumatoid lesions in axial plain in a female population. Clin Rheumatol. 1997;16(1):80–6.
37. Dang AC, Rodner CM. Unusual compression neuropathies of the forearm, part II: median nerve. J Hand Surg Am. 2009;34(10):1915–20.
38. Jabaley M, Wallace W, Heckler F. Internal topography of major nerves of the forearm and hand: a current view. J Hand Surg Am. 1980;5(1):1–18.
39. Sunderland S. The intraneural topography of the radial, median and ulnar nerves. Brain. 1945;68:243–99.
40. Belcher HJ, Varma S, Schonauer F. Endoscopic carpal tunnel release in selected rheumatoid patients. J Hand Surg Br. 2000;25(5):451–2.
41. Ertel AN, Millender LH, Nalebuff EA, et al. Flexor tendon ruptures in patients with rheumatoid arthritis. J Hand Surg Am. 1988;13(6):860–6.
42. Louie DL, Earp BE, Collins JE, et al. Outcomes of open carpal tunnel release at a minimum of ten years. J Bone Joint Surg Am. 2013;95(12):1067–73.
43. Adkinson JM, Chung KC. Minimal-incision in situ ulnar nerve decompression at the elbow. Hand Clin. 2014;30(1):63–70.
44. Mainard D, Saury P, Delagoutte JP. Ulnar nerve compression at the elbow caused by synovial cyst of rheumatoid origin. Rev Rhum Mal Osteoartic. 1991; 58(9):611–4.
45. Cho C-H, Kim B-S, Bae K-C, et al. Attritional rupture of ulnar nerve in a patient with rheumatoid arthritis. J Rheum Dis. 2012;19(6):348–50.
46. Nakagawa N, Abe S, Saegusa Y, et al. Giant geode at the olecranon in the rheumatoid elbow—two case reports. Clin Rheumatol. 2004;23(4):358–61.
47. Waugh RP, Zlotolow DA. In situ decompression of the ulnar nerve at the cubital tunnel. Hand Clin. 2007;23(3):319–27. vi.
48. McGowen A. The results of transposition of the ulnar nerve for traumatic ulnar neuritis. J Bone Joint Surg Br. 1950;32(3):293–301.
49. Posner MA. Compressive neuropathies of the ulnar nerve at the elbow and wrist. Instr Course Lect. 2000;49:305–17.
50. Idler RS. General principles of patient evaluation and nonoperative management of cubital syndrome. Hand Clin. 1996;12(2):397–403.
51. Minami M, Kato S, Kondo M, et al. Posterior interosseous nerve palsy secondary to rheumatoid cyst of the elbow joint: case report. Mod Rheumatol. 2004;14: 191–5.
52. Ogawa H. Posterior interosseous nerve palsy related to rheumatoid synovitis of the elbow. Mod Rheumatol. 2007;17:327–9.

53. Polatsch DB, Melone Jr CP, Beldner S, et al. Ulnar nerve anatomy. Hand Clin. 2007;23(3):283–9.
54. Kalaci A, Aslan B, Yanat AN. Spontaneous rupture of ulnar nerve due to neglected cubital tunnel syndrome associated with rheumatoid arthritis. J Clin Rheumatol. 2007;13(4):217–8.
55. Moore JR, Weiland AJ. Bilateral attritional rupture of the ulnar nerve at the elbow. J Hand Surg Am. 1980;5:358–60.
56. Ochi K, Ikari K, Momohara S. Attrition rupture of ulnar nerve in an elbow of a patient with rheumatoid arthritis. J Rheumatol. 2014;41(10):2085.
57. Feldon P, Terrono AL, Nalebuff EA, et al. Rheumatoid arthritis and other connective tissue diseases. In: Wolfe SW, Hotchkiss RN, Pederson WC, Kozin SH, editors. Green's operative hand surgery. 6th ed. Philadelphia, PA: Elsevier; 2011. p. 1993–2065.
58. Kishner S, Biundo Jr JJ. Posterior interosseous neuropathy in rheumatoid arthritis. J Clin Rheumatol. 1996;2(1):29–32.
59. Millender LH, Nalebuff EA, Holdsworth DE. Posterior interosseous-nerve syndrome secondary to rheumatoid synovitis. J Bone Joint Surg Am. 1973;55(4):753–7.
60. Malipeddi A, Reddy VR, Kallarackal G. Posterior interosseous nerve palsy: an unusual complication of rheumatoid arthritis: case report and review of the literature. Semin Arthritis Rheum. 2011;40(6):576–9.
61. Hirachi K, Kato A, Minami T, et al. Clinical features and management of traumatic posterior interosseous nerve palsy. J Hand Surg Br. 1998;23(3):413–7.
62. Hanna BD, Robertson FW, Ansell BM, et al. Nerve entrapment at the elbow in rheumatoid arthritis. Rheumatol Rehabil. 1975;14(4):212–7.
63. Chan JK, Kennett R, Smith G. Posterior interosseous nerve palsy in rheumatoid arthritis: case report and literature review. J Plast Reconstr Aesthet Surg. 2009;62(12):e556–60.
64. Dang AC, Rodner CM. Unusual compression neuropathies of the forearm, part I: radial nerve. J Hand Surg Am. 2009;34(10):1906–14.
65. Abrams RA, Ziets RJ, Lieber RL, et al. Anatomy of the radial nerve motor branches in the forearm. J Hand Surg Am. 1997;22(2):232–7.
66. Thomas SJ, Yakin DE, Parry BR, et al. The anatomical relationship between the posterior interosseous nerve and the supinator muscle. J Hand Surg Am. 2000;25(5):936–41.
67. Eaton CJ, Lister GD. Radial nerve compression. Hand Clin. 1992;8(2):345–57.
68. Naam NH, Nemani S. Radial tunnel syndrome. Orthop Clin North Am. 2012;43(4):529–36.
69. Ishikawa H, Hirohata K. Posterior interosseous nerve syndrome associated with rheumatoid synovial cysts of the elbow joint. Clin Orthop Relat Res. 1990; 254:134–9.
70. Westkaemper JG, Varitimidis SE, Sotereanos DG. Posterior interosseous nerve palsy in a patient with rheumatoid synovitis of the elbow: a case report and review of the literature. J Hand Surg Am. 1999; 24(4):727–31.
71. Roth AI, Stulberg BN, Fleegler EJ, et al. Elbow arthrography in the evaluation of posterior interosseous nerve compression in rheumatoid arthritis. J Hand Surg Br. 1986;11(1):120–2.
72. Muratmatsu K, Kojima T, Yoshida K. Peripheral neuropathies associated with rheumatoid synovial cysts of the elbow joint: three case reports. J Clin Rheumatol. 2006;12:287–90.
73. Hall HC, Mackinnon SE, Gilbert RW. An approach to the posterior interosseous nerve. Plast Reconstr Surg. 1984;74(3):435–7.
74. Kahlenberg JM, Fox DA. Advances in the medical treatment of rheumatoid arthritis. Hand Clin. 2011; 27(1):11–20.

Current Treatment Outcomes Among Patients with Rheumatoid Hand and Wrist Deformities

6

Jennifer F. Waljee

Introduction

Rheumatoid arthritis (RA) is the most common inflammatory arthropathy, causing substantial pain and disability for over one million individuals in the USA [1–5]. To date, there is no cure for RA, and its etiology remains unknown. Advances in medical treatment have alleviated many of the severe disease manifestations among patients with RA. The early, targeted treatment to achieve low disease activity is considered the current standard of care. However, for nearly 20 % of patients, joint destruction, pain, and disability persist, and the chronic inflammation associated with RA is correlated with an increased risk of systemic complications, including cardiovascular disease [6]. Identifying patients who may not respond to medical regiments remains elusive, and prophylactic and therapeutic surgical procedures continue to play an important role in the management of RA to alleviate chronic joint-related pain and deformity. Prophylactic surgical procedures include synovectomy and off-loading procedures (e.g., radiolunate fusion, distal ulna resection), whereas therapeutic surgical procedures include joint replacement, joint arthrodesis, tendon transfer, and tendon rebalancing procedures [7]. This review will explore the current state of outcomes among patients with RA and future directions that focus on streamlining surgical decision-making and the cost efficiency of care in order to better direct patients to the treatments that best align with their goals and priorities.

Medical Management of RA

In the early stages of RA, physical therapy can significantly reduce pain and increase ability to perform activities of daily living. In this early stage, nonoperative management is indicated [8]. Traditional medical therapy includes nonsteroidal anti-inflammatory drugs (NSAIDs), steroids, and analgesics. Although these agents cannot stop disease progression, they can minimize inflammation and pain [9]. In the 1980s, disease-modifying antirheumatic drugs (DMARDs), such as methotrexate, leflunomide, and sulfasalazine, were introduced. For example, methotrexate can slow disease progression and is safe for long-term use [10–12]. Today, the majority of patients are initiated on DMARDs within 3 months of diagnosis and are now standard of care for newly diagnosed patients [13–15]. In 1998, biologic DMARDs were approved by the FDA for use

J.F. Waljee, MD, MS (✉)
Comprehensive Hand Center, Section of Plastic Surgery, Department of Surgery, The University of Michigan Health System, 1500 E. Medical Center Drive, 2130 Taubman Center, SPC 5340, Ann Arbor, MI 48109-5340, USA
e-mail: filip@med.umich.edu

K.C. Chung (ed.), *Clinical Management of the Rheumatoid Hand, Wrist, and Elbow*,
DOI 10.1007/978-3-319-26660-2_6

among patients with RA and can effectively slow disease progression and sustain remission over time. Although numerous biologic DMARDs exist, all inhibit a common pathway directed toward proinflammatory cytokines including TNF (TNFα), interleukin-1 (IL-1), interleukin-6 (IL-6), or T or B cells. For example, etanercept is a soluble TNFα receptor that competes with native receptors in order to block the proinflammatory effect of TNFα. Multiple studies have demonstrated that when combined with methotrexate, biologics rapidly improve symptoms and halt joint erosion [16–23]. The use of biologics among patients within the first 2 years of diagnosis of RA has increased markedly over time, rising from 3 % in 1999 to 26 % in 2006 [24, 25].

Current guidelines now advocate the use of DMARDs with a "treat to target" approach. The principles of this tailored strategy include reaching disease remission as the best target, particularly for patients with early disease, and low-disease activity as an alternative target for patients with longer-standing disease [26]. Low disease activity is defined by several measures. For example, the disease activity score (DAS) is a quantitative index that includes the number of swollen joints, tender joints, acute-phase response, and patient self-report of general health [27]. Using the DAS-28, a score of <3.2 is considered LDA or <2.4 for the DAS-44. Alternatively, the Simplified or Clinical Disease Activity Indices (SDAI, CDAI) can be used to estimate disease activity. In general, LDA is defined as the state at which progression of joint damage is minimal and physical function, quality of life, and work capacity are preserved. Disease activity is assessed at regular intervals, and therapy is modified at least every 3 months until the treatment target (remission or low disease activity) is reached, ideally within 6 months [28]. Once the desired outcome has been achieved, reducing the dose or expanding the interval between doses is a feasible approach that enables maintenance of the outcome in most patients.

Despite their popularity and promise, several unanswered questions remain regarding biologics. First, biologics are powerful immunosuppressants, and their long-term risks are unknown. Furthermore, biologics are administered by either intravenous infusion or subcutaneous injection. The extent to which eligible patients are capable of administering this independently or have the resources to receive therapy at a facility is unknown but varies by patient sociodemographic attributes. Physician attributes may also influence receipt of biologic therapy, and in the USA, a relative shortage of rheumatologists exists [29]. Many RA patients are managed by primary care providers who may be unfamiliar with complex RA treatment regimens, and clinical decision-making may vary by physician specialty [30, 31]. Finally, patient response to DMARD therapy is not uniform and is dependent on important factors, including the chronicity of disease and prior medication exposure [6].

Surgical Management of RA

In contrast to medical therapy, surgery cannot alter disease progression but can provide predictable and effective relief from joint pain and deformity [32]. Knee replacement remains the most common initial procedure among RA patients. However, upper extremity procedures are performed earlier, in general, compared with lower extremity procedures, suggesting the impact that joint pain, deformity, and disability have on the activities of daily living among patients with RA [33]. Surgical outcomes are generally poorer among patients with RA compared with osteoarthritis, but many patients experience sustained pain relief and can return to many of their usual activities of daily living [34–36]. For example, among patients with upper extremity disability, total wrist fusion (TWF) and silicone metacarpophalangeal arthroplasty (SMPA) remain two of the most predictably effective surgical interventions [37]. An ongoing, prospective multicenter study of RA patients has consistently demonstrated that SMPA enhances self-reported hand function, restores anatomic finger position, and improves arc and range of motion, even for severe deformities [38–41] (Figs. 6.1 and 6.2). These improvements are sustained in 5-year follow-up, and even patients with severe ulnar drift

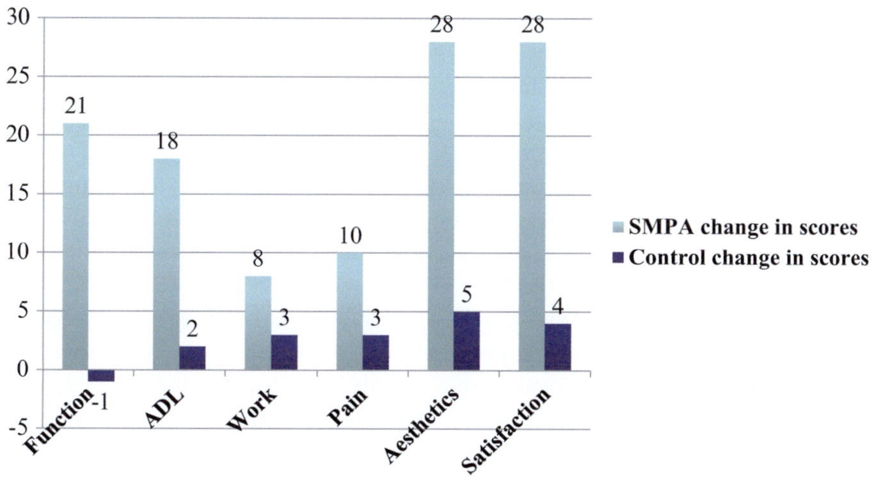

Fig. 6.1 MHQ scores improve significantly 3 years following SMPA

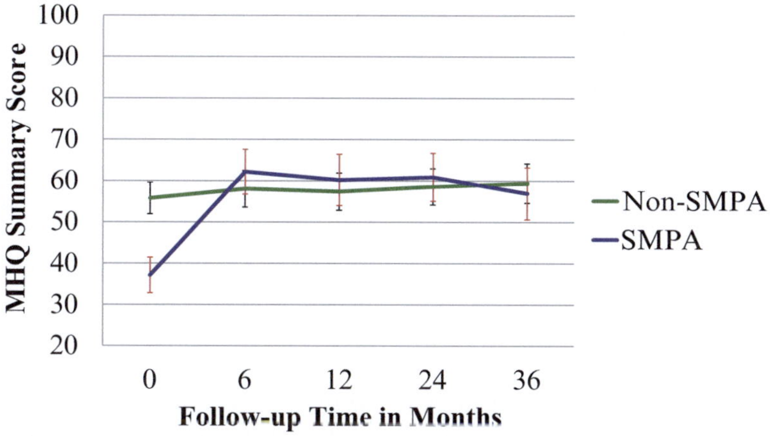

Fig. 6.2 MHQ scores maintained at 3 year FU. From Chung KC, et al. Long-term follow-up for rheumatoid arthritis patients in a multicenter outcomes study of silicone metacarpophalangeal joint arthroplasty. *Arthritis Care Res (Hoboken)*. 2012; 64(9):1292–300. Reprinted with permission from John Wiley and Sons

or extension lag achieve benefit comparable to patients with less advanced deformity [40, 41].

Similarly, for patients with debilitating radiocarpal arthritis, TWF remains a cornerstone of treatment. Technological advances in implant reconstruction have spurred interest in the possibility of implant wrist arthroplasty to preserve motion. A large systematic review of 20 studies and over 800 procedures revealed that functional outcomes and range of motion following wrist fusion were similar compared with arthroplasty [42]. Although wrist arthroplasty offers the possibility of greater wrist range of motion, wrist arthroplasty is technically challenging and expensive with a greater risk of implant complications. Clinical studies have not demonstrated a substantial overall benefit with arthroplasty over wrist fusion for patients with RA [42–45].

Despite the benefits of surgery, procedures for RA have declined following the introduction of DMARDs [46]. For example, in Japan, an analysis of data drawn from the Institute of Rheumatology,

Rheumatoid Arthritis (IORRA) study, between 2000 and 2007, reveals that synovectomy procedures have diminished fivefold following the introduction of methotrexate in 1999 [47]. Moreover, patients undergoing surgery present with milder disease compared with patients in previous years [47–54]. Recent studies in Sweden and Denmark also report a decline in large joint arthroplasty and synovectomy [47, 55–57]. In the USA, regional studies have identified similar trends [50, 58]. Taken together, these findings suggest that medical therapy is supplanting surgical intervention, despite the costs associated with newer biologic agents and the predictability of surgical outcomes.

Current Treatment Patterns among Patients with Rheumatoid Arthritis

Although numerous studies have examined the effectiveness of medical and surgical therapy for RA, a comprehensive approach to integrate medical regimens and surgical reconstruction has not been described [59]. For example, rheumatologists are skeptical of the efficacy of prophylactic and therapeutic surgery for RA (Table 6.1). Many prefer to treat patients pharmacologically for as long as possible and perceive surgery as an end-stage, salvage option [59, 60]. Furthermore, rheumatologists feel that hand surgeons may be overly aggressive in their approach to patients and too optimistic regarding the benefits of surgery [60–62]. In contrast, surgeons feel that patients are referred too late for surgery to prevent further joint destruction. Many perceive that medical therapy is extended into advanced stages of disease, and the possibility of reconstructing functionally and aesthetically acceptable hands becomes impossible.

Interestingly, surgeons and rheumatologists agree that evidence regarding the relative effectiveness of medical and surgical therapy is lacking. Over half of the surgeons feel that there is high-quality research to support the usefulness of rheumatoid hand surgical procedures; yet, far fewer rheumatologists feel that there is high-quality data to affirm the value of surgical reconstruction [59]. Both rheumatologists and surgeons feel that the other's knowledge of surgical options and outcomes is suboptimal and overestimate their ability to communicate with one another. As such, the indications for hand and upper extremity reconstructive procedures for RA-related deformities remain controversial among rheumatologists and surgeons, and rates of surgery vary widely across the USA [2, 59].

These differences have measurable effects on the delivery of care to RA patients. For example, less than 20 % of hand surgeons and rheumatologists treat RA patients in a multidisciplinary setting, despite strong evidence that supports this approach. On a population level, controversy regarding the relative effectiveness of medical and surgical therapy translates into differences in care across the country [63]. For example, an analysis of administrative data reveals a 9- to 12-fold difference in the rates of upper extremity joint fusion, tenosynovectomy, and arthroplasty by geographic location, irrespective of the number of hand surgeons, disease prevalence, or the sociodemographic profile of the region [64]. In a recent analysis of Medicare beneficiaries

Table 6.1 Hand surgeons' and rheumatologists' attitudes toward the effectiveness of MCP joint arthroplasty for RA

	Responded usually/always (%)			
	Hand surgeons	Rheumatologists	p-value	OR
Improves function	82.5	34.1	<0.001	10.1
Decreases pain	91.8	59.2	<0.001	8.1
Improves aesthetics	95.0	66.5	<0.001	11.8
Improves pain	33.1	23.6	<0.001	1.6

From: Alderman AK, Chung KC, Kim HM et al. 2003. Effectiveness of Rheumatoid Hand Surgery: Contrasting Perceptions of Hand Surgeons and Rheumatologists. Journal of Hand Surgery: 28A: 3–11. Reprinted with permission from Elsevier Limited diagnosed with RA, rates of surgery also varied ninefold across hospital referral regions in the USA; younger, female, white patients were more likely to undergo surgery. Treatment is also dependent on access to subspecialty physicians, and rates of surgery are higher in regions with greater numbers of orthopedic surgeons. Similarly, rates of surgery are lower in areas of higher rheumatologist density [33, 65]. It is possible that in regions with fewer practicing rheumatologists, patients have less access to DMARDs and aggressive medical regiments, which in turn leading these patients to progress more quickly toward advanced deformities, resulting in higher rates of surgery. Alternatively, these findings may reflect differences in referral patterns for surgery among rheumatologists who are uncertain regarding the effectiveness of joint reconstruction [60–62].

The utilization of DMARDs for RA also demonstrates substantial variation at the geographic and patient level [30, 66]. For example, older patients, patients of lower educational and socioeconomic levels, and African-American patients are less likely to receive DMARDs [67]. Financial barriers also contribute to the differences in access to DMARDs, and federal programs to subsidize medication costs, such as Medicare Part D, do not ameliorate this burden [24, 48, 68–73]. To date the relative cost-effectiveness analysis of medical and surgical therapy remains unknown. Although surgical intervention is often thought of as a salvage option for patients who have failed medical therapy, patients experience predictable relief with durable outcomes from joint reconstruction. For example, RA patients with lower extremity joint destruction gain considerable improvement of pain and function following knee and hip arthroplasty, despite the increased risk of short- and long-term complications, compared with patients undergoing joint replacement for osteoarthritis [74, 75]. Similarly, a recent cost-effectiveness analysis of patients undergoing SMPA demonstrates that favorable outcomes are maintained for several years, and associated costs are far less compared with DMARD regimens, even in the setting of complications and revision procedures [76].

Summary

In light of accelerating healthcare expenditures and an increasing incidence of RA, current research efforts and funding must be directed toward identifying those practices that most efficiently and effectively benefit patients. Executing research among patients with RA remains challenging. RA is rare enough that accruing sufficient patient samples in a prospective manner can be expensive and challenging, and the manifestations and clinical presentation of RA are variable. Robust evidence to support surgical intervention is sparse and often limited by small study sample sizes, retrospective study design, and heterogeneous outcome measurements. Nonetheless, clinical outcomes research will continue to play a pivotal role going forward to identify the relative effectiveness of current treatment options and strategies to create a tailored approach to each patient.

Acknowledgment This research was supported by a Mentored Clinical Investigator Award to Dr. Waljee through the Agency for Healthcare Research and Quality (1K08HS023313-01) and a Clinical Arthritis Research Grant from the American Foundation for Surgery of the Hand.

Financial disclosures and conflicts of interest: The author has nothing to disclose.

References

1. Helmick CG, Felson DT, Lawrence RC, et al. Estimates of the prevalence of arthritis and other rheumatic conditions in the United States. Part I. Arthritis Rheum. 2008;58:15–25.
2. O'Dell JR. Therapeutic strategies for rheumatoid arthritis. N Engl J Med. 2004;350:2591–602.
3. Sherrer YS, Bloch DA, Mitchell DM, Young DY, Fries JF. The development of disability in rheumatoid arthritis. Arthritis Rheum. 1986;29:494–500.
4. Ward MM, Javitz HS, Yelin EH. The direct cost of rheumatoid arthritis. Value Health. 2000;3:243–52.
5. Rat AC, Boissier MC. Rheumatoid arthritis: direct and indirect costs. Joint Bone Spine. 2004;71: 518–24.
6. Felson DT, Klareskog L. The genetics of rheumatoid arthritis: new insights and implications. JAMA. 2015;313:1623–4.
7. Chung KC, Pushman AG. Current concepts in the management of the rheumatoid hand. J Hand Surg Am. 2011;36:736–47. quiz 47.

8. Buljina AI, Taljanovic MS, Avdic DM, Hunter TB. Physical and exercise therapy for treatment of the rheumatoid hand. Arthritis Care Res. 2001;45:392–7.
9. Kahlenberg JM, Fox DA. Advances in the medical treatment of rheumatoid arthritis. Hand Clin. 2011;27(1):11–20.
10. Kremer JM, Lee JK. The safety and efficacy of the use of methotrexate in long-term therapy for rheumatoid arthritis. Arthritis Rheum. 1986;29:822–31.
11. Weinblatt ME, Coblyn JS, Fox DA, et al. Efficacy of low-dose methotrexate in rheumatoid arthritis. N Engl J Med. 1985;312:818–22.
12. Rheumatoid Arthritis. http://ww2.arthritis.org/conditions/diseasecenter/RA/default.asp. Accessed 18 Jan 2008.
13. American College of Rheumatology Subcommittee on Rheumatoid Arthritis Guidelines. Guidelines for the management of rheumatoid arthritis: 2002 update. Arthritis Rheum. 2002;46:328–46.
14. Klippel JH. Biologic therapy for rheumatoid arthritis. N Engl J Med. 2000;343:1640–1.
15. Smolen JS, Landewé R, Breedveld FC, et al. EULAR recommendations for the management of rheumatoid arthritis with synthetic and biological disease-modifying antirheumatic drugs. Ann Rheum Dis. 2010;69:964–75.
16. Weinblatt ME, Keystone EC, Furst DE, et al. Adalimumab, a fully human anti-tumor necrosis factor alpha monoclonal antibody, for the treatment of rheumatoid arthritis in patients taking concomitant methotrexate: the ARMADA trial. Arthritis Rheum. 2003;48:35–45.
17. Bathon JM, Martin RW, Fleischmann RM, et al. A comparison of etanercept and methotrexate in patients with early rheumatoid arthritis. N Engl J Med. 2000;343:1586–93.
18. Lipsky PE, van der Heijde DM, St Clair EW, et al. Infliximab and methotrexate in the treatment of rheumatoid arthritis. Anti-tumor necrosis factor trial in rheumatoid arthritis with concomitant therapy study group. N Engl J Med. 2000;343:1594–602.
19. Breedveld FC, Emery P, Keystone EC, et al. Infliximab in active early rheumatoid arthritis. Ann Rheum Dis. 2004;63:149–55.
20. den Broeder AA, Joosten LAB, Saxne T, et al. Long term anti-tumour necrosis factor [alpha] monotherapy in rheumatoid arthritis: effect on radiological course and prognostic value of markers of cartilage turnover and endothelial activation. Ann Rheum Dis. 2002; 61:311–8.
21. Weinblatt ME, Kremer JM, Bankhurst AD, et al. A trial of etanercept, a recombinant tumor necrosis factor receptor:Fc fusion protein, in patients with rheumatoid arthritis receiving methotrexate. N Engl J Med. 1999;340:253–9.
22. Wolfe F, Michaud K. The loss of health status in rheumatoid arthritis and the effect of biologic therapy: a longitudinal observational study. Arthritis Res Ther. 2010;12:R35.
23. Scott DL, Kingsley GH. Tumor necrosis factor inhibitors for rheumatoid arthritis. N Engl J Med. 2006; 355:704–12.
24. Yazici Y, Shi N, John A. Utilization of biologic agents in rheumatoid arthritis in the United States: analysis of prescribing patterns in 16,752 newly diagnosed patients and patients new to biologic therapy. Bull NYU Hosp Jt Dis. 2008;66:77–85.
25. Hjardem E, Hetland ML, Ostergaard M, Krogh NS, Kvien TK. Prescription practice of biological drugs in rheumatoid arthritis during the first 3 years of post-marketing use in Denmark and Norway: criteria are becoming less stringent. Ann Rheum Dis. 2005;64: 1220–3.
26. Guidelli GM, Barskova T, Brizi MG, et al. One year in review: novelties in the treatment of rheumatoid arthritis. Clin Exp Rheumatol. 2015;33:102–8.
27. van Riel PL. The development of the disease activity score (DAS) and the disease activity score using 28 joint counts (DAS28). Clin Exp Rheumatol. 2014; 32:S-65–74.
28. Smolen JS, Aletaha D. Rheumatoid arthritis therapy reappraisal: strategies, opportunities and challenges. Nat Rev Rheumatol. 2015;11:276–89.
29. Deal CL, Hooker R, Harrington T, et al. The United States rheumatology workforce: supply and demand, 2005–2025. Arthritis Rheum. 2007;56:722–9.
30. Neovius M, Simard JF, Askling J, Group AS. Nationwide prevalence of rheumatoid arthritis and penetration of disease-modifying drugs in Sweden. Ann Rheum Dis. 2011;70:624–9.
31. Neovius M, Sundstrom A, Simard J, et al. Small-area variations in sales of TNF inhibitors in Sweden between 2000 and 2009. Scand J Rheumatol. 2011; 40:8–15.
32. Jonsson B, Larsson SE. Functional improvement and costs of hip and knee arthroplasty in destructive rheumatoid arthritis. Scand J Rheumatol. 1991;20:351–7.
33. Waljee J, Zhong L, Baser O, Yuce H, Fox DA, Chung KC. The incidence of upper and lower extremity surgery for rheumatoid arthritis among medicare beneficiaries. J Bone Joint Surg Am. 2015;97:403–10.
34. Ravi B, Escott B, Shah PS, et al. A systematic review and meta-analysis comparing complications following total joint arthroplasty for rheumatoid arthritis versus for osteoarthritis. Arthritis Rheum. 2012;64: 3839–49.
35. Kirwan JR, Currey HL, Freeman MA, Snow S, Young PJ. Overall long-term impact of total hip and knee joint replacement surgery on patients with osteoarthritis and rheumatoid arthritis. Br J Rheumatol. 1994;33:357–60.
36. Clement ND, Breusch SJ, Biant LC. Lower limb joint replacement in rheumatoid arthritis. J Orthop Surg Res. 2012;7:27.
37. Ghattas L, Mascella F, Pomponio G. Hand surgery in rheumatoid arthritis: state of the art and suggestions for research. Rheumatology (Oxford). 2005;44: 834–45.

38. Chung KC, Kowalski CP, Myra Kim H, Kazmers IS. Patient outcomes following Swanson silastic metacarpophalangeal joint arthroplasty in the rheumatoid hand: a systematic overview. J Rheumatol. 2000; 27:1395–402.
39. Chung KC, Kotsis SV, Kim HM. A prospective outcomes study of Swanson metacarpophalangeal joint arthroplasty for the rheumatoid hand. J Hand Surg Am. 2004;29:646–53.
40. Chung KC, Burke FD, Wilgis EF, Regan M, Kim HM, Fox DA. A prospective study comparing outcomes after reconstruction in rheumatoid arthritis patients with severe ulnar drift deformities. Plast Reconstr Surg. 2009;123:1769–77.
41. Chung KC, Burns PB, Wilgis EF, et al. A multicenter clinical trial in rheumatoid arthritis comparing silicone metacarpophalangeal joint arthroplasty with medical treatment. J Hand Surg Am. 2009;34: 815–23.
42. Cavaliere CM, Chung KC. Total wrist arthroplasty and total wrist arthrodesis in rheumatoid arthritis: a decision analysis from the hand surgeons' perspective. J Hand Surg Am. 2008;33:1744–55. 55e1–2.
43. Cavaliere CM, Chung KC. A systematic review of total wrist arthroplasty compared with total wrist arthrodesis for rheumatoid arthritis. Plast Reconstr Surg. 2008;122:813–25.
44. Cavaliere CM, Chung KC. A cost-utility analysis of nonsurgical management, total wrist arthroplasty, and total wrist arthrodesis in rheumatoid arthritis. J Hand Surg Am. 2010;35:379–91. e2.
45. Cavaliere CM, Oppenheimer AJ, Chung KC. Reconstructing the rheumatoid wrist: a utility analysis comparing total wrist fusion and total wrist arthroplasty from the perspectives of rheumatologists and hand surgeons. Hand (NY). 2010;5(1):9–18.
46. Skytta ET, Honkanen PB, Eskelinen A, Huhtala H, Remes V. Fewer and older patients with rheumatoid arthritis need total knee replacement. Scand J Rheumatol. 2012;41:345–9.
47. Momohara S, Ikari K, Mochizuki T. Declining use of synovectomy surgery for patients with rheumatoid arthritis in Japan. Ann Rheum Dis. 2009;68:291–2.
48. Tanaka E, Inoue E, Mannalithara A, et al. Medical care costs of patients with rheumatoid arthritis during the prebiologics period in Japan: a large prospective observational cohort study. Mod Rheumatol. 2010; 20:46–53.
49. Momohara S, Inoue E, Ikari K, et al. Risk factors for wrist surgery in rheumatoid arthritis. Clin Rheumatol. 2008;27:1387–91.
50. da Silva E, Doran MF, Crowson CS, O'Fallon WM, Matteson EL. Declining use of orthopedic surgery in patients with rheumatoid arthritis? Results of a long-term population-based assessment. Arthritis Rheum. 2003;2003:216–20.
51. Ward MM. Decreases in rates of hospitalizations for manifestations of severe rheumatoid arthritis, 1983–2001. Arthritis Rheum. 2004;50.
52. Weiss RJ, Stark A, Wick MC, Ehlin A. Orthopaedic surgery of the lower limbs in 49802 rheumatoid arthritis patients: results from the Swedish national inpatient registry during 1987–2001. Ann Rheum Dis. 2006;65:335–41.
53. Fevang BT, Lie SA, Havelin LI, Engasaeter LB, Furnes O. Reduction in orthopedic surgery among patients with chronic inflammatory joint disease in Norway, 1994–2004. Arthritis Rheum. 2004;57: 529–32.
54. Yamanaka H, Inoue E, Singh G, Tanaka E, Nakajima A, Taniguchi A. Improvement of disease activity of rheumatoid arthritis patients from 2000 to 2006 in a large observational cohort study IORRA in Japan. Mod Rheumatol. 2007;17:283–9.
55. Fevang BT, Lie SA, Havelin LI, Engesaeter LB, Furnes O. Reduction in orthopedic surgery among patients with chronic inflammatory joint disease in Norway, 1994–2004. Arthritis Rheum. 2007;57: 529–32.
56. Pedersen AB, Johnsen SP, Overgaard S, Soballe K, Sorensen HT, Lucht U. Total hip arthroplasty in Denmark: incidence of primary operations and revisions during 1996–2002 and estimated future demands. Acta Orthop. 2005;76:182–9.
57. van Vollenhoven RF, Askling J. Rheumatoid arthritis registries in Sweden. Clin Exp Rheumatol. 2005;23: S195–200.
58. Louie GH, Ward MM. Changes in the rates of joint surgery among patients with rheumatoid arthritis in California, 1983–2007. Ann Rheum Dis. 2010;69: 868–71.
59. Alderman AK, Chung KC, Kim HM, Fox DA, Ubel PA. Effectiveness of rheumatoid hand surgery: contrasting perceptions of hand surgeons and rheumatologists. J Hand Surg Am. 2003;28:3–11. discussion 2–3.
60. Glickel SZ. Commentary: effectiveness of rheumatoid hand surgery. J Hand Surg. 2003;28:12–3.
61. Alderman AK, Ubel PA, Kim HM, Fox DA, Chung KC. Surgical management of the rheumatoid hand: consensus and controversy among rheumatologists and hand surgeons. J Rheumatol. 2003;30: 1464–72.
62. Burke FD, Miranda SM, Owen VM, Bradley MJ, Sinha S. Rheumatoid hand surgery: differing perceptions amongst surgeons, rheumatologists and therapists in the UK. J Hand Surg Eur Vol. 2011;36: 632–41.
63. Alderman AK, Chung KC. Measuring outcomes in hand surgery. Clin Plast Surg. 2008;35:239–50.
64. Alderman AK, Chung KC, Demonner S, Spilson SV, Hayward RA. The rheumatoid hand: a predictable disease with unpredictable surgical practice patterns. Arthritis Rheum. 2002;47:537–42.
65. Zhong L, Chung KC, Baser O, Fox DA, Yuce H, Waljee JF. Variation in rheumatoid hand and wrist surgery among medicare beneficiaries: a population-based cohort study. J Rheumatol. 2015;42:429–36.

66. Edwards CJ, Campbell J, van Staa T, Arden NK. Regional and temporal variation in the treatment of rheumatoid arthritis across the UK: a descriptive register-based cohort study. BMJ Open. 2012;2: e001603.
67. Schmajuk G, Trivedi AN, Solomon DH, et al. Receipt of disease-modifying antirheumatic drugs among patients with rheumatoid arthritis in medicare managed care plans. JAMA. 2011;305:480–6.
68. Polinski JM, Mohr PE, Johnson L. Impact of medicare Part D on access to and cost sharing for specialty biologic medications for beneficiaries with rheumatoid arthritis. Arthritis Rheum. 2009;61:745–54.
69. Wailoo AJ, Bansback N, Brennan A, Michaud K, Nixon RM, Wolfe F. Biologic drugs for rheumatoid arthritis in the medicare program: a cost-effectiveness analysis. Arthritis Rheum. 2008;58:939–46.
70. Doshi JA, Li P, Puig A. Impact of the medicare modernization act of 2003 on utilization and spending for medicare part B-covered biologics in rheumatoid arthritis. Arthritis Care Res (Hoboken). 2010;62:354–61.
71. DeWitt EM, Lin L, Glick HA, Anstrom KJ, Schulman KA, Reed SD. Pattern and predictors of the initiation of biologic agents for the treatment of rheumatoid arthritis in the United States: an analysis using a large observational data bank. Clin Ther. 2009;31:1871–80. discussion 58.
72. Zhang J, Xie F, Delzell E, et al. Trends in the use of biologic therapies among rheumatoid arthritis patients enrolled in the US medicare program. Arthritis Care Res (Hoboken). 2013;65(11):1743–51.
73. Bonafede MM, Fox KM, Johnson BH, Watson C, Gandra SR. Factors associated with the initiation of disease-modifying antirheumatic drugs in newly diagnosed rheumatoid arthritis: a retrospective claims database study. Clin Ther. 2012;34:457–67.
74. Goodman SM, Ramsden-Stein DN, Huang WT, et al. Patients with rheumatoid arthritis are more likely to have pain and poor function after total hip replacements than patients with osteoarthritis. J Rheumatol. 2014;41:1774–80.
75. Stundner O, Chiu YL, Sun X, et al. Perioperative outcomes in patients with rheumatoid versus osteoarthritis for total hip arthroplasty: a population-based study. Clin Exp Rheumatol. 2013;31:889–95.
76. Squitieri L, Chung KC, Hutton DW, Burns PB, Kim HM, Mahmoudi E. A 5-year cost-effectiveness analysis of silicone metacarpophalangeal arthroplasty in patients with rheumatoid arthritis. Plast Reconstr Surg. 2015;136:305–14.

7 Application of Patient-Rated Questionnaires in Rheumatoid Hand Outcomes Research

Erika D. Sears

With pressures to slow the rising costs of health care, there has been a persistent and intense emphasis on measuring outcomes of medical treatments. The science of outcomes measurement has evolved over the past 30 years and is currently instrumental to support the practice of evidence-based medicine, improve health-care delivery, and evaluate the impact of newer technologies. Outcomes research has been especially critical in understanding the effectiveness of hand surgery for patients with rheumatoid arthritis (RA). Prior to the development of standardized outcomes instruments, reported results of rheumatoid hand surgery were mixed. Thus, many rheumatologists were in doubt of the benefits of surgery to improve their patients' hand function, leading to variable collaborative care between rheumatologists and hand surgeons [1, 2]. However, with improved outcomes measurement in RA research, rheumatologists and hand surgeons are increasingly convinced of the benefits of hand surgery to improve patient outcomes and quality of care. All clinicians should have an intimate understanding of the intricacies of outcomes measurement due to the eventual impact on future research, clinical decision-making, and health policy.

E.D. Sears, MD, MS (✉)
Comprehensive Hand Center, Section of Plastic Surgery, Department of Surgery, The University of Michigan Health System, 1500 E. Medical Center Drive, 2130 Taubman Center, SPC 5340, Ann Arbor, MI 48109-5340, USA
e-mail: endavis@med.umich.edu

The Case for Patient-Rated Outcome Measurement

Objective outcomes, such as grip strength, range of motion, extensor lag measurements, and radiographic assessments were the primary outcomes of rheumatoid hand surgery research of the distant past [3]. As the outcomes movement in medicine has evolved, there has been a shift from utilization of objective clinical measures toward inclusion of outcomes from the patient's perspective. With increasing utilization of patient-reported outcomes, a discrepancy between objective measures (impairment) and patient-rated measures (disability) has become apparent [4–9]. Initially, objective measures were thought to be a reliable surrogate of overall patient function. However, it is now widely accepted that objective impairment measures result in varying level of disability based on a variety of patient factors [10–15]. The ultimate goal of hand surgery in patients with RA is to improve hand function and quality of life rather than to improve specified degrees of motion or amount of grip strength. Thus, patient-reported outcomes are now the primary method to measure success of RA surgery or any other medical intervention in

K.C. Chung (ed.), *Clinical Management of the Rheumatoid Hand, Wrist, and Elbow*,
DOI 10.1007/978-3-319-26660-2_7

which quality of life is the main focus. The addition of patient-rated measures has allowed patients' voices to be included in the assessment of outcomes in research and clinical practice. These types of outcomes are often referred to as subjective, patient-reported, or patient-rated outcome (PRO) measures.

PRO questionnaires are used to measure general health, specific symptoms, or domains of health status from the patient's perspective. Although health status and health-related quality of life (HRQOL) are terms often used interchangeably, they are separate entities. Health status is a specific domain of health, such as a scale that rates pain, satisfaction, or work ability. HRQOL is the impact that health status has on overall physical, emotional, and social well-being. PRO questionnaires are used to measure health status, HRQOL, or both. These instruments are classified as generic, region-specific, or disease-specific, based on the intended outcome for which the questionnaire was designed to measure.

Generic questionnaires are used for patients with any diagnosis and are designed to measure general domains of health, such as HRQOL, that are relevant to all patients. These broad domains of health are typically measured by using multiple relevant subscales. In general, researchers have greater familiarity with generic instruments because they are more widely applied across medical disciplines. Furthermore, scores can be compared across patients having different diagnoses and treatments. However, generic questionnaires will not capture all relevant domains of health that patients care about in the treatment for specific clinical problems, such as RA. Region-specific and disease-specific questionnaires have been developed to address these limitations. Region-specific instruments are administered to assess domains of health relevant to a specific anatomic region, such as the hand, wrist, or entire upper extremity. Disease-specific questionnaires measure patient-rated symptoms or aspects of health status relevant to a particular disease process, such as RA. These specific instruments are better able to capture health domains that are influenced by a given disease processes. In addition, region- or disease-specific measures are typically more responsive to change after treatment. However, these measurements are unable to be compared to patients with unrelated diagnoses to evaluate relative societal impact and there is less familiarity across the research community with utilization of more specialized questionnaires.

Quality Assessment of Patient-Rated Questionnaires

Creation of patient-rated questionnaires for clinical and health services research requires a rigorous development process. Upon realizing the variable quality in reporting PROs in the literature, a panel of experts in the measurement science field [the Consensus-Based Standards for the Selection of Health Status Measurement Instruments (COSMIN) study group] devised consensus language and recommendations (Table 7.1) to allow researchers and clinicians to systematically evaluate the quality of questionnaires and studies utilizing patient-reported outcomes [16–18]. At a minimum, scientifically sound PRO instruments undergo a lengthy process of reliability, validity, and responsiveness testing for the desired target patient population.

Reliability

Reliability is assurance that questionnaires are measuring intended health domains in a reproducible manner. Types of reliability include reliability of repeated measures (test–retest), estimation of measurement error, and internal consistency. Intraclass correlation coefficients (ICC) are calculated to measure test–retest reliability. Instruments have acceptable reliability with an ICC greater than 0.9. Measurement error is represented by standard error of measurement (SEM) calculation, which can be translated to calculation of the smallest detectable change (SDC). The SDC is the change above measurement error that can be interpreted as real ($SDC = 1.96 \times \sqrt{2} \times SEM$). Internal consistency testing is

Table 7.1 Questionnaire measurement properties, definitions, and quality criterion

Domain	Property	Definition	Quality criterion
Reliability	Reliability	Extent to which patients can be distinguished from one another despite measurement errors (relative measurement error)	ICC > 0.7
	Measurement error	Extent to which scores on repeated measures are close to one another (absolute measurement error)	SDC < MCID
	Internal consistency	Extent to which items within a scale are intercorrelated and measuring the same construct	0.7 < Cronbach α < 0.95
Validity	Content validity	The domain of interest is comprehensively represented by items in the questionnaire	Clear description of measurement aim, target population, concepts being measured, item selection, and involvement of target population in item selection
	Criterion validity	Extent to which scores of questionnaire relate to gold standard comparison	Correlation > 0.7
	Construct validity	Extent to which scores of questionnaire relate to other measures based on hypotheses of concepts being measured	Specific hypotheses are formulated and >75 % results in accordance with hypotheses
Responsiveness	Responsiveness	Ability of questionnaire to detect clinically important change	AUC > 0.7 or MCID > SDC

ICC intraclass correlation, *SDC* smallest detectable change, *MCID* minimal clinically important difference, *AUC* area under the curve represented by calculation of Cronbach α and determines whether items within a given scale are appropriately related to one another. Cronbach α greater than 0.7 indicates that items grouped to measure a given phenomenon have acceptable internal consistency. However, a Cronbach $\alpha > 0.95$ is undesired and indicates that items within the scale are excessively redundant in measuring the given phenomenon [18].

Validity

Validity testing assures that health domains of interest are measured accurately. It is important to note that validity is not an all-or-nothing concept specific to a given questionnaire. However, instruments are validated to measure a desired outcome for a specific patient population. The instrument can often be applied to many different types of patient groups, but the application of a questionnaire for each patient population must be demonstrated through a series of studies over time.

There are several types of validity testing that are utilized to verify that an instrument measures what is intended, including content validity, criterion validity, and construct validity. Criterion validity refers to comparison of the instrument relative to a gold standard. However, gold standard measures rarely exist in the context of measurement of patient-reported outcomes. For example, there is no single test that is widely accepted as the best method to measure disease severity in patients with rheumatoid arthritis. If such a gold standard existed, then there would likely not be a reason to develop a new instrument.

Content validity and construct validity are more commonly utilized to demonstrate measurement accuracy. Content validity refers to a qualitative assessment of whether the questionnaire adequately covers all health domains that are relevant to the measured phenomenon. This requires input of all individuals with an interest in the phenomenon, including patients, clinicians, and experts. Instruments must undergo pilot testing, and methods for item selection and reduction should be reported. Construct validity is a quantitative assessment to verify that an instrument behaves in the way that is intended. This is often done through hypothesis testing in which the patient-rated instrument is compared to objective or subjective measures, with verification that the instrument behaves as expected. The instruments of comparison are not necessarily gold standard measurement tools. However, evaluation of the questionnaire of interest relative to other assessment tools helps to build experience in the manner in which the questionnaire behaves for various circumstances for patient populations of interest.

Cross-culture adaption of the questionnaire is another component of validity checking. Instruments are commonly translated to languages other than the language in which they were originally developed. Once these instruments are translated to another language, researchers must make sure the questionnaire is conceptually equivalent in the translated language through a process of forward translation, backward translation, and cognitive interviews.

Lastly, floor and ceiling effects are noted when assessing validity in specific patient populations. Floor and ceiling effects occur when instruments are unable to be responsive to patients who cluster at the lower or upper ends of the measurement scale. For example, for a questionnaire assessing overall functional ability, an athlete may always report a score indicating high functioning ability despite having an injury. Inability to detect this change in an athlete would constitute a ceiling effect. Scores should be scattered across the spectrum of the measurement scale with less than 15 % of respondents noted with the maximum or minimum score for a given subset of patients [18].

Responsiveness

Responsiveness is the sensitivity in which a questionnaire is able to detect change over time or after an intervention. Demonstration of responsiveness is considered a form of longitudinal validity testing. Effect size (ES) and standardized response mean (SRM) are the most commonly used parameters of responsiveness that compares changes in scores over time to variability in scores. ES is calculated from the change in a given patient-rated score divided by the standard deviation of the score at baseline. SRM is calculated from the change in score divided by the standard deviation of the change score.

Although ES and SRM are historically accepted methods to measure responsiveness, the COSMIN panel has recommended alternative methods. Rather than attributing degree of responsiveness to the absolute value of ES or SRM, the COSMIN panel recommends assessment of responsiveness in a similar manner in which validity testing is performed, given that responsiveness is a form of longitudinal validity [17, 18]. Thus, changes in scores should be compared to changes in reference clinical measures relative to predefined hypotheses. One method of testing the ability of a questionnaire to detect change relative to a comparison criterion is through calculation of area under the curve (AUC) for a receiver operating characteristic (ROC) curve. For example, in order to construct an ROC curve to assess a questionnaire's responsiveness in detecting patient satisfaction, the change in questionnaire score is compared to a binary reference standard for satisfaction. The change in score is evaluated relative to the reference standard to determine how well a given threshold of change predicts satisfaction. The ROC curve is a plot of the true positive rate and false positive rate across the spectrum of thresholds that are tested to predict satisfaction. AUC greater than 0.7 demonstrates adequate responsiveness of a measure to detect change relative to the comparison criteria [18]. It should be noted that the COSMIN panel takes the position that previously published studies with traditional measures of responsiveness still constitute some degree of responsiveness evidence. However, to make the evidence of responsiveness stronger, the panel recommends establishing and testing hypotheses of treatment effects (similar to validity testing), whether analyzed retrospectively or prospectively [19].

Most importantly, clinically important change should be distinguished from measurement error. The minimal clinically important difference (MCID) is defined as the minimal change in a given domain score that is detectible by the patient, also termed clinically significant change. The MCID varies among differing patient populations for which an instrument is applied. In order to assure that clinically significant change is outside of the measurement error of an instrument, the SDC (see reliability) must be smaller than the MCID [17, 18]. If this is not the case, then the MCID cannot be distinguished from measurement error.

Commonly Used Patient-Rated Questionnaires for the Rheumatoid Hand Patient

Several generic and extremity-specific questionnaires have undergone extensive testing and have been utilized to measure rheumatoid arthritis outcomes. Brief details of commonly employed instruments in rheumatoid hand research are outlined in Table 7.2. However, researchers are encouraged to thoroughly evaluate studies of the development process of any instrument being considered for use in research in order to fully assess rigor of testing, comprehensiveness of health domains, the patient population on which the instrument was validated, and other administration details that will impact utilization of the questionnaire in a given research setting. RA is one of the few disease processes treated by hand surgeons that has great impact on both hand function and overall health status. Therefore, outcomes measured by both generic and extremity-specific patient-rated questionnaires may have relevance to clinicians and researchers interested in RA treatment outcomes.

Medical Outcomes Study 36-Item Short-Form Health Survey (SF-36)

The SF-36 is one of the most well-known generic PRO questionnaires. The 36-item survey is utilized to measure overall well-being and global functioning represented by eight health domains [20].

Table 7.2 Common patient-rated questionnaires utilized in rheumatoid hand research

Name	Type	Characteristics
Arthritis Impact Measurement Scale 2 (AIMS-2)	Disease-specific	Forty-five items Nine health status domains, measuring overall patient impact of rheumatoid arthritis Scored 1–10 (10 = worst health status)
Disability of the Arm, Shoulder, and Hand (DASH)	Region-specific	Thirty items Optional 4-item module for athletes or musicians Function and symptom domains, measuring overall upper extremity disability Both extremities assessed together Scored 0–100 (100 = maximum disability) Shortened 11-item QuickDASH version available
Medical Outcomes Study Short Form-36 (SF-36)	Generic	Thirty-six items Eight health domains, measuring overall well-being and global functioning Widely used across all medical specialties Scored 0–100 (100 = best health status) Shortened 12-item version available
Michigan Hand Outcomes Questionnaire (MHQ)	Region-specific	Fifty-seven items Six domains of hand function, measuring hand function, ADLs, work performance, pain, appearance, and satisfaction Mean domain scores (including inverse of pain score) represents composite hand function Each extremity assessed separately Scored 0–100 (100 = best health status) Shortened 12-item brief MHQ version available
Patient-Reported Outcomes Measurement Information System (PROMIS)	Generic or region-specific	Variety of item banks exist based on domain of interest physical function or upper extremity function subscale applicable to RA studies Administered via uniform set of items or computerized adaptive testing for a given domain
Visual analog scale	Symptom-specific, disease-specific, or region-specific	Single item Most common used pain assessment tool Scored 0–10 (10 = maximal pain or disability) Similarly utilized to assess overall disability or hand disability

Each domain is scored from 0 to 100, with 100 representing no disability. A shortened version exists, the SF-12, which may be utilized in situations when researchers are concerned with responder burden.

Arthritis Impact Measurement Scale 2 (AIMS-2)

The AIMS-2 is a 45-item questionnaire that was developed and validated to measure disease activity in patients with rheumatoid arthritis [21]. The AIMS-2 questionnaire evaluates the impact of RA on the patient as a whole within nine health status domains, including mobility, physical activity, dexterity, household activities, activities of daily living, anxiety, depression, social activity, and pain. AIMS-2 scores range from 1 to 10, with lower scores indicating better health status.

Visual Analog Scales

The visual analog scales (VAS) is often used to quantify pain for both research and clinical purposes. To administer the VAS, a 10 cm straight line with a verbal or written description at each extreme of pain (no pain at the lower end and worst pain ever at the upper end) is shown to the respondent. Patients mark the position between the two endpoints that corresponds to their level of pain. The scale takes very little time to administer and is easily utilized in the clinical and research setting. VAS has been shown to have acceptable test–retest reliability and responsiveness to change over time [22]. A recent systematic review found VAS to be the most commonly utilized method of pain evaluation in musculoskeletal clinical trials [23]. Similarly, VAS instruments have also been developed and validated to measure hand disability and overall disability due to rheumatoid arthritis [24].

Michigan Hand Outcomes Questionnaire

The Michigan Hand Outcomes Questionnaire (MHQ) is a 57-item questionnaire developed to evaluate six domains of hand function, including overall hand function, activities of daily living, work performance, pain, hand appearance, and patient satisfaction with hand function [25]. These domains are assessed for each hand individually for comparison, which is unique among other PRO questionnaires for upper extremity conditions. The MHQ also evaluates the impact of appearance on overall hand function, which is often neglected with other commonly used questionnaires. Scores for each domain range from 0 to 100. Higher scores indicate better health status, with the exception of the pain scale in which a higher score indicates greater pain. After reversing the pain score, an overall MHQ score is calculated from the mean of the domain scores. A 12-item brief MHQ version was developed for clinical practice, whereas the full version is recommended for research [26].

Disability of the Arm, Shoulder, and Hand/Upper Extremity Function Scale (DASH)

The DASH is a 30-item questionnaire that has been validated for a variety of upper extremity conditions, including RA [27]. The survey items address physical function, symptoms, and social role function. There is an optional module with four additional questions for musicians or athletes. Respondents are asked to rate difficulty of completing each task on a 6-point ordinal scale. Thus, the disability score is related to the function of both upper extremities as a single unit. The final score ranges from 0 to 100, with a higher score indicating greater disability [28]. A shorter version, the QuickDASH, was developed utilizing 11 of the most sensitive items and is highly correlated with the full DASH version [29].

Patient-Reported Outcomes Measurement Information System

Patient-Reported Outcomes Measurement Information System (PROMIS), developed by the National Institutes of Health, is a thoroughly vetted bank of questionnaire items divided into many different key domains of interest, including physical function, pain, or fatigue, among others. Reliable and valid item banks are developed using item response theory, which make it possible to estimate a given trait based on any subset of items in the survey bank that are appropriate for the respondent's trait level. A trait can be estimated through a uniform set of questions in the item bank for all participants in a given study. Alternatively, pools of questions can be administered as computerized adaptive tests (CAT) for greater efficiency. When a pool of questions is administered via CAT, subsequent items given to the respondent are adjusted based on responses to earlier questions in the survey. For example, if a respondent reports that he has difficulty completing a simple task, the respondent will then not be asked to rate difficulty in completing a more complex task. CAT reduces survey burden by eliminating irrelevant questions and minimizes floor and ceiling effects by adjusting items according to the respondent's previous responses. The physical function item bank can be administered to evaluate overall functioning of the patient. A specific upper extremity function subscale also exists to allow more specific evaluation of PROs relevant to treatment of upper extremity disorders [30–32].

Considerations in Questionnaire Selection and Administration

A single perfect questionnaire for the measurement of hand outcomes simply does not exist. Researchers must verify that the questionnaire has demonstrated validity, reliability, and responsiveness for the study population of interest. The investigator's comfort level with the strengths, administration, and interpretation of a given PRO questionnaire will also have some influence on selection. However, selection of the appropriate instrument is ultimately determined by the research question at hand and the desired health domains to be measured. The interests of the study population are paramount, and the researcher must consider whether domains of health that respondents care most about are assessed. In addition, likelihood of floor or ceiling effects should be weighed relative to patient characteristics and capabilities of the study questionnaire.

Rheumatoid arthritis is unique in that therapies have potential to influence overall patient well-being and hand function. Often, more than one questionnaire is utilized for a given study due to the varying domains of health that are measured for each available instrument. For example, if a researcher is interested in studying whether hand surgery improves both hand disability and overall quality of life, respondents should be given questionnaires that reliably measure both hand disability and overall quality of life. In this case, an extremity-specific questionnaire, such as the DASH or MHQ, would be responsive to measure hand disability. In addition, a generic instrument, such as the SF-36 would be needed to estimate changes in overall quality of life. Furthermore, if an investigator desires to study the impact of rheumatoid hand surgery compared to the contralateral hand as a control, the MHQ would be the best selection given its ability to assess each hand independently. Thus, the specific study question should be the primary influence on questionnaire selection.

Researchers should resist the urge to administer a battery of multiple questionnaires simply with the goal of capturing as much information as possible. Administering too many study questionnaires to a given patient will increase the likelihood of respondent burden, poor data quality, and missing responses. There is no set threshold of an ideal number of questions a researcher can ask before causing respondent burden. Rather, instrument selection should be based on careful consideration of domains of health required to evaluate a given study hypothesis. Only those questionnaires that directly address domains of health needed for the study should be administered to participants.

The feasible sample size of the proposed study relative to the measurement error of a questionnaire being considered also impacts instrument selection. For example, if two potential questionnaires are determined to measure similar domains of health but one has a much larger SDC, then selection of the questionnaire with the smaller SDC will require a smaller sample size in power calculations. The impact of SDC and MCID on the sample size required for group comparisons should be considered prior to questionnaire selection to reduce the chance of type II error and allow greater efficiency in planning costly research trials.

The method of questionnaire delivery must also be considered. Many PRO questionnaires can be administered via pen and paper, computer, tablet, or verbal communication. Selection of the mode of administration may depend on the respondent's comfort with technology, associated costs, and ease of data entry and analysis. Ultimately, the investigator must assure that the questionnaire is validated for the preferred mode of administration. In addition, time points of measurement must be performed with sufficient follow-up time in order to capture adequate outcomes. Lastly, investigators must assure that the study protocol does not interfere with validity of the utilized instrument. Questionnaire items should not be altered, and the instrument must be administered to respondents with similar characteristics as the study sample in which validity testing was performed.

Future Directions

With time, patient-rated measures have become the primary outcome in many clinical trials and outcomes studies. The field of measurement science has grown tremendously, and the quality of PRO questionnaires has continued to improve along the way. Development of sound assessment tools requires time and patience in demonstrating the reliability, validity, and responsiveness in patient populations of interest. Use of these tested questionnaires further increases experience with application of these measurement tools.

PRO instruments are particularly important in rheumatoid hand research given the impact of surgical intervention on quality of life and the discord between patient-rated and objective clinical measures. Although PROs are ubiquitous in research, they are rarely utilized in routine clinical practice. With continued rising costs of health care, there will be increasing pressure for providers to justify the value of their treatments. Measurement of patient-reported outcomes in everyday practice will be instrumental in building evidence of outcomes associated with medical treatments relative to the costs of those treatments. Increased utilization of item response theory and computerized adaptive testing formats will allow patient-reported outcomes to be measured with improved granularity and greater efficiency. Establishing accurate and efficient measurement of important clinical domains will be critical in persuading clinicians to regularly use these instruments for quality improvement and individual patient evaluation.

References

1. Alderman AK, Chung KC, Kim HM, Fox DA, Ubel PA. Effectiveness of rheumatoid hand surgery: contrasting perceptions of hand surgeons and rheumatologists. J Hand Surg. 2003;28(1):3–11. discussion 2–3. PubMed.
2. Alderman AK, Ubel PA, Kim HM, Fox DA, Chung KC. Surgical management of the rheumatoid hand: consensus and controversy among rheumatologists and hand surgeons. J Rheumatol. 2003;30(7):1464–72. PubMed.
3. Chung KC, Kowalski CP, Myra Kim H, Kazmers IS. Patient outcomes following Swanson silastic metacarpophalangeal joint arthroplasty in the rheumatoid hand: a systematic overview. J Rheumatol. 2000; 27(6):1395–402. PubMed.
4. Chung KC, Kotsis SV. Outcomes of hand surgery in the patient with rheumatoid arthritis. Curr Opin Rheumatol. 2010;22(3):336–41. PubMed Pubmed Central PMCID: 2898123.
5. Chung KC, Burns PB, Wilgis EF, Burke FD, Regan M, Kim HM, et al. A multicenter clinical trial in rheumatoid arthritis comparing silicone metacarpophalangeal joint arthroplasty with medical treatment. J Hand Surg. 2009;34(5):815–23. PubMed Pubmed Central PMCID: 4381953.
6. Chung KC, Burns PB, Kim HM, Burke FD, Wilgis EF, Fox DA. Long-term follow-up for rheumatoid

arthritis patients in a multicenter outcomes study of silicone metacarpophalangeal joint arthroplasty. Arthritis Care Res. 2012;64(9):1292–300. PubMed Pubmed Central PMCID: 3422446.
7. Heald AE, Fudman EJ, Anklesaria P, Mease PJ, Team GS. Single-joint outcome measures: preliminary validation of patient-reported outcomes and physical examination. J Rheumatol. 2010;37(5):1042–8. PubMed.
8. Malcus Johnsson P, Sandqvist G, Sturesson AL, Gulfe A, Kopylov P, Tagil M, et al. Individualized outcome measures of daily activities are sensitive tools for evaluating hand surgery in rheumatic diseases. Rheumatology. 2012;51(12):2246–51. PubMed.
9. Waljee JF, Chung KC. Objective functional outcomes and patient satisfaction after silicone metacarpophalangeal arthroplasty for rheumatoid arthritis. J Hand Surg. 2012;37(1):47–54. PubMed.
10. Badalamente M, Coffelt L, Elfar J, Gaston G, Hammert W, Huang J, et al. Measurement scales in clinical research of the upper extremity, part 1: general principles, measures of general health, pain, and patient satisfaction. J Hand Surg. 2013;38(2):401–6. quiz 6. PubMed.
11. Badalamente M, Coffelt L, Elfar J, Gaston G, Hammert W, Huang J, et al. Measurement scales in clinical research of the upper extremity, part 2: outcome measures in studies of the hand/wrist and shoulder/elbow. J Hand Surg. 2013;38(2):407–12. PubMed.
12. Giladi AM, Chung KC. Measuring outcomes in hand surgery. Clin Plast Surg. 2013;40(2):313–22. PubMed.
13. MacDermid JC. Patient-reported outcomes: state-of-the-art hand surgery and future applications. Hand Clin. 2014;30(3):293–304. v. PubMed.
14. Sears ED, Chung KC. A guide to interpreting a study of patient-reported outcomes. Plast Reconstr Surg. 2012;129(5):1200–7. PubMed Pubmed Central PMCID: 3340576.
15. Waljee JF, Chung KC. Outcomes research in rheumatoid arthritis. Hand Clin. 2011;27(1):115–26. PubMed.
16. Mokkink LB, Terwee CB, Patrick DL, Alonso J, Stratford PW, Knol DL, et al. The COSMIN study reached international consensus on taxonomy, terminology, and definitions of measurement properties for health-related patient-reported outcomes. J Clin Epidemiol. 2010;63(7):737–45. PubMed.
17. Mokkink LB, Terwee CB, Patrick DL, Alonso J, Stratford PW, Knol DL, et al. The COSMIN checklist for assessing the methodological quality of studies on measurement properties of health status measurement instruments: an international Delphi study. Qual Life Res. 2010;19(4):539–49. PubMed Pubmed Central PMCID: 2852520.
18. Terwee CB, Bot SD, de Boer MR, van der Windt DA, Knol DL, Dekker J, et al. Quality criteria were proposed for measurement properties of health status questionnaires. J Clin Epidemiol. 2007;60(1):34–42. PubMed.
19. Angst F. The new COSMIN guidelines confront traditional concepts of responsiveness. BMC Med Res Methodol. 2011;11:152. author reply PubMed Pubmed Central PMCID: 3231875.
20. Ware Jr JE, Sherbourne CD. The MOS 36-item short-form health survey (SF-36): I. Conceptual framework and item selection. Med Care. 1992;30(6):473–83. PubMed.
21. Meenan RF, Mason JH, Anderson JJ, Guccione AA, Kazis LE. AIMS2. The content and properties of a revised and expanded arthritis impact measurement scales health status questionnaire. Arthritis Rheum. 1992;35(1):1–10. PubMed.
22. Clark P, Lavielle P, Martinez H. Learning from pain scales: patient perspective. J Rheumatol. 2003;30(7): 1584–8. PubMed.
23. Litcher-Kelly L, Martino SA, Broderick JE, Stone AA. A systematic review of measures used to assess chronic musculoskeletal pain in clinical and randomized controlled clinical trials. J Pain. 2007;8(12):906–13. PubMed Pubmed Central PMCID: 2691574.
24. Massy-Westropp N, Ahern M, Krishnan J. A visual analogue scale for assessment of the impact of rheumatoid arthritis in the hand: validity and repeatability. J Hand Ther. 2005;18(1):30–3. PubMed.
25. Chung KC, Pillsbury MS, Walters MR, Hayward RA. Reliability and validity testing of the Michigan hand outcomes questionnaire. J Hand Surg. 1998; 23(4):575–87. PubMed.
26. Waljee JF, Kim HM, Burns PB, Chung KC. Development of a brief, 12-item version of the Michigan hand questionnaire. Plast Reconstr Surg. 2011;128(1):208–20. PubMed Pubmed Central PMCID: 3124660.
27. Chiari-Grisar C, Koller U, Stamm TA, Wanivenhaus A, Trieb K. Performance of the disabilities of the arm, shoulder and hand outcome questionnaire and the Moberg picking up test in patients with finger joint arthroplasty. Arch Phys Med Rehabil. 2006;87(2):203–6. PubMed.
28. Beaton DE, Katz JN, Fossel AH, Wright JG, Tarasuk V, Bombardier C. Measuring the whole or the parts? Validity, reliability, and responsiveness of the disabilities of the arm, shoulder and hand outcome measure in different regions of the upper extremity. J Hand Ther. 2001;14(2):128–46. PubMed.
29. Beaton DE, Wright JG, Katz JN, Upper Extremity Collaborative Group. Development of the QuickDASH: comparison of three item-reduction approaches. J Bone Joint Surg Am. 2005;87(5):1038–46. PubMed.
30. Khanna D, Krishnan E, Dewitt EM, Khanna PP, Spiegel B, Hays RD. The future of measuring

patient-reported outcomes in rheumatology: patient-reported outcomes measurement information system (PROMIS). Arthritis Care Res. 2011;63 Suppl 11: S486–90. PubMed.
31. Doring AC, Nota SP, Hageman MG, Ring DC. Measurement of upper extremity disability using the patient-reported outcomes measurement information system. J Hand Surg. 2014;39(6):1160–5. PubMed.
32. Tyser AR, Beckmann J, Franklin JD, Cheng C, Hon SD, Wang A, et al. Evaluation of the PROMIS physical function computer adaptive test in the upper extremity. J Hand Surg. 2014;39(10):2047–51.e4. PubMed.

Part II

Rheumatoid Wrist

Biomechanics of the Rheumatoid Wrist Deformity

8

Gregory Ian Bain, Thomas Clifton, John J. Costi, and Jeganath Krishnan

Introduction

Rheumatoid arthritis (RA) is a common systemic inflammatory disease that is associated with progressive disability, significant morbidity, early death, and significant socioeconomic costs [1]. Although it can affect any synovial joint, the wrist is the most frequently involved. Chronic synovitis and pannus expansion result in degradation of articular cartilage and bone, ligamentous laxity, and significant deformity. This in part follows a predictable pattern of change and therefore targeted early operative intervention can be achieved, ranging from arthroscopic synovectomy to complete wrist arthrodesis.

Electronic supplementary material: The online version of this chapter (doi:10.1007/978-3-319-26660-2_8) contains supplementary material, which is available to authorized users. Videos can also be accessed at http://link.springer.com/chapter/10.1007/978-3-319-26660-2_8.

G.I. Bain, MBBS, FRACS, PhD (✉)
J. Krishnan, MBBS, FRACS, PhD
Department of Orthopaedic Surgery, Flinders University, Adelaide, SA, Australia
e-mail: greg@gregbain.com.au

T. Clifton, MBBS, BA
Orthopaedics, Royal Adelaide Hospital, Adelaide, SA, Australia

J.J. Costi, BEng (Mech, Hons), PhD, FIEAust
Biomechanics and Implants Research Group, The Medical Device Research Institute; School of Computer Science, Engineering and Mathematics, Flinders University, Adelaide, SA, Australia

Multiple Ring Concept of the Wrist Stability

The wrist has three synovial spaces: the radiocarpal, midcarpal, and distal radioulnar joint (DRUJ). However, there are four articulating joints because the ulnar-carpal articulation should not be ignored. Another way to conceptualize the joints of the wrist is to consider it as a series of conjoined rings, which operate in concert with each other. This forms the basis of the "multiple ring concept of the wrist." The structure, stability, and borders of the rings are defined by the intrinsic ligamentous attachments. The sites where the rings are linked form major stability points of the carpus. The wrist joint is unique in that it provides movement in all three planes and must provide a stable platform for the function of the hand in all positions in space. The rings provide stability, while allowing transmission and dissipation of force throughout the range of motion. This is particularly important at the extremes of motion, where the stability is threatened. Disruption of these ligaments creates instability within the ring, which can then impart a *global* instability to the wrist.

K.C. Chung (ed.), *Clinical Management of the Rheumatoid Hand, Wrist, and Elbow*,
DOI 10.1007/978-3-319-26660-2_8

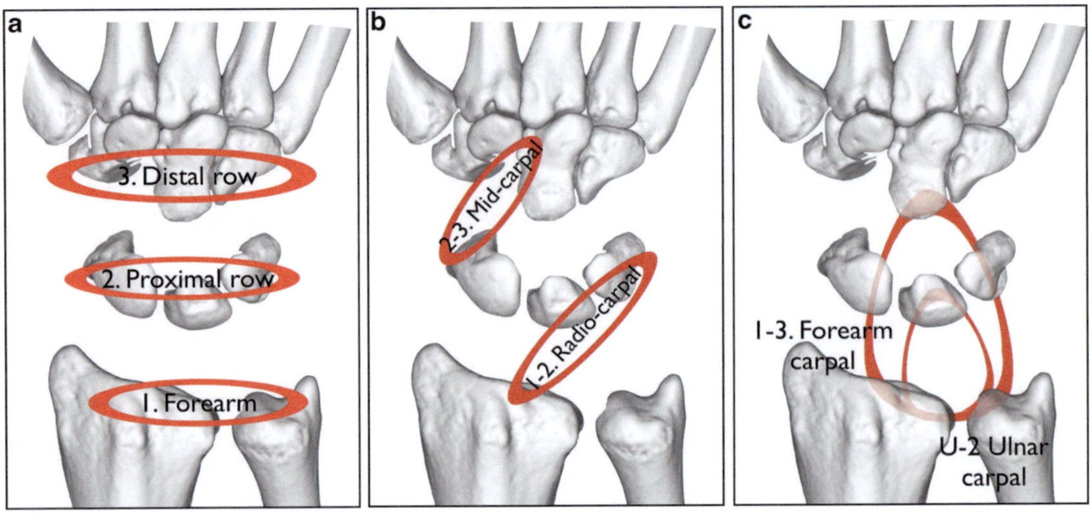

Fig. 8.1 Multiple ring concept of the wrist: (**a**) rows of rings; (**b**) inter-row rings, radiocarpal and midcarpal; (**c**) arcuate carpal rings, greater and lesser. Published with permission of © Dr. Gregory Bain 2015. All Rights Reserved

Rows of Rings

There are three rows of rings of the wrist: the DRUJ, proximal carpal row, and distal carpal row (Fig. 8.1a).

1. The DRUJ ring is stabilized by the radioulnar ligaments, with failure causing DRUJ instability.
2. The proximal carpal row is stabilized by the dorsal intercarpal ligament and the volar scaphotriquetral ligaments. Failure examples include scapholunate and lunotriquetral instability.
3. The distal carpal row is stabilized by the volar and dorsal interosseous ligaments, failure of which causes axial instability.

Inter-row Rings

These are the rings that link and provide stability between the individual rows (Fig. 8.1b, c).

1. The radiotriquetral ring, which has been referred to as the Kuhlman's sling [2], includes the dorsal radiocarpal ligament and the volar radiotriquetral ligament, preventing ulnar translocation.
2. The scaphoid-trapezium-trapezoid (STT) ring is a simple hinge joint, consisting of the scaphotrapezoid and scaphocapitate ligaments. Failure of the STT ring causes midcarpal instability.
3. The **lesser arcuate ring** consists of the ulnar-lunate and radiolunate ligaments, which stabilizes the lunate to the forearm to prevent volar subluxation of the carpus.
4. The **greater arcuate ring** consists of the radioscaphocapitate and the ulnar capitate ligaments, which stabilizes the distal carpal row to the forearm, to prevent distraction of the wrist (Fig. 8.1c).

Variability in Carpal Morphology

Finally it should be noted that there can be significant variation in the morphology of carpal bones, which can affect the movement at the joints. At the midcarpal joint, the lunate type [3] has been shown to alter the pattern and range of motion at the radiocarpal joint (Fig. 8.2) [4]. Variations have also been identified in the morphology of the capitate [5], triquetrohamate joint [6], and scaphoid [7], which also have an effect on the carpal motion.

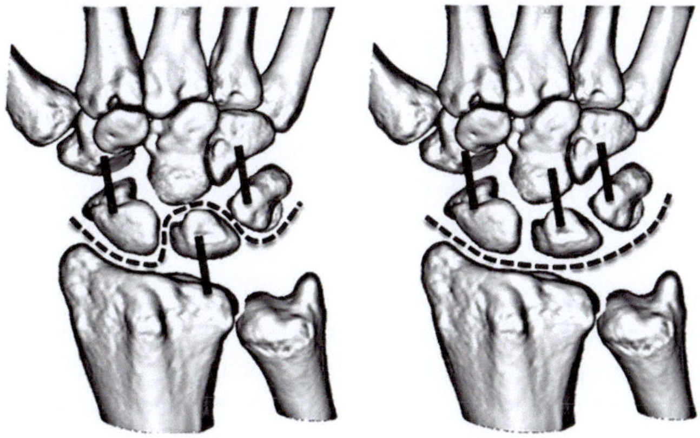

Fig. 8.2 Effect of lunate morphology on plane of motion during wrist flexion/extension. Note that the type of lunate morphology significantly affects the plane of motion of the wrist (*dotted lines*) and those joints with a restricted motion (*solid bar*). Reproduced from The Effect of Lunate Morphology on the 3-Dimensional Kinematics of the Carpus JHS (Am) 20154, Copyright G I Bain

Pathophysiology: Rheumatoid Arthritis at the Wrist

Rheumatoid arthritis (RA) is a common autoimmune disease characterized by synovial inflammation and hyperplasia, autoantibody production, cartilage and bone destruction, as well as many other systemic features. Although the exact cause is unknown, the pathogenesis has been well described.

Adrian Flatt reported that there are three stages in the rheumatoid process [8]:

1. *Synovitis*, which typically occurs at the sites of capsular attachments
2. *Destruction* of the periarticular cartilage, which is often at the bare areas and capsular attachments
3. *Deformity*, which is due to the osseous and ligamentous destruction

Synovitis

Synovitis occurs when leukocytes infiltrate the synovial compartment, causing a profound reorganization of synovial architecture and an expansion of synovial inflammatory tissue or pannus. The change in the architecture of the synovium, caused by complex change in immune-modulated signaling pathways and cytokines, eventuates in chronic inflammation of the joint. This causes a loss of the lubricating effects of the synovium and, together with the activation of fibroblasts, permits the growth of hyperplastic synovium or pannus [9]. The hyperplastic synovium is the major contributor to cartilage and joint damage in RA.

Joint Destruction

Cartilage

The joint destruction that occurs is a result of both chronic inflammation and mechanical forces. The normal wrist joint is a synovial joint with a negative pressure environment and well-hydrated articular cartilage. In RA, there is destruction of the articular cartilage at the pannus-cartilage junction. The cartilage is degraded by invasion of synovial cells and immune cells causing chondrolysis and collagen breakdown, frequently at the edge of the joint capsule.

Bone

Bony erosion also occurs rapidly in RA, affecting 80 % of patients 1 year after diagnosis [10]. The chronic inflammatory state results in hyperemia and increased bone resorption with increase in the activity of osteoclasts, without a compensatory increase in osteoblasts. Osteopenia and osteoporosis are later sequelae as the arthritis creates a painful joint, with disuse osteopenia, creating further bone loss. Areas of high contact pressure will develop bony eburnation and osteophytes, similar to degenerative osteoarthritis. These may result in sharp bone edges that may lead to joint capsule breach and tendon rupture. Examples include the Mannerfelt lesion and extensor tendon ruptures over the ulnar head.

Ligaments

The concept of "pseudo-laxity" is of major importance (Fig. 8.3). Pseudo-laxity occurs with a loss of the height of the articular cartilage, which creates a *relative* lengthening of ligament. This results in a greater and pathological range of movement and contributes to the joint instability and abnormal joint mechanics.

The expansive synovium also creates laxity of the *intrinsic and extrinsic ligaments* in the wrist, by both mechanical force and chronic inflammation. The growing pannus in the wrist joint puts mechanical strain on the ligaments, stretching them beyond the point of elastic compliance (elastic modulus). The chronic inflammatory pannus also degrades the ligaments directly by similar cellular mechanisms described above. Laxity of the ligaments in the wrist results in an altered and pathological range of movement about the joint, creating increased articular contact pressures and contributing further to degradation of cartilage and bone (Fig. 8.4).

Load and Articular Contact Pressure

In the rheumatoid wrist, there are also abnormal joint contact pressures and a loss of efficiency of synovial fluid. In a finite element analysis, Bajuri and colleagues simulated advanced RA wrist changes such as cartilage and bone destruction, dislocation, and carpal collapse and assessed the change in load born by the carpus [11]. The authors demonstrated a three times increase in contact pressures at all articulations and a loss of the uniform distribution of stress, owing largely to a loss of articular cartilage. They further stipulated that bony erosion contributed to the increased contact pressure, via articulation with sharper edges. This can be explained by the principle that a constant force (F) with a decreased surface area of contact (A) results in increased pressure (P):

$$P = F / A$$

Bajuri and colleagues also showed a shift in the load bearing of the wrist from the radius to the ulna as the carpus collapses and slides down the distal radius (Fig. 8.5). The alteration in load modeled by the authors is based on the common carpal deformities found in the RA wrist.

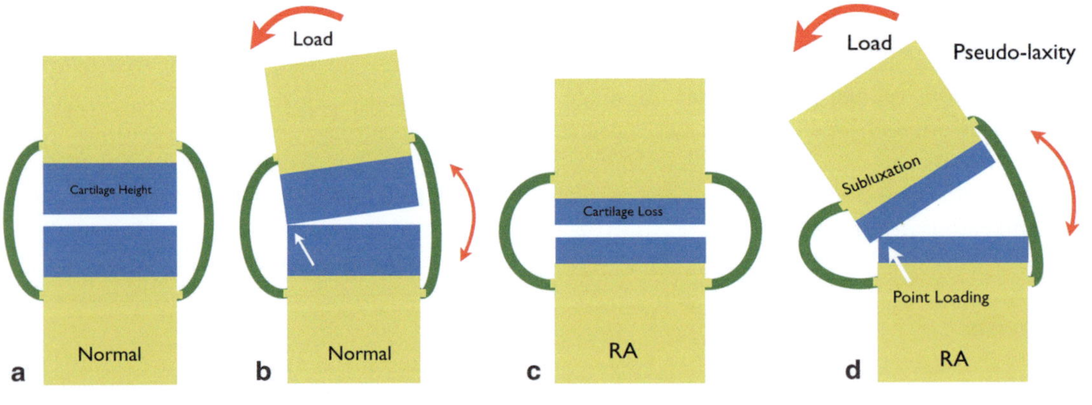

Fig. 8.3 Pseudo-laxity. In the normal joint (**a**) the articular cartilage height is seen as "joint space" on the X-rays. With loading (**b**) the joint will tilt until the collateral ligament is tight. In RA there is loss of articular cartilage (**c**), which is seen as "joint space narrowing" on plain radiographs. The collateral ligaments are the normal length but are relatively lax. With loading (**d**) the joint will tilt until the collateral ligament is tight. The loss of articular cartilage allows the joint to tilt further, which appears to be joint laxity (pseudo-laxity). Note the other effects including abnormal loading and a tendency to joint subluxation. Published with kind permission of © Dr. Gregory Bain 2015. All Rights Reserved

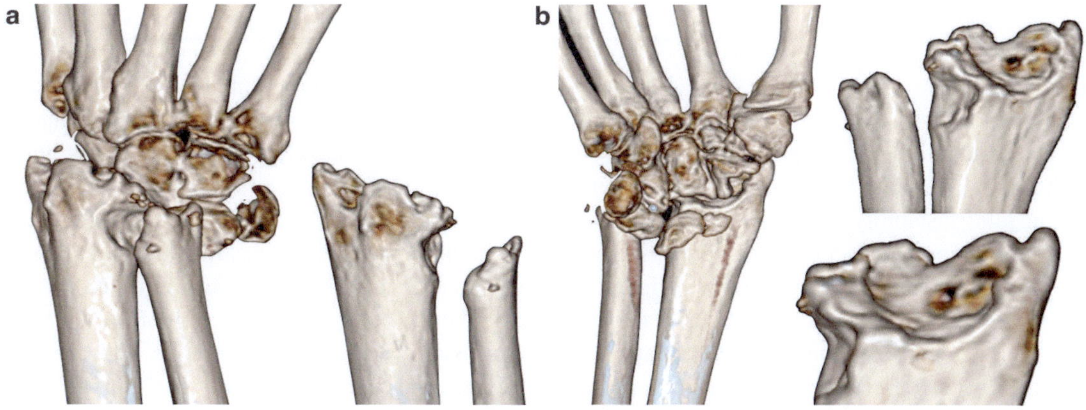

Fig. 8.4 Erosive arthropathy of the wrist. (**a**, **b**) Dorsal aspect of the wrist, demonstrating that the distal ulnar is dislocated dorsally and the carpus is dislocated in a volar, ulnar, supination, and proximal direction. Note the extensive erosion of the sigmoid notch. Published with kind permission of © Dr. Gregory Bain 2015. All Rights Reserved

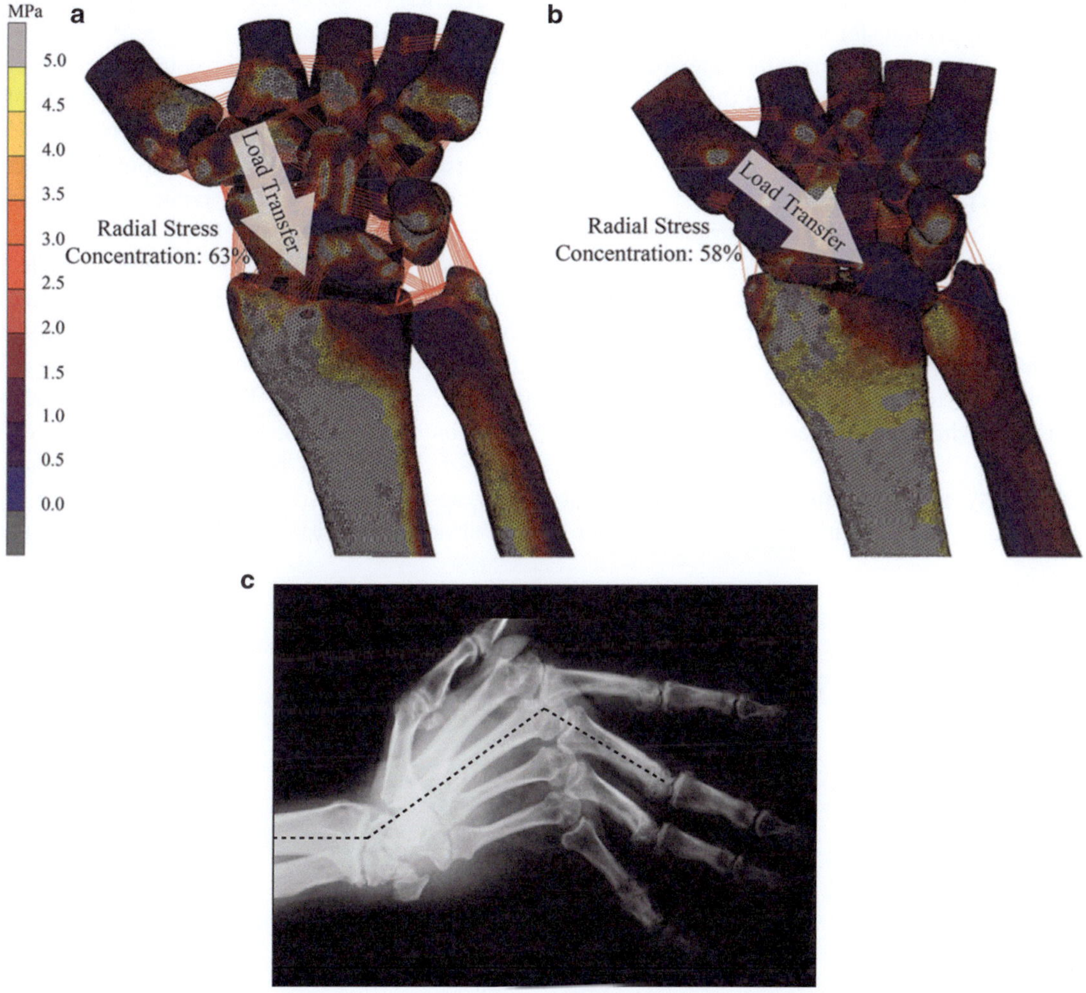

Fig. 8.5 Von Mises stress distribution for the palmar aspect of the (**a**) healthy model and (**b**) RA model (Used with permission from MN Bajuri et al. J Engineering in Medicine, 2012 [11]). (**c**) Characteristic "*Z*" deformity of the hand. Ulnar translocation and radial deviation of the wrist are commonly associated with ulnar drift of the fingers (Published with kind permission of © Dr. Gregory Bain 2015. All Rights Reserved)

Deformity

In the rheumatoid wrist, ligamentous laxity and destruction of articular cartilage and bone eventuate in joint instability and significant deformity. The most important factor in the deforming process is the laxity of ligaments. Of all the ligaments in the wrist, the loss of palmar and dorsal radiotriquetral ligaments and palmar radiolunate ligaments has been described as the most crucial [5].

Adjacent joints may compromise each other, producing a characteristic "Z" deformity (Fig. 8.5b). Ulnar translocation and radial deviation of the wrist are commonly associated with ulnar drift of the fingers. When performing multiple MCP joint arthroplasties in RA, we use the ECRL to ECU transfer as a prophylactic reconstructive procedure to correct the other side of the "Z" deformity, thereby reducing the incidence of recurrent ulnar drift deformity.

Radiocarpal Deformity

Due to the degradation of articular cartilage and ligamentous laxity, the carpus as a whole tends to translocate in the direction of the articular slope of the radius. The distal radius has a mean radial inclination of 24° and volar tilt of 11° [12]. Carpus tends to "slide" down the slope of the distal radius, which is potentiated by the force of the flexors and extensors of the wrist and fingers. Resultantly, the most common deformity is that the carpus translocates in an *ulnar*, *volar*, *supination*, and *proximal* direction [12, 13]. This carpal translocation may also result in tendon imbalance and leads to secondary deformity such as ulnar deviation of the fingers.

In the coronal plane, there is loss of the radiocarpal alignment with the carpus translocating in an ulnar direction. This deformity has been described to be due to destruction of the articular disk and the internal ligamentous structures of the radiocarpal joint [14]. The scapholunate ligament is prone to weakening from the synovitis, leading to flexion of the scaphoid and an increase in the scapholunate angle, promoting collapse of the radial column [15]. Unhinged from the scaphoid, the lunate translocates in a volar direction and dorsiflexes. Videos 8.1 and 8.2 show a patient with advanced rheumatoid changes of the wrist with volar, ulnar, and proximal translocation of the carpus. Video 8.1 demonstrates the laxity of ligaments at the wrist created by rheumatoid changes. Video 8.2 shows the pronounced effect of rheumatoid changes on the range of movement in the flexion/extension axis at the wrist.

These findings have been recently modeled using three-dimensional CT scan reconstructions. Arimitsu and colleagues studied carpal kinematics using three-dimensional CT scans of patients with advanced RA of the wrist [12]. They confirmed that the centroids (center of volume) of each carpal bone shifted in an ulnar, volar, and proximal direction along the slope of the surface of the distal radius (Fig. 8.6).

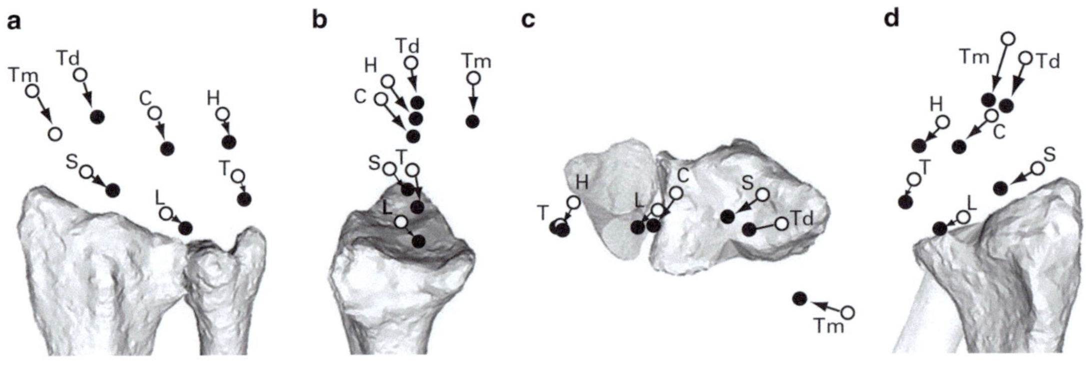

Fig. 8.6 Diagrams showing centroid translocation from (**a**) a dorsal view, (**b**) ulnar view, (**c**) distal view, and (**d**) radiopalmar view. All the centroids translocated in an ulnar, proximal, and volar direction (Used with permission from Aramitsu et al., J Bone Joint Surg Br. 2007 [12])

Distal Radioulnar Joint

The DRUJ is often the first compartment of the wrist involved in the rheumatoid process. The static restraints are the triangular fibrocartilaginous complex (TFCC) and interosseous membrane, and the dynamic restraints are the extensor carpi ulnaris (ECU) tendon and the pronator quadratus muscle. Destruction of the distal radius and the adjacent ligaments, and collapse and translation of the carpus, predispose to the *ulnar-carpal abutment*. The destruction of the TFCC by the synovitic process destabilizes the DRUJ articulation and causes the ulnar head to move dorsally [13]. The extrinsic stabilizers are inadequate to resist the natural collapse pattern, and what follows is the sequence of events leading to *caput ulnae syndrome* (Backdahl 1963) [16].

Video 8.3 gives some insight into the etiology of tendon ruptures. The sigmoid notch of the distal radius has a sharp hardened area of bone due to abnormal loading and erosion from the synovitis in the DRUJ.

As the forearm rotates, the sharp hard bone of the sigmoid notch sculptures the ulnar head, like a chisel sculptures wood on a lathe. Interestingly, it can be appreciated that as they push into each other, they subsequently sharpen each other. Once the ulnar head develops a sharp ridge around its head, it can then have an effect on other adjacent structures. In this case, as the forearm rotates, the sharp edge of the ulna head cuts through the dorsal capsule and then subsequently through the extensor tendons. It is our experience that tendon ruptures only occur with abrasion from sharpened bone (or metallic implants). Tendon ischemia and synovial invasion may weaken the tendon and predispose it to injury. But it is the sharp bone that divides the tendon.

Treatment of Rheumatoid Arthritis Wrist Deformity

Synovectomy

In the early stages of synovitis, prior to the development of significant destruction or deformity, a synovectomy can be a useful treatment option. Though the standard has been open synovectomy, which allows for inspection of all compartments and the extensor tendons, arthroscopic synovectomy is also being performed with success [17, 18]. The arthroscopic approach has the advantage of reduced joint capsule and ligament damage, allowing for earlier mobilization and reduced hospital stay [19]. It has been shown that if the procedure is performed before joint destruction occurs, the natural history can be improved, although disease progression can still occur [20–22]. Recent studies have demonstrated that there can also be benefits for patients who have later stages of the disease (e.g., Larsen stage III) [23].

Radiocarpal Joint

An intact midcarpal joint and localized pathology within the radiocarpal joint are common findings in the early stages of the RA wrist [24]. As we have seen, the carpus tends to translocate in proximal, volar, and ulnar directions, causing radial deviation of the radiocarpal joint. In these cases, partial wrist fusion may be beneficial to relieve pain and prevent instability and deformity, while maintaining a functional range of motion [25].

Radiolunate Fusion

Radiolunate (RL) fusion is a well-established technique that was developed from the observation that spontaneous radiolunate ankylosis will stabilize the joint, minimize further joint deterioration, and improve pain. Chamay and colleagues demonstrated that surgical fusion of the radiolunate joint served as a block to further carpal translocation [13]. Several authors have reported successful outcomes [26, 27], whereas others have reported a high incidence of radiolunate nonunion [13, 15]. A surgical prerequisite is that the adjacent joints (radioscaphoid and midcarpal) are free of disease. Unfortunately the radioscaphoid joint is often involved [25].

Radioscapholunate Fusion

If the radioscaphoid joint is involved in the inflammatory process, then a radioscapholunate (RSL) fusion is indicated. Like the RL fixation, an absolute prerequisite for RSL fusion is a functional midcarpal joint to maintain painless movement. The long-term outcomes of RSL fusion have demonstrated a high complication rate and a range of motion of 33–40 % of the normal wrist [28–31]. There is an increasing trend to perform a distal scaphoidectomy to increase range of movement at the midcarpal joint [31, 32].

Authors' Technique: RSL Fusion

In cadaveric studies, we have also demonstrated that excision of the triquetrum improves the range of ulnar deviation and extension [32]. We have also performed this technique in a clinical series with good results [33]. The excision of the triquetrum provides good bone graft for the fusion mass and minimizes the risk of ulnar-carpal impaction (Fig. 8.7).

The authors' technique is to debride the articulation between the distal radius and the reciprocal articular surfaces of the scaphoid and the lunate. Two 1.1 mm *K*-wires are advanced between the scaphoid and the lunate with the distal articulation in view, ensuring that it is perfectly reduced. *K*-wires are then passed from the proximal pole of the scaphoid and the lunate into the distal radius. This will often provide adequate stability but if there is concern, then pin plates or locking plates can be used. Cancellous bone graft harvested from the excised triquetrum and distal pole of the scaphoid is then packed around the fusion sites. Alternatively, memory staples may be placed between the distal radius and proximal pole of the scaphoid and between the distal radius and lunate to achieve a stable fixation with compression. Following the stabilization, the position is confirmed to be satisfactory with the aid of fluoroscopy.

Distal Radioulnar Joint

For patients with rheumatoid arthritis involving the DRUJ, there are several surgical options. The standard was traditionally the Darrach procedure, which is resection of the distal 1–2 cm of the ulna [34]. However, this is most often complicated by instability of the proximal stump as the TFCC is destabilized. Alternatives to the Darrach procedure include

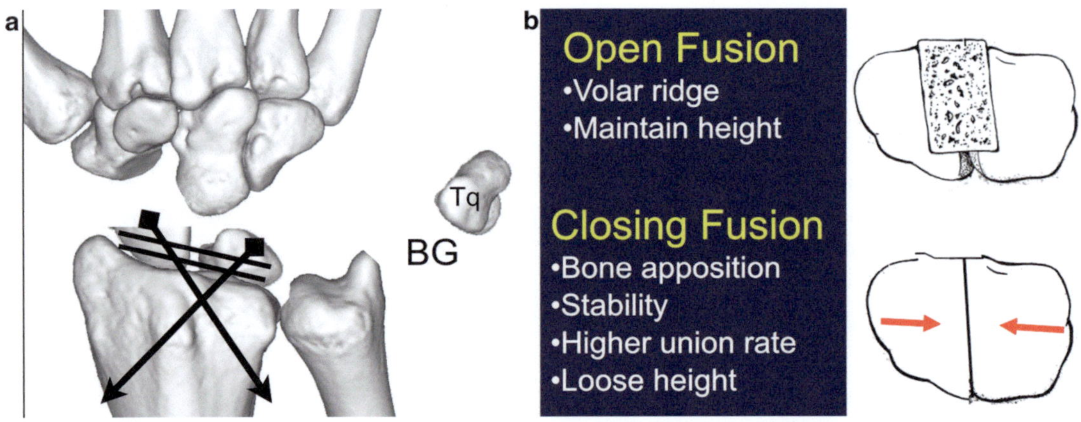

Fig. 8.7 (**a**) The authors' preferred technique for RSL fusion. The distal scaphoid excision increases radial deviation and flexion. Excision of the triquetrum increases ulnar deviation and extension, provides excellent bone graft, and prevents ulnar-carpal impaction. The scaphoid and lunate are anatomically reduced under direction vision and held with the 2 × 1.1 mm *K*-wires. The proximal row is then stabilized to the radius with cannulated screws or *K*-wires. (**b**) The authors utilize a closing fusion technique, as it provided greater stability, increases the contract area, and is therefore more likely to lead to a successful fusion (Published with kind permission of © Dr. Gregory Bain 2015. All Rights Reserved)

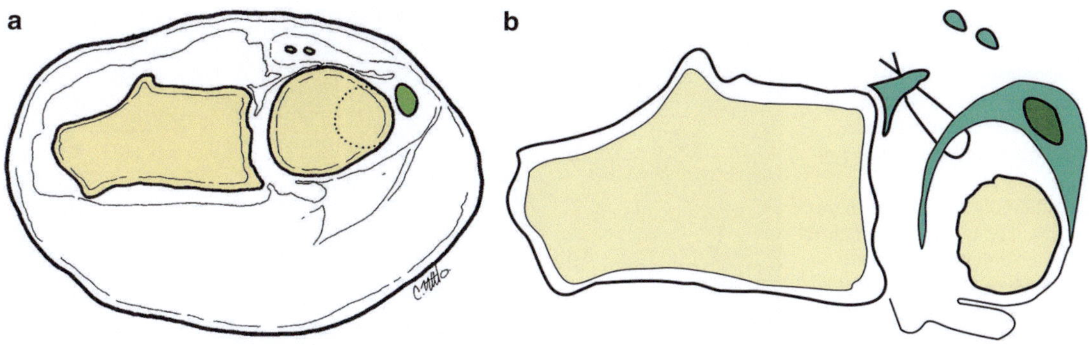

Fig. 8.8 Matched hemi-resection of the distal ulna. Note how the capsular-retinacular flap acts as an interposition and brings the captured ECU tendon over the top of the distal ulna to provide stability. From Bain, Roth et al. *J Hand Surg* 1995 [38], reproduced with permission

the hemi-resection techniques described by Bowers in 1985 and Watson in 1986 [35, 36]. These procedures seek to preserve the TFCC by resecting the ulnar articular cylinder while maintaining the shaft, styloid, and TFCC. If DRUJ instability is considered a problem, some surgeons prefer a Sauvé-Kapandji procedure, as it will stabilize the DRUJ. Unfortunately the instability will continue but is just transferred more proximally [37].

Authors' Technique: Matched Hemi-resection

For patients with rheumatoid arthritis involving the DRUJ, with an unstable and deformed distal ulna, the authors' preferred technique is the matched hemi-resection developed by the late Dr. Jim Roth [38]. The extensor retinaculum is divided over the fifth extensor compartment. The dorsal radioulnar joint capsule and the adherent infra-tendinous portion of the extensor retinaculum are divided 1 mm from their attachment to the sigmoid notch. No attempt is made to separate the dorsal capsule from the retinaculum, and the ECU is not removed from the retinacular flap. An oblique osteotomy of the distal ulna is performed and the distal ulna shaped to match the contour of the distal radius throughout forearm rotation. Care is taken to ensure that there is adequate resection and no impingement between the ulnar and radius and the ulnar styloid and carpus.

The joint is also examined with intraoperative fluoroscopy throughout supination and pronation. The ulnar-based retinacular flap is undermined from the adjacent ulna and tendons, allowing it to be mobilized and used as an interposition graft (Fig. 8.8). The technique helps to stabilize the distal ulna, as the ECU tendon is stabilized over the top of the distal ulnar stump. The ulnar-based retinacular flap is sutured to the 1 mm stump. The supra-tendinous portion of the retinaculum is repaired distally to prevent bowstringing of the extensor digiti minimi tendon.

Case Discussion: Arthroplasty of the Wrist

The case presented in Fig. 8.4 and Videos 8.1, 8.2, 8.3, 8.4, 8.5, 8.6, 8.7, and 8.8 is a complex total wrist arthroplasty case, as the long-term dislocation makes it difficult to reduce the new articulation. As a consequence, we set out to perform an arthroplasty, but if an adequate reduction could not be obtained, we would revert to an arthrodesis. To decompress the joint, we excised more of the carpus than usual and shortened the radius and ulna. We could then insert the trial prosthesis but it was tight, and the wrist had a fixed flexion deformity of approximately 20°.

After shortening of the radius by an extra few millimeters, excising of the volar wrist capsule, and fractional lengthening of the FRC and FCU, we were able to reduce the joint and obtain extension with the trial prosthesis in situ. We consider at that point an arthroplasty was a viable option,

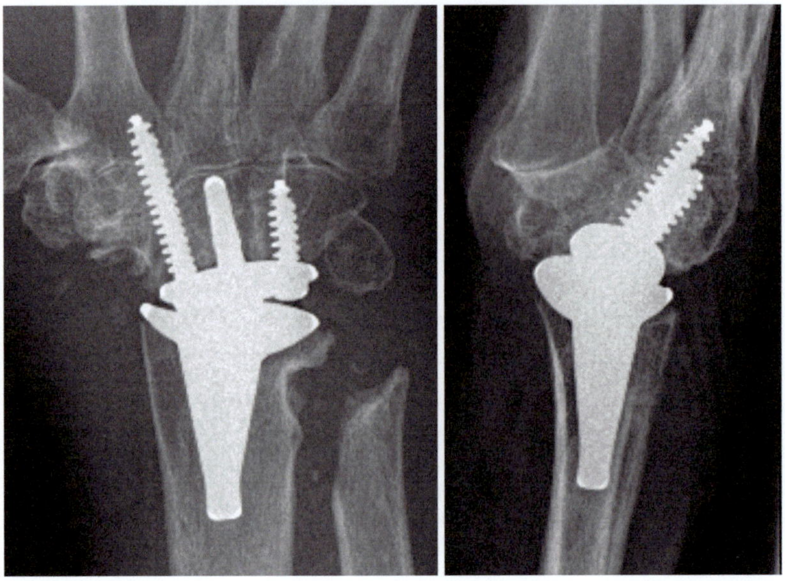

Fig. 8.9 Postoperative radiographs of total wrist arthroplasty. The radius and ulnar have been shortened and the anterior capsule excised with fractional lengthening of FCR and FCU, and the prosthesis is well seated in the radius. The wrist is maintained in extension until the soft tissues have stabilized. The distal ulna was managed with a matched hemi-resection

and a definitive prosthesis was inserted. The wrist could be extended to 20° but would naturally assume a posture in 20° of flexion. As the wrist had been in the flexion posture for some years, we were concerned that with the usual early active motion rehabilitation, she may never extend the wrist and be left with a permanent fixed flexion deformity. We therefore applied a volar slab and held the wrist in the extension arc for 4 weeks, followed by a resting extension splint at night for 3 months. She has subsequently maintained functional motion of the wrist (Fig. 8.9).

Case Discussion: Arthroplasty of the DRUJ

Arthroplasty of the DRUJ is beyond the scope of this manuscript; however, an interesting case worthy of discussion is a 35-year-old lady with RA who had painful dorsal instability of the DRUJ and attrition ruptures of the extensor tendons (Fig. 8.10a, b). The patient was still active, so an ulnar head replacement was preferred to a matched hemi-resection. However the dorsal sigmoid notch was eroded, so it would not contain the ulnar head. A dorsal sigmoid notch osteoplasty redirected the sigmoid notch, so that it would contain the ulnar head arthroplasty (Fig. 8.10c). The patient has maintained a functional range of motion.

Conclusion

The pathological process of rheumatoid arthritis in the wrist joint results in significant pain and loss of function. The chronic inflammation causes articular cartilage loss, pseudo-laxity, true ligamentous laxity, joint destruction, and deformity. Targeted surgical intervention can stabilize the joint, halt the progression of disease, and alleviate the symptoms, while maintaining an adequate range of motion.

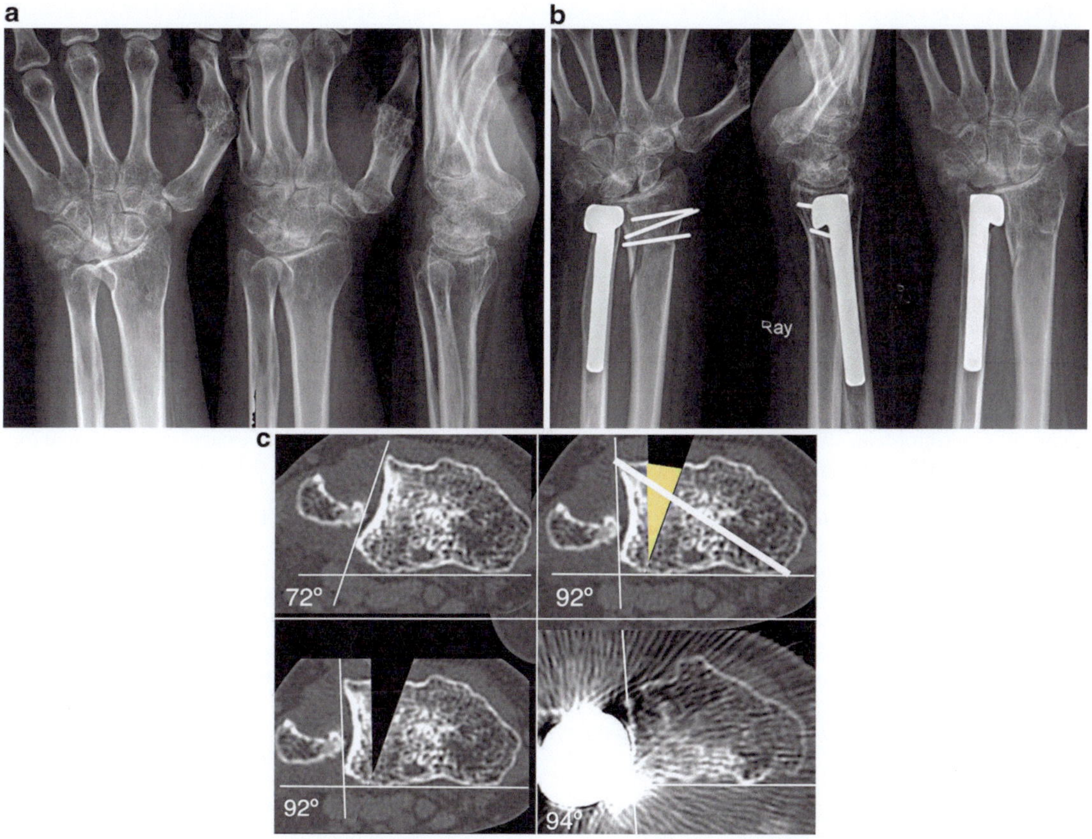

Fig. 8.10 Rheumatoid arthritis with advanced DRUJ destruction, managed with sigmoid notch osteoplasty. (**a**) At time of surgery, the dorsal aspect of the sigmoid notch was clearly eroded and would not contain the native head or a trial ulnar component. A dorsal sigmoid notch osteoplasty was performed with the aim of stabilizing the component. (**b**) The ulnar head arthroplasty is well contained due to the sigmoid notch osteoplasty. Note that on the lateral view the ulnar head is now reduced. (**c**) Sigmoid notch osteoplasty. (i) Preoperative CT scan with abnormal shaped sigmoid notch. (ii) The aim was to perform a 200 sigmoid notch osteotomy, to better contain the ulnar head. (iii) The osteotomy is supported with bone graft and stabilized with *K*-wires. (iv) Follow-up CT scan demonstrates that the osteotomy united and that the ulnar prosthesis remained stable. We have added the measured angles but do acknowledge sampling and interpretation errors. However the important point is that the osteotomy did unite and contained the ulnar head and allowed her to return to functional activities. Published with kind permission of © Dr. Gregory Bain 2015. All Rights Reserved

References

1. Boonan A, Severens JL. The burden of illness of rheumatoid arthritis. Clin Rheumatol. 2011;30 Suppl 1:S3–8.
2. Tubiana R, Thomine J, Mackin E. Examination of the hand and wrist. 2nd ed. London: Martin Kunitz; 1996.
3. Viegas SF, Wagner K, Patterson R, Peterson P. Medial (hamate) facet of the lunate. J Hand Surg Am. 1990;15(4):564e571.
4. Bain GI, Clitherow HD, Millar S, Fraysse F, Costi JJ, Eng K, McGuire DT, Thewlis D. The effect of lunate morphology on the 3-dimensional kinematics of the carpus. J Hand Surg Am. 2015;40(1):81–9.
5. Yazaki N, Burns ST, Morris RP, Andersen CR, Patterson RM, Viegas SF. Variations of capitate morphology in the wrist. J Hand Surg Am. 2008;33(5):660–6.
6. McLean J, Eames MA, Fogg QA, Pourgiezis N, Bain GI. An anatomical study of the Triquetrum-Hamate joint. J Hand Surg Am. 2006;31(4):601–7.
7. Watts AC, McLean JM, Fogg Q, Bain GI. Scaphoid anatomy. In: Slutsky DJ, Slade III JF, editors. The scaphoid. New York: Thieme; 2011. p. 3–10.

8. Flatt A. The care of the arthritic hand. 5th ed. St. Louis: Quality Medical Publishing; 1995.
9. McInnes I, Schett G. The pathogenesis of rheumatoid arthritis. New Engl J Med. 2011;365:2205–19.
10. Van Der Heijde DM. Joint erosions and patients with early rheumatoid arthritis. Br J Rheumatol. 1995;34:74–8.
11. Bajuri M, Kadir M, Amin I, Öchsner A. Biomechanical analysis of rheumatoid arthritis of the wrist joint. J Eng Med. 2012;226(7):510–20.
12. Arimitsu S, Murase T, Hashimoto J, Oka K, Sugamoto K, Yoshikawa H, Moritomo H. A three dimensional quantitative analysis of carpal deformity in rheumatoid wrists. J Bone Joint Surg Br. 2007;89:490–4.
13. Chamay A, Della Santa D, Vilaseca A. Radiolunate arthrodesis. Factor of stability for the rheumatoid wrist. Ann Chir Main. 1983;2(1):5–17.
14. McMurtry RH, Youm Y, Flatt A, Gillepsie TE. Kinematics of the wrist. Clinical applications. J Bone Joint Surg. 1978;60A:955–9.
15. Chung KC, Pushman AG. Current concepts in the management of the rheumatoid hand. J Hand Surg. 2011;36A:736–47.
16. Backdahl M. The caput ulnae syndrome in rheumatoid arthritis: a study of the morphology, abnormal anatomy and clinical picture. Acta Rheumatol Scand. 1963;5:1–75.
17. Adolfsson L, Nylander G. Arthroscopic synovectomy of the rheumatoid wrist. J Hand Surg [Br]. 1993;18:92–6.
18. Bain G, Munt J, Turner PC. New advances in wrist arthroscopy. Arthroscopy. 2008;24(3):355–67.
19. Kim S, Jung K. Arthroscopic synovectomy in rheumatoid arthritis of the wrist. Clin Med Res. 2007;5(4):244–50.
20. Adolfsson L, Frisen M. Arthroscopic synovectomy of the rheumatoid wrist. A 3.8 year follow-up. J Hand Surg [Br]. 1997;22:711–3.
21. Adolfsson L. Arthroscopic synovectomy of the wrist. Hand Clin. 2011;27:395–9.
22. Adolfsson L, Nylander G. Arthroscopic synovectomy of the rheumatoid wrist. J Hand Surg. 1993;18B: 92–6.
23. Kim SJ, Jung KA, Kim JM, Kwun JD, Kang HJ. Arthroscopic synovectomy in wrists with advanced rheumatoid arthritis. Clin Orthop Relat Res. 2006;449:262–6.
24. Arimitsu S, Murase T, Hashimoto J, Yoshikawa H, Sugamoto K, Moritomo H. Three-dimensional kinematics of the rheumatoid wrist after partial arthrodesis. J Bone Joint Surg Am. 2009;91:2180–7.
25. Bain G, McGuire D. Decision making for partial carpal fusions. J Wrist Surg. 2012;01(02):103–14.
26. Honkanen PB, Makela S, Konttinen YT, Lehto MU. Radiocarpal arthrodesis in the treatment of the rheumatoid wrist. A prospective midterm follow-up. J Hand Surg Eur Vol. 2007;32:368–76.
27. Ishikawa H, Murasawa A, Nakazono K. Long-term follow-up study of radiocarpal arthrodesis for the rheumatoid wrist. J Hand Surg Am. 2005;30:658–66.
28. Nagy L, Büchler U. Long-term results of radioscapholunate fusion following fractures of the distal radius. J Hand Surg. 1997;22B:705–10.
29. Bach AW, Almquist EE, Newman DM. Proximal row fusion as a solution for radiocarpal arthritis. J Hand Surg. 1991;16A:424–31.
30. Bain GI, Ondimu P, Hallam P, Ashwood N. Radioscapholunate arthrodesis—a prospective study. Hand Surg. 2009;14(2–3):73–82.
31. Garcia-Elias M, Lluch A, Ferreres A, Papini-Zorli I, Rahimtoola ZO. Treatment of radiocarpal degenerative osteoarthritis by radioscapholunate arthrodesis and distal scaphoidectomy. J Hand Surg Am. 2005;30:8–15.
32. Bain G, Sood A, Yeo CJ. RSL fusion with excision of distal scaphoid and triquetrum: a cadaveric study. J Wrist Surg. 2014;3(1):37–41.
33. Bain G, Ondimu P, Hallam P, Ashwood N. Radioscapholunate arthrodesis – a prospective study. Hand Surg (Asian). 2009;14:73–82.
34. De Smet L. The distal radio-ulnar joint in rheumatoid arthritis. Acta Orthop Belg. 2006;72:381–6.
35. Bowers WH. Distal radioulnar arthroplasty: the hemiresection interposition technique. J Hand Surg. 1985;10A:169–17878.
36. Watson HK, Ryu J, Burgess RC. Matched distal ulna resection. J Hand Surg. 1986;11A:812–7.
37. Sauvé L, Kapandji M. Nouvelle technique de traitement chirurgical des luxations récidivantes isolées de l'extré- mité inferieure du cubitus. J Chir. 1936;47:589–94.
38. Bain G, Roth J, Pugh D, MacDermid J. Matched hemiresection interposition arthroplasty of the distal radioulnar joint. J Hand Surg. 1995;20A(6):944–50.

Concepts and Indications of Rheumatoid Wrist Surgery

9

Marco Rizzo

Introduction

Rheumatoid arthritis (RA) is the most commonly encountered inflammatory arthropathy that affects the wrist. The precise mechanism of disease remains debated, but RA is generally understood to be an autoimmune process that targets the synovium, tenosynovium, and cartilage. The HLA-II locus appears to be a factor associated with genetic activation of the disease [1]. This leads to stimulation of a neutrophil infiltration that causes free radical and lysosomal enzyme release resulting in local tissue destruction.

Within 2 years from diagnosis, greater than 50 % of patients will have wrist pain, and greater than 90 % will have disease within 10 years [2]. Uncontrolled and/or aggressive RA can often result in pain, limited motion, severe joint destruction, and deformity. When compared to osteoarthritis, severe RA can result in markedly greater joint destruction, bone loss, and deformity. Sequelae of disease can also result in soft-tissue problems such as tendon irritation and rupture. Severe involvement can also result in adjacent soft-tissue disease as in conditions like Vaughan–Jackson syndrome or Mannerfelt lesions which are due to attritional rupture of extensor and flexor tendons at the wrist [3, 4]. The degree of wrist involvement and collapse remains important because it can predict outcomes of more distal surgery [5].

It is important to appreciate that in addition to musculoskeletal involvement, systemic manifestations of rheumatoid arthritis can occur. Organ systems including the skin, lungs, eyes, vasculature, and heart may also be affected. Felty syndrome is defined as RA associated with splenomegaly and a low white blood cell count. Still syndrome results in fevers, rash, and arthritis and may affect children or adults.

Clinical Presentation and Evaluation

Pain and functional limitation are typically the primary reasons patients present to their physician for evaluation. Occasionally they are concerned about deformity and general appearance of the wrist and hand. Obtaining a complete medical history including that of their rheumatoid disease is essential. A history of previous surgery and all medications should be included in the evaluation. If the patient has had prior surgeries for their disease, past surgical experiences can be helpful in giving prognosis and avoiding previous pitfalls. A complete examination from the neck to the hand is essential, and one must understand

M. Rizzo, MD (✉)
Department of Orthopedic Surgery, Mayo Clinic, 200 First St. SW, Rochester, MN 55905, USA
e-mail: Rizzo.marco@mayo.edu

K.C. Chung (ed.), *Clinical Management of the Rheumatoid Hand, Wrist, and Elbow*, DOI 10.1007/978-3-319-26660-2_9 that cervical spine disease is common in RA and needs to be evaluated in individuals as part of their preoperative assessment. The workup should include X-rays of the cervical spine and electromyography (EMG) in patients with radicular or neurologic symptoms. Systemic evaluation of the musculoskeletal system will round out an appropriate workup of these often complex patients. Establishing a relationship with the patient's rheumatologist is important to better understand the patient, their disease, and the operative planning when necessary. Rheumatologists can also advise on perioperative management of the patient's anti-inflammatory medications.

A comprehensive evaluation of the patient should include functional, anatomical, radiological, psychological, medical, financial, and surgical assessments. The functional assessment is aimed at quantifying and prioritizing their problem list in the context of their lifestyle and their environment. An anatomical assessment, which has already been alluded to, must appreciate the complex interaction of joints and their variable degree of disease involvement. As a result, isolated surgery is rarely appropriate in the context of treating rheumatoid arthritis of the wrist. In addition to confirming the degree of arthritis and assessing deformity, a radiological assessment is critical not only in helping identify the quality and quantity of residual bone stock but in establishing what can as well as cannot be done from a surgical reconstruction. A psychological assessment helps identify the hopes, desires, fears, and anxieties of the patient and is critical in establishing a mutual understanding and expectation of the outcomes of surgery. Rheumatoid patients are often complicated and require multiple visits to establish a relationship and trust. It is important to engage the patient to define their priorities and goals of potential surgery. The medical status of the patient and their disease is critical in determining the risks and optimal timing of surgery. Their degree of disease control has a significant bearing on success of surgery. Associated systemic disease such as pneumonitis, pericarditis, and vasculitis has a particular bearing on optimal patient selection and timing of surgery. The financial assessment is applicable to both the patient and to the medical community in general. The direct cost of care as well as the cost of time away from work can have a significant impact on a patient's ability to undergo treatment(s). In addition, general health-care costs may need to be justified in the future as the health-care community evolves to evidence-based medicine.

Synovitis and swelling reflecting the inflammatory process are common and can be appreciated on physical exam. It is important to keep in mind that the disease is diffuse and pain and synovitis of the elbow can affect the proximal and distal radioulnar joints and the forearm axis of rotation. In addition, synovitis of the elbow may result in posterior interosseous nerve dysfunction which can mimic tendon ruptures of the hand. Synovitis of the wrist impacts the appearance of the hand, is painful, and limits function. Dorsal synovitis is generally easier to appreciate than volar synovitis due to the more superficial position of the dorsal synovium. The pre-styloid recess of the ulna is a hypervascular area and is commonly affected in RA, leading to cartilage destruction and attenuation of the stabilizing ligaments. As the disease progresses at the distal radioulnar joint, dorsal displacement of the ulna, or more accurately palmar decent of the radius as the ulna is a fixed structure, occurs resulting in the caput ulna syndrome causing pain, limiting pronosupination, and potentially rupturing the extensor tendons [6]. Although less obvious, volar wrist synovitis and inflammation may be quite severe. Unfortunately, the initial presenting sign may be attritional flexor tendon rupture caused by synovitis, bony destruction, and osteophytosis of the carpus—this is most common at the scaphotrapeziotrapezoid joint and affects mainly the flexor pollicis longus tendon (Fig. 9.1) [3]. In addition, volar synovitis can contribute to significant compression neuropathies such as carpal tunnel syndrome. In long-standing or severe disease, the supporting soft tissues of the wrist become progressively incompetent, and the wrist will deform in a predictable pattern. The carpus translates ulnarly and supinates resulting in radial deviation of the wrist. This wrist deformity significantly contributes to a downstream compensatory ulnar deviation tendency of the digits leading to the classic zigzag deformity of the wrist–hand complex (Fig. 9.2) [7].

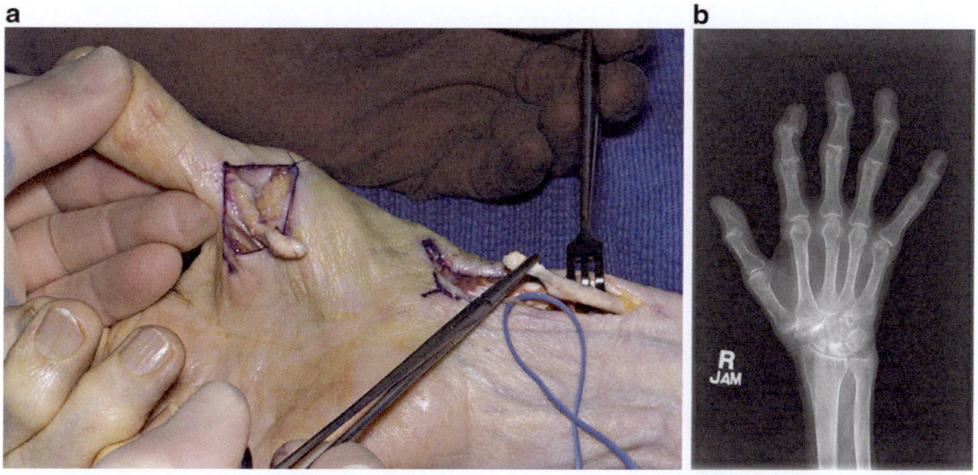

Fig. 9.1 (**a**) A patient with attritional rupture of the flexor pollicis longus secondary to synovitis and arthritis. (**b**) AP radiograph demonstrating severe scaphotrapeziotrapezoid (STT) arthritis

Fig. 9.2 The typical appearance of the rheumatoid wrist. The carpus translates ulnarly, supinates, and radially deviates. This can lead to MCP joint ulnar deviation distally

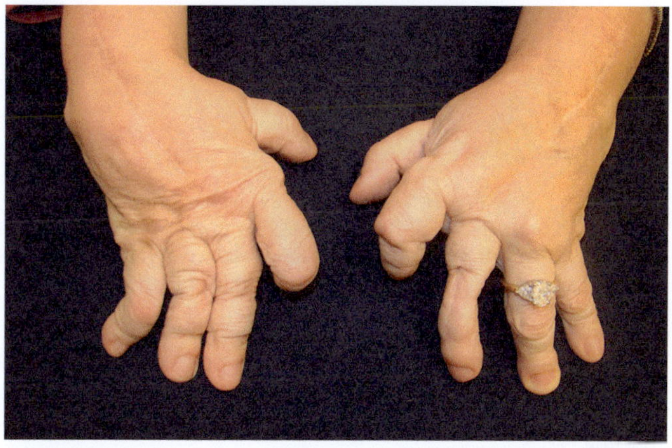

Physical examination of the wrist assesses the degree of pain to palpation and motion and amount of swelling. Most patients have more pain with palpation at areas of increased swelling. One should determine the range of motion in flexion extension, radioulnar deviation, and pronosupination, as well as grip and pinch strength. Pain with resisted flexion and extension is helpful. It will not only reflect joint disease but may also suggest tenosynovitis and potential "tendons at risk." Comparing passive motion versus active motion is necessary and may reflect the source of pathology. For example, failure to actively extend a digit may be secondary to tendon rupture, such as that seen in a caput ulna or Vaughan–Jackson syndrome (Fig. 9.3) [8]. However, other circumstances may be the culprit including volar subluxation of the metacarpophalangeal (MP) joint, extensor tendon subluxation due to sagittal band insufficiency, or posterior interosseous neuropathy at the elbow. These etiologies for limited MP extension can be differentiated through a good and thorough physical examination. Patients with MP joint subluxation will lack passive extension of the joint. Extensor tendon subluxation secondary to ulnar drift of the digits and radial sagittal band insufficiency have passive extension but not active extension of the MP joint. Posterior interosseous neuropathy is often associated with swelling at the elbow and will likely also have

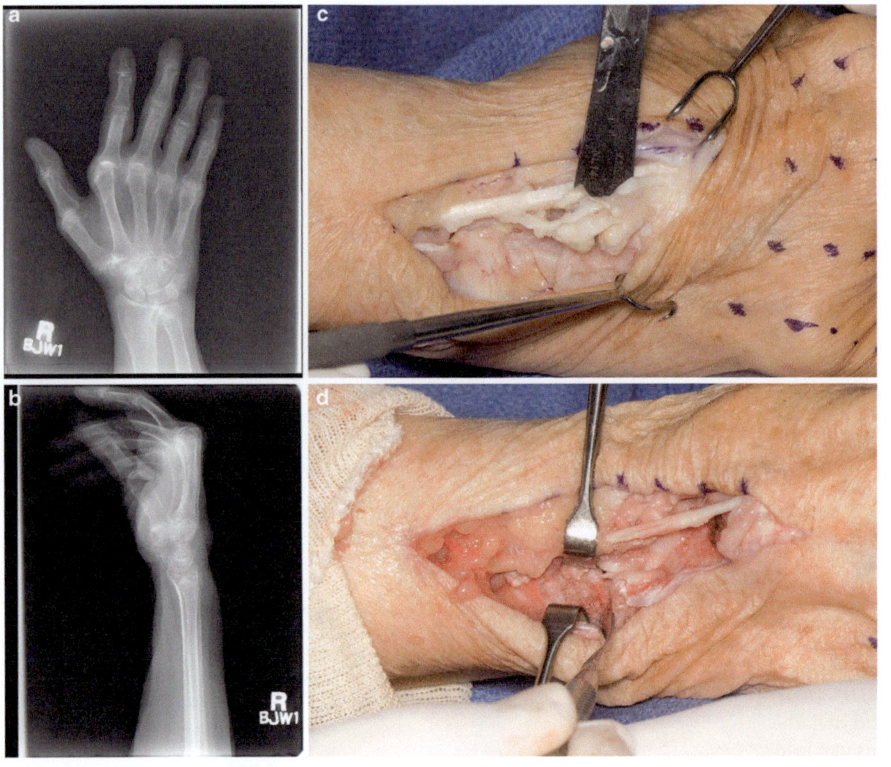

Fig. 9.3 (**a** and **b**) PA and lateral of right wrist/hand of a patient who presented with loss of extension of the ring and small finger and pain at the ulnar side of the wrist. (**c**) Intraoperative photograph demonstrates attritional rupture of the extensor tendons secondary to synovitis and irritation from the osteophytes/irregularity of the distal radioulnar joint (**d**)

limited thumb interphalangeal joint extension. Patients with tendon rupture will often have pain and deformity at the distal radioulnar joint and lack a tenodesis extension effect with wrist flexion.

Compression neuropathy of the wrist, such as carpal tunnel syndrome, can result from direct inflammatory influence on the nerve as well as tenosynovitis, synovitis, and joint destruction of the carpus (Fig. 9.4). Carpal tunnel release usually combined with flexor tenosynovectomy in patients with rheumatoid arthritis has been shown to yield good results and generally carries a favorable prognosis [9]. Patients with bilateral involvement and multiple upper extremity joint involvement pose special challenges and prioritization of the patient's complaints and dysfunction are important. The skin in patients with RA is typically thin and carries a higher risk of delayed wound healing or dehiscence, which predisposes to infection. Rheumatoid nodules may be present and can often be painful and associated with joint deformity.

Radiographs of the wrist are important in the evaluation of patients with rheumatoid arthritis and discerning the degree of bony destruction and arthritis. They are essential for operative planning and help delineate what can and cannot be done from a surgical standpoint. Early disease with joint space narrowing is typically seen initially at the distal radioulnar and the radioscaphoid joints [10, 11]. Mid-carpal disease is typically a later finding [12, 13]. Radiographs help define the more commonly utilized classification systems [14, 15]. Although not specific to the wrist, the Larsen classification is commonly used [15]. It is based on stages 0–5, with stage 0 being a normal joint. Stage 1 demonstrates periarticular swelling, osteoporosis, and slight narrowing of the joint. Stage 2 includes erosions and mild joint space narrowing. Stage 3 involves moderate destructive changes and joint space narrowing. Stage 4 reveals end-stage destruction with preservation of the articular surface, and stage 5 shows a mutilated or ankylosed joint with destruction of

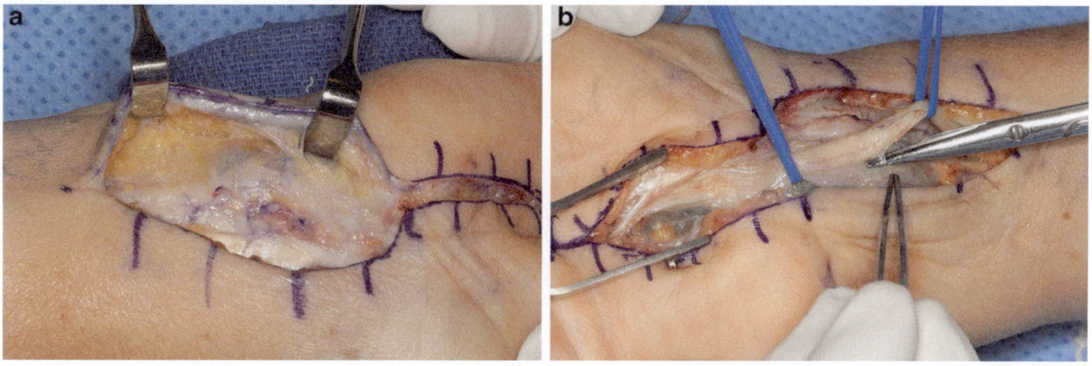

Fig. 9.4 (**a**) Intraoperative photograph of a patient with severe carpal tunnel syndrome associated with synovitis and tenosynovitis. (**b**) Note the hourglass compression of the nerve proximal to the vessel loop

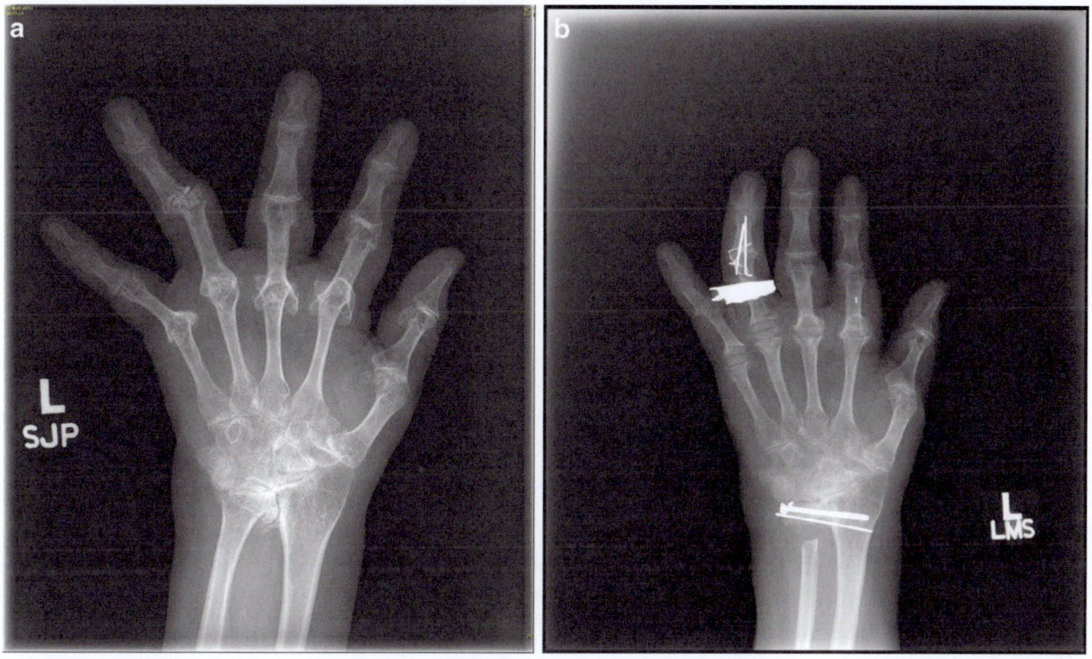

Fig. 9.5 (**a**) PA radiograph of a Wrightington three wrist. Note the severe subluxation and ulnar drift of the carpus. (**b**) This patient was treated with a Sauve–Kapandji procedure

the articular surfaces. The Wrightington classification is more specific for the wrist, and the system outlines treatment recommendations based on the stage of disease [14]. The stages range from 1 to 4. Stage 1 radiographs reveal osteoporosis, with cysts and erosions, and the recommended treatment is synovectomy. In stage 2 disease, the radiographs demonstrate carpal instability; the recommended treatment is soft-tissue stabilization or partial arthrodesis of the wrist. By stage 3, the wrist has frank destruction and subluxation, and these patients will likely best be surgically treated with an arthroplasty or arthrodesis (Fig. 9.5). Stage 4 disease radiographs show severe radial destruction, and arthrodesis is likely the only feasible surgical option. Simmen and Huber proposed an alternate classification system, based more on the natural course of the disease rather than their radiographic appearance [16]. There are three types,

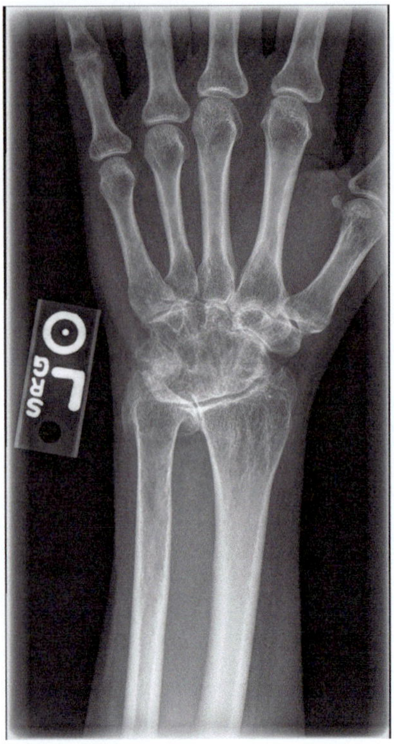

Fig. 9.6 Type 1 Simmen classification wrist. This patient has spontaneous ankyloses of the carpus

and type 1 is defined as the ankylosing type and is characterized by spontaneous fusion of the wrist (Fig. 9.6). Type 2 is defined as the osteoarthritic type and has characteristics of osteoarthritis and osteoporosis. These patients tend to have some inherent wrist stability, which may afford more surgical reconstructive options. Type 3 patients have the disintegrative type and have significant bone loss and instability, and they are subdivided into 3a (more ligamentous instability) and 3b (more bony resorption).

Computed tomography can be helpful in providing a more precise measure of the degree of arthritis and joint involvement. Magnetic resonance imaging (MRI) studies provide an excellent delineation of the soft tissues about the wrist including the degree of synovitis and tenosynovitis, thickness and integrity of the cartilage, and bone marrow changes. Studies have demonstrated that MRI can reveal improvement in tenosynovitis in response to treatment [17]. Scoring systems based on MRI have defined to grade the cartilage changes in patients with early RA [18]. In addition, bone edema on MRI has been shown, in patients with early disease, to predict who goes on to develop radiographic damage and may help identify patients who could benefit from a more aggressive treatment [19].

Nonoperative Treatment

Pharmacologic treatments aimed at minimizing the inflammatory process are an established mainstay in the management of rheumatoid arthritis. Corticosteroids and methotrexate have been used for years. Some surgeons prefer stopping non-corticosteroid anti-inflammatory medications, such as methotrexate, for a period prior to and following surgery to help avoid delayed healing and infection [20]. However, other studies have shown that continuing methotrexate does not increase the risk of perioperative infection [21]. Newer generation pharmaceuticals including antitumor necrosis factor agents have gained acceptance and are effective in reducing the synovitis and disease progression of RA. This has fortuitously resulted in fewer patients requiring surgical intervention and also suggests that improved outcomes after surgery can be seen in these patients. Unfortunately, these newer generation medications have been shown to increase generalized infection rates especially in the lower respiratory tract and soft tissues, particularly in patients who are also on corticosteroids [22]. Previous studies suggest no increased risk of infection with the use of infliximab in patients undergoing surgery for Crohn's disease [23]. The impact of these medications on perioperative morbidity, if any, has yet to be fully realized. The medications have a widely variable clearance time from the bloodstream including 8 days for etanercept, 15 days for adalimumab, and 57 days for infliximab. Due to the lack of hard science, many surgeons will consult with the patient and their rheumatologist regarding perioperative cessation/resumption of these medications.

Static and dynamic splinting is an established treatment for RA and can provide pain relief, functional improvement, and hopeful correction of deformity. However, a Cochrane database review showed that although patients appear to prefer wearing splints to not wearing them, there is no proven benefit with respect to pain or range of motion [24]. In contrast, Veehof et al. showed that wearing wrist splints for as little as four weeks can significantly help with pain [25]. Despite the pain relief, function- and patient-related outcome measures were not significantly different when compared to controls. Adams et al. prospectively evaluated static splinting in the treatment of early RA and noted that it does not significantly improve function and pain or retard deformity progression when compared to placebo [26].

Intra-articular injections of steroid have been utilized for many years in the treatment of RA and can improve swelling, pain, and patient-perceived outcomes [27]. Konai et al. demonstrated that intra-articular steroid injection was superior to systemic corticosteroid in the treatment of monoarticular RA of the knee [28]. In contrast, Weitoft and Ronnblom prospectively evaluated the use of splinting as an adjunct following steroid injection of the wrist and found no difference in outcomes between groups [29]. They concluded that other joints affected by RA may not respond in a similar fashion to knees. Other more recent investigations examined the use of intra-articular injection of anti-TNF agents and have determined that it is generally safe [30]. Bliddal et al. performed a randomized comparison of the use of intra-articular wrist injections of 25 mg of etanercept versus 40 mg of methylprednisolone [31]. There was no significant difference in outcomes. The authors concluded that, because of the increased cost of etanercept, it should be reserved primarily for patients who have adverse effects to steroid injections.

Indications/Contraindications for Surgery

When considering surgery of the rheumatoid wrist, a thoughtful assessment of many factors is necessary. These patients require a comprehensive evaluation. Persons affected by RA may be malnourished as a result of their disease as well as the medications used for treatment. Thus, nutritional assessment and optimization is important. It is also important to appreciate that the poor pharmacologic control of the disease can undermine the outcome following surgery. Anesthetic risk is higher in patients with cervical spine disease. Because many patients are on immunosuppressive medications, surgery carries higher risk of wound- and tissue-healing problems and infection.

The timing and indication for surgery remains somewhat controversial [32]. Persistent symptoms, synovitis, or swelling despite a 3–6 month course of conservative treatment can be viewed by most physicians as an indication for surgery [33, 34]. Exceptions include cases in which surgery would be prophylactic against irreversible soft-tissue injury or damage such as seen in tendon ruptures. Deformity or progression of deformity of the wrist, such as a zigzag deformity, has been advocated by some surgeons as requiring prophylactic intervention [35, 36]. Frank tendon rupture itself is generally an indication for surgery.

Contraindications for surgery include significant comorbidities and poor general health. Poor or insufficient proximal arm function that is not correctable is a relative contraindication to wrist surgery. Relative contraindications for wrist arthroplasty (including total wrist replacement) include history of previous infection, insufficient bone stock and long-standing fixed wrist deformity.

Surgical Considerations

In assessing patients with RA who have multiple joints affected, it is generally preferred, whenever possible, to surgically treat from proximal to distal and address the lower extremities first, as many patients will require crutches and weight bear on their upper extremities following lower extremity surgery.

A thoughtful approach from the surgeon will help optimize the treatment plan for each patient. It is important to identify the problem list, including clarifying the patient's goals prior to agreeing to surgery. This will help establish a mutual understanding and temper expectations. Operate for specific goals and agree to those goals preoperatively. Plan the least surgery for the most benefit and keep it as simple as possible. Communicate with the occupational therapists to minimize delays or confusion about the protocol and have a program that is synergistic.

When applicable, surgical priorities can also be established. The nerves are priority one and should take precedent. Flexor tendon injuries/rupture would follow, and these typically may be treated at the same time as wrist reconstruction or synovectomy. The following priority would be the thumb. A winning procedure in rheumatoid surgery is the thumb metacarpophalangeal joint arthrodesis. It can provide a stable pain-free post and markedly improves function. The MCP joints are the next priority; followed by the extensor tendons. The final priorities are the proximal interphalangeal (PIP) and distal interphalangeal (DIP) joints, respectively.

Surgical treatments for the rheumatoid wrist generally include synovectomy, tenosynovectomy, tendon repair/reconstruction, treatment of the arthritic distal radioulnar joint, partial and complete arthrodesis of the radiocarpal joint, and wrist arthroplasty. Multiple procedures are commonly done in the same setting.

Summary

Rheumatoid arthritis of the wrist is common and can lead to significant deformity and dysfunction of not just the wrist, but also the hand. Patients often present with swelling, pain, and limited function. As the disease progresses, a typical pattern of wrist deformity will ensue, resulting in supination of the carpus, volar translation, and radial deviation. This position of the wrist can contribute to the typical ulnar drift of the digits seen commonly in patients with RA. Physical exam findings demonstrate pain with palpation, limited range of motion, and crepitus. Nonoperative treatments, especially pharmacologic therapies, hold promise in managing the disease progression. Surgery should be considered when nonoperative treatments fail. Surgical considerations in patients with RA require a thoughtful approach with a comprehensive understanding of the patient's overall disease and its severity. Surgical intervention should be based on a mutual understanding of the patient's goals. Decisions for surgery are often best made in conjunction with the patient's rheumatologist in addition to the patient themselves. We try to do the simplest surgeries for the most gain; therapy programs need to be available and synergistic. With this thoughtful and patient-centered approach, pain relief, patient satisfaction, and improvement of function can be realized.

References

1. Crilly A, Maiden N, Capell HA, Madhok R. Genotyping for disease associated HLA DR beta 1 alleles and the need for early joint surgery in rheumatoid arthritis: a quantitative evaluation. Ann Rheum Dis. 1999;58(2):114–7.
2. Trieb K. Treatment of the wrist in rheumatoid arthritis. J Hand Surg [Am]. 2008;33(1):113–23.
3. Mannerfelt L, Norman O. Attrition ruptures of flexor tendons in rheumatoid arthritis caused by bony spurs in the carpal tunnel. A clinical and radiological study. J Bone Joint Surg. 1969;51(2):270–7.
4. Vaughan-Jackson OJ. Rupture of extensor tendons by attrition at the inferior radio-ulnar joint; report of two cases. J Bone Joint Surg Am. 1948;30B(3):528–30.
5. Taleisnik J. Rheumatoid synovitis of the volar compartment of the wrist joint: its radiological signs and its contribution to wrist and hand deformity. J Hand Surg [Am]. 1979;4(6):526–35.
6. Backdahl M. The caput ulnae syndrome in rheumatoid arthritis. A study of the morphology, abnormal anatomy and clinical picture. Acta Rheumatol Scand. 1963;5:1–75.
7. Stack HG, Vaughan-Jackson OJ. The zig-zag deformity in the rheumatoid hand. Hand. 1971;3(1):62–7.
8. Wilson RL, DeVito MC. Extensor tendon problems in rheumatoid arthritis. Hand Clin. 1996;12(3):551–9.
9. Shinoda J, Hashizume H, McCown C, Senda M, Nishida K, Doi T, et al. Carpal tunnel syndrome grading system in rheumatoid arthritis. J Orthop Sci. 2002;7(2):188–93.
10. Bywaters EG. The early radiological signs of rheumatoid arthritis. Bull Rheum Dis. 1960;11:231–4.
11. Martel W, Hayes JT, Duff IF. The pattern of bone erosion in the hand and wrist in rheumatoid arthritis. Radiology. 1965;84:204–14.
12. Taleisnik J. Combined radiocarpal arthrodesis and midcarpal (lunocapitate) arthroplasty for treatment of

rheumatoid arthritis of the wrist. J Hand Surg [Am]. 1987;12(1):1–8.
13. Hindley CJ, Stanley JK. The rheumatoid wrist: patterns of disease progression. A review of 50 wrists. J Hand Surg. 1991;16(3):275–9.
14. Hodgson SP, Stanley JK, Muirhead A. The Wrightington classification of rheumatoid wrist X-rays: a guide to surgical management. J Hand Surgery (Edinb). 1989;14(4):451–5.
15. Larsen A, Dale K, Eek M. Radiographic evaluation of rheumatoid arthritis and related conditions by standard reference films. Acta Radiol Diagn. 1977;18(4): 481–91.
16. Simmen BR, Huber H. The wrist joint in chronic polyarthritis—a new classification based on the type of destruction in relation to the natural course and the consequences for surgical therapy. Handchir Mikrochir Plast Chir. 1994;26(4):182–9.
17. Lisbona MP, Maymo J, Perich J, Almirall M, Carbonell J. Rapid reduction in tenosynovitis of the wrist and fingers evaluated by MRI in patients with rheumatoid arthritis after treatment with etanercept. Ann Rheum Dis. 2010;69(6):1117–22.
18. McQueen F, Clarke A, McHaffie A, Reeves Q, Williams M, Robinson E, et al. Assessment of cartilage loss at the wrist in rheumatoid arthritis using a new MRI scoring system. Ann Rheum Dis. 2010;69: 1971–5.
19. Haavardsholm EA, Boyesen P, Ostergaard M, Schildvold A, Kvien TK. Magnetic resonance imaging findings in 84 patients with early rheumatoid arthritis: bone marrow oedema predicts erosive progression. Ann Rheum Dis. 2008;67(6): 794–800.
20. James D, Young A, Kulinskaya E, Knight E, Thompson W, Ollier W, et al. Orthopaedic intervention in early rheumatoid arthritis. Occurrence and predictive factors in an inception cohort of 1064 patients followed for 5 years. Rheumatology (Oxford). 2004;43(3):369–76.
21. Jain A, Witbreuk M, Ball C, Nanchahal J. Influence of steroids and methotrexate on wound complications after elective rheumatoid hand and wrist surgery. J Hand Surg [Am]. 2002;27(3):449–55.
22. Favalli EG, Desiati F, Atzeni F, Sarzi-Puttini P, Caporali R, Pallavicini FB, et al. Serious infections during anti-TNFalpha treatment in rheumatoid arthritis patients. Autoimmun Rev. 2009;8(3):266–73.
23. Marchal L, D'Haens G, Van Assche G, Vermeire S, Noman M, Ferrante M, et al. The risk of post-operative complications associated with infliximab therapy for Crohn's disease: a controlled cohort study. Aliment Pharmacol Ther. 2004;19(7):749–54.
24. Egan M, Brosseau L, Farmer M, Ouimet MA, Rees S, Wells G, et al. Splints/orthoses in the treatment of rheumatoid arthritis. Cochrane Database Syst Rev. 2003;(1):CD004018.
25. Veehof MM, Taal E, Heijnsdijk-Rouwenhorst LM, van de Laar MA. Efficacy of wrist working splints in patients with rheumatoid arthritis: a randomized controlled study. Arthritis Rheum. 2008;59(12):1698–704.
26. Adams J, Burridge J, Mullee M, Hammond A, Cooper C. The clinical effectiveness of static resting splints in early rheumatoid arthritis: a randomized controlled trial. Rheumatology. 2008;47(10):1548–53.
27. Lopes RV, Furtado RN, Parmigiani L, Rosenfeld A, Fernandes AR, Natour J. Accuracy of intra-articular injections in peripheral joints performed blindly in patients with rheumatoid arthritis. Rheumatology (Oxford). 2008;47(12):1792–4.
28. Konai MS, Vilar Furtado RN, Dos Santos MF, Natour J. Monoarticular corticosteroid injection versus systemic administration in the treatment of rheumatoid arthritis patients: a randomized double-blind controlled study. Clin Exp Rheumatol. 2009;27(2):214–21.
29. Weitoft T, Ronnblom L. Randomised controlled study of postinjection immobilisation after intra-articular glucocorticoid treatment for wrist synovitis. Ann Rheum Dis. 2003;62(10):1013–5.
30. Bliddal H, Terslev L, Qvistgaard E, Recke P, Holm CC, Danneskiold-Samsoe B, et al. Safety of intra-articular injection of etanercept in small-joint arthritis: an uncontrolled, pilot-study with independent imaging assessment. Joint Bone Spine. 2006;73(6):714–7.
31. Bliddal H, Terslev L, Qvistgaard E, Konig M, Holm CC, Rogind H, et al. A randomized, controlled study of a single intra-articular injection of etanercept or glucocorticosteroids in patients with rheumatoid arthritis. Scand J Rheumatol. 2006;35(5):341–5.
32. Alderman AK, Chung KC, Kim HM, Fox DA, Ubel PA. Effectiveness of rheumatoid hand surgery: contrasting perceptions of hand surgeons and rheumatologists. J Hand Surg [Am]. 2003;28(1).3–11. discussion 2–3.
33. Millender LH, Nalebuff EA. Preventive surgery – tenosynovectomy and synovectomy. Orthop Clin North Am. 1975;6(3):765–92.
34. Ryu J, Saito S, Honda T, Yamamoto K. Risk factors and prophylactic tenosynovectomy for extensor tendon ruptures in the rheumatoid hand. J Hand Surg (Edinb). 1998;23(5):658–61.
35. Mannerfelt L. On surgery of the rheumatoid hand: consensus and controversy. J Hand Surg (Edinb). 1989;14(3):259–60.
36. Shapiro JS. The wrist in rheumatoid arthritis. Hand Clin. 1996;12(3):477–98.

Management of the Distal Radioulnar Joint in Rheumatoid Arthritis

10

Brian D. Adams

History

The distal radioulnar joint (DRUJ) is frequently involved in rheumatoid arthritis (RA), but the amount of derangement is quite variable [1]. Occasionally, the DRUJ is the first joint affected by RA, with pain, swelling, and possibly joint subluxation occurring before other joints in the wrist and hand are affected. Conversely, a patient can present later with extensor tendon ruptures of the small and ring fingers, referred to as the Vaughan–Jackson lesion, with minimal history of pain and swelling of the DRUJ [2]. In most patients with radiocarpal arthritis symptoms, the DRUJ will also typically show arthritis by both physical and radiographic examinations; however, the only complaint may be a bump on the back of the wrist that represents dorsal prominence of the distal ulna.

Pathophysiology and Physical Examination Findings

The ulnar head is covered mostly by articular surface. The DRUJ capsule, and its synovial lining, is large and redundant to permit large amount of motion. The large articular surface is inflamed causing swelling, tenderness, and ultimately joint destruction. A synovial reflection is present near the fovea of the ulnar head, which is the bony depression at the base of the ulnar styloid and the primary ulnar insertion site of the triangular fibrocartilage complex (TFCC) and the ulnocarpal ligaments (UCL). Chronic inflammation of this synovium results in damage to these important stabilizing ligaments [1, 2].

Physical examination demonstrates prominence of the distal ulna that is caused by joint swelling from synovitis occurring early in the disease but later results from a combination of synovitis and dorsal subluxation of the distal ulna, which is referred to as the caput ulnae syndrome. Distal ulna prominence is often accentuated by concurrent disease and deformity at the ulnocarpal joint in which the carpus supinates and volarly subluxates, resulting in substantially increased distance between the ulnar head and carpus.

Despite advanced DRUJ arthritis and deformity, forearm rotation is typically maintained because of excessive laxity in the joint caused by the disease. DRUJ crepitus is common but is often not associated with pain, even in severe disease. Crepitus is commonly associated with osteophytes that can contribute to mechanical damage of the overlying extensor tendons, resulting in tendon ruptures, especially of the small and ring fingers.

B.D. Adams, MD (✉)
Department of Orthopedic Surgery,
Baylor College of Medicine, 7200 Cambridge,
Suite 10A, Houston, TX 77030, USA
e-mail: bdm.adams@gmail.com

K.C. Chung (ed.), *Clinical Management of the Rheumatoid Hand, Wrist, and Elbow*,
DOI 10.1007/978-3-319-26660-2_10

Extensor carpi ulnaris (ECU) tenosynovitis is another frequent concurrent process that exacerbates the DRUJ deformity [2, 3]. The tenosynovitis causes weakening of the ECU subsheath and the overlying extensor retinaculum that results in volar subluxation of the tendon from its normal position in the osseous groove of the dorsal ulna head. The tendon subluxation substantially changes its action from wrist extension and ulnar deviation to wrist ulnar deviation alone. The ECU also loses its normal depressive action on the ulnar head. If the ECU tendon subluxates more volarly, the tendon may actually produce wrist flexion and exacerbate ulnar translocation and supination deformity of the radiocarpal joint.

Treatment Options

After ensuring the disease is being optimally treated by appropriate medications, early management of DRUJ synovitis includes corticosteroid injection into the joint and splinting of the wrist. An ulnar gutter splint or distal forearm band can be made to partially stabilize the DRUJ and partially restrict forearm rotation without substantially impeding finger or thumb motion. However, these devices may not be tolerated because they can restrict wrist motion, and, therefore, splints are typically worn intermittently for arthritic flares. Because of the risk of tendon ruptures associated with chronic DRUJ synovitis, examinations should be repeated regularly until the synovitis is confirmed to be substantially improved by medications and splinting.

If synovitis persists despite nonoperative treatment, especially if associated with dorsal ulnar head subluxation and crepitus, surgical treatment is considered before extensor tendon ruptures occur. The surgical options are similar to those used for arthritis of the DRUJ from other causes. However, when contemplating reconstruction, one needs to consider other concerns such as treating ECU tenosynovitis and subluxation, severe dorsal subluxation of the ulna, finger extensor tenosynovitis or ruptures, and ulnar translocation of the carpus. Furthermore, options may be influenced or limited by current overall disease control, concurrent treatment requirement for the radiocarpal joint, previous surgical procedures that altered the local tissues typically used for a reconstruction, as well as the patient's rehabilitation capacity.

The three primary traditional treatment options are the Darrach resection, Sauvé–Kapandji procedure, and hemiresection of the distal ulna. Each of these procedures is often combined with a stabilization of the distal ulna using a local tenodesis or capsular flap and a soft tissue interposition between the distal ulna and radius to reduce ulna impingement against the radius. In some patients in whom the overall rheumatoid disease is quiescent and well controlled, the DRUJ is not subluxated, the bone quality is adequate, and an implant arthroplasty can be considered. Although there are many specific anatomic factors associated with the indications for each of these procedures, there are some that are considered more important, which will be emphasized during the description of each procedure.

Darrach Procedure

Rheumatoid disease remains one of the main indications for the Darrach procedure because it is simple, alleviates pain, provides cosmetic improvement, and removes the cause for extensor tendon injury [4–6]. However, it has been reported to increase the risk of initiating or worsening ulnar translocation of the carpus, which is a common malady of the rheumatoid wrist. After a Darrach procedure, a younger patient may complain of reduced power grip, which is likely caused by the reduced support of the carpus. Almost all patients claim to have some crepitus during forearm rotation caused by rubbing between the ulnar stump and radius, but unlike nonrheumatoid patients, this is typically not symptomatic, especially in the lower-demand elderly patient.

A wide variation of technical modifications has been described, including level of ulnar resection, retention of ulnar styloid, mechanism of ulnar stump stabilization, and use of soft tissue

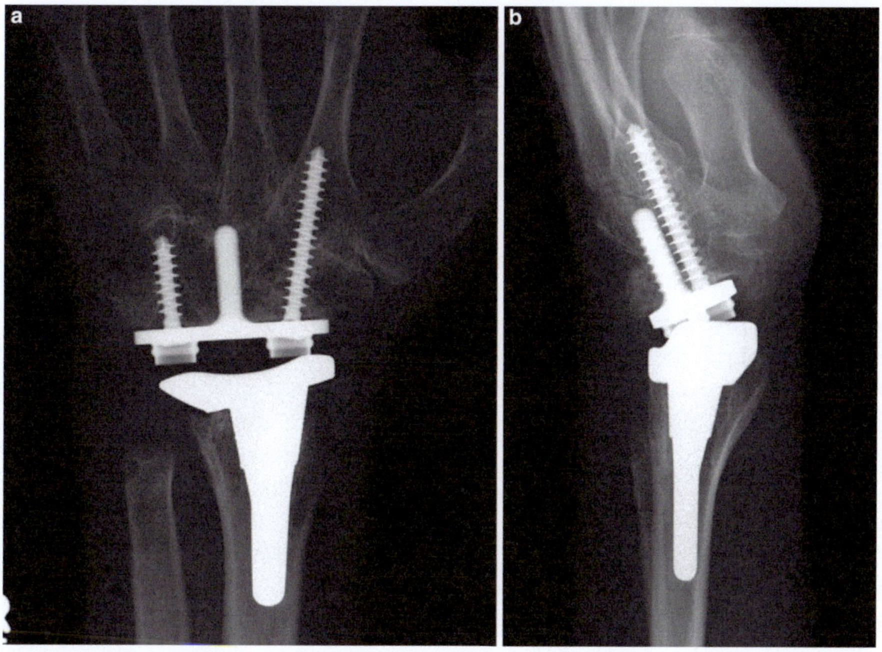

Fig. 10.1 Darrach procedure performed in combination with a total wrist arthroplasty. Note the remodeling of the distal ulna that has occurred

interposition [6]. The severity of the bone destruction, joint subluxation, and soft tissue attenuation often limits the potential modifications that can be used. In most rheumatoid cases, the ulnar resection is performed at the level just proximal to the sigmoid notch without retaining the ulnar styloid, the ulnar stump is slightly contoured to remove sharp edges, and a flap of volar capsule is transferred to the stump and secured by sutures placed through small holes in the stump [7]. In younger more active patients, alternative stump stabilization using either an ECU or flexor carpi ulnaris (FCU) tenodesis along with soft tissue interposition using capsule or pronator quadratus is often performed [8–11].

In patients with active radiocarpal synovitis and evidence of ulnar translocation of the carpus, a Darrach may increase the translocation by removing the buttressing effect of the distal ulna. A combined procedure maybe required if such cases, which includes a radiolunate or radioscapholunate fusion to stabilize the carpus. Because the Darrach procedure is typically an uncomplicated procedure, it can be combined with more complex procedures such as total wrist replacement that also stabilizes the radiocarpal joint (Fig. 10.1). ECU subluxation can be treated at the same time by relocating the tendon over the dorsal aspect of the ulnar stump and stabilizing the tendon in this position by reefing the extensor tendon retinaculum or creating a sling using a strip of the retinaculum [3]. Relocating the ECU tendon will help stabilize the ulnar stump, reduce its deforming force on the wrist, and possibly improve wrist extension. Some surgeons prefer to stabilize the ECU by performing an extensor carpi radialis longus (ECRL) to ECU tendon transfer, which may also provide some dynamic counter to the deforming forces across the wrist.

A dorsal surgical approach over the ulnar head is typically used to preserve any remaining TFCC components; however, some variation is dependent on concurrent procedures. If the ECU tendon does not require repositioning, then an approach through the fifth extensor compartment or between the fifth and sixth compartments is most efficient and allows closure by directly repairing the capsule and retinaculum together. If the ECU tendon requires repositioning, then a radially based extensor retinaculum flap can be raised first in order to be used as a sling for the ECU tendon, followed by an approach through the floor of the sixth compartment. This approach also allows access to the fifth extensor compartment for tenosynovectomy; the fifth compartment tendons are typically left superficial to the retinaculum at time of repair. If there is severe ulnar translocation of the carpus and a radiolunate fusion is also planned, then the capsulotomy can be extended distally to include the ulnocarpal joint and lunate fossa for joint preparation.

Hemiresection of the Distal Ulna

Because instability is associated with the Darrach procedure, hemiresection (HR) of the distal ulna, which removes the articular surface and a few millimeters of the underlying cancellous bone but when possible retains the ulnar attachments of the TFCC, has the potential advantages of preserving some stabilizers of the distal ulna, and the exposed cancellous bone encourages healing to the surrounding soft tissue sleeve (Fig. 10.2) [12, 13]. Although its primary indications are post-traumatic or degenerative arthritis because the procedure is designed to have a functioning TFCC, the procedure can be useful in select rheumatoid patients, usually younger, whose primary problem at the DRUJ is articular surface degeneration with minimal joint subluxation. Because some convergence of the radius and ulna will occur after partial resection of the ulnar head, ulnar-positive variance is a relative contraindication because it increases the likelihood of impingement between the ulnar styloid and triquetrum; however, a concurrent ulna shortening through the cancellous portion of the ulnar head can be performed to reduce this risk. However, ulnar shortening increases the complexity of the procedure and thus reduces its relative benefit over other options. Irreparable damage to the TFCC and ulnar carpal translocation are relative contraindications because the resection may exacerbate the translation and because the procedure has minimal benefit over a Darrach procedure. However, the HR procedure can be combined with ECU tendon repositioning and stabilization procedures. Unlike the Darrach procedure, HR nearly always includes a soft tissue interposition using local capsule, pronator quadratus, or allograft tissue.

The surgical approach is similar to that described above for the Darrach procedure. Because this procedure will typically be used for a stable DRUJ, performing the exposure through the fifth extensor compartment allows the best preservation of the stabilizing soft tissues and optimum closure using combined repair of the capsule and extensor retinaculum. The tissue

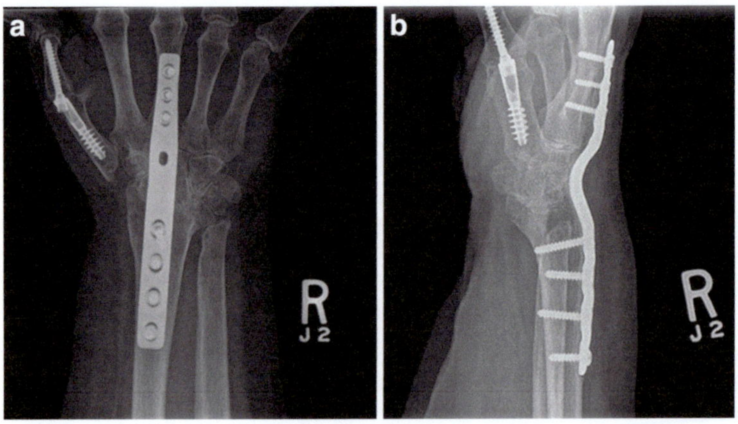

Fig. 10.2 A hemiresection arthroplasty was performed in conjunction with a total wrist arthrodesis and an arthrodesis of the thumb MCP joint

used for interposition is often determined at the time of surgery, which depends on its quality and mobility for transferring into the space. In case the local tissue is not adequate for interposition, having allograft or other commercial biologic substitute available at surgery is desirable.

Sauvé–Kapandji Procedure

The Sauvé–Kapandji (SK) procedure consists of a radioulnar joint fusion and creation of a pseudoarthrosis proximal to the fusion by resecting the ulnar neck (Fig. 10.3) [14–17]. The procedure may include a stabilization technique for the ulnar stump and a soft interposition between the stump and distal radius [18]. Although the indications are similar to those for the Darrach and HR procedures, it has a potential advantage because it retains support for the ulnar carpus and thus reduces the risk of ulnar carpal translocation, which is common in rheumatoid arthritis. However, it has the same disadvantage of the Darrach procedure regarding instability of the ulnar stump.

Either a dorsal or ulnar surgical approach can be used, which may depend on the necessity for concurrent procedures. Preparation of the fusion site is easier through a dorsal exposure similar to that described above for a Darrach or HR, whereas fixation is usually easier when using an ulnar approach. The periosteum is excised around the ulnar neck and approximately 1 cm of the neck is resected with an oscillating saw. If there is ulnar-positive variance, a correspondingly greater segment of ulna is removed so that when

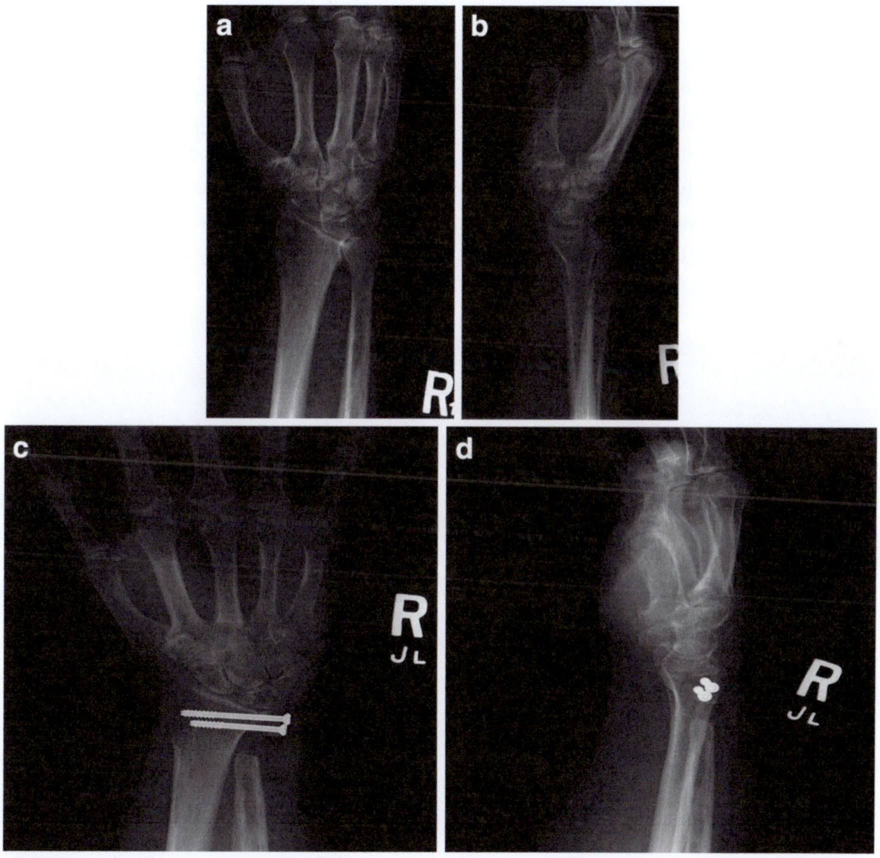

Fig. 10.3 Sauvé–Kapandji procedure performed using two screws for fixation. (**a** and **b**) Preoperative X-rays and (**c** and **d**) postoperative X-rays

the head is recessed to neutral variance, the resulting gap will be 1 cm. The opposing articular surfaces of the ulnar head and sigmoid notch are denuded to cancellous bone. The ulnar head is held against the sigmoid notch in neutral rotation and at the proper longitudinal position. Two parallel guide wires are inserted into the head just beneath the ECU sheath and into the radius; their positions are confirmed with fluoroscopy. The choice of fixation depends on the size and quality of the bone. If the ulnar head is sufficient, the use of two cannulated screws for fixation is optimal but cannot always be achieved. Do not allow the head to tilt while tightening the screws to avoid stylocarpal impingement. If the pronator quadratus muscle is to be used for interposition, it can be detached from its ulnar insertion and advanced into the osteotomy site and sutured in place to the ECU sheath. To gain additional stability of the proximal ulnar stump in a younger patient, I use the FCU tenodesis technique described by Lamey and Fernandez, in which a distally based strip of FCU tendon is raised and passed into the exposed medullary canal of the ulnar stump and out through a hole drilled in the stump; it is then sutured back onto itself under tension.

A modified technique was described by Fujita that is particularly useful for patients with advance rheumatoid disease of the DRUJ in whom the ulnar head is severely eroded and therefore could not be used successfully for a standard SK procedure [19]. In this modification, the ulnar osteotomy is made approximately 2 cm proximal to the head, the head–neck piece is rotated 90° from its normal orientation, and then the neck is inserted into a large hole drilled in the sigmoid notch. A screw is inserted through the head and down the medullary canal of the neck and into the distal radius to gain fixation of the construct. Although the technique creates an articular surface with the nonarticular part of the ulna, it does construct a strong support for the ulnar carpus.

Implant Arthroplasty

Although distal ulnar implant arthroplasty is gaining popularity for a variety of arthritic conditions involving the DRUJ because it reproduces near-normal kinematics of the joint, there are greater challenges when using this technique for rheumatoid arthritis (Fig. 10.4) [20, 21]. The two primary concerns are joint stability and bone quality. With the exception of using a constrained implant, implant arthroplasty relies on soft tissue con-

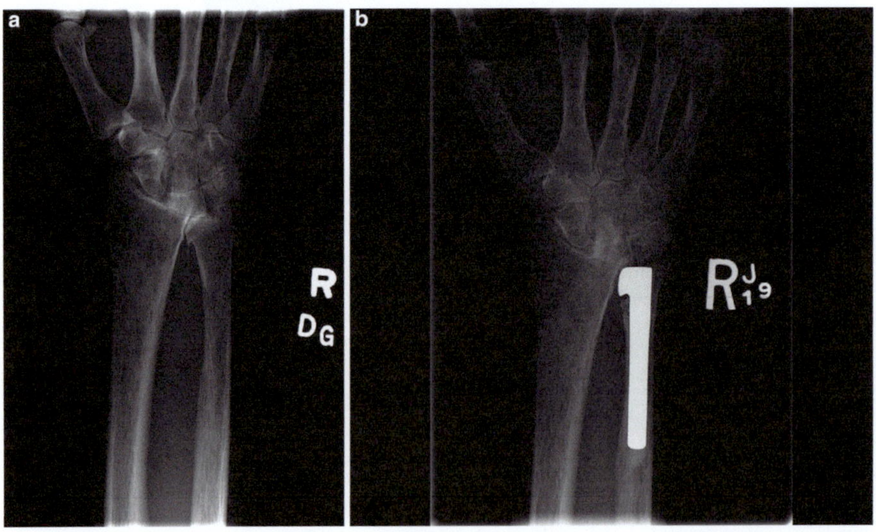

Fig. 10.4 A partial ulnar head replacement was implanted in combination with a radiolunate arthrodesis in an active female with minimal active rheumatoid disease

straints, which are typically attenuated or eventually affected in rheumatoid arthritis, and thus the risk of developing joint instability is substantial. Because bone quality is affected by the rheumatoid disease and its medical treatment, progressive and excessive erosion of the sigmoid notch following total or partial ulnar head replacement is a concern. A total joint replacement, either constrained or unconstrained, may initially obviate some of these concerns; however, the relative functional benefits of these more complex and costly procedures compared to traditional procedures in this patient population are small, particularly because the potential complications of implant loosening and infection are higher. Therefore, implant arthroplasty should likely be reserved for younger, active rheumatoid patients with a painful DRUJ due to articular degeneration but who have a relatively stable and well-aligned joint and adequate bone quality (Fig. 10.4).

Outcomes

The results of the three traditional procedures are generally good for relief of pain, elimination of offending mechanical reasons for tendon ruptures, and aesthetic improvement by reducing or eliminating the prominence of the ulnar head. Fortunately, radioulnar impingement with associated crepitus is rarely painful or substantially noticeable and typically improves as the distal ulna remodels. The distal radius also frequently remodels at the site of the pseudo-articulation between the radius and ulnar stump following a Darrach or SK procedure. The distal ulna also remodels following an HR procedure but the radius is often not affected.

The overall improvement in pain and function may be affected by concurrent procedures depending on the severity of the conditions necessitating these procedures. For example, a younger patient with severe ulnar translocation of the carpus that is treated by a Darrach or HR procedure and concurrent radiolunate fusion will likely require a longer recovery and rehabilitation and be more affected by the change in wrist motion than the distal ulna procedure. Similarly, a distal ulna procedure will often have less impact on recovery and ultimate hand function than concurrent finger joint reconstructions or tendon transfers.

With the exception of possible progressive ulnar translocation of the carpus following a Darrach or HR procedure, there is little risk of functional deterioration of these traditional procedures despite pseudo-joint formation with possible narrowing of the distal ulna and remodeling of the radius. Although there is no clear evidence that one of the three traditional procedures provides a better long-term functional outcome, selecting a given procedure based on local anatomical deformity, systemic disease activity, and patient goals may provide some benefits toward better wrist function, lower risk, and more rapid recovery.

References

1. O'Donovan TM, Ruby LK. The distal radioulnar joint in rheumatoid arthritis. Hand Clin. 1989;5:249–56.
2. Backdahl M. The caput ulnae syndrome in rheumatoid arthritis: a study of the morphology, abnormal anatomy and clinical picture. Acta Rheumatol Scand Suppl. 1963;5:1–75.
3. Spinner M, Kaplan EB. Extensor carpi ulnaris: its relationship to the stability of the distal radio-ulnar joint. Clin Orthop. 1970;68:124–9.
4. DiBenedetto MR, Lubbers LM, et al. Long-term results of the minimal resection Darrach procedure. J Hand Surg [AM]. 1991;16:445–50.
5. Nolan 3rd WB, Eaton RG. A Darrach procedure for distal ulnar pathology derangements. Clin Orthop. 1992;275:85–9.
6. Tulipan DJ, Eaton RG, et al. The Darrach procedure defended: technique redefined and long-term follow-up. J Hand Surg [Am]. 1991;16:438–44.
7. Blatt G, Ashworth C. Volar capsule transfer for stabilization following resection of the distal end of the ulna. Orthop Trans. 1979;3:13–4.
8. Tsai TM, Shimizu H, et al. A modified extensor carpi ulnaris tenodesis with the Darrach procedure. J Hand Surg [Am]. 1993;18:697–702.
9. Breen TF, Jupiter JB. Extensor carpi ulnaris and flexor carpi ulnaris tenodesis of the unstable distal ulna. J Hand Surg [Am]. 1989;14:612–7.
10. Leslie BM, Carlson G, et al. Results of extensor carpi ulnaris tenodesis in the rheumatoid wrist undergoing a distal ulnar excision. J Hand Surg [Am]. 1990;15:547–51.
11. Johnson RK. Stabilization of the distal ulna by transfer of the pronator quadratus origin. Clin Orthop. 1992;275:130–2.

12. Bowers WH. Distal radioulnar joint arthroplasty: the hemiresection-interposition technique. J Hand Surg [Am]. 1985;10:169–78.
13. Watson HK, Gabuzda GM. Matched distal ulna resection for posttraumatic disorders of the distal radioulnar joint. J Hand Surg [Am]. 1992;17: 724–30.
14. Kapandji IA. The Kapandji-Sauve procedure. J Hand Surg [Br]. 1992;17:125–6.
15. Millroy P, Coleman S, et al. The Sauve-Kapandji operation: technique and results. J Hand Surg [Br]. 1992;17:411–4.
16. Rothwell AG, O'Neill L, et al. Sauve-Kapandji procedure for disorders of the distal radioulnar joint: a simplified technique. J Hand Surg [Am]. 1996;21: 771–7.
17. Nakamura R, Tsunoda K, et al. The Sauve-Kapandji procedure for chronic dislocation of the distal radioulnar joint with destruction of the articular surface. J Hand Surg [Br]. 1992;17:127–32.
18. Vincent KA, Szabo RM, et al. The Sauve-Kapandji procedure for reconstruction of the rheumatoid distal radioulnar joint. J Hand Surg [Am]. 1993;18: 978–83.
19. Fujita S, Masada K, et al. Modified Sauve-Kapandji procedure for disorders of the distal radioulnar joint in patients with rheumatoid arthritis. J Bone Joint Surg. 2005;87-A:134–9.
20. Willis AA, Berger RA, Cooney III WP. Arthroplasty of the distal radioulnar joint using a new ulnar head endoprosthesis: preliminary report. J Hand Surg Am. 2007;32(2):177–89.
21. Yen Shipley N, Dion GR, Bowers WH. Ulnar head implant arthroplasty: an intermediate term review of 1 surgeon's experience. Tech Hand Up Extrem Surg. 2009;13(3):160–4.

Soft Tissue Reconstructive Procedures in the Rheumatoid Wrist, Including Tendon Transfer Procedures

11

Philippe Bellemère

Flexor Tenosynovectomy

Tenosynovectomy of the flexor tendons is performed when symptoms persist in spite of 3–6 months of conservative treatment. These symptoms may be the starting point of the disease. They cause pain and stiffness of the fingers, often in the morning. The clinical examination reveals crepitus when the flexor tendons are palpated between the proximal and distal palmar creases. Due to tenosynovitis, adhesion of the flexor profundus and superficialis tendons limits finger flexion. Tenosynovitis in the wrist may cause carpal tunnel syndrome and forms a mass in the carpal tunnel.

The aim of surgery is symptom relief and preventing tendon rupture.

Technique

The incision must allow the surgeon to perform a tenosynovectomy extending from proximal to distal. In order to treat tenosynovitis in the palm and the wrist, the classic volar approach to the carpal tunnel is generally sufficient. If there is a synovial pannus proximal to the carpal tunnel, the incision is extended proximally with a Z incision between the two flexion creases of the wrist (Fig. 11.1). The median nerve and the branches are located and released (Fig. 11.2). Tenosynovectomy must be performed tendon by tendon by removing any tenosynovitis surrounding each tendon. A number 15 scalpel blade is initially used. Manipulation of the tendon with forceps should be as atraumatic as possible. A fine rongeur is useful to carefully extract any intratendinous synovium (Fig. 11.3). If the tendon is torn or partly ruptured, it must be repaired with a 4/0 PDS suture. The carpal tunnel must be thoroughly explored, and any protruding bone in contact with the tendons must be removed from the floor of the carpal tunnel. Capsular perforations must be sutured or covered with a capsular flap.

Early postoperative mobilization is required to avoid adhesion around the tendons. Physiotherapy must aim to dissociate the actions of the superficial and the profundus flexors. Tenosynovectomy is a procedure that devascularizes the tendons, and there is a potential risk of secondary rupture, particularly when the tendon has been damaged by synovial infiltration. The surgeon must convey to the therapist to initiate more gentle therapy when the tendons are frayed.

P. Bellemère, MD (✉)
Clinique Jeanne d'Arc, Institut de la Main Nantes Atlantique, 21, rue des Martyrs, Nantes 44100, France
e-mail: philippe.bellemere@me.com

K.C. Chung (ed.), *Clinical Management of the Rheumatoid Hand, Wrist, and Elbow*,
DOI 10.1007/978-3-319-26660-2_11

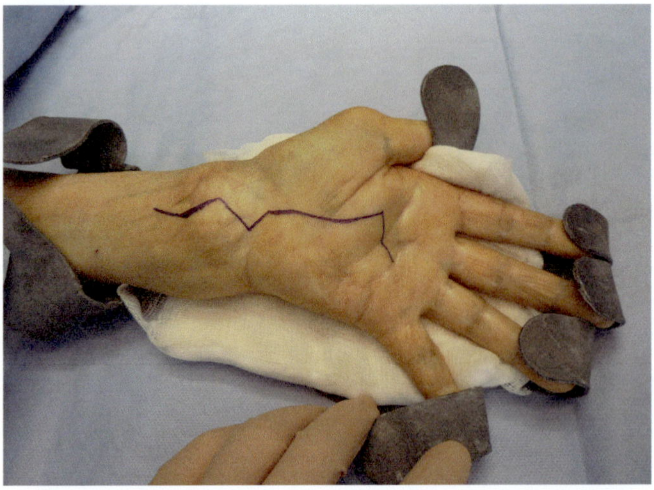

Fig. 11.1 Carpal tunnel approach extended proximally and distally

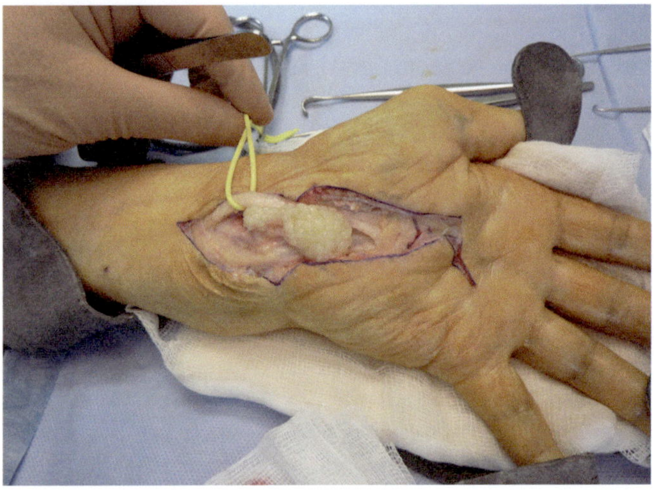

Fig. 11.2 Synovial pannus with rice-like foreign bodies. The median nerve is protected

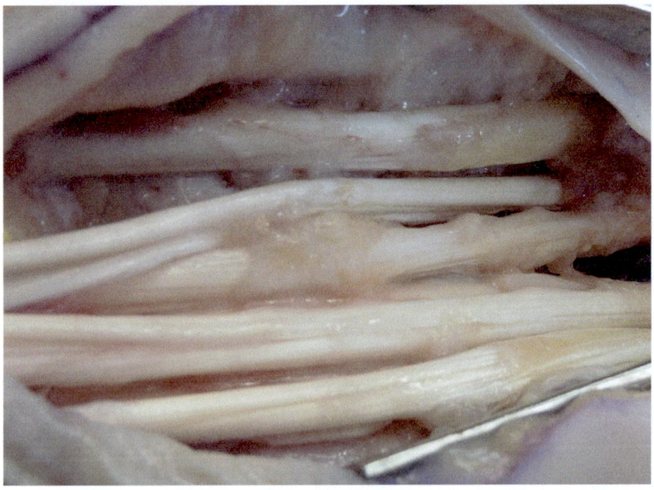

Fig. 11.3 Intratendinous synovitis should be removed

Results

The results of flexor tenosynovectomies are generally good and relapses or repeat tenosynovectomies are rare [1–5]. Pain relief is quite predictable; however, as Duché emphasizes [3], the mobility always improves after 4 months and then deteriorates over time to return to its preoperative level at a follow-up of 8 years. Nevertheless, a tenosynovectomy in the early stages of the disease would appear to protect the patient from the risk of subsequent tendon rupture.

Flexor Tendon Ruptures

Although these are less common than extensor tendon ruptures, flexor tendon ruptures are no less serious, due to their effect on function. Two thirds of all flexor tendon ruptures occur in the carpal tunnel [6, 7]. Ruptures in zone IV of the flexor pollicis longus (FPL) tendon and the index flexor tendons are the most common. The main cause is attrition of the tendon on the volarly subluxed distal scaphoid (Mannerfelt syndrome for rupture of FPL tendon), the lunate in the DISI position, the anterior radius (due to carpus malposition), or a prominent metal device used for partial or total wrist fusion or arthroplasty [8] (Fig. 11.4). The palmar edge of the trapezium, hamate, and ulnar head may also be the cause of the rupture, but proliferative synovitis is frequently seen in the ruptured tendon. It affects the flexor tendons by infiltration, causes nodule formation, changes their ultrastructure, and eventually leads to tendon necrosis and spontaneous rupture (Fig. 11.5).

The indication for surgery depends mainly on the patient's demands, the number of tendons ruptured, and the status of the distal joints. If the distal joints are stiff, destroyed, and painful, fusion should be considered rather than tendon repair.

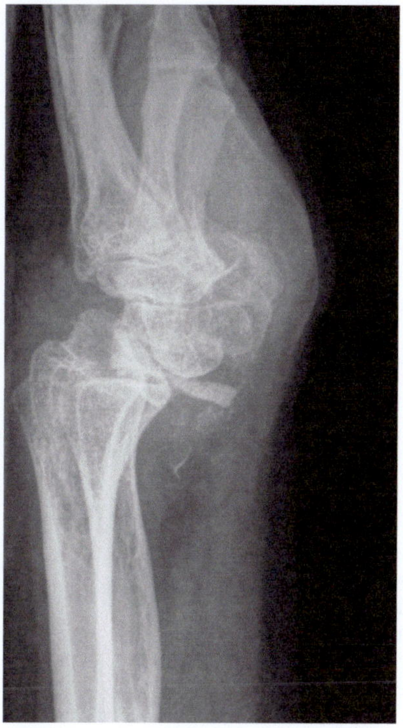

Fig. 11.4 Volarly subluxed carpus and palmar bony spurs may cause flexor tendon rupture

Technique

The option for surgery depends on the time of presentation. It is best to intervene if the rupture is detected within 4–6 weeks before myostatic contracture of the flexor muscle hinders recovery of muscle function. Even in its early presentation, direct suture is rarely possible due to attrition and loss of substance at each end of the tendon, and tendon reconstruction is necessary. The tendon ends are retrieved and debrided to healthy tissue.

For the thumb, a direct tendon graft using the palmaris longus (PL) is the best option for FPL tendon rupture. When PL is not present, a strip of flexor carpi radialis (FCR) can be used as a graft. It is better not to sacrifice an intact FDS tendon to restore FPL function so as to avoid instability of the digital chain and keep later reconstruction options open [9]. If there are associated ruptured FDS tendons, one of the FDS tendon can be used as graft to repair the FPL. When the palmaris longus is not present or the rupture is very old, an FDS tendon from the ring or the middle finger is used as a tendon transfer. However, when MP joint has good motion, repair of FPL tendon is not always necessary and IP fusion may be an option.

One proximal tendon can be used to power ruptured flexor tendons of two fingers. When

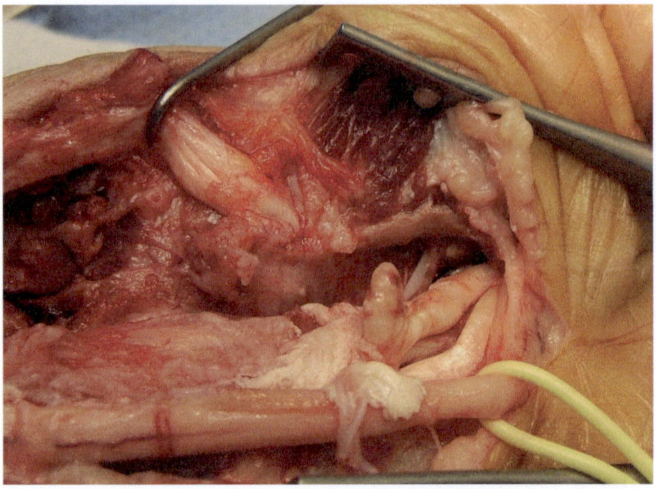

Fig. 11.5 Flexor tendon ruptures in the carpal tunnel with marked tendon infiltration and necrosis

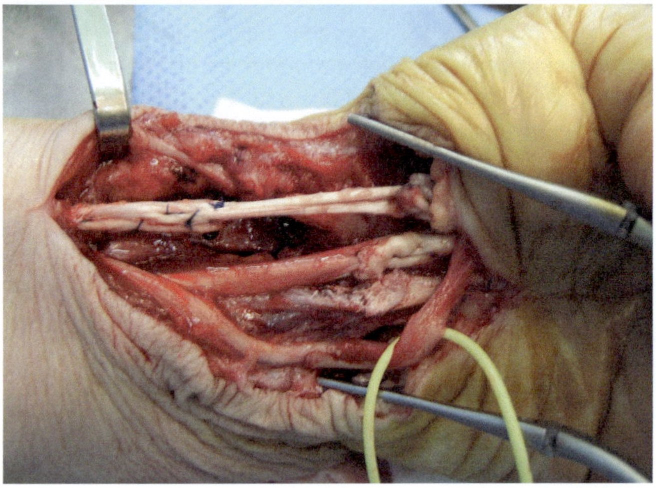

Fig. 11.6 Ruptures of FPL and index FDS and FDP tendons repaired with intercalated grafts (PL for FPL, index FDS for index FDP)

both the FDS and FDP tendons are ruptured, a segment of superficialis tendon can be used as an intercalated graft to reconstruct the profundus tendon (Fig. 11.6).

Tension of the graft is set so that the MCP joint and IP joints are in flexion when the wrist is in extension and in complete extension when the wrist is in flexion. A slight overtension of 15° of flexion for the IP joints is recommended to strengthen the muscle especially if the rupture is old. The graft is secured proximally and distally to tendon stumps using a Pulvertaft weave. For 6 weeks after the operation, the tendon reconstruction is protected with a dorsal wrist splint. Early mobilization is guided by passive and active flexor tendon repair rehabilitation protocol.

In cases of multiple flexor tendon rupture, the aim is first to restore a functional thumb with a PL graft and index pinch at FDS transfer. One can then restore the overall flexion of the ulnar fingers with an FDS to FDP transfer.

Results

Good results can be achieved if a single finger tendon rupture is treated early, but usually results are mediocre and overall finger flexion is poor [6, 10]. Synovial invasion and multiple flexor tendon rupture have a bad prognosis. Prevention with early tenosynovectomy is the best treatment to avoid flexor tendon rupture.

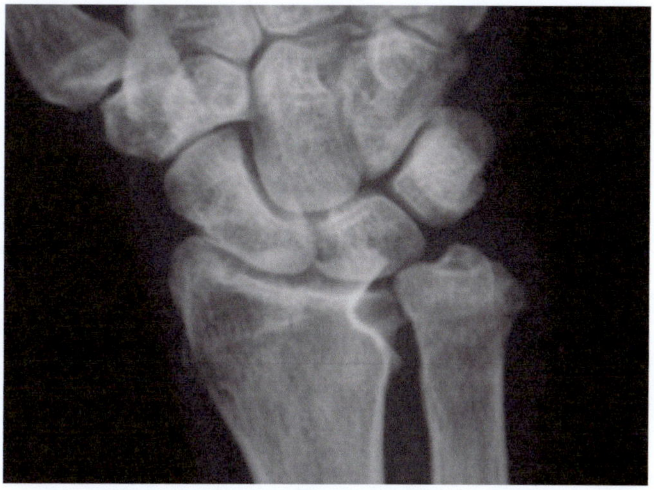

Fig. 11.7 PA radiological view of the wrist showing the Freiberg's scallop sign of the ulnar border of the radius

Extensor Tenosynovectomy

Extensor synovitis is more visible than flexor synovitis and may be treated earlier. The indication for tenosynovectomy should be considered when pain and swelling are not relieved in spite of 3–6 months of conservative treatment. The aim of treatment is to relieve symptoms and prevent tendon rupture. Apart from the duration of symptoms, Ryu identified two radiological prognostic factors for the risk of tendon rupture [11]: the scallop sign as described by Freiberg and dorsal dislocation of the distal ulna (Fig. 11.7). When one of these radiological signs is present, early prophylactic tenosynovectomy should be considered.

Three-dimensional computed tomography (3DCT) imaging is interesting to quantify the risk of extensor tendon rupture for cases of caput ulnae syndrome. Cutoff values for extensor tendon rupture have been determined by Ishikawa for when the dorsal subluxation ratio is 32 % and the carpal supination angle is 14° [12]. Over these values, early prophylactic tenosynovectomy should be considered.

Technique

A dorsal longitudinal incision is made along the axis of the radius and the third metacarpal. This incision is best because it respects venous drainage and the dorsal sensory branches of the radial and ulnar nerve. There is a risk of hematoma or skin necrosis in rheumatoid patients when oblique or zigzag incisions are used (Fig. 11.8). The extensor retinaculum must be preserved despite the aggressive nature of the disease because it can serve three roles: stabilization of the ulnar head, prevention of bowstringing of the extensor tendon, and reinforcement of the dorsal capsule. The extensor retinaculum is incised vertically over the ECU tendon. A radial-based rectangular flap is carefully raised from the sixth compartment to the second (Fig. 11.9). The first compartment rarely requires tenosynovectomy and is not opened. Exposing the tendons can be difficult with a big synovial pannus. There is a risk of damaging the dorsal retinaculum and cutting the EDM at the distal part of the flap. The knife should cut the septum between the compartments from proximal to distal with a subperiosteal detachment over Lister tubercle. Tenosynovectomy is performed on each tendon, and partial rupture must be reinforced with a PDS suture as described for flexor tendon tenosynovectomy. Lister tubercle is removed to avoid further erosion of the extensor tendons.

If there is pain or carpal synovitis, the posterior interosseous nerve is usually removed about 4–5 cm proximally with its branch to the distal radioulnar joint (DRUJ).

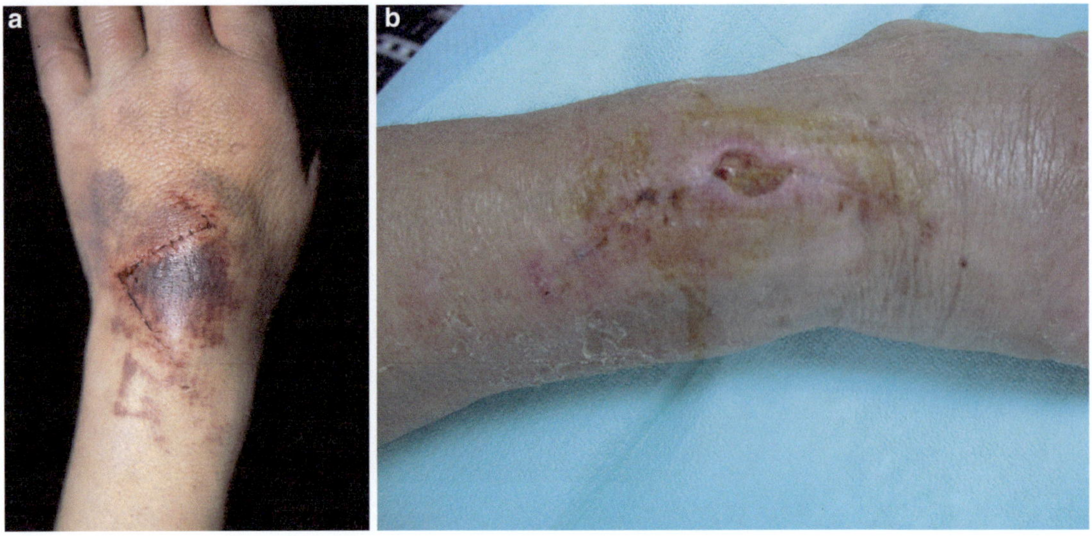

Fig. 11.8 Skin complications with dorsal wrist approach in RA. (**a**) Hematoma with a zigzag incision. (**b**) Skin necrosis

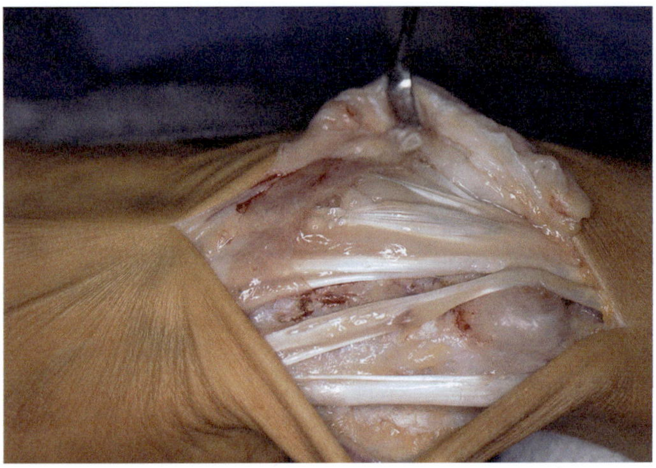

Fig. 11.9 Extensor tendon synovitis. The dorsal retinaculum is reflected radially from the ulnar side of ECU tendon

After the operation, a palmar wrist splint is worn for 3 weeks. Early finger mobilization with full passive and active flexion and extension is encouraged.

Results

Results of extensor tenosynovectomy are usually good; recurrence of synovitis and reoperation are rare. The rate of postoperative extensor tendon rupture is low, about 1 % according to many authors [12, 13]. The main causes of rupture are attrition over the distal ulna, synovial invasion, and weakening of the tendon.

Wrist Synovectomy

Within 2 years of RA being diagnosed, more than half of patients will have wrist pain, and over 90 % will have wrist disease within 10 years [14].

When obvious carpal synovitis is present, with relative absence or mild joint destruction, synovectomy of the radiocarpal and midcarpal joint is indicated.

Technique

This procedure is frequently combined with extensor tenosynovectomy and is performed through an approach with a distally U-shaped flap as described by Tubiana [15] (Fig. 11.10). The ulnar border of the flap is incised in line with the lunotriquetral joint and the radial border in the line with the radial styloid. Synovectomy is performed with the wrist pulled by the assistant. It may be possible to remove the synovitis from the palmar side and the ulnar and radial recess with a fine rongeur. Preservation of the intrinsic and extrinsic ligaments during the synovectomy is paramount, especially during midcarpal synovectomy. Strong attachment of the dorsal flap must be meticulous at the end of the procedure. Bone anchors in the radius may help capsule attachment.

The DRUJ may have synovitis requiring DRUJ synovectomy. Dorsal instability of the ulnar head is frequently associated with a distension of the dorsal capsule by the synovial pannus. The DRUJ is exposed from the sixth compartment. The ECU tendon is subluxed ulnarly and palmarly. The capsule is incised vertically over the DRUJ line. Care must be taken not to divide the triangular fibrocartilage complex (TFCC) or ulnocarpal ligaments. Synovectomy is then performed with the help of a fine rongeur. In the early stages, when the joint is not destroyed, the ulnar head is preserved and must be stabilized with a strong attachment of the DRUJ dorsal capsule to the ulnar margin of the radius. Bone anchors may help at this critical stage.

After wrist synovectomy, a palmar splint with the wrist in neutral position is worn day and night for 3 weeks, and then gentle mobilization is started. A splint is worn for daily activities and at night until 6 weeks postoperatively.

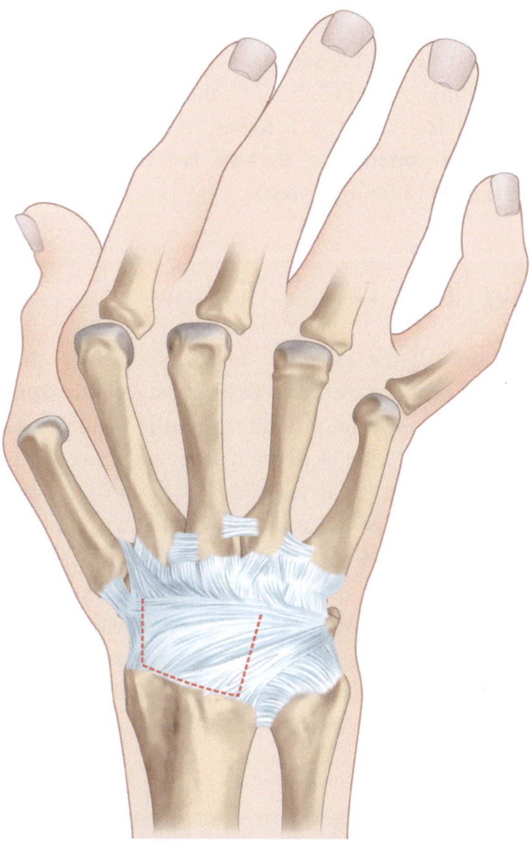

Fig. 11.10 Tubiana's capsular flap (Adapted from Merle [9])

Results

Surgical wrist synovitis in RA has been shown to provide pain relief and improve wrist function despite postoperative joint stiffness for certain patients. It may slow down the rheumatoid destruction process; however, there is no study that conclusively demonstrates that surgical synovectomy changes the natural course of rheumatoid arthritis by delaying joint destruction [16–19].

Nowadays, arthroscopic techniques allow better visualization and accessibility in the multiarticulated complex wrist joint and have the advantages of reduced postoperative morbidity and, more importantly, less postoperative joint stiffness compared with conventional open synovectomy [17, 18]. In the small series in the literature, long-term results have not shown that the radiological course of the disease was stopped. Adolfsson, in his series of 11 RA wrists treated with arthroscopic synovectomy, found nine cases in which radiographic progression does not correlate with the patients' symptoms [20].

Lee [21] reported the long-term clinical results after arthroscopic synovectomy for RA wrists refractory to medication. The rates of clinical remission, without recurrence of synovitis, were

75 % and 65 % at 5 and 10 years of follow-up, respectively. In his series, as in certain open synovectomy series [18, 22, 23], the rate of synovitis control for wrists at a lower radiological stage was not superior to that of wrists at a more advanced radiologic stage.

Rupture of Extensor Tendons

Rupture of the extensor tendon should be suspected when there is no pain but a slight extension lag, especially with the little finger and thumb (Fig. 11.11). Rupture occurs most commonly on the ulnar side due to synovitis of the DRUJ and wrist deformity as in the "caput ulnae syndrome" first described by Backdahl in 1963. Rupture of the extensor pollicis longus (EPL) tendon is also a frequent event in RA patients due to attrition of the tendon over the Lister tubercle. Isolated tendon ruptures of the extensor digiti minimi (EDM) or EPL can be misdiagnosed because the functional loss is slight and often overlooked by more severe RA involvements. Loss of finger extension can also be the consequence of other differential diagnoses in rheumatoid patients: extensor tendon subluxation over the MCP joint, palmar MCP joint dislocation, or posterior interosseous nerve palsy.

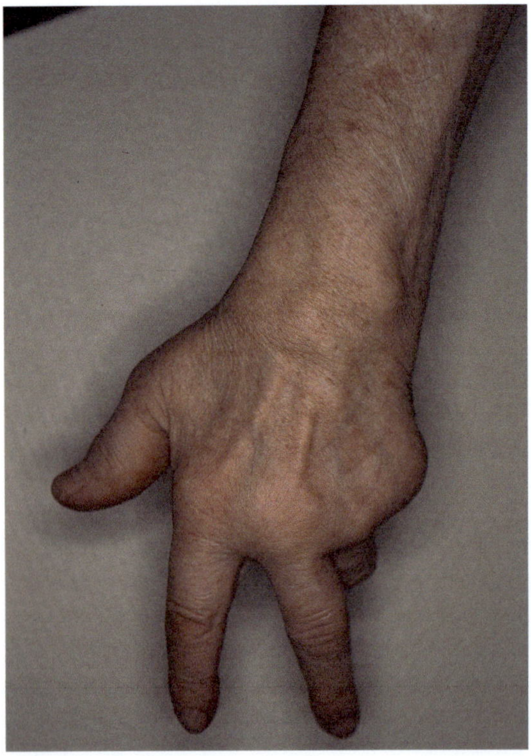

Fig. 11.11 Extensor tendon ruptures over the wrist of the ring and little finger

Once extensor tendon rupture has been diagnosed, prompt surgery is indicated. The number of ruptured tendons is correlated with preoperative surgical delay [24].

Tendon reconstruction should not be performed without first addressing function of the MCP joints. Stiff, painful, destroyed, or subluxed joints should be treated specifically in order to maximize the tendon reconstruction.

Technique

Reconstruction of digital extension may use three procedures:

- Side-to-side or end-to-side suture
- Tendon graft from palmaris longus (PL), strip of ECRB or ECRL, plantaris tendon, or extensor of the fourth toe
- Tendon transfer from extensor indicis proprius (EIP) or flexor digiti superficialis (FDS) of the middle or ring finger

Surgical options depend on the number of tendon ruptures and numerous strategies have been described [8, 9].

For the fingers, when there is a single tendon rupture, side- or end-to-side suture with one tendon for two fingers is a frequent option.

Rupture of the EPL can be treated by an EIP transfer or a tendon graft with the PL when the EIP cannot be used. Tendon grafting runs the risk of adhesions in RA, and survival of the graft may be compromised when wound dehiscence or skin necrosis occurs. Furthermore grafting requires good contractility of the proximal muscle that cannot be achieved beyond 3 months following the rupture [25, 26]. Muscle retraction with a passive excursion of less than 2 cm is not recommended for grafting. For all these reasons, tendon transfers are usually favored over tendon grafts.

For rupture of both extensors in the little finger, there are two options: transfer of the EIP to the stump of the little finger extensor digitorum communis (EDC) or grafting the EDC using the EDM, especially if there is a doubt about the functionality of the EIP. Alternative, end to side repair of the little finger extensor tendon to the intact ring finger extensor tendon is a good, simple option.

Tendon ruptures involving the ring and little fingers can be treated as described above for the little finger and with a side-to-side suture of the EDC IV to the EDC III (Fig. 11.12).

Tendon rupture involving the middle and the ring finger can be treated with a side-to-side suture of each tendon to its adjacent EDC.

When there are three or more digital extension losses to treat, multiple intercalated grafts may have a risk of massive adhesions. A tendon transfer using a flexor superficialis of the ring finger is often preferred. For example, rupture involving the middle, the ring, and the little finger can be treated with a side-to-side suture of the EDC III to EDC II and transferring FDS III to EDC IV and V. Another option is an EIP to EDC IV and V transfer.

Tendon rupture involving the whole finger can be treated by transferring two flexor superficialis tendons [27]: FDS III to EDC II and III and FDS IV to EDC IV and V. The FDS tendons are harvested with an incision at the base of the finger. This will minimize the risk of a swan neck deformity of the finger in case of a floppy PIP joint. The tendons are extracted from the middle of the forearm and subcutaneously tunneled around the radial side of the forearm or through the interosseous membrane (with potential scarring), to reach the distal stumps of the tendon over the hand (Fig. 11.13).

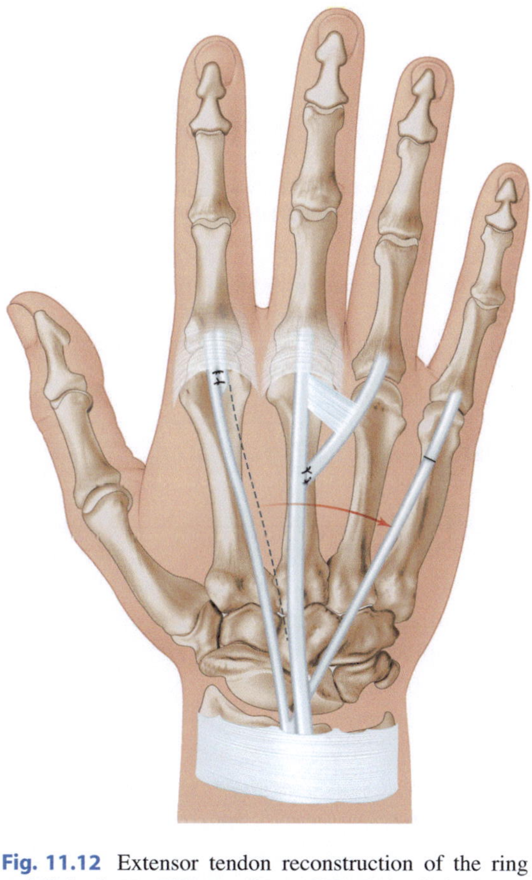

Fig. 11.12 Extensor tendon reconstruction of the ring and little finger. EIP transfer to EC of the little finger. Side-to-side suture of EC IV to EC III

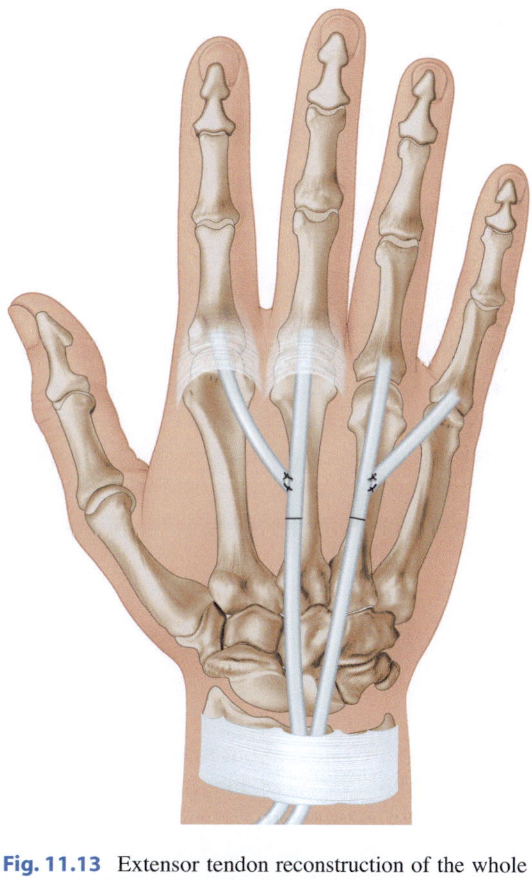

Fig. 11.13 Extensor tendon reconstruction of the whole finger with double FDS tendon transfer through the interosseous membrane

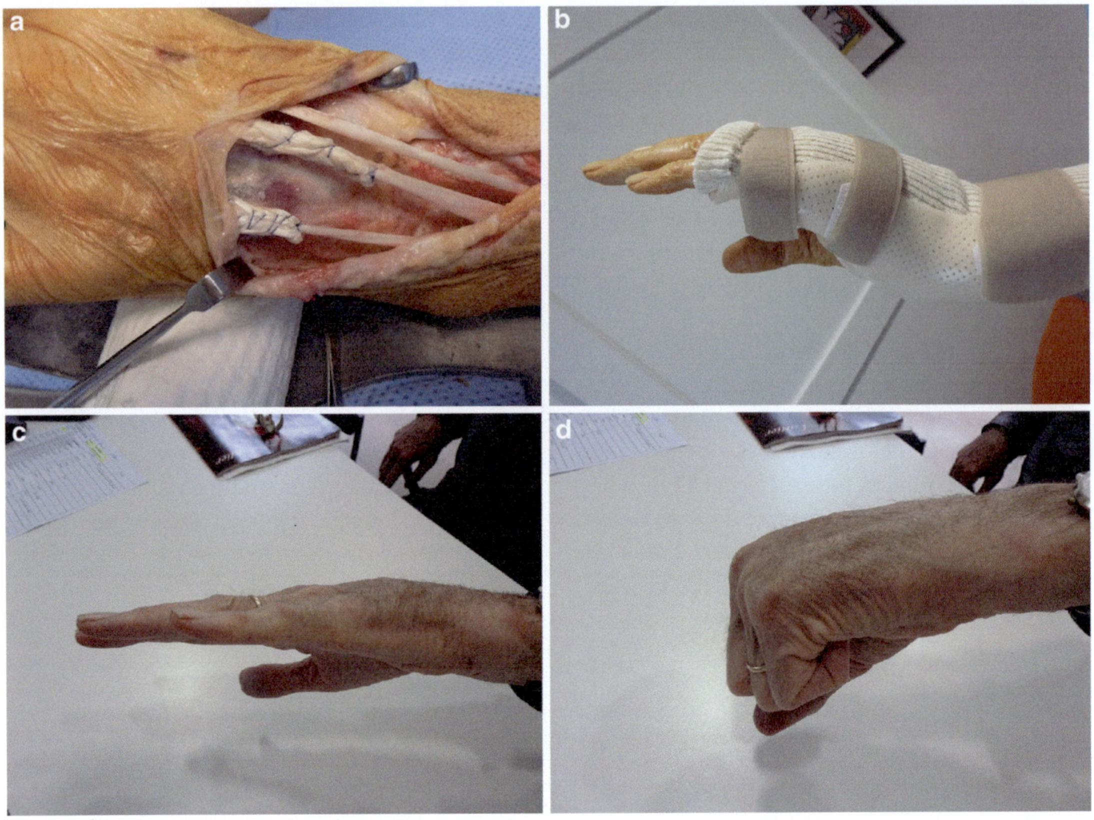

Fig. 11.14 Clinical case: rupture of EDC III, IV, and V tendons over the wrist. (**a**) EIP transfer to the EDCV and FDS transfer to EDC IV and EDC III. (**b**) Postoperative splint allowing early finger active mobilization. (**c**) and (**d**) result

Postoperative protocol after extensor tendon reconstruction requires a palmar splint for 4 weeks with 30° of wrist extension and 40° of MP joint flexion. The DIP and PIP joints are free for early passive and active mobilization (Fig. 11.14). Full digital flexion is encouraged. A dynamic splint may be used to protect the double-sided weave sutures (Pulvertaft) of the intercalated graft.

Results

As with flexor tendon repair, the results of extensor tendon repair are usually good when one or two tendons are repaired but may be disappointing when three or more tendons are ruptured, even if solid repair and early mobilization are performed. Patient satisfaction is correlated with the MP joint extension lag but not with pulp-to-palm distance [28].

Once again, prevention with early synovectomy is the best treatment to avoid tendon rupture.

Wrist Balancing Procedures

The aim of these procedures is to prevent, correct, or limit the deformities of the rheumatoid wrist, which is dorsal subluxation of the ulnar head, carpal supination, radial inclination, and ulnar displacement of the wrist. These deformities must be reducible for the balancing procedure to be effective.

Technique

Wrist balancing procedures (WBP) are frequently or systematically performed concurrently with

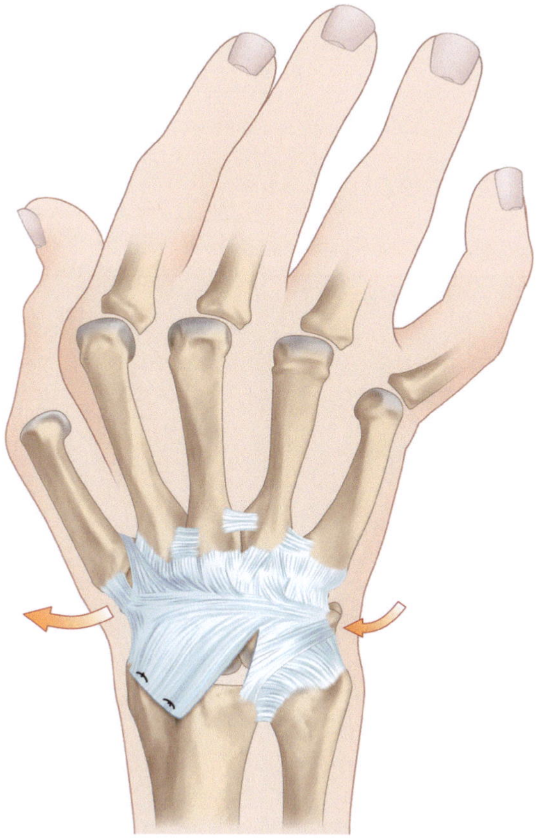

Fig. 11.15 Reattachment under tension of the Tubiana's capsular flap on the dorsal radial edge of the radius (Adapted from Merle [9])

tenosynovectomy of extensor tendons, radiocarpal and midcarpal synovectomy or any DRUJ procedure. For example, after radio- and midcarpal synovectomy, the U-shaped flap of the dorsal capsule can be reattached under tension with the wrist placed in mild extension, while the assistant reduces the ulnar translation and carpal supination [9, 15] (Fig. 11.15).

However, most WBPs are focused on the dorsal and ulnar edge of the wrist, especially around the ECU, to place it in a dorsal and radial position over the ulnar head.

Realignment of the ECU according to Spinner–Kaplan uses a plasty of the dorsal retinaculum divided into three parts (Fig. 11.16). The proximal part is left dorsally to the extensor tendon to avoid a bowstringing effect. The intercalary flap wraps and places the ECU tendon over the ulnar head. It is strongly attached to the ulnar edge of the radius. The distal flap is left palmarly to the tendons to protect them from the bone spurs and reinforce the dorsal capsule. Some authors divide the retinaculum into two parts with the distal one left palmarly to the extensor tendons and wrapping the ECU [29].

Radial deviation and ulnar displacement of the wrist can be treated by transferring the ECRL as proposed initially by Clayton and Ferlic [30]. The ECRL transfer is attached either on the ulnar border of the ECRB in a mild deformity [29] or into the insertion of the ECU with a strong attachment (side-to-side or with a Pulvertaft weave or with a bone anchor onto the base of the fifth metacarpal). In cases of severe deviation, the ECU is lassoed by the ECRL which is attached to the ulnar border of the ECRB as described by Merle [9] (Fig. 11.17).

Another possibility to reduce radial deviation and supination of the carpus and prevent its ulnar deviation is Tubiana's procedure [15]. This uses the distal palmar oblique portion of the extensor retinaculum which is attached to the palmar aspect of the pisiform. For this procedure this structure is passed palmarly to the ECU and firmly attached with tension to the posteroulnar border of the distal radius (Fig. 11.16).

Results

It is difficult to evaluate the efficacy of WBP procedures because they are associated with many other procedures, especially those involving the DRUJ. Furthermore, the results depend on medical treatment and the patient's activity and needs.

According to the series of 32 wrists operated on by Ito [31], when combined with wrist synovectomy, an ECRL to ECU transfer can provide effective stabilization on the X-rays at over 5 years (mean, 8.8 y). Despite a progression in the radiologic stages of radiocarpal joints, radial angulation of the wrist decreased significantly, but ulnar slippage of the carpus did not change.

In a series of 78 wrists treated by dorsal synovectomy, Sauvé–Kapandji procedure, and wrist

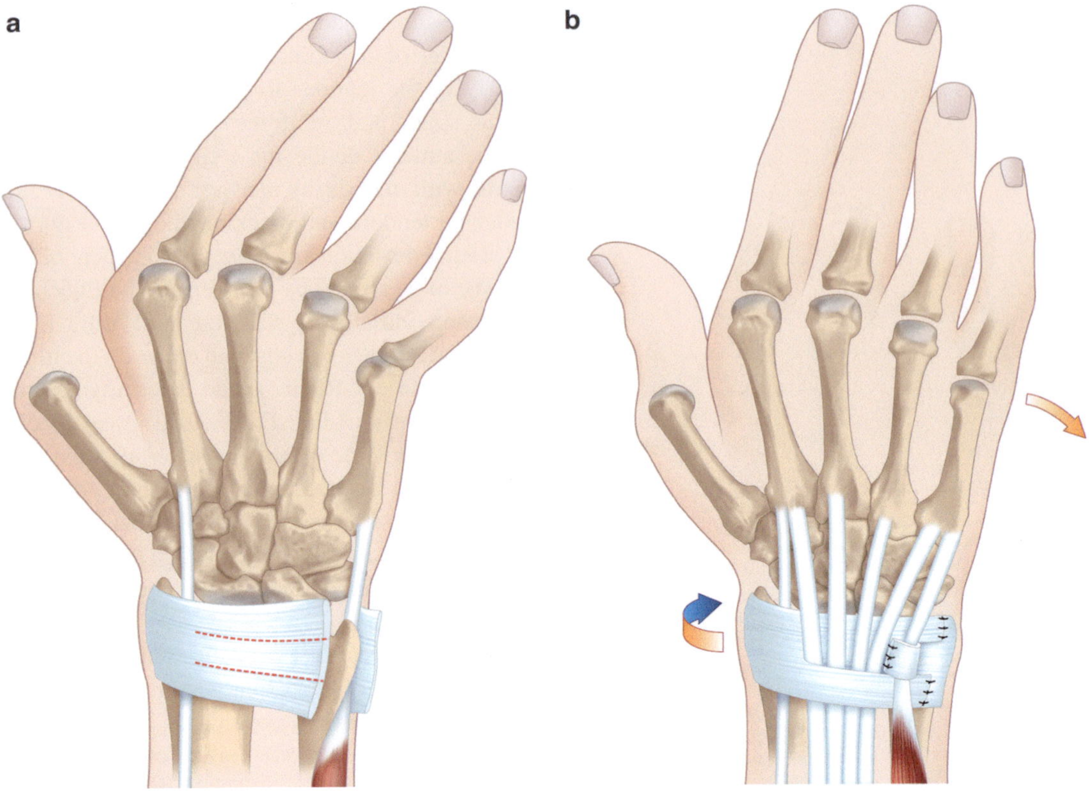

Fig. 11.16 Realignment of the ECU (Spinner–Kaplan procedure). (**a**) The dorsal retinaculum is divided in three parts. (**b**) ECU tendon is wrapped and dorsally stabilized over the ulnar head (Adapted from Merle [9])

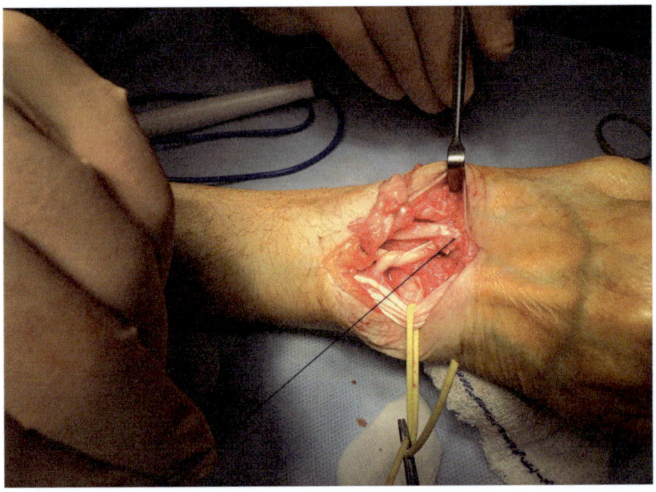

Fig. 11.17 ECRL distally detached is transferred to the ECU

balancing procedure, Alnot found good results on pain relief, a 28° loss of range of motion and 1 postoperative re-rupture of the extensor tendon, at a mean follow-up of 7.2 years [32].

Radiographically, 72 % of wrists remained stable according to Larsen's classification, but carpal height decreased in all cases and ulnar slippage increased in 11 %.

Conclusion

None of these soft tissue procedures (STP), even when they are combined with each other, seem to have any radical effect on the natural course of the disease. Indeed, this varies from one patient to another and depends mainly on the medical treatment prescribed. In fact, the number of STPs used by surgeons for the RA wrist have decreased over these last 10 years due to improvements in medical treatment [33]. Early surgical treatment should therefore be considered when symptoms are not relieved before 3–6 months [34, 35] of medical treatment or when imaging prognosis factors are present. STPs may help the patient to relieve pain and symptoms, protect the tendons, correct wrist deformity, and slow down the disease's progression.

References

1. Ferlic DC, Clayton ML. Flexor tenosynovectomy in the rheumatoid finger. J Hand Surg. 1978;3A:364–7.
2. Dahl E, Mikkelsen OA, Sorensen JU. Flexor tendon synovectomy of the hand in rheumatoid arthritis. A follow-up study of 201 operated hands. Scand J Rheumatol. 1976;5:103–7.
3. Duché R, Canovas F, Thaury MN, Bouges S, Allieu Y. Tenosynovectomy of the flexors in rheumatoid polyarthritis. Analytic study of short term and long term mobility of the fingers. Ann Chir Main Memb Super. 1993;12:85–92. French.
4. Tolat AR, Stanley JK, Evans RA. Flexor tenosynovectomy and tenolysis in longstanding rheumatoid arthritis. J Hand Surg Br. 1996;21:538–43.
5. Eiken O, Haga T, Sälgeback S. Volar tenosynovectomy in the rheumatoid hand. Scand J Plast Reconstr Surg. 1976;10:59–63.
6. Ertel AN, Millender LH, Nalebuff E, McKay D, Leslie B. Flexor tendon ruptures in patients with rheumatoid arthritis. J Hand Surg Am. 1988;13:860–6.
7. Ertel AN. Flexor tendon ruptures in rheumatoid arthritis. Hand Clin. 1989;5:177–90.
8. Schindele SF, Herren DB, Simmen BR. Tendon reconstruction for the rheumatoid hand. Hand Clin. 2011;27:105–13.
9. Merle M. Rheumatoid Wrist. In: Merle M, Lim A, editors. Elective hand surgery: rheumatological and degenerative conditions, nerve compression syndromes. London: World Scientific; 2011. p. 121–78.
10. Aubert JP, Mattei JP, Legre R, Roux H, Magalon G. Ruptures of the tendons of the hand and wrist in rheumatoid arthritis. J Chir (Paris). 1994;131:420–2. French.
11. Ryu J, Saito S, Honda T, Yamamoto K. Risk factors and prophylactic tenosynovectomy for extensor tendon ruptures in the rheumatoid hand. J Hand Surg Br. 1998;23:658–61.
12. Brumfield Jr R, Kuschner SH, Gellman H, Liles DN, Van Winckle G. Results of dorsal wrist synovectomies in the rheumatoid hand. J Hand Surg Am. 1990;15:733–5.
13. Benoit O, Limousin M, Chantelot C, Cordonnier D, Fontaine C, Polveche G. Extensor tendon rupture after dorsal surgery of the rheumatoid wrist: analysis of nine reviewed cases. Chir Main. 2003;22:24–9. French.
14. Trieb K. Treatment of the wrist in rheumatoid arthritis. J Hand Surg Am. 2008;33:113–23.
15. Tubiana R. Technique of dorsal synovectomy of the rheumatoid wrist. Ann Hand Chir. 1990;9:138–45.
16. Dumontier C. Synovectomies du poignet rhumatoïde. In: Allieu Y, editor. La main et le poignet rhumatoïdes. Paris: Expansion scientifique française; 1996. p. 21–34.
17. Böhler N, Lack N, Schwägerl W, Sollermann C, Teigland J, Thabe H, Tillmann K. Late results of synovectomy of wrist, MP and PIP joints: multicenter study. Clin Rheumatol. 1985;4:23–5.
18. Vahranen V, Patiala H. Synovectomy of the wrist in rheumatoid arthritis and related diseases. A follow-up study of 97 consecutive cases. Arch Orthop Trauma Surg. 1984;102:230–7.
19. Allieu Y, Daussin PA, Chammas M, Asencio G, Canovas F, Lussiez B, Brahin B. Results of rheumatoid wrist surgery (arthrodesis excepted): 16 patients with more than 20 year follow-up. Rev Chir Orthop. 2005;91:24–33. French.
20. Adolfsson L. Arthroscopic synovectomy of the wrist. Hand Clin. 2011;27:395–9.
21. Lee HI, Lee KH, Koh KH, Park MJ. Long-term results of arthroscopic wrist synovectomy in rheumatoid arthritis. J Hand Surg Am. 2014;39:1295–300.
22. Thirupathi RG, Ferlic DC, Clayton ML. Dorsal wrist synovectomy in rheumatoid arthritis – a long-term study. J Hand Surg. 1983;8A:848–56.
23. Chalmers PN, Sherman SL, Raphael BS, Su EP. Rheumatoid synovectomy: does the surgical approach matter? Clin Orthop Relat Res. 2011;469:2062–71.
24. Sakuma Y, Ochi K, Iwamoto T, Saito A, Yano K, Naito Y, et al. Number of ruptured tendons and surgical delay as prognostic factors for the surgical repair of extensor tendon ruptures in the rheumatoid wrist. J Rheumatol. 2014;41:265–9.
25. Mountney J, Blundell CM, McArthur P, Stanley D. Free tendon interposition grafting for the repair of ruptured extensor tendons in the rheumatoid hand. J Hand Surg Br. 1998;23:662–5.
26. Nakamura S, Katsuki M. Tendon grafting for extensor tendon ruptures of fingers in rheumatoid hands. J Hand Surg Br. 2002;27:326–8.
27. Nalebuff EA, Patel MR. Flexor digitorum sublimis transfer for multiple extensor tendon ruptures in rheumatoid arthritis. Plast Reconstr Surg. 1973;52:530–3.

28. Chung US, Kim JH, Seo WS, Lee KH. Tendon transfer or tendon graft for ruptured finger extensor tendons in rheumatoid hands. J Hand Surg Eur. 2010;35:279–82.
29. Alnot JY, Fauroux L. Synovectomy in the realignment-stabilization of the rheumatoid wrist. Apropos of a series of 104 cases with average follow-up of 5 years. Rev Rhum Mal Osteoartic. 1992;59:196–206. French.
30. Clayton ML, Ferlic DC. Tendon transfer for radial rotation of the wrist in rheumatoid arthritis. Clin Orthop Relat Res. 1974;100:176–85.
31. Ito J, Koshino T, Okamoto R, et al. Radiologic evaluation of the rheumatoid hand after synovectomy and extensor carpi radialis longus transfer to extensor carpi ulnaris. J Hand Surg Am. 2003;28:585–90.
32. Welby F, Alnot JY. Acromelic arthritis: a new entity. Rev Chir Orthop. 2007;93:571–81. French.
33. Fontaine C. Rheumatoid arthritis surgery has not disappeared! Chir Main. 2014;33:311–4.
34. Kozlow JH, Chung KC. Current concepts in the surgical management of rheumatoid and osteoarthritic hands and wrists. Hand Clin. 2011;27:31–41.
35. Rizzo M, Cooney III WP. Current concepts and treatments for the rheumatoid wrist. Hand Clin. 2011;27: 57–72.

12 Advances in Total Wrist Arthroplasty

Guillaume Herzberg and Michel E.H. Boeckstyns

Introduction

Much has been written on the history of the use of total wrist arthroplasty (TWA) to treat rheumatoid patients [1]. TWA for rheumatoid patients is still a controversial issue [2–5]. For this reason, the reader should keep in mind that total wrist fusion (TWF) remains the standard in which all wrist arthroplasty procedures are judged. TWA is a challenger of TWF. It is a more ambitious procedure because patients always prefer motion [6], but failures can occur despite recent improvements. Because TWA is a relatively new procedure, only time and experience will provide more consistent outcomes when TWA is chosen for a particular patient.

The purpose of this chapter was to provide current concepts about the indications, contraindications, and current results of TWA for end-stage rheumatoid arthritis.

G. Herzberg, MD, PhD (✉)
Orthopaedics, Herriot Lyon France,
5 Place Arsonval, Lyon 69437, France
e-mail: guillaume.herzberg@chu-lyon.fr

M.E.H. Boeckstyns, MD
Clinic for Hand Surgery, Gentofte Hospital,
University of Copenhagen, Hellerup, Denmark

Indications and Contraindications

The indication for TWA in RA is a painful pancarpal arthritic wrist. This means a stage IV or V according to Larsen's classification [7] or a stage II according to Simmen and Herren's classification [8]. We prefer to use Simmen's classification because it highlights the "arthrosis" type 2 stage (Fig. 12.1) compared with the "ankylosing" type 1 stage (Fig. 12.2) and the "destructive" type 3 stage (Fig. 12.3).

Volar carpal subluxation in type 2 RA wrists should not be considered as a contraindication. However, the surgeon should not expect good results with TWA for Simmen type 1 or 3 RA wrists.

The use of walking aids or nonfunctional/irreparable wrist motors are contraindications to TWA as well as severe stiffness of both wrists especially if non-reducible flexion deformity is present. Active infection is the classic contraindication to any implant surgery. Active RA with difficulties in medical treatment adjustments is a contraindication to any major wrist surgery.

Specifications and Current Results of Recent TWA Designs

The use of the Maestro total wrist system (Biomet, Warsaw, IN) was recently reported by Nydick [9] in 5 RA wrists within a series of 23

K.C. Chung (ed.), *Clinical Management of the Rheumatoid Hand, Wrist, and Elbow*,
DOI 10.1007/978-3-319-26660-2_12

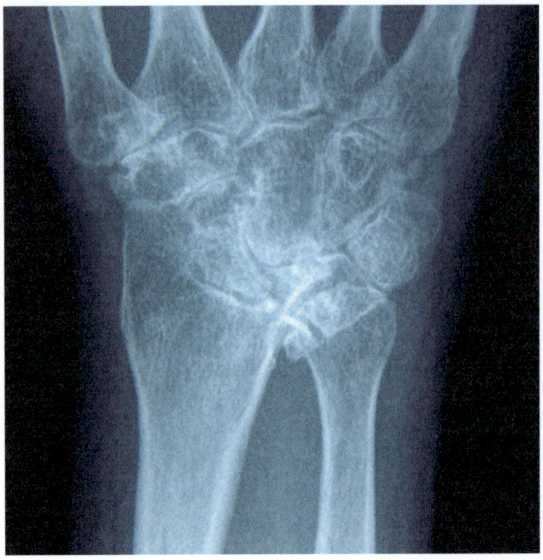

Fig. 12.1 Simmen stage II end-stage rheumatoid wrist is a good indication for TWA in a compliant patient understanding the risk–benefit issue of TWA compared with TWF

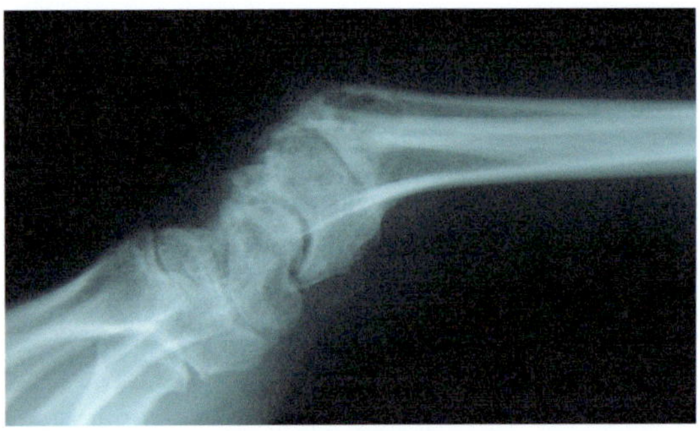

Fig. 12.2 Simmen stage I ankylosing rheumatoid wrist may not be currently considered as a good candidate for TWA

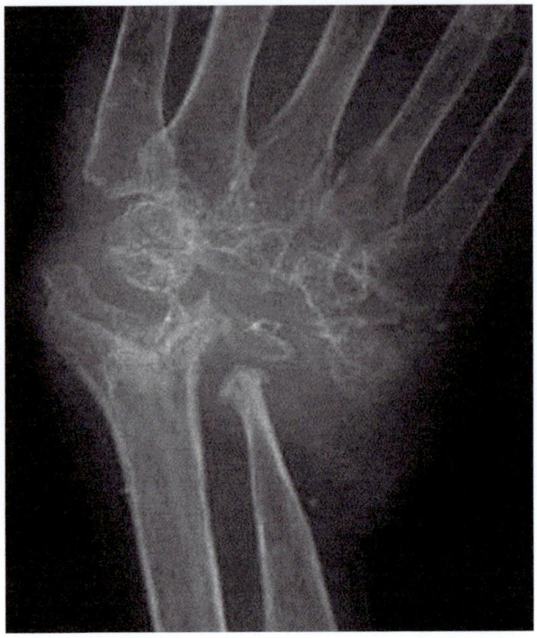

Fig. 12.3 Simmen stage III osteolytic unstable rheumatoid wrist should still be treated with total wrist fusion

TWA. The Maestro TWA comprises of press-fit radial and carpal components. The carpal component fixation is augmented with non-locking screws into the second metacarpal and hamate, with care being taken not to cross the fourth and fifth carpometacarpal joints. Distal ulna resection was associated in 3 of these 5 Maestro cases. Nydick et al. reported the results of their five RA wrists at a mean follow-up of 28 months. The average VAS pain improved by seven points, and postoperative wrist motion gain was 4° meaning that wrist motion was essentially maintained. The average postoperative DASH score was 54 points, and the average postoperative Mayo wrist score was 49 % (poor according to Cooney's stratification). The postoperative forearm rotation arc was not reported. A total of two complications (40 %) were reported within the five RA wrists. One patient had persistent wrist flexion contracture with loss of extension (0° of extension, 60° of flexion) despite flexor carpi radialis tenotomy and flexor carpi ulnaris lengthening. One patient had a volar wrist dislocation that occurred from a fall shortly after surgery and was successfully treated with closed reduction and extension splinting for 2 weeks. Nydick's study was not specifically aimed at rheumatoid patients. Thus, the numbers are very small, and it is too early to get valid conclusions about the use of this new implant to treat the end-stage rheumatoid wrist.

The use of the first-generation UTW TWA (KMI) was reported by Ward [10] using the technique described by Menon [11]. The radial component and the central stem of the carpal component were fixed with cement. The carpal component was further secured with two screws into the carpus. The distal part of the ulna was resected in all cases. Ward et al. reported the results of a prospective series of 19 "UTW1" TWA in 15 patients with rheumatoid arthritis disease at a mean follow-up of 7.3 years. The DASH score improvement was 22 points, ranging from 62 pts preoperatively to 40 pts postoperatively. The mean improvement in wrist flexion–extension arc was 14°. The postoperative forearm rotation arc and VAS pain were not specifically reported. A total of nine wrists (47 %) underwent revision surgery because of carpal component loosening. A total of two additional wrists had radiographic evidence of carpal component subsidence at the time of latest follow-up. The implant survival rate at follow-up was 60 %. These results with the UTW1 implant were far from satisfactory regarding the revision rate. In our opinion, this series should be considered as historical since this implant is no longer available and has been replaced by the UTW2 implant.

The use of the UTW2 TWA (Integra LifeSciences, Plainsboro, NJ) was reported by Ferreres in 2011 [12] in 21 wrists of which 14 had rheumatoid arthritis. The mean follow-up was 5.5 years. The distal part of the ulna was resected in all cases. Pain during activities of daily living was absent or slight in 81 % of the patients. The postoperative PRWE averaged 24 %. Looking specifically at the results of the rheumatoid patients in this series, the average postoperative wrist flexion–extension arc was 69°. Mean postoperative PRWE for pain was 14. Mean postoperative PRWE for pain was 16. A total of five patients were very satisfied, eight patients were satisfied, and one was not satisfied. Ferreres reported two minor postoperative complications and one ulnar subsidence with periprosthetic osteolysis. These results were by far superior to those reported by Ward. These results confirm how important TWA design and instrumentation are with respect to clinical outcomes and implant survival.

We reported in 2011 [13] the use of the Remotion (SBI) TWA in a single-center study of 13 RA wrists at a mean follow-up of 32 months. VAS pain improvement was 6/10 points. The average postoperative wrist flexion–extension arc was 53°, which is a 12° decrease from preoperative measurements but still a functional range of active motion. Grip strength improved from 7 kg preoperatively to 11 kg postoperatively. A total of 11 patients subjectively felt much improved and two felt improved. There were no reoperations or dislocations at this short-term evaluation, but we observed two loosenings, one carpal and one radial, none of which symptomatic enough to warrant revision. The fact that true loosening with implant subsidence could be well tolerated was a new finding that in our opinion was directly related to the implant design regarding its primary stability.

A European multicentre study using the Remotion (SBI) TWA at a much larger scale (75 patients at mean follow-up of 4 years) provided similar results [14]. VAS pain improvement was 4.8/10 points. The average postoperative wrist flexion–extension arc was 58°. Postoperative grip strength improvement reached 40 %. The mean quick DASH improvement was 20 pts. There were 5 % complications requiring implant revision and 2 % minor complications not requiring revision. We observed a 12 % rate of periprosthetic radiological loosening. The survival rate at a mean of 4-year follow-up was 96 %. These results were confirmed in a subsequent analysis with longer follow-up [15]. Currently the Remotion (SBI) TWA has the largest reported outcomes compared with other implants. These results make it easier when discussing with a patient about the outcome he or she can expect if operated on with TWA for complete wrist destruction from rheumatoid disease. This does not mean that this implant is better than any other last-generation TWA since no paper reported any comparative study between different implants. Here are some tips and tricks about the Remotion surgical technique.

Preoperative templating with scaled X-rays is very important to make sure that rheumatoid carpal collapse does not preclude the TWA insertion. The implant should not be oversized. A Darrach procedure is most often combined with TWA. The combined use of ulnar head implant and TWA has seldom been reported and cannot be recommended at this time. The capsulotomy should allow satisfactory view of the destroyed carpus, provide access to the ulnar head, and allow for closure at the end of the procedure so that the implant is covered and not in direct contact with the extensor tendons. We currently recommend a "Z" capsulotomy of the wrist combined with an extension toward the ulnar neck. In order to properly orient radial and carpal stems, the wrist should be flexed 90° once bony resections are done. Because proper rotation of the components is critical, we recommend the surgeon to be seated at the end of the upper extremity. Fluoroscopy should be available in the OR so that proper stem positioning can be checked. The stem of the carpal component should be aligned with the third metacarpal. The carpal implant should be seated into a fused distal carpus. If the fusion is not completed by the disease at the time of the operation, it should be performed simultaneously around the carpal component using the cancellous part of the resected bone. It is our opinion that the second and third CMC joints should ideally not be crossed by any part of the carpal component of the implant (stem or screws) in order to keep some carpometacarpal micromotion. This micromotion may act as a shock absorber to compensate for the modified biomechanics of the prosthetic wrist. This remark is not valid if the second and third CMC joints are already fused by the disease, but in any event the stem should not go too far into the third metacarpal. The dorsal retinaculum should be anatomically closed at the completion of the procedure.

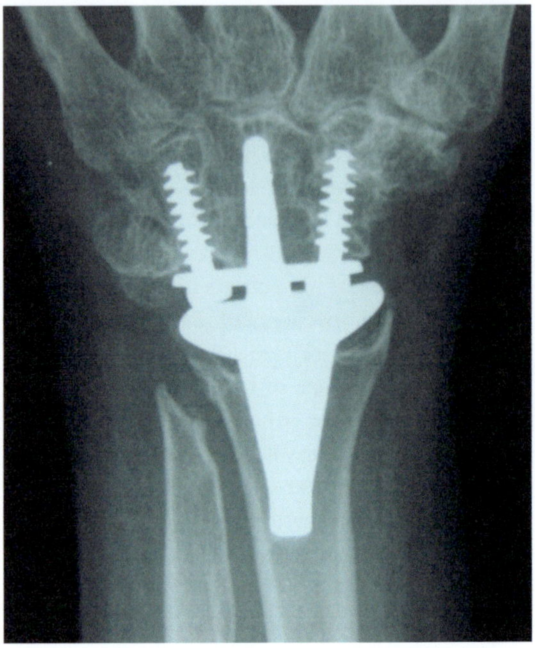

Fig. 12.4 Example of Remotion TWA in the nondominant rheumatoid wrist of a 44-year-old female 3 years after surgery. The patient was much improved compared to her preoperative status and very satisfied. Her postoperative PRWE was 7pts; Quick DASH was 14 pts. Active flexion–extension arc was 45°

Conclusions

There has been a major breakthrough about the use of TWA to treat rheumatoid wrists since 2000 [13–16]. Several new designs have been proposed, all featuring smaller implants. When compared with the older-generation metal on polyethylene TWA, the results and survival rates with the current designs are much better. Experience and follow-ups are gradually increasing. Arthroplasty surgery using new-generation TWA designs has become a reliable procedure (Fig. 12.4) for most rheumatoid patients with stage II Simmen "osteoarthritic-like" wrists even if there is a volar subluxation of the carpus with respect to the radius. The procedure is even more justified if the rheumatoid involvement is bilateral and if a TWF is chosen on the other side [5, 17]. When dealing with rheumatoid Simmen stage II panarthritis of the wrist, the patient's and surgeon's decision-making should consider several factors. First of all, TWF for end-stage rheumatoid arthritis for whatever Simmen's stage is a time-honored standard procedure with reliable long-term results. However, complete loss of wrist motion has obvious negative consequences on wrist function [18]. This is particularly true if there is multiple joint involvement of the ipsilateral upper extremity [6]. In this situation or when dealing with a patient who wishes to keep some active motion or if there is bilateral wrist involvement, it is now possible to consider TWA. Given the still limited experience with the above-described new-generation implants, the patient must be aware that complications and revision cannot be excluded. Among complications of these new TWA designs, periprosthetic osteolysis

[19, 20] is a concern and is currently under investigation. The patient should be informed of this potential complication before surgery is undertaken. In other words, because revision of failed TWA usually consists of TWF, TWA can now be considered as a motion-preserving option before eventual TWF in a compliant and motivated patient who is well aware of the potential complications. In our opinion, given the fact that we are now more confident with the use of Remotion TWA, arthroplasty is our first choice in a compliant patient presenting with a Simmen 2 rheumatoid wrist whether the involvement is bilateral or not. We consider TWA as an option "before" TWF and TWF as a revision option should the TWA fail. In this situation, conversion of the TWA to TWF can be done in one or two stages. If two stages are required, there is a need for a temporary cement spacer for 3 months before TWF. In any event, in rheumatoid patients, the TWF does not require a massive bone graft since implant's volume was limited. Fixation of TWF with a dorsal pre-contoured plate is seldom possible in our experience because of the wrist distortion and skin fragility, and we prefer to use temporary K-wires.

References

1. Cooney WP, Rizzo M. Total wrist replacement: a retrospective comparative study. J Wrist Surg. 2012; 1(2).165–72.
2. Cavaliere CM, Chung KC. A systematic review of total wrist arthroplasty compared with total wrist arthrodesis for rheumatoid arthritis. Plast Reconstr Surg. 2007;122:813–25.
3. Cavaliere CM, Chung KC. TWA and total wrist arthrodesis in RA: a decision analysis from the hand surgeon's perspective. J Hand Surg Am. 2008;33A: 1744.
4. Cavaliere CM, Chung KC. A cost-utility analysis of nonsurgical management: TWA, and total wrist arthrodesis in RA. J Hand Surg Am. 2010;35A:379.
5. Trieb K. Treatment of the wrist in RA. J Hand Surg Am. 2008;33A:113–23.
6. Adams BD. Total wrist arthroplasty. J Am Soc Surg Hand. 2001;1:236–48.
7. Larsen A, Dale K, Eek M, Pahle J. Radiographic evaluation of rheumatoid arthritis by standard reference films. J Hand Surg Am. 1983;8:667–9.
8. Herren DB, Simmen BR. Limited and complete fusion of the rheumatoid wrist. J Am Soc Surg Hand. 2002;2:21–32.
9. Nydick JA. Clinical outcomes of arthrodesis and arthroplasty for the treatment of post traumatic wrist arthritis. J Hand Surg Am. 2013;38(5):899–903.
10. Ward CM, Adams BD. Five to ten year outcomes of the universal total wrist arthroplasty in patients with rheumatoid arthritis. J Bone Joint Surg Am. 2011;93A(10):914–9.
11. Menon J. Total wrist arthroplasty for rheumatoid arthritis. In: Saffar P, Amadio PC, Foucher G, editors. Current practice in hand surgery. London: Martin Dunitz; 1997. p. 209–14.
12. Ferreres A, Lluch A. Universal total wrist arthroplasty: midterm follow-up study. J Hand Surg Am. 2011;36A(6):967–73.
13. Herzberg G. Prospective study of a new total wrist arthroplasty. Chir Main. 2011;30:20–5.
14. Herzberg G, Boeckstyns MEH, Sorensen AI, Axelsson P, Kroener K, Liverneaux P, et al. "Remotion" total wrist arthroplasty: preliminary results of a prospective international multicenter study of 215 cases. J Wrist Surg. 2012;1(1):17–21.
15. Boeckstyns MEH, Herzberg G, Merser S. Favorable results after total wrist arthroplasty. Acta Orthop. 2013;84(4):415–9.
16. Boeckstyns MEH, Herzberg G, Sorensen AI, Axelsson P, Kroner K, Liverneaux P, et al. Can TWA be an option in the treatment of the severely destroyed post traumatic wrist? J Wrist Surg. 2013;2(4).324–9.
17. Herzberg G. Management of bilateral advanced rheumatoid wrist destruction. J Hand Surg Am. 2008; 33A:1192–5.
18. Barbier O, Saels P, Thonnard JL, Rombouts JJ. Long-term functional results of wrist arthrodesis in rheumatoid arthritis. J Hand Surg Br Eur. 1999;24B(1):27–31.
19. Boeckstyns MEH, Herzberg G. Periprosthetic osteol ysis after total wrist arthroplasty. J Wrist Surg. 2014;3(2):101–6.
20. Boeckstyns MEH, Toxvaerd A, Bansal M, Vadstrup LS. Wear particles and osteolysis in patients with TWA. J Hand Surg Am. 2014;39A(12):2396.

Total Wrist Fusion and Limited Wrist Fusion Procedures in Rheumatoid Arthritis

13

Hajime Ishikawa

Introduction

The wrist is a "keystone" of hand function [1]. Pain-free stability of the wrist is a prerequisite for the rheumatoid wrist to maintain power and perform various manual tasks. To prevent wrist deterioration, tight medical control of disease activity is essential. Severe extensor tenosynovitis, dorsal subluxation of the ulnar head, carpal supination, and dislocated ECU tendon were associated with finger extensor tendon ruptures. Synovectomy of the extensor tendons and the wrist joint combined with a Darrach procedure was recommended for the treatment of painful rheumatoid wrist. Clinical results were satisfactory, but over time, ulnar shift and palmar subluxation of the carpus with progressive deterioration could occur. For the moderately deteriorated wrist, limited wrist radiolunate (RL), radioscapholunate (RSL), and radiolunotriquetral (RLT) fusion provides pain relief, stability, and some motion through the midcarpal joint. In the wrist, in which both the radiocarpal and the midcarpal joints were damaged, midcarpal arthroplasty using a tendon ball combined with limited wrist fusion at the radiocarpal was one of the options for wrist reconstruction. For the highly deteriorated wrist with dislocation, total wrist fusion using an intramedullary wrist fusion rod (WFR) fixation is the most reliable procedure to provide long-lasting pain relief and stability with gain in grip power.

H. Ishikawa, MD, PhD (✉)
Rheumatology, Niigata Rheumatic Center,
1-2-8 Honcho, Shibata, Niigata 957-0054, Japan
e-mail: med@ra-center.com

Natural Course of Rheumatoid Wrist Disease

Rheumatoid arthritis (RA) is a systemic disease with chronic inflammation of synovial joints. Persistent joint inflammation frequently leads to destructive lesions of the cartilage and bone. The wrist is frequently involved in RA, even in the early stage of the disease. The cumulative incidence for the onset of wrist symptoms is higher than that of elbow and shoulder symptoms. Hämäläinen reported a cumulative incidence of wrist involvement in RA was over 70 % at 3 years and 95 % at 11 years after onset of the disease [2].

Disease Activity and Wrist Deterioration

A retrospective study was performed on 122 wrists in 66 patients, who started treatment using disease modifying antirheumatic drugs (DMARDs) within the first year of the disease

K.C. Chung (ed.), *Clinical Management of the Rheumatoid Hand, Wrist, and Elbow*,
DOI 10.1007/978-3-319-26660-2_13

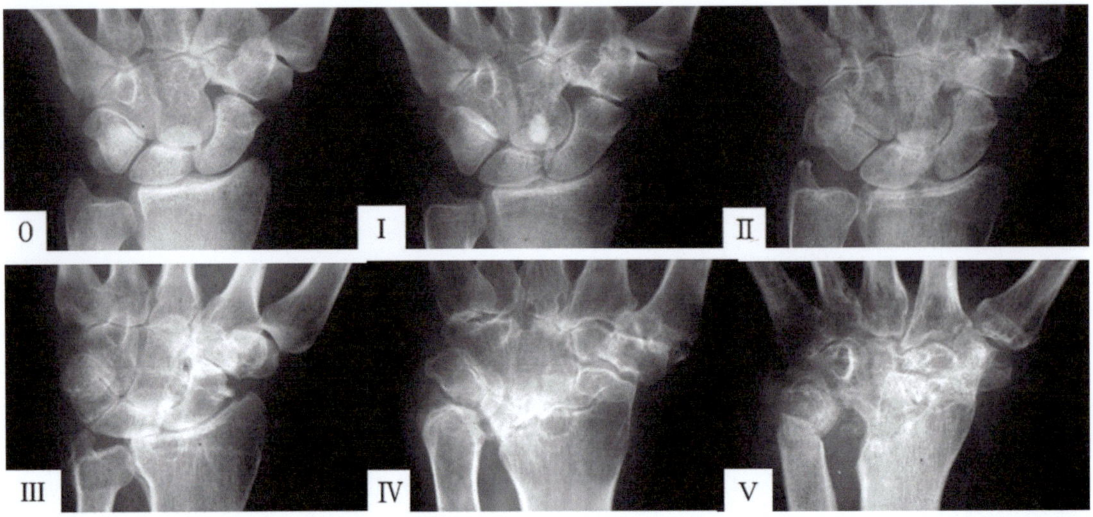

Fig. 13.1 Larsen grade of the wrist (degree of deterioration) [4, 5]. Grade 0, normal; Grade I, bone atrophy, erosion (<1 mm), joint space narrowing; Grade II, one or several erosions (≧1 mm); Grade III, marked erosions; Grade IV, loss of joint space; partial remaining of joint contour; Grade V, mutilating change, complete destruction of joint contour

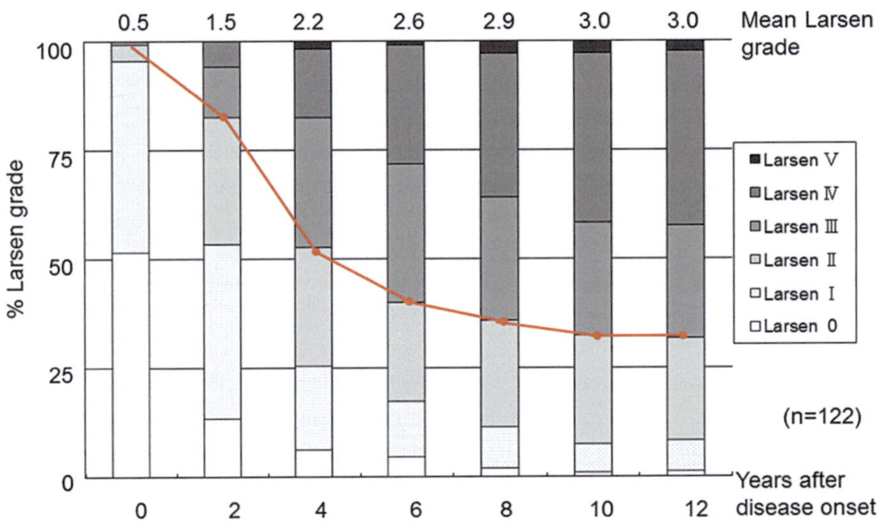

Fig. 13.2 Distribution of Larsen grade. At 10 years, Larsen grade III or more settled in 69 % of the whole

onset and followed for more than 10 years without surgical intervention [3]. Analysis of distribution of Larsen grade, i.e., degree of joint deterioration [4, 5] showed that Larsen grade III or more settled in 69 % of the series at 10 years (Figs. 13.1 and 13.2). The mean disease activity score (DAS) 28-C reactive protein (CRP) [3] was high during the first 2 years, followed by a decrease and a flattening of the curve of disease activity in the wrists with Larsen grades IV and V at year 10. Generally, carpal collapse [6] progressed more in early stage and decreased linearly over 10 years. Individually, continuous high disease activity and progression in radiographic damage were observed in the carpal collapsed group (Larsen grades IV and V at year 10) from

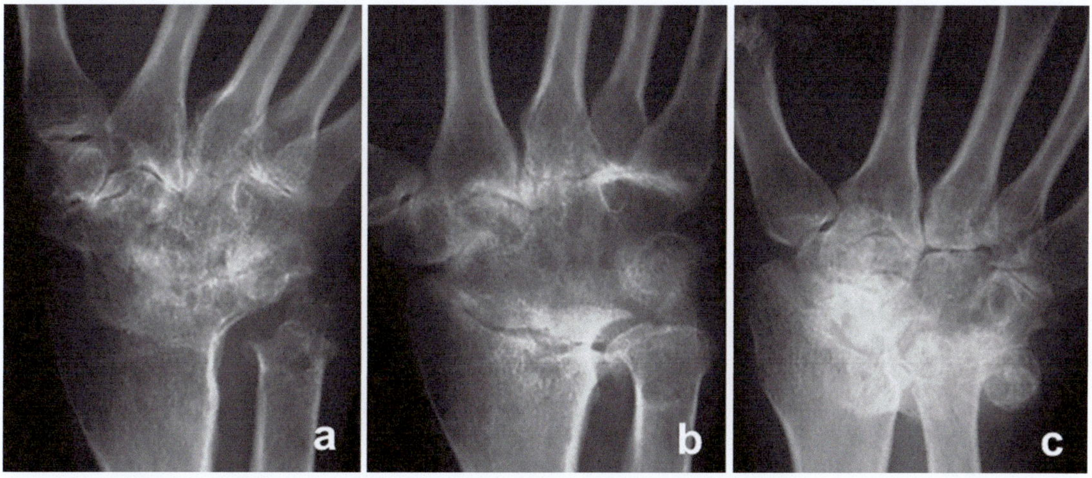

Fig. 13.3 Schulthess classification (type of deterioration) [7]. (**a**) Type I, ankyloses. (**b**) Type II, osteoarthritis. (**c**) Type III, disintegration

early stage of the disease. The cutoff values of the mean DAS 28-CRP(3) during year 0–2, which indicated progression to Larsen grade III or more at year 10, and Schulthess type I (ankylosis) or III (disintegration) [7, 8] at year 10 were 3.34 (sensitivity 70.9 % and specificity 72.1 %) and 3.63 (sensitivity 74.3 % and specificity 77.0 %), respectively (Fig. 13.3). In patients with RA, deterioration of the wrist joint was influenced by disease activity. Identifying this activity and the course of wrist progression may be useful in predicting wrist deterioration.

Deformity at the Wrist Joint Affected by RA

Wrist deformity is composed of six factors: carpal collapse, dorsal subluxation of the ulnar head, carpal supination, ulnar carpal shift, palmar carpal subluxation, and radial carpal deviation [9, 10] (Fig. 13.4). Taleisnik stated they were contributed by loss of stability of the palmar compartment of the wrist joint [9] (Fig. 13.5). The radiological signs of rheumatoid synovitis that suggests involvement of the palmar compartments of the wrist include grooving of the scaphoid, pseudocysts of the distal radius, and scapholunate dissociation. These changes weaken the radiocarpal ligamentous support. This leads to loss of stability of the scaphoid, which goes into a volar-flexed position, contributing to shortening the radial carpal height and favoring rotation of the carpus into supination, radial deviation of the metacarpals, and ulnar drift of the fingers. Other important changes are erosions of the dorsal-ulnar corner of the radius and of the triquetrum, indicating involvement of the ulnocarpal complex and a potential for palmar subluxation of the ulnar carpus. Dorsal subluxation of the ulnar head is caused by disruption of ulnocarpal (UC) ligament and triangular fibrocartilage (TFC). Palmar subluxation of extensor carpi ulnaris (ECU) tendon and carpal supination also contribute this subluxation. Eventually the whole carpal bones slip along the slope of articular surface of the distal radius ulnopalmarly owing to loss of ligamentous support.

Wrist Deformity and Extensor Tendon Rupture

Extensor tendon rupture on the dorsum of the wrist is commonly seen in the RA patient. It causes immediate dysfunction of the hand and surgical reconstruction is usually required [11].

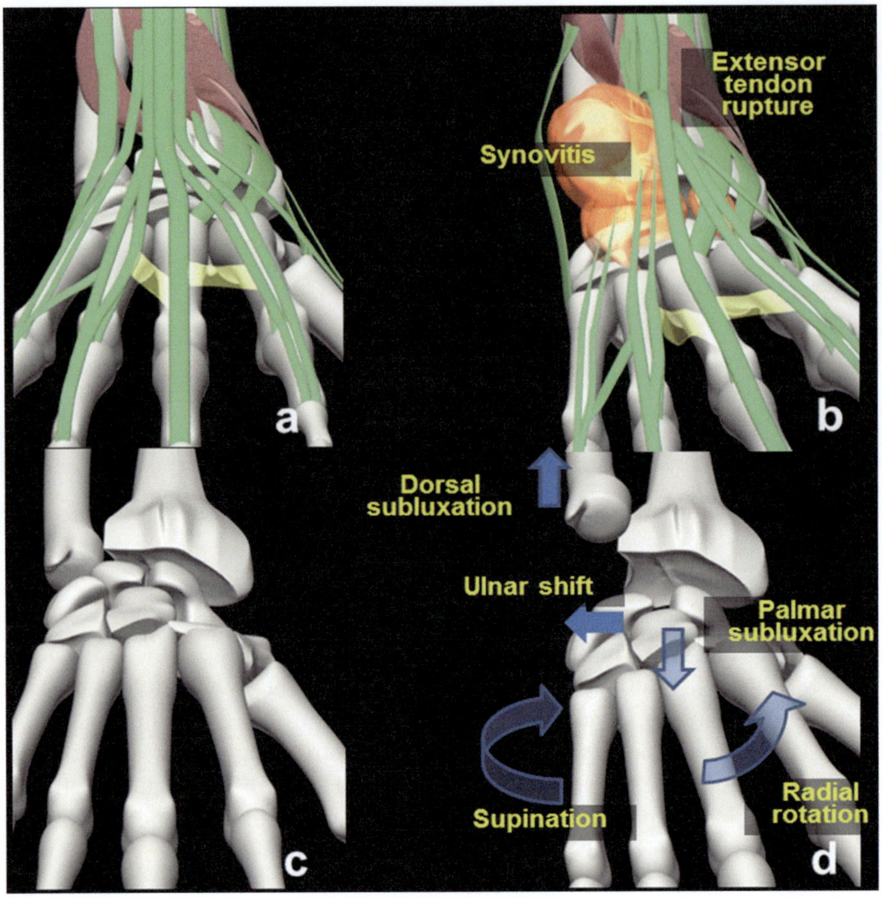

Fig. 13.4 Wrist deformity and extensor tendon rupture (*right hand*). (**a**, **c**) Normal wrist and (**b**, **d**) wrist affected by RA

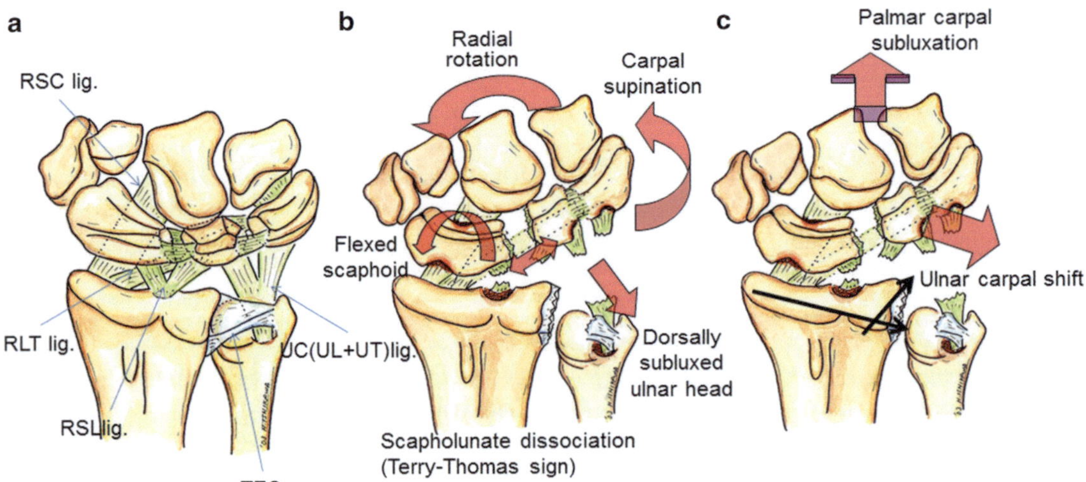

Fig. 13.5 Mechanism of wrist deformity. *RSC* radioscaphocapitate ligament, *RLT* radiolunotriquetral ligament, *RSL* radioscapholunate ligament, *UC* ulnocarpal ligament, *UL* ulnolunate ligament, *UT* ulnotriquetral ligament, *TFC* triangular fibrocartilage

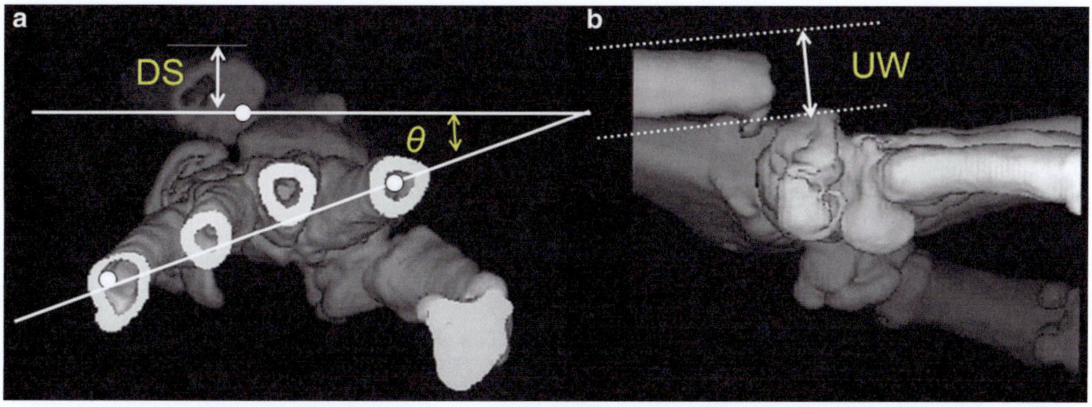

Fig. 13.6 Measurement of carpal supination and dorsal subluxation of ulnar head [12]. Three-dimensional computed tomography (3DCT) images of the wrist. (**a**) The image of the wrist viewing a cross section of the third metacarpal 10° from the distal dorsal side to the proximal palmar side. DS = the distance between the most protruded point of ulnar head and the tangential line of the plateau of fourth dorsal compartment, passing the level of the contact point (*white dot*) of both bones. θ = the angle formed between the connecting line of the center of the second and the fifth metacarpal cross sections and the tangential line of the dorsal surface of the distal radius; this angle is carpal supination angle (CSA). (**b**) The image from the ulnar side. UW = the width of the ulnar head; dorsal subluxation ratio (DSR) was calculated by DS/UW × 100 (%)

Three-dimensional computed tomography (3DCT) images of 108 wrists in 102 patients with RA and 38 wrists in 38 healthy volunteers were analyzed retrospectively [12]. All of the rheumatoid wrists had persistent pain for more than 6 months despite ongoing medical treatment. Extensor tendon rupture was noted in 49 wrists in 47 patients, and no rupture was noted in 59 wrists in 56 patients. The dorsal subluxation ratio (DSR) of the ulnar head and the carpal supination angle (CSA) were measured utilizing a new technique (Fig. 13.6). The average DSR and CSA in the rupture group ($n = 49$), the non-rupture group ($n = 59$), and the normal wrist group ($n = 38$) were 37 %, 19 %, and 26 % and 15°, 11°, and 6°, respectively. The cutoff values for extensor tendon rupture in the wrists of patients with RA were 32 % (sensitivity, 70 %; specificity, 75 %) in the DSR and 14° (71 %, 68 %) in the CSA. By utilizing 3DCT imaging of the rheumatoid wrist, these parameters of wrist deformity can help improve our ability to predict extensor tendon rupture.

In another research, palmar dislocation of ECU tendon was evaluated from 3DCT images with a soft tissue window [13]. 3DCT images of 102 wrists from 96 patients with RA were analyzed. Extensor tendon rupture was found in 43 of 102 wrists (42 %). Dislocation of the ECU tendon was found in 35 of 102 wrists (34 %), and it was a strong risk factor for extensor tendon rupture with odds ratio of 22.2 (95 % confidence interval 7.6–65.1, $p < 0.001$) (Fig. 13.7). Therefore, along with severe extensor tenosynovitis [14] and scallop sign (not significant in this study) in the radiograph [15], early recognition of wrist deformity and palmar dislocation of ECU tendon may "potentially" decrease the rate of unsuspected extensor tendon ruptures in RA (Table 13.1).

Synovectomy and Darrach Procedure

For the painful wrists with persistent synovitis and limited forearm rotation due to disorder at the distal radioulnar joint (DRUJ), synovectomy and Darrach procedure (ulnar head resection) [16] had been recognized as a classic but reliable method to provide favorable results. In our previous study, 43 rheumatoid wrists in 43 patients with bilateral wrist involvement were treated with synovectomy of the extensor tendons and the

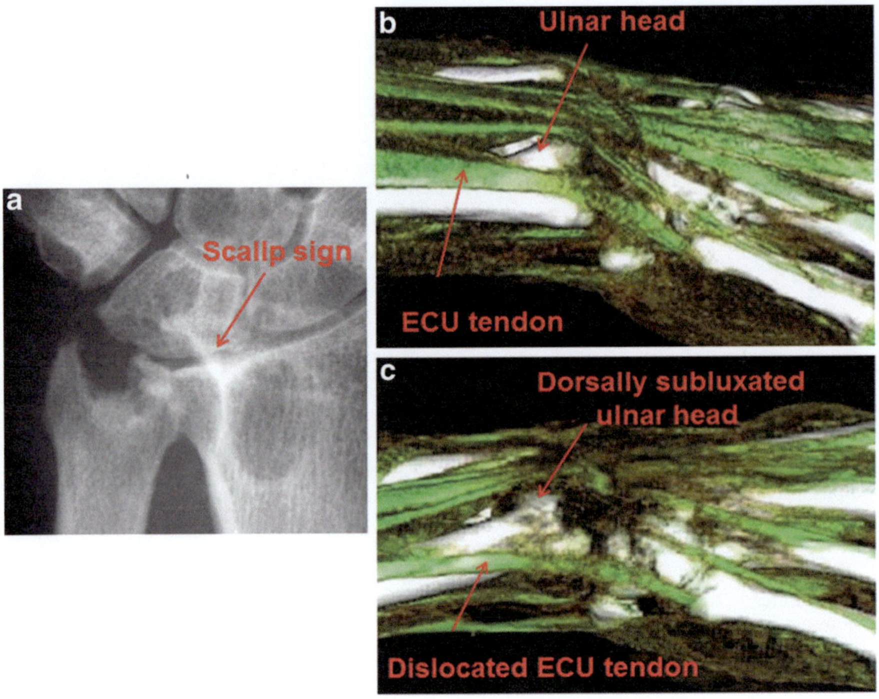

Fig. 13.7 Scallop sign and dislocation of ECU tendon. (**a**) Scallop sign. (**b**) Normal wrist (3DCT). (**c**) Dislocated ECU tendon in the wrist affected by RA (3DCT). *ECU* extensor carpi ulnaris

Table 13.1 Risk of extensor tendon rupture

	Odds ratio	95 % confidence interval	*p*-value
Extensor tenosynovitis			
Mild	1.7	0.3–8.9	0.504
Moderate	4.5	0.9–22.5	0.065
Severe	19.4	3.2–117.1	0.001
Scallop sign	1.7	0.8–3.9	0.177
Wrist deformity			
Dorsal subluxation of ulnar head[a]	3.9	1.6–65.1	<0.001
Carpal supination[b]	4.0	1.7–9.4	<0.001
Dislocation of ECU tendon	22.2	7.6–65.1	<0.001

ECU extensor carpi ulnaris
[a]Dorsal subluxation ratio (DSR) ≥32 %
[b]Carpal supination angle (CSA) ≥14°

wrist joint combined with a Darrach procedure in the period from 1966 to 1986 [17]. Clinical and radiologic assessment of the wrists were carried out after an average follow-up period of 11 years, with comparison of the treated and the opposite untreated wrists. The authors confirmed what others have concluded regarding the operation: pain was generally decreased, forearm rotation increased, and wrist extension and palmar flexion changed little. Radiologically, carpal collapse and palmar carpal subluxation progressed nearly parallel to the opposite wrists, but ulnar carpal shift was much greater in the surgically treated wrists (Fig. 13.8). Therefore, it was suggested that some measure to prevent ulnar carpal shift, such as radiolunate (RL) fusion [19, 20] or Clayton's tendon transfer [transfer of extensor carpi radialis longus (ECRL) tendon to ECU tendon] [21], should be included in this operation. If ulnar carpal shift progressed, it might affect imbalance of the fingers and loss of grip power.

Concept of Limited Wrist Fusion

Stack and Vaughan-Jackson [22] reported on the wrist of a rheumatoid patient in whom ulnar drift of the fingers was prevented by spontaneous RL fusion in 1971. In addition, Chamay and

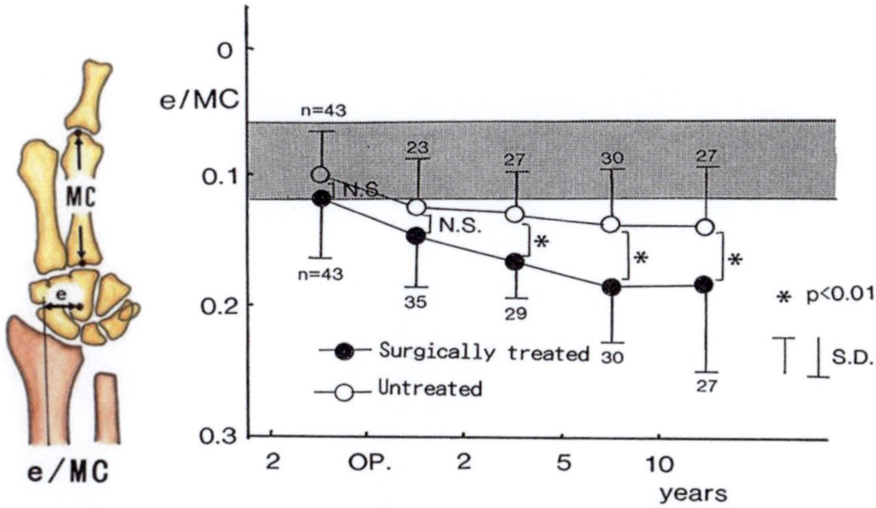

Fig. 13.8 Ulnar carpal shift after Darrach procedure [17]. Speed of ulnar carpal shift was accelerated in the surgically treated wrists compared to that in the untreated wrists 2 years after the surgery. Measurement of the ulnar carpal shift ratio (*e*/MC). *e*, The perpendicular distance from the center of rotation proposed by Youm et al. [18], which is located on the proximal one-fourth of the capitate in the midline to the extension of the midaxial line of the radius. For cases of a collapsed capitate for which the center of rotation cannot be identified, the middle point of the third metacarpal base is used as a reference point. MC, the length of the third metacarpal. The *shaded area* indicates the normal range (mean ± SD), *NS* not significant, *SD* standard deviation

Della-Santa [19] observed that spontaneous RL fusion occurred for 13 % of rheumatoid wrists, which remained mobile and stable, and they called this physiological phenomenon "the natural mode of cure." In 1983, they reported on the results of four surgical RL fusions, and this procedure has since been used as a method of preventing ulnar shift and palmar subluxation of the carpus (Fig. 13.9) [19, 20]. In the wrist with advanced disease, relying only on RL fusion is insufficient for obtaining stability, and thus we included the scaphoid or triquetrum at the site of fusion as part of our treatment area [23, 24]. Several authors have reported favorable results for sole RL fusion with short- to medium-term follow-up [25–27].

Surgical Technique Limited Wrist Fusion [17, 25]

A straight oblique skin incision was made along the dorsum of the wrist, where the extensor retinaculum was split longitudinally at the ulnar border of the sixth extensor compartment and raised as a radially based flap. Synovectomy of the extensor tendons was then carried out, and the terminal branch of the posterior interosseous nerve was resected. The distal end of the ulna was resected 1.5–2 cm in length and proliferated synovium in the wrist joint was removed. The lunate fossa of the radius and proximal articular surface of the lunate were exposed with the wrist in flexion by inserting an elevator into the notch at the origin of the radioscapholunate (RSL) ligament. Using a bur, degenerated cartilage and sclerotic bone were removed from the lunate fossa and proximal articular surface of the lunate. Bone chips harvested from the resected ulnar head were packed into the lunate fossa and the lunate was moved into its neutral position as much as possible. Two parallel Kirschner wires 1.2 mm in diameter were then inserted from the triquetrum obliquely through the lunate to the radius, and using a staple gun (powered metaphyseal stapler, Linvatec Corp., FL, USA), two staples (width × length of 13 × 15 mm) were inserted between the lunate and the radius, and the Kirschner wires were removed. If the lunate had severely collapsed, the cartilage between the lunate and the triquetrum was removed, and the Kirschner wires were left in position. The pronator quadratus (PQ) muscle was then raised as a

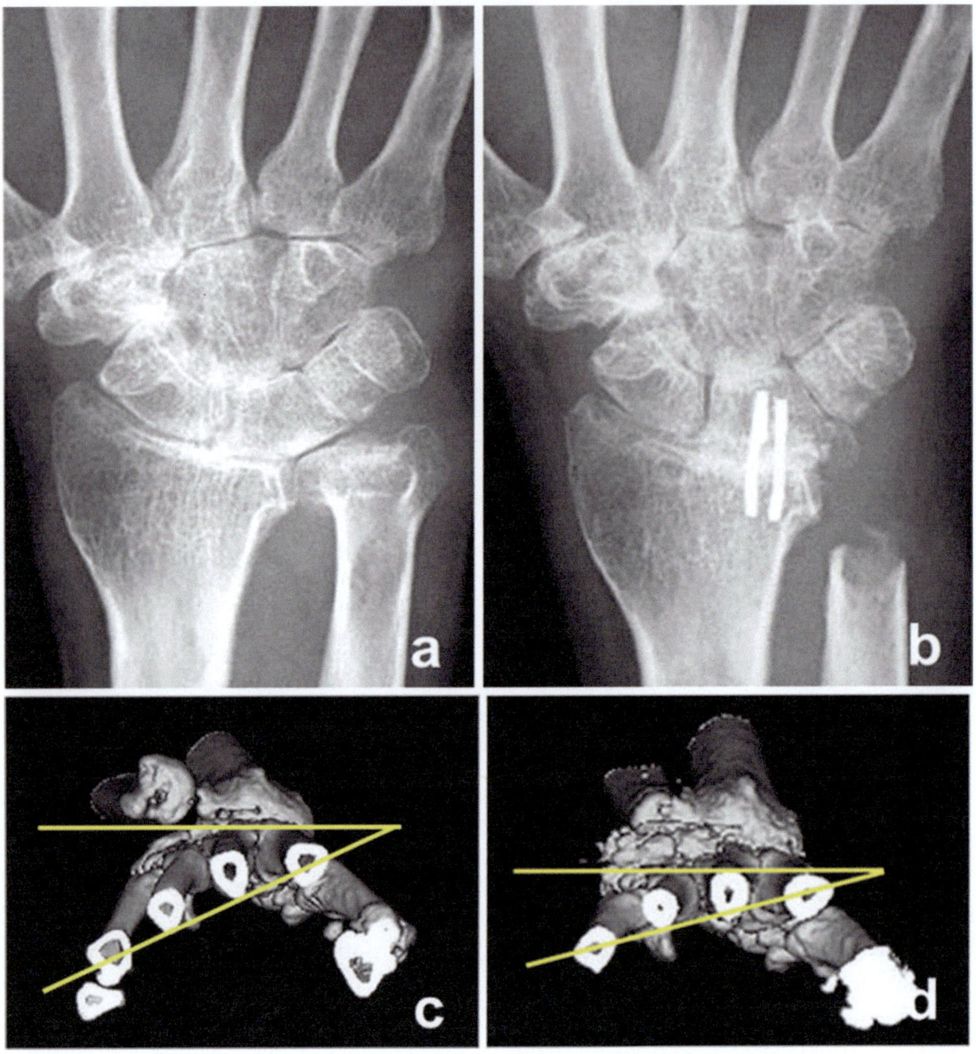

Fig. 13.9 Radiolunate (RL) fusion and Darrach procedure. (**a**) Preoperative radiograph. (**b**) Postoperative radiograph. (**c**) Preoperative 3DCT. (**d**) Postoperative 3DCT. Dorsal subluxation of the distal ulna and carpal supination were corrected

flap and sutured to the dorsal periosteum and fascia around the ulnar stump. If dorsal subluxation of the distal ulna remained, a distal-based strip of one-half of ECU tendon [28] or flexor carpi ulnaris (FCU) tendon [29] was used as a stabilizer by passing it through a drill hole made in the ulnar stump (Fig. 13.10). A short arm cast was applied for 4 weeks and an elastic wrist support (dj Orthopaedics, CA, USA) was then applied for 4 weeks after this.

Long-Term Result of Limited Wrist Fusion

A retrospective review was performed on 25 wrists of 25 rheumatoid patients who underwent limited (RL, RSL, RLT) wrist fusion [23]. All patients underwent synovectomy of the extensor tendons and the wrist joint combined with Darrach procedure. The indication for limited

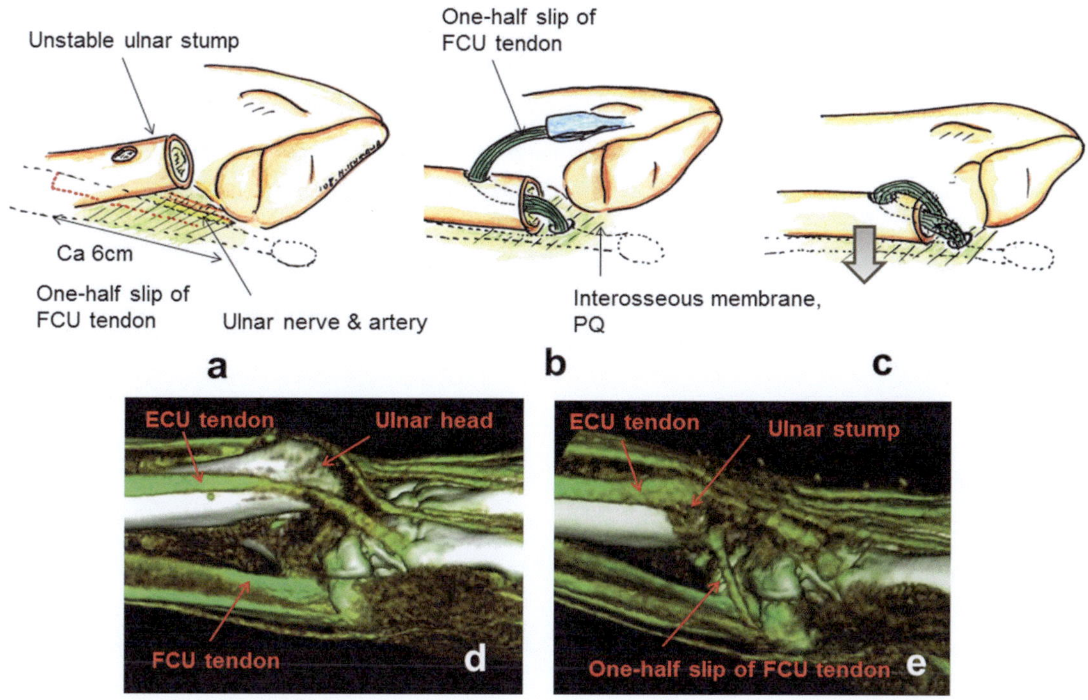

Fig. 13.10 Stabilization of ulnar stump using FCU tendon. (**a**, **b**, **c**) Surgical technique. (**d**) Dorsally subluxated ulnar head (3DCT). (**e**) Stabilized ulnar stump using one-half slip of FCU tendon (3DCT). *ECU* extensor carpi ulnaris, *FCU* flexor carpi ulnaris, *PQ* pronator quadratus

wrist fusion included radiographic changes in the Larsen grades II–IV, midcarpal joint space of greater than 1 mm, and ulnar shift or palmar subluxation of the carpus (Fig. 13.11). The presence of scapholunate dissociation was another optional indication. The mean follow-up period was 12.5 (10–18) years, and radiographs taken just before the operation, 0–2 years, 2–5 years, 5–10 years, and more than 10 years after the operation, were evaluated. At the time of follow up, wrist pain was resolved for 88 % of the wrists, whereas 12 % experienced occasional mild pain. Swelling generally decreased and grip power significantly increased, and flexion decreased and forearm rotation significantly increased. The complication rate was low. Radiographically, carpal collapse initially improved but returned to the preoperative level by the time of the 5-year follow-up. Ulnar shift and palmar subluxation initially improved and were maintained by the time of the 10-year follow-up (Figs. 13.12, 13.13, and 13.14). The midcarpal joint space was preserved in 16 wrists (64 %), and all except one wrist in a patient with mutilating type of the disease remained stable. We concluded that limited wrist fusion for treatment of the rheumatoid wrist results in good stability with preservation of some motion despite radiographic progression of the disease. However, significant decrease in flexion was noted postoperatively (Table 13.2). It was an unfavorable outcome. In our retrospective review of this series, in the wrists with postoperative loss of flexion [30], articular cartilage was eroded or fibrously fused at the lunocapitate (LC) joint at the time of operation, which contributed to the loss of motion.

Midcarpal Arthroplasty (Capitate Head Replacement) with Limited Wrist Fusion

To avoid loss of motion after wrist fusion, midcarpal arthroplasty by replacing the damaged capitate head with a tendon ball was combined

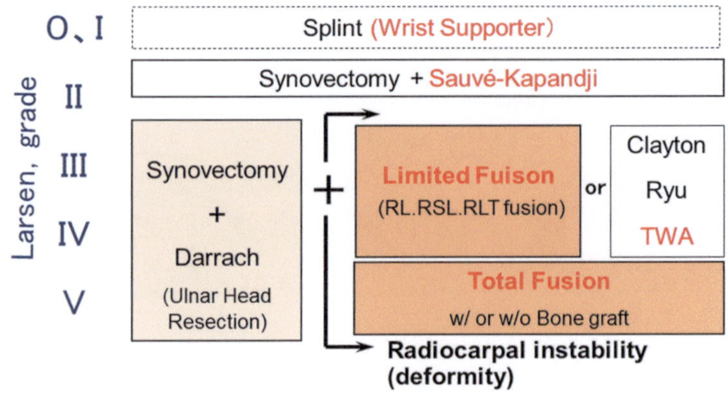

Fig. 13.11 Surgical reconstruction for the rheumatoid wrist. Clayton = Clayton's tendon transfer, transfer of extensor carpi radialis longus (ECRL) tendon to extensor carpi ulnaris (ECU) tendon; Ryu = fibrous nonunion, *TWA* total wrist arthroplasty, *RL* radiolunate, *RSL* radioscapholunate, *RLT* radiolunotriquetral

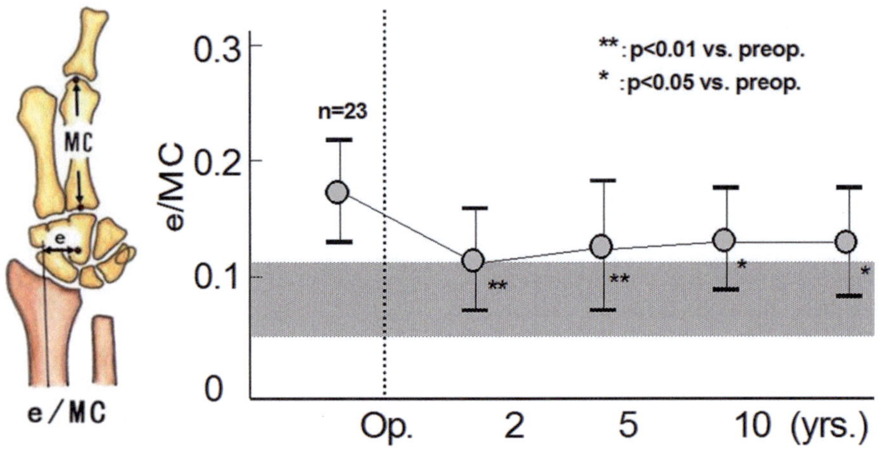

Fig. 13.12 Ulnar carpal shift after limited (RL, RSL, RLT) fusion [24]. Ulnar shift was corrected and no significant progression was noted. *e*/MC = ulnar carpal shift ratio. The *shaded area* indicates the normal range (mean ± SD)

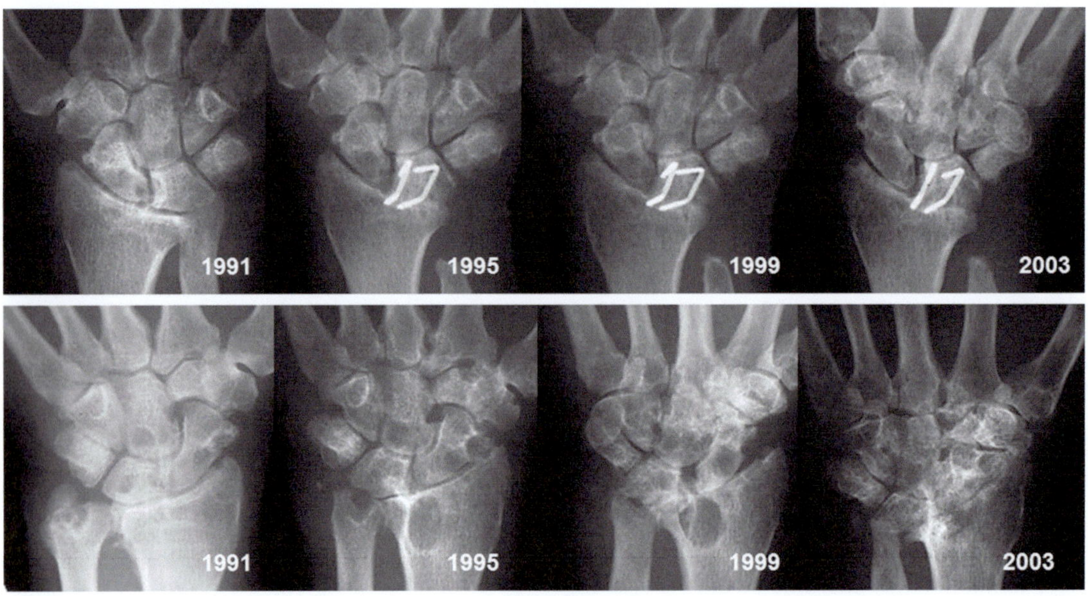

Fig. 13.13 Serial radiographs of the wrist with RL fusion (*upper row*) and the wrist without surgical treatment (*lower row*) in the same patient with RA. *RL* radiolunate

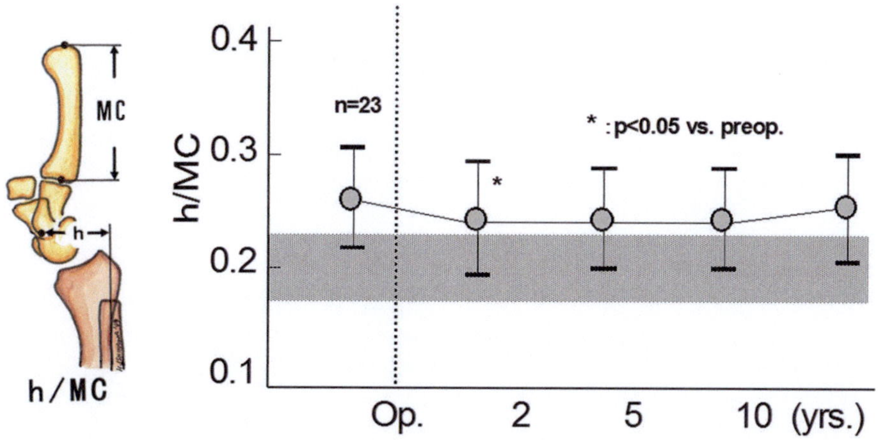

Fig. 13.14 Palmar carpal subluxation after limited (RL, RSL, RLT) fusion [24]. There was not a significant change in the palmar subluxation. Measurement of the palmar carpal subluxation ratio (*h*/MC). *h* = the perpendicular distance from the rotation center of the carpus proposed by Youm et al. [18], which is located on the *middle point* of the most proximal border of the capitate to the extended line along the dorsal cortex of the radial diaphysis. MC = the length of the third metacarpal. The *shaded area* indicates the normal range (mean±SD), *NS* not significant, *SD* standard deviation. *h*/MC = palmar carpal subluxation ratio

Table 13.2 Clinical results of limited wrist fusion

	Grip power (mmHg)		Extension/flexion (°)		Radial/ulnar deviation (°)		Supination/pronation (°)	
Site of fusion	Pre-op	Post-op	Pre-op	Post-op	Pre-op	Post-op	Pre-op	Post-op
RL (*n*=16)	104	143*	30/27	25/14**	7/21	1*/13	72/66	84*/79*
RLT (*n*=3)	119	206	21/24	30/8*	−8/22	−5/13	87/73	77/83
RSL (*n*=6)	81	102	18/32	13/13*	−1/21	−4/18	80/60	86/66
Total (*n*=25)	100	141**	26/28	22/13**	3/21	−1/14	76/65	83*/76*

RL radiolunate, *RLT* radiolunotriquetral, *RSL* radioscapholunate (*$p<0.05$, **$p<0.01$)

with limited wrist fusion. This procedure was indicated to the wrists in Larsen grade III or IV with deterioration and joint space narrowing both at the radiocarpal and the midcarpal joints. In 1987, Taleisnik stated that stability should be secured at the radiocarpal joint and mobility should be secured at the midcarpal joint and the capitate head replaced with a silicone implant [31]. Palmaris longus (PL) tendon of 10 cm in length was harvested and it was spread out and wrapped around (Fig. 13.15) the resected capitate head. The tendon ball was inserted in the lunocapitate (LC) joint and its ears were sutured to the capsule. This procedure was performed on 40 wrists, and radiological change was investigated with an average follow-up of 4 years (Fig. 13.16). Bony fusion at the RL joint occurred in most of the wrists. Widening of the joint space was observed in 80 % of the wrists at the LC joint, 50 % at the triquetrohamate (TH) joint, and 40 % at the radioscaphoid (RS) joint, maintaining motion without progression of arthritis. However, ankylosis occurred in five wrists (Table 13.3). Preoperative 30° of average extension and 27° of average flexion changed to 22° and 19°, respectively, at the time of follow-up.

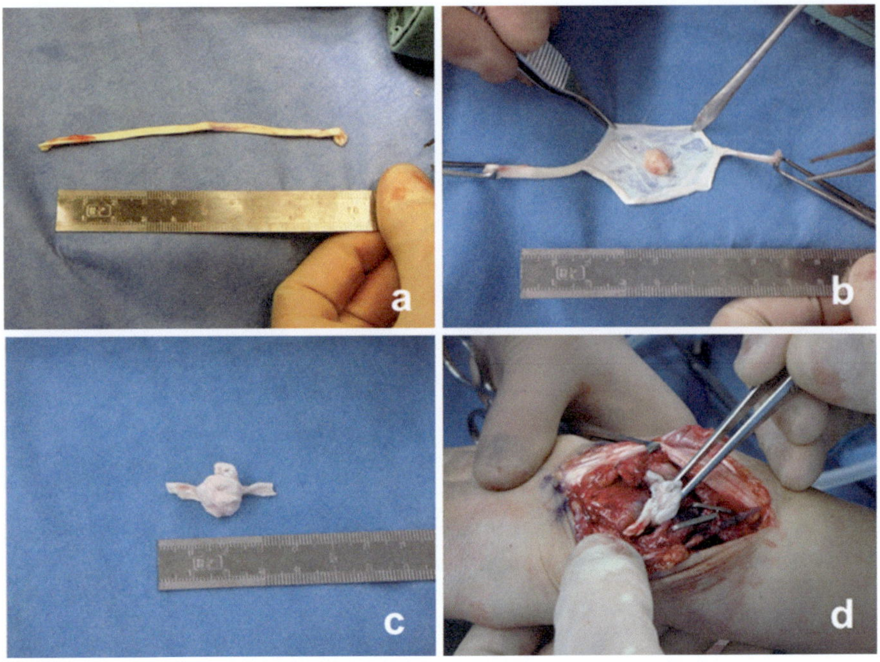

Fig. 13.15 Surgical technique of capitate head replacement with a tendon ball. (**a**) Palmaris longus (PL) tendon (ca. 10 cm). (**b**) Bone nucleus (resected capitate head) and PL tendon. (**c**) Tendon ball (ca. 4 mm diameter). (**d**) Insertion of a ball in the lunocapitate (LC) joint

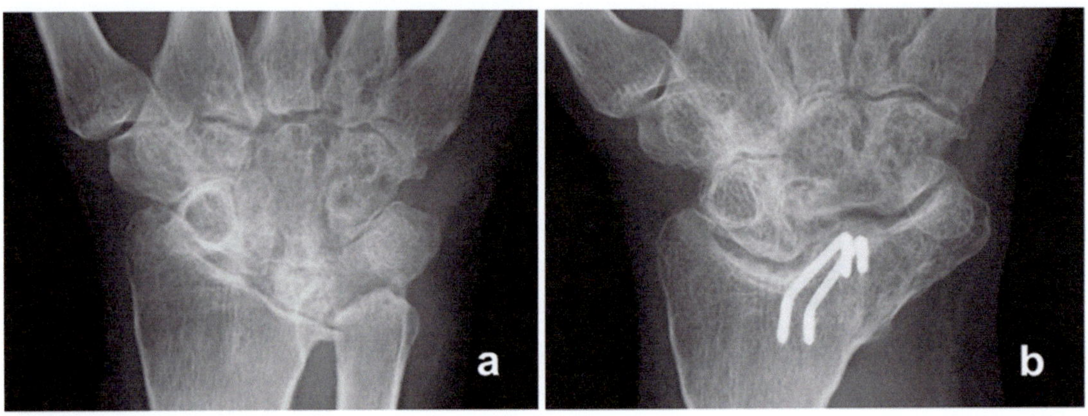

Fig. 13.16 Radiolunotriquetral (RLT) fusion and capitate head replacement (CHR) with a tendon ball. (**a**) Preoperative radiograph. (**b**) Postoperative radiograph

Table 13.3 Radiological change after capitate head replacement (CHR) (n=40)

[Wrists (%)]	Radiolunate (RL) joint	Lunocapitate (LC) joint	Triquetrohamate (TH) joint	Radioscaphoid (RS) joint
Widening	0 (0)	42 (80)	20 (50)	16 (40)
No change	0 (0)	7 (17.5)	18 (45)	18 (45)
Narrowing	1 (2.5)	1 (2.5)	2 (5)	6 (15)
Disappeared	39 (97.5)	0 (0)	0 (0)	0 (0)

Indication of Total Wrist Fusion

Total wrist fusion is the last resort for the severely deteriorated wrist joint. It is indicated for the wrist in Larsen grade IV or V with ulnopalmar subluxation or dislocation (Fig. 13.11). Total fusion is the most reliable procedure to provide a long-lasting pain relief and stability to achieve gain in grip power [32]. In mutilans RA, intercalated iliac crest grafting is used to restore carpal height [33] (Figs. 13.17 and 13.18). However, the wrist loses its mobility by the fusion, and range of finger motion might be reduced because of loss of dynamic tenodesis effect and extensor tendon adhesion after a wrist fusion procedure.

There are various surgical procedures for total wrist fusion (Fig. 13.19). Several procedures for total wrist fusion using bone grafts without hardware [34] for internal fixation had been reported since Abbott's paper in 1942 [42]. He used grafts of cancellous bone from the ilium. Procedures using materials for internal fixation such as metal pin and wire [35, 36, 38, 40, 41], screw [37, 43], metal plate [39], staple, and bioabsorbable poly-L-lactide rod [44] have been reported since Robinson's paper in 1952 [43]. He fixed the capitate to the radius using a screw. Clendenin reported major complications of total wrist fusion including pseudoarthrosis (6 in 31 patients), deep wound infection (1 in 31 patients), neuroma (1 in 31 patients), fracture of healed fusion (2 in 31 patients), and impingement of Steinmann pin on metacarpophalangeal joint (1 in 31 patients) [45]. Wrist fusion today is often performed using a dorsal plate, with the AO wrist arthrodesis plate (Synthes GmbH, Switzerland) probably being the most popular. Although plate fixation may provide good stability, prominent plates occasionally need to be removed [46]. Fracture through screw holes following plate removal has been reported [47], and nonunion at the third carpometacarpal joint has been described [48].

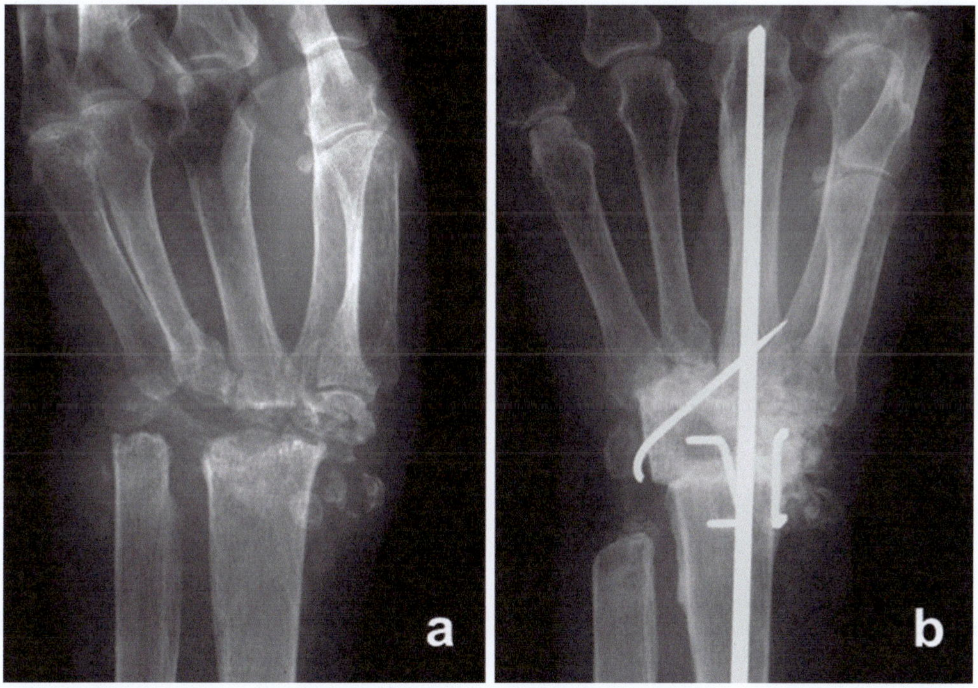

Fig. 13.17 Total wrist fusion with intercalated iliac bone graft. (**a**) Preoperative radiograph. (**b**) Postoperative radiograph

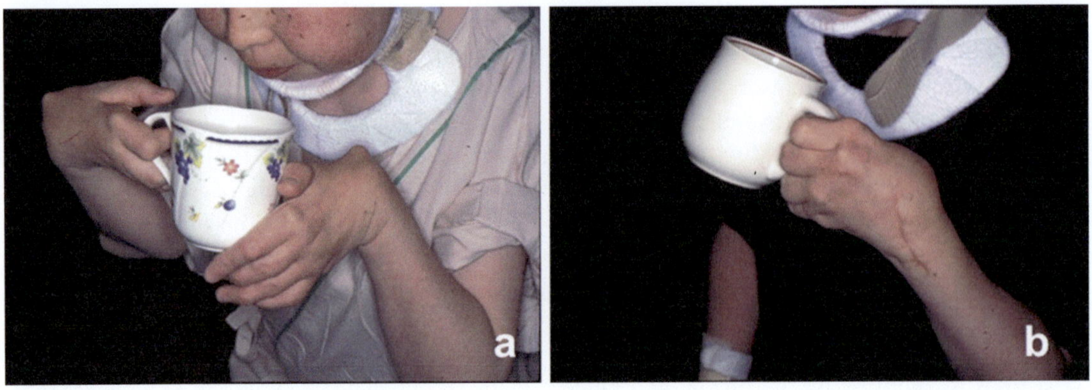

Fig. 13.18 Total wrist fusion with intercalated iliac bone graft (the same patient in Fig. 13.17). (**a**) Preoperative wrist with mutilans rheumatoid arthritis. (**b**) Postoperative radiograph

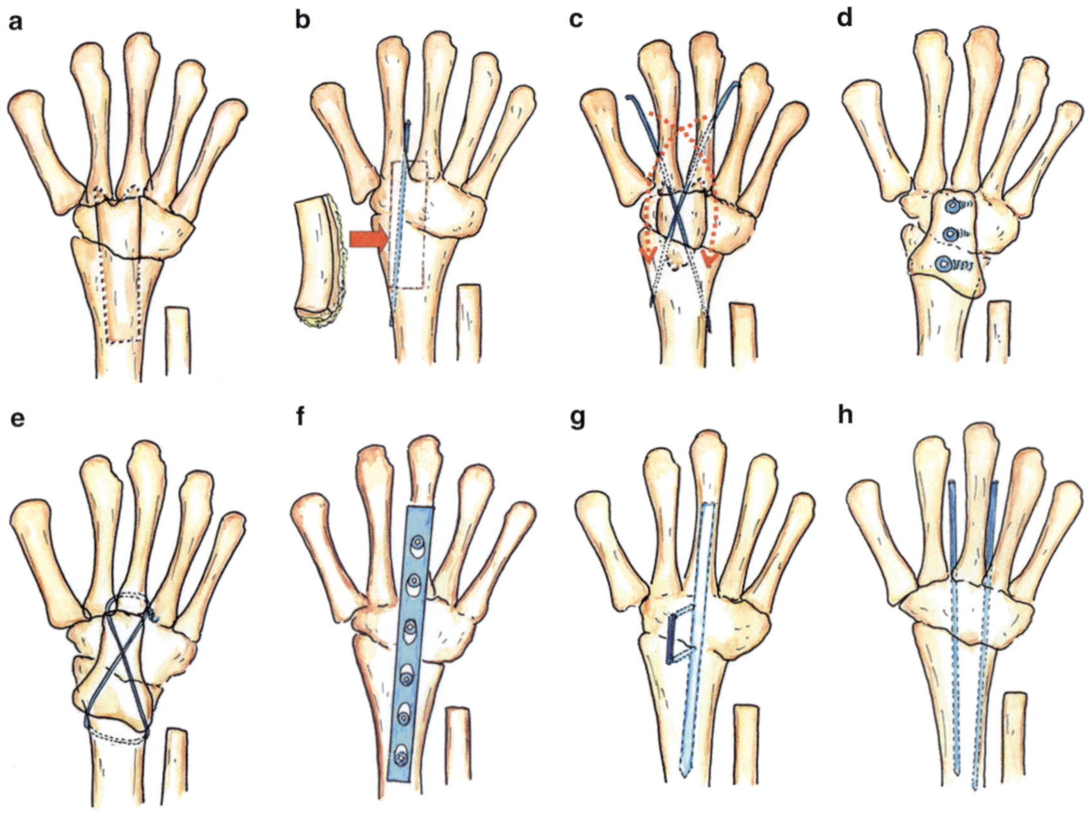

Fig. 13.19 Method of total wrist fusion. (**a**) No internal fixation (bone grafting), Carroll [34]. (**b**) Kirschner wire fixation with an iliac bone grafting from the radial side, Haddad and Riordan [35]. (**c**) Bowed crossed Kirschner wires, Minami [36]. (**d**) Screw fixation, Tannenbaum [37]. (**e**) Intraosseous wiring, Wood [38]. (**f**) Plate fixation, Wright and McMurtry [39]. (**g**) Intramedullary rod fixation, Clayton [1], Mannerfelt and Malmsten [40], Millender and Nalebuff [41]. (**h**) Double intermedullary fixation, Feldon [32]

Comparison between Total Wrist Fusion And Total Wrist Arthroplasty

In the systematic review of total wrist fusion and total wrist arthroplasty, Cavaliere and Chung reported that outcomes of total wrist fusion were comparable and possibly better than those for total wrist arthroplasty in rheumatoid patients [49]. Total wrist fusion provides more reliable pain relief than total wrist arthroplasty. Satisfaction was high in both groups, but complications and revision rates were higher for total wrist arthroplasty. In utility survey, there was the minimal increase in utility for arthroplasty over fusion because of its preserved motion, but surgeons did not view arthroplasty as superior to fusion [50].

Position for Total Wrist Fusion

The optimal position for total fusion is controversial (Table 13.4). It appears that a position of 10–30° of extension and of 0–15° of ulnar flexion is best in most cases [51]. If the bilateral wrists are to be fused, each wrist needs to be fused in a different position. Clayton recommended fusion in a neutral position, which is defined as 0° on the lateral with about 10° ulnar deviation [52]. The arc of pronation and supination substituted for flexion and extension without shoulder and elbow substitution. In a neutral position, finger pinch of the thumb and index finger is about 7.5 cm below the axis in pronation. Supination will give an arc of elevation of 15 cm without awkward moving of the shoulder and elbow. Field in 1996 suggested a period of immobilization before wrist fusion by having the patient wear a splint to determine the best individual position and also to allow the patient to become accustomed to an immobilized wrist to simulate wrist fusion [53].

Inclusion of the Carpometacarpal Joints in Total Wrist Fusion

Haddad and Riordan in 1967 [35] and Rauhaniemi in 2005 [54] recommended that the second and the third carpometacarpal (CM) joints should be included in the fusion to prevent development of painful motion and instability at these joints. However, Abbott in 1942 [42] and Nagy in 2002 [48] stated that the CM joint should be spared to preserve some motion at the CM joint. When the wrist was fused by including the third CM joint with the AO wrist arthrodesis plate, nonunion rate was high at the CM joint after plate removal [48].

Table 13.4 Position for total wrist fusion

	Ipsilateral	Bilateral
Dupont and Vainio (1968)	0–15° of extension, slight ulnar flexion	Dominant hand, neutral; nondominant hand, 10° of flexion
Haddad and Riordan (1967)	10–15° of extension and ulnar flexion, aligning the shaft of the second metacarpal with the distal end of the radius	
Milford (1982)	10–20° of extension, aligning the shaft of the third metacarpal with the distal end of the radius	
Dick (1982)	15–20° of extension	Dominant hand, 20° of extension; nondominant hand, neutral
Clayton (1984)	Neutral (0° of extension/flexion), 10° of ulnar flexion	
Nalebuff (1988)	5–10° of extension, 5° of ulnar flexion	Dominant hand, same as ipsilateral arthrodesis; nondominant hand, neutral
Volz (1980)	15° of extension good to perform ADL, 20° of ulnar flexion is not recommended	
Pryce (1980)	Grip power is stronger in 15° of extension and 15° of ulnar flexion than in neutral	

Inter- or Intramedullary Pin Fixation for Total Wrist Fusion

The method of intramedullary fixation was presented first by Clayton in 1965 [1] using a Steinmann pin. This modified method was presented by Mannerfelt and Malmusten in 1971 [40, 55] and by Millender and Nalebuff in 1973 [41, 56]. In the method of Mannerfelt and Malmusten, a flexible Rush rod was used to fuse in different degrees of flexion or extension. In the method of Millender and Nalebuff, a large Steinmann pin and staples were used with small bone grafts from the distal end of the ulna through a smaller skin incision. Also, Nalebuff and Feldon [32] modified intermedullary single-pin fixation to dual-pin technique to provide rotational stability as well as anteroposterior and lateral stability. We have performed wrist fusions using the method of Millender and Nalebuff and clinical results were satisfactory. However, we realized several technical problems and tricks in the method of inter- or intramedullary pin fixation: (1) migration of the pin distally or proximally, (2) in case with intermedullary pin fixation, widening of the intermetacarpal space and the pin sticking out, (3) rotation of the pin and the carpus, and (4) risk of fracture of the third metacarpal, when the pin was inserted directly from the metacarpal shaft proximally. After considering these problems described above, in 1999, we developed a wrist fusion rod (WFR, Teijin Nakashima Medical Co., Ltd. Okayama, Japan), a cannulated titanium rod, 4.5 mm in diameter, which could be buried into the third metacarpal and the radius with proximal fins and a transverse locking screw to prevent the rod migration and rotation of the rod in the medullary canal (Fig. 13.20). The length of the rod is ranging from 140 to 200 mm (140, 160, 180, and 200 mm). Using a special bender, the desired position of the wrist could be obtained at the operation.

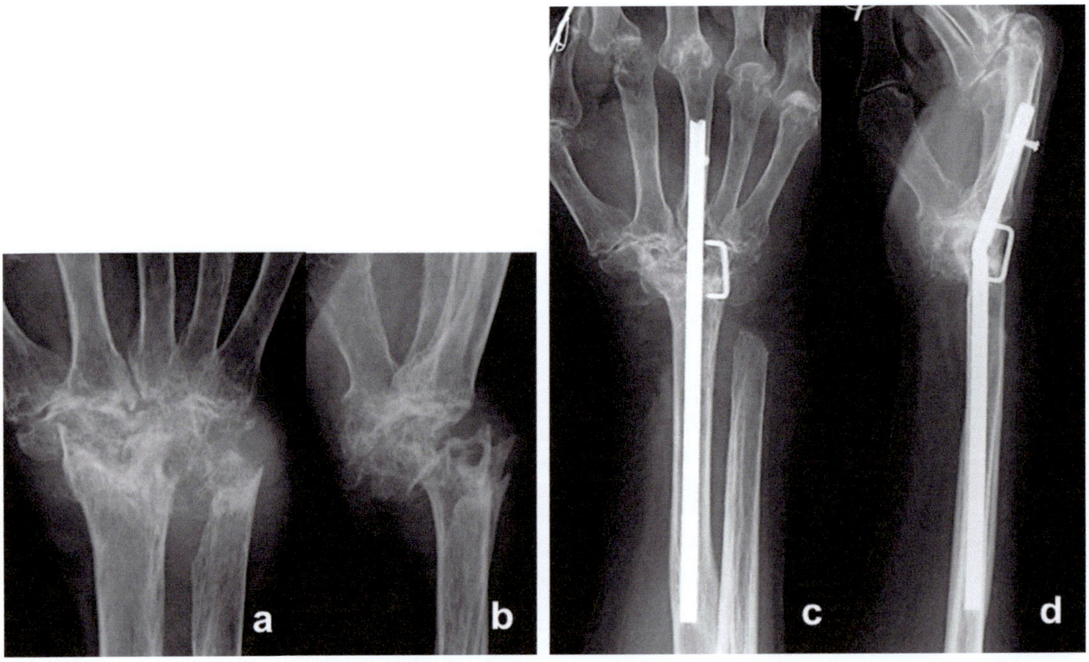

Fig. 13.20 Total wrist fusion using a new intramedullary rod, WFR. (**a**, **b**) Preoperative radiograph. (**c**, **d**) Postoperative radiograph

Surgical Technique of Total Wrist Fusion Using Wrist Fusion Rod

After bone preparation, a Kirschner wire 3 mm in diameter was inserted into the radius manually and measured its length (M mm). From the carpal side, a guide wire was inserted through the third metacarpal shaft so as to emerge from the dorsal cortex of the metacarpal neck. The length of the carpal side (L mm) was measured. After reaming, the rod ($M+L-25$ mm) was inserted in antegrade fashion from the carpus to the third metacarpal distally. After emerging the rod from the dorsum of the metacarpal neck, the rod was inserted through a guide pin in the retrograde fashion from the carpus into the radius proximally. The rod was countersunk until the distal end of the rod reached the metacarpal isthmus. After removing the guide wire, the rod was bent to a desired angle using a special bender. The gap between the fragments was packed with morselized bone grafts obtained from resected bones. After the distal part of the rod was fixed by inserting a transverse locking screw, supplemental fixation with a staple or a Kirschner wire was added. Postoperative immobilization using a short arm cast or a wrist splint was continued for 8 weeks.

Results of Total Wrist Fusion Using WFR

Total wrist fusion using WFR was performed in 39 wrists in 33 patients with RA. The mean age at the operation was 60 (28–75) years old and the mean follow-up period was 39 (5–76) months. Intercalated iliac bone grafting was performed in eight wrists. Bony fusion occurred in 87 % of the wrists in a reduced position. Breakage of the rod (the old version of the rod, 4 mm in diameter) occurred in four wrists (11 %) due to overuse of the hand or fall before completion of bony fusion,

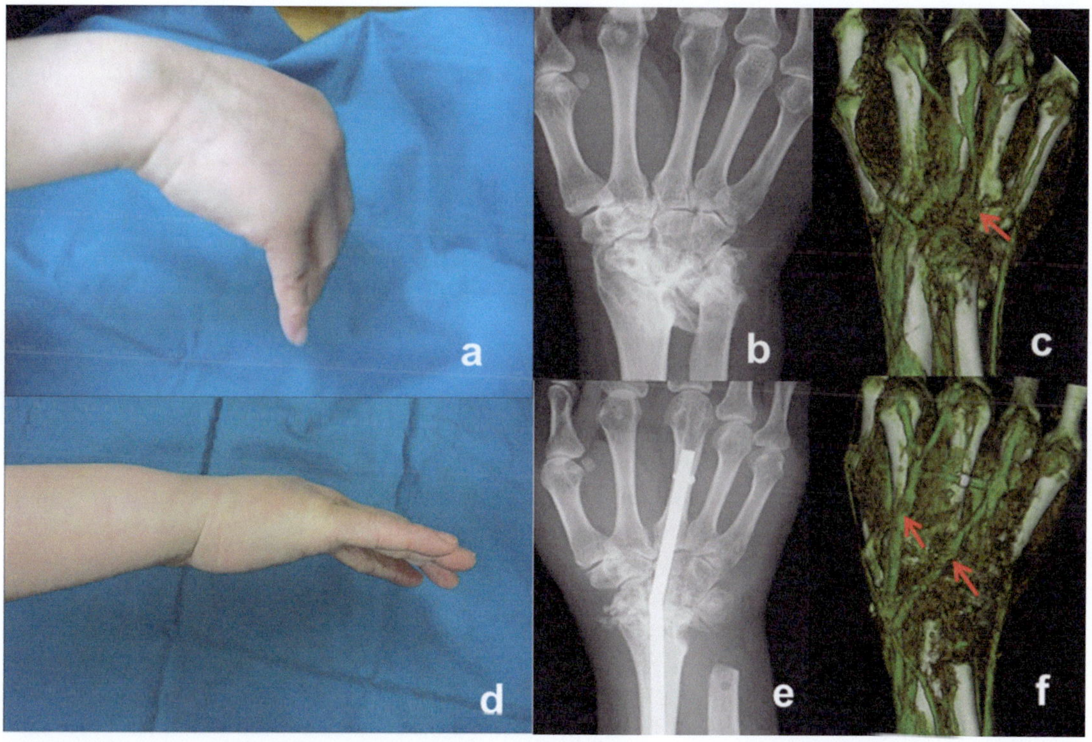

Fig. 13.21 Total wrist fusion and reconstruction of multiple finger extensor tendon ruptures. A 49-year-old female patient with RA. (**a**) Preoperative state of the hand. (**b**) Preoperative radiograph. (**c**) Preoperative 3DCT. The *arrow* shows tendon ruptures. (**d**) Postoperative 4 months. (**e**) Postoperative radiograph. (**f**) Postoperative 3DCT. The *arrow* shows transferred tendons

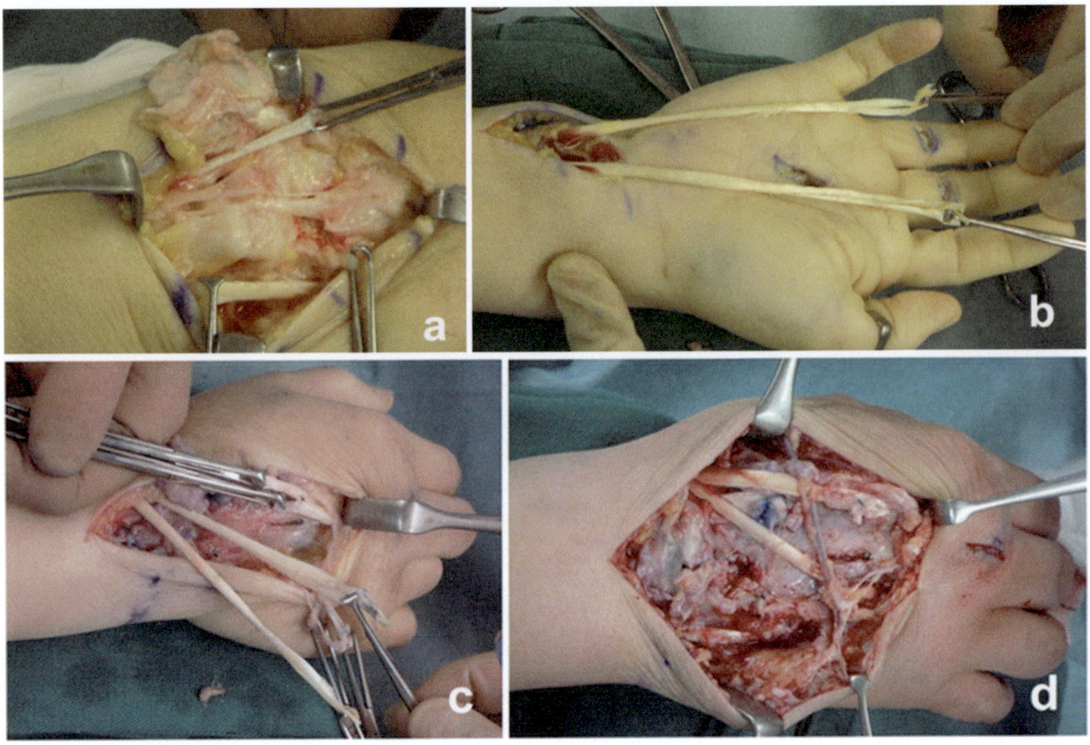

Fig. 13.22 Total wrist fusion and reconstruction of multiple finger extensor tendon ruptures (the same patient in Fig. 13.21). (**a**) Rupture of EDC II-V, EIP, and EDM tendons. (**b**) FDS III and FDS IV tendons. (**c**, **d**) Subcutaneous transfer of finger flexor tendons. *EDC* extensor digitorum communis, *EIP* extensor indicis proprius, *EDM* extensor digiti minimi, *FDS* flexor digitorum superficialis

but the patients did not complain of pain. Three rods were removed and one rod was still in the bone. In the new version of the rod, its diameter increased to 4.5 mm and reinforced. There were no major complications. Preoperative pain and swelling disappeared in all operated wrists. Grip power increased to 77 % (30 wrists), and average gain was 2.5 kg (pre-op, 7.7 kg; post-op, 10.2 kg). Subluxated wrist was reduced to its anatomical position and fused in slight extension (pre-op, 14°; post-op, 10°) and slight ulnar deviation (pre-op, 8°; post-op, 7°). Patients' satisfaction scale from 5 (most satisfying) to 1 (unsatisfying) was 4.9 in 16 patients. In the radiological assessment, ulnar carpal shift ratio, *e*/MC, was corrected significantly (pre-op, 0.17; post-op, 0.07; $p<0.01$). Palmar carpal subluxation ratio, *h*/MC, was also corrected significantly (pre-op, 0.22; post-op, 0.14; $p<0.01$).

A Case with Total Wrist Fusion and Reconstruction of Multiple Extensor Tendon Ruptures (Figs. 13.21 and 13.22)

A 49-year-old female patient with RA had extension loss in the index through the little fingers. She could not grasp a large object (a cylinder of 85 mm in diameter) and pick up a small object (a peg of 20 mm in diameter). The cause of this multiple extensor tendon ruptures was considered to be (1) weakness of the tendon due to extensor tenosynovitis, (2) attrition by the bony edge of the deformed wrist, and (3) overuse of the hand after remission of the disease by using biological agent. Synovectomy of the extensor tendons and the wrist joint combined with a Darrach procedure, ulnar stump stabilization using one-half of FCU tendon, total wrist arthrodesis using WFR, transfer of flexor digitorum superficialis (FDS) III tendon to the ruptured extensor digitorum communis (EDC) II and EDC III tendons, and transfer of FDS IV tendon to the ruptured EDC IV, V and extensor digiti minimi (EDM) tendons passing the FDS tendons subcutaneously on the radial side of the wrist were performed. Four months after the operation, she was satisfied with this operation, because of (1) complete pain relief, (2) gain in grip power (15.7–18.4 kg) and pinch power (0.6–1.6 kg), (3) improved hand function including grasping a large object and picking up a small object, and (4) good appearance of the hand.

References

1. Clayton ML. Surgical treatment at the wrist in rheumatoid arthritis. A review of thirty-seven patients. J Bone Joint Surg. 1965;47A:741–50.
2. Hämäläinen M, Kammonen M, Lehtimäki M, Nurmi V-M, Repo A, Ikävalko M, et al. Epidemiology of wrist involvement in rheumatoid arthritis. In: Simmen BR, Hagena F-W, editors. The wrist in rheumatoid arthritis, vol. 17. Basel: Karger; 1992. p. 1–7.
3. Toyohara I, Ishikawa H, Abe A, Nakazono K, Murasawa A. Disease activity and the course of wrist deterioration over 10 years in the patients with rheumatoid arthritis. Mod Rheumatol. 2009;19:47–52.
4. Larsen A, Dale K, Eek M. Radiographic evaluation of rheumatoid arthritis and related conditions by standard reference films. Acta Radiol Diagn. 1977;18:481–91.
5. Larsen A. How to apply Larsen score in evaluating radiographs of rheumatoid arthritis in long-term studies. J Rheumatol. 1995;22:1974–5.
6. Trentham DE, Masi AT. Carpometacarpal ratio. A new quantitative measure of radiologic progression of wrist involvement in rheumatoid arthritis. Arthritis Rheum. 1976;19:939–44.
7. Simmen BR, Huber H. The rheumatoid wrist: a new classification related to the type of the natural course and its consequences for surgical therapy. In: Simmen BR, Hagena F-W, editors. The wrist in rheumatoid arthritis, 17. Basel: Karger; 1992. p. 13–25.
8. Flury MP, Herren DB, Simmen BR. Rheumatoid arthritis of the wrist, classification related to the natural course. Clin Orthop Relat Res. 1999;366:72–7.
9. Taleisnik J. Rheumatoid synovitis of the volar compartment of the wrist joint: its radiological signs and its contribution to wrist and hand deformity. J Hand Surg. 1979;4:526–35.
10. Shapiro JS. The wrist in rheumatoid arthritis. Hand Clin. 1996;12:477–98.
11. Moore JR, Weiland AJ, Valdata L. Tendon ruptures in the rheumatoid hand: analysis of treatment and functional results in 60 patients. J Hand Surg. 1987;12A:9–14.
12. Ishikawa H, Abe A, Murasawa A, Nakazono K, Horizono H, Ishii K, et al. Rheumatoid wrist deformity and risk of extensor tendon rupture evaluated by 3DCT imaging. Skeletal Radiol. 2010;39:467–72.
13. Seki E, Ishikawa H, Murasawa A, Nakazono K, Abe A, Horizono H, et al. Dislocation of the extensor carpi ulnaris tendon in rheumatoid wrists using three-dimensional computed tomographic imaging. Clin Rheumatol. 2013;32:1627–32.
14. Ryu J, Saito S, Honda T, Yamamoto K. Risk factors and prophylactic tenosynovectomy for extensor tendon ruptures in the rheumatoid hand. J Hand Surg. 1998;23B:658–61.
15. Freiberg RA, Weinstein A. The scallop sign and spontaneous rupture of extensor tendons in rheumatoid arthritis. Clin Orthop Relat Res. 1972;83:128–30.
16. Darrach W. Anterior dislocation of the head of the ulna. Ann Surg. 1912;56:802–3.
17. Ishikawa H, Hanyu T, Tajima T. Rheumatoid wrists treated with synovectomy of the extensor tendons and the wrist joint combined with a Darrach procedure. J Hand Surg. 1992;17A:1109–17.
18. Youm Y, McMurtry RY, Flatt AE, Gillespie TE. Kinematics of the wrist. I. An experimental study of radial-ulnar deviation and flexion-extension. J Bone Joint Surg. 1978;60A:423–31.
19. Chamay A, Della Santa D, Vilaseca A. Radiolunate arthrodesis. Factor of stability for the rheumatoid wrist. Ann Chir Main. 1983;2:5–17.
20. Chamay A, Della SD. Radiolunate arthrodesis in rheumatoid wrist (21 cases). Ann Chir Main Memb Super. 1991;10:197–206.
21. Clayton ML, Felic DC. Tendon transfer for radial rotation of the wrist in rheumatoid arthritis. Clin Orthop Relat Res. 1974;100:176–85.
22. Stack HG, Vaughan-Jackson OJ. The zig-zag deformity in the rheumatoid hand. Hand. 1971;3:62–7.
23. Ishikawa H, Murasawa A, Nakazono K. Long-term follow-up study of radiocarpal arthrodesis for the rheumatoid wrist. J Hand Surg. 2005;30A:658–66.
24. Herren DB, Ishikawa H. Partial arthrodesis for the rheumatoid wrist. Hand Clin. 2005;21:545–52.
25. Ishikawa H, Hanyu T, Saito H, Takahashi H. Limited arthrodesis for the rheumatoid wrist. J Hand Surg. 1992;17A:1103–9.
26. Borisch N, Haussmann P. Radiolunate arthrodesis in the rheumatoid wrist: a retrospective clinical and radiological longterm follow-up. J Hand Surg. 2002;27B:61–72.
27. Motomiya M, Iwasaki N, Minami A, Matsui Y, Urita A, Funakoshi T. Clinical and radiological results of radiolunate arthrodesis for rheumatoid arthritis: 22 wrists followed for an average of 7 years. J Hand Surg. 2013;38A:1484–91.

28. Leslie BM, Carlson G, Ruby LK. Results of extensor carpi ulnaris tenodesis in the rheumatoid wrist undergoing a distal ulnar excision. J Hand Surg. 1990;15A:547–51.
29. Tsai T, Stillwell JH. Repair of chronic subluxation of the distal radioulnar joint (ulnar dorsal) using flexor carpi ulnaris tendon. J Hand Surg. 1984;9B:289–93.
30. Arimitsu S, Sugamoto K, Hashimoto J, Murase T, Yoshikawa H, Morimoto H. Analysis of radiocarpal and midcarpal motion in stable and unstable rheumatoid wrists using 3-dimensional computed tomography. J Hand Surg. 2008;33A:189–97.
31. Taleisnik J. Combined radiocarpal arthrodesis and midcarpal (lunocapitate) arthroplasty for treatment of rheumatoid arthritis of the wrist. J Hand Surg. 1987;12A:1–8.
32. Nalebuff EA, Terrono AL, Feldon P. Arthrodesis of the wrist: indications and surgical technique. In: Lichtman DM, Alexander AH, editors. The wrist and its disorders. Philadelphia: W.B. Saunders Company; 1997. p. 671–81.
33. Fontaine C, Mouliade S, Wavreille G, Chantelot C. Wrist arthrodesis with intercalated iliac crest graft in mutilans rheumatoid arthritis. Chir Main. 2014;33:336–43.
34. Carroll RE, Dick HM. Arthrodesis of the wrist for rheumatoid arthritis. J Bone Joint Surg. 1971;53A:1365–9.
35. Haddad Jr RJ, Riordan DC. Arthrodesis of the wrist. A surgical technique. J Bone Joint Surg. 1967; 49A:950–4.
36. Minami A, Kato H, Iwasaki N. Total wrist arthrodesis using bowed crossed K-wires. J Hand Surg. 1999;24B:410–5.
37. Tannenbaum DA, Louis DS. The Stein and Gill technique for wrist arthrodesis. Tech Hand Up Extrem Surg. 1999;3:181–4.
38. Wood MB. Wrist arthrodesis using dorsal radial bone graft. J Hand Surg. 1987;12A:208–12.
39. Wright CS, McMurtry RY. AO arthrodesis in the hand. J Hand Surg. 1983;8A:932–5.
40. Mannerfelt L, Malmsten M. Arthrodesis of the wrist in rheumatoid arthritis. A technique without external fixation. Scand J Plast Reconstr Surg. 1971;5: 124–30.
41. Millender LH, Nalebuff EA. Arthrodesis of the rheumatoid wrist. An evaluation of sixty patients and a description of a different surgical technique. J Bone Joint Surg. 1973;55A:1026–34.
42. Abbott LC, Saunders JBDM, Bost FC. Arthrodesis of the wrist with the use of grafts of cancellous bone. J Bone Joint Surg. 1942;24A:883–98.
43. Robinson RF, Kayfets DO. Arthrodesis of the wrist; preliminary report of a new method. J Bone Joint Surg. 1952;34A:64–70.
44. Voutilainen N, Juutilainen T, Pätiälä H, Rokkanen P. Arthrodesis of the wrist with bioabsorbable fixation in patients with rheumatoid arthritis. J Hand Surg. 2002;27B:563–7.
45. Clendenin MB, Green DP. Arthrodesis of the wrist-complications and their management. J Hand Surg. 1981;6A:253–7.
46. Zachary SV, Stern PJ. Complications following AO/ ASIF wrist arthrodesis. J Hand Surg. 1995;20A: 339–44.
47. Deluca PA, Lindsey RW, Ruwe PA. Refracture of bones of the forearm after the removal of compression plates. J Bone Joint Surg. 1988;70A:1372–6.
48. Nagy L, Büchler U. AO-wrist arthrodesis: with and without arthrodesis of the third carpometacarpal joint. J Hand Surg. 2002;27A:940–7.
49. Cavaliere CM, Chung KC. Total wrist arthroplasty and total wrist arthrodesis in rheumatoid arthritis: a decision analysis from the hand surgeons' perspective. J Hand Surg. 2008;33A:1744–55.
50. Cavaliere CM, Chung KC. A cost-utility analysis of nonsurgical management, total wrist arthroplasty, and total wrist arthrodesis in rheumatoid arthritis. J Hand Surg. 2010;35A:379–91.
51. Louis DS, Hankin FM. Arthrodesis of the wrist: past and present. J Hand Surg. 1986;11A:787–9.
52. Clayton ML, Ferlic DC. Arthrodesis of the arthritic wrist. Clin Orthop Relat Res. 1984;187:89–93.
53. Field J, Herbert TJ, Prosser R. Total wrist fusion. A functional assessment. J Hand Surg. 1996;21B: 429–33.
54. Rauhaniemi J, Tiusanen H, Sipola E. Total wrist fusion: a study of 115 patients. J Hand Surg. 2005; 30B:217–9.
55. Kluge S, Schindele S, Henkel T, Herren D. The modified Clayton-Mannerfelt arthrodesis of the wrist in rheumatoid arthritis: operative technique and report on 93 cases. J Hand Surg. 2013;38A:999–1005.
56. Kobus RJ, Turner RH. Wrist arthrodesis for treatment of rheumatoid arthritis. J Hand Surg. 1990; 15A:541–6.

Application of Arthroscopy in the Treatment of Rheumatoid Wrist

14

Clara Wong Wing Yee and Pak-cheong Ho

Introduction

Rheumatoid arthritis is a common autoimmune systemic inflammatory disease affecting approximately 1 % of the worldwide population [1]. Wrist joints are commonly involved. Within 2 years of diagnosis, more than half of patients will have wrist pain, and more than 90 % will have wrist disease by 10 years [2]. The pain, swelling, instability, and deformity cause significant disability. Symptomatic relief of pain; improvement of function; protection of the capsular, ligamentous, and tendinous structures; and possible systemic amelioration of the disease after open synovectomy were well reported [3–8]. Rewarding results of arthroscopic synovectomy were also demonstrated in previous studies [9–15]. With the additional advantages of minimal invasiveness and relative benignity, arthroscopic procedures are replacing open procedures. The advancement of surgical techniques and skills of operation now extend the role of arthroscopy beyond synovectomy to more complicated reconstructive surgeries in rheumatoid wrists. The role of arthroscopy, analysis of our long-term results of 13 years (6–17.5 years), surgical techniques, and other applications of arthroscopy in patients with rheumatoid wrists are discussed here in detail.

Wrist Arthroscopic Synovectomy

Indications and Limitations

With the advancement of surgical techniques in wrist arthroscopy, arthroscopic synovectomy can be safely performed in almost all wrist arthritic conditions. Rheumatoid wrist has inherent ligamentous laxity. This makes portal site development and arthroscope insertion easier and gives a better space for the arthroscope to work into (Fig. 14.1). Moreover, this operation is performed under portal site local anesthesia (PSLA) [16], which obviates the potential risks of general anesthesia for rheumatoid patients who may have associated cervical instability or other medical comorbidities. In general, continued wrist pain and refractory synovitis of 3–6-month duration are indications for arthroscopic synovectomy.

However, difficulties may be encountered when there is local scarring due to previous surgery, significant extra-articular pathologies

Electronic supplementary material: The online version of this chapter (doi:10.1007/978-3-319-26660-2_14) contains supplementary material, which is available to authorized users. Videos can also be accessed at http://link.springer.com/chapter/10.1007/978-3-319-26660-2_14.

C.W.W. Yee, FRCSEd(Orth), FHKCOS, FHKAM(Orth)
P.-c. Ho, FHKCOS, FHKAM(Orth), FRCS(Edin) (✉)
Department of Orthopaedics and Traumatology,
Prince of Wales Hospital, 30-32 Ngan Shing Street,
Shatin, Hong Kong, SAR, China
e-mail: clara.wongclara@gmail.com;
clarawong@ort.cuhk.edu.hk; pcho@ort.cuhk.edu.hk

K.C. Chung (ed.), *Clinical Management of the Rheumatoid Hand, Wrist, and Elbow*,
DOI 10.1007/978-3-319-26660-2_14

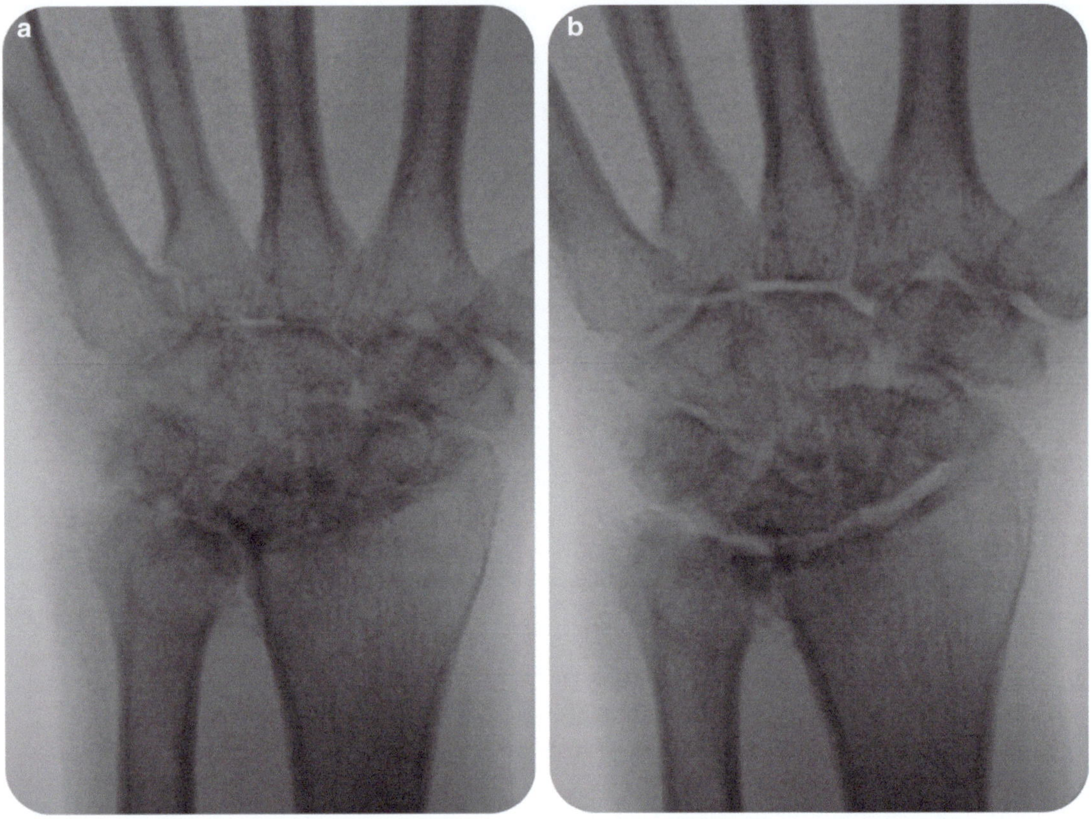

Fig. 14.1 (**a**) X-rays are deceptive in rheumatoid wrists. There seems to have no joint space from this X-ray for the arthroscope to go into. (**b**) After traction is applied. The joint spaces are shown up in this traction view

such as extensor tendon subluxation, and significant joint deformity with altered anatomy. Tendon injuries can be avoided by making a bigger incision and careful dissection before introducing the arthroscopic instruments. In associated extensor tenosynovitis, arthroscopic synovectomy can then be performed after open tenosynovectomy, or the procedure is converted to open. Local skin infection is an absolute contraindication for the procedure.

Role

Performing arthroscopy in a wrist with inflammatory arthritis does not only have a therapeutic role of removing the inflamed synovium. It also bears an invaluable diagnostic role.

Arthroscopy Helps in Early Diagnosis

Rheumatoid arthritis is considered an autoimmune disease [17, 18]. Autoimmunity and the overall systemic and articular inflammatory load drive the destructive progression of the disease. It has been recognized that early intervention improves clinical outcomes and reduces accrual of joint damage and disability [19–21]. Undoubtedly, treating patients at a stage at which evolution of joint destruction can still be prevented would be ideal. In 2010, the American College of Rheumatology and the European League Against Rheumatism (ACR/EULAR) refocused attention on the important need for earlier diagnosis and treatment and therefore developed new classification criteria for rheumatoid arthritis [22]. It is designed to be more sensitive to define "definitive" rheumatoid arthritis in early

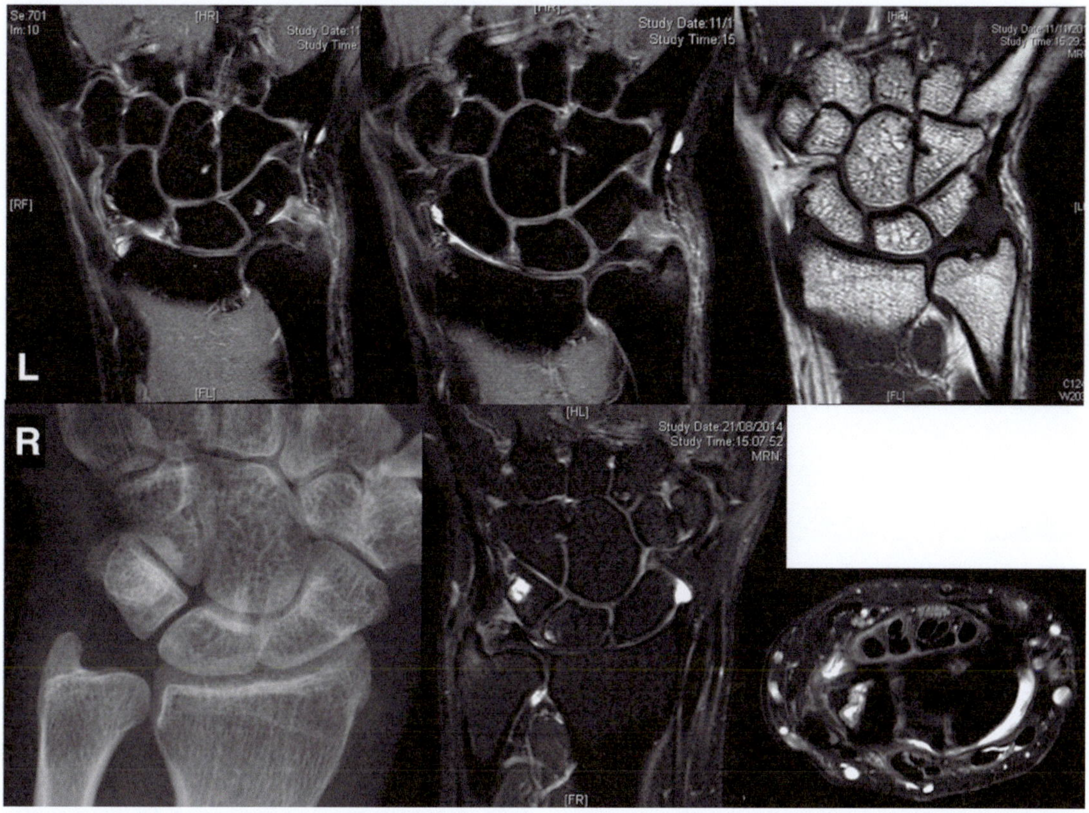

Fig. 14.2 MRI of a 50-year-old lady who presented with unprovoked on and off bilateral whole wrist pain, mild swelling, and increase in temperature for 3 months. X-ray of her right wrist showed tiny calcification at the tip of ulnar styloid and over the region of TFCC. Radiologist commented that there was mild focal synovitis at the ulnocarpal and radiocarpal interval, mild erosive changes of the carpus, and ECU tenosynovitis suggestive of rheumatologist disease. Her rheumatoid factor and anti-citrullinated antibodies were negative, inflammatory markers were mildly elevated, and serum urate level was high. She was then started with DMARDs by rheumatologist. Arthroscopy would be helpful to differentiate whether this was a rheumatoid arthritis, crystal deposition disease, degeneration, erosive changes, or benign subchondral carpal bone cysts

disease than the 1987 ACR classification criteria, so that more patients in early disease can benefit from starting disease-modifying antirheumatic drugs (DMARDs) or biologics. In the ACR/EULAR classification criteria, "joint involvement" refers to "any swollen or tender joint on examination." This can be arbitrary to identify a diseased joint by physical examination, and therefore the criteria also include "may be confirmed by imaging evidence of synovitis." Structural changes of the joint, which can be visualized by conventional radiography or sophisticated imaging techniques, help identify and distinguish rheumatoid arthritis from other arthritic diseases [23]. However, in early disease, these changes are rarely apparent and difficult to be interpreted with limited interobserver reliability [24–28] (Fig. 14.2).

In our experience, arthroscopy plays a prominent diagnostic role in rheumatoid arthritis. Wrist arthroscopy gives a direct visualization and full access to almost all areas within the joint, which may be more thorough and comprehensive than an open approach. Any abnormal synovitis can be detected in early cases. Severity, location, and appearance of the synovitis are better evaluated. The appearance of the inflamed synovium is inspected under a magnified view. The images showed villonodular in rheumatoid arthritis, seronegative arthritis, and psoriatic arthritis

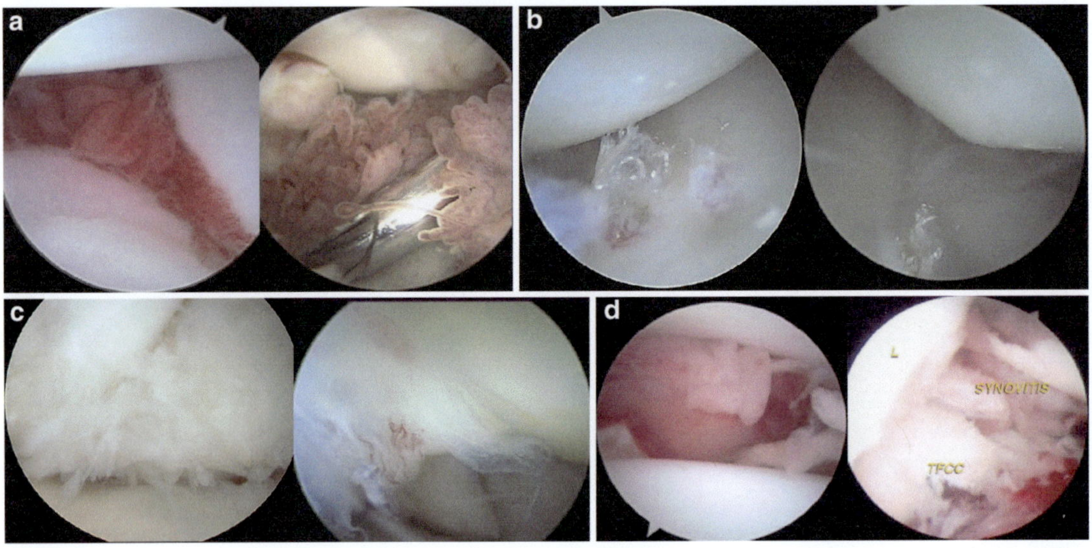

Fig. 14.3 Appearance of synovium in the arthroscopic view of the radiocarpal joint. (**a**) *S* scaphoid, *R* radius. The synovitis appeared villonodular, which can happen in rheumatoid arthritis, seronegative arthritis, and psoriatic arthritis. The synovium would appear less engorged with vasculature if the disease is not active. (**b**) The whitish, chalky tophaceous materials overlying the synovium and cartilage. (**c**) The synovium appears fibrillated in osteoarthritis and post-traumatic arthritis. (**d**) The synovium appears fibrinoid in septic arthritis

(Fig. 14.3a), and they also showed tophaceous in gouty arthritis (Fig. 14.3b), fibrillated in osteoarthritis and post-traumatic arthritis (Fig. 14.3c), and fibrinoid in infective arthritis (Fig. 14.3d). These morphological features of the synovium help to give additional clues for the early diagnosis of rheumatoid arthritis and differentiate it from other arthritic disorders.

Arthroscopy Facilitates Synovial Biopsy for Histopathological and Microbiological Analysis

Wrist arthroscopy allows for synovial biopsy for histopathological and microbiological analysis [29]. Infective or neoplastic conditions can be excluded [29]. It permits biopsy regions not accessible to percutaneous biopsy needle, e.g., at the cartilage-pannus junction, where joint erosion commonly begins with characteristic microscopic and immunohistological features of rheumatoid arthritis [30–32]. Studies also indicated that synovial histopathology had a high diagnostic prediction and positive predictive values for the diagnosis of inflammatory arthritis especially in patients with an atypical presentation [31–33]. Clinical outcome, prognosis of disease progression, and response to therapeutic intervention can also be predicted [30–34].

Arthroscopy Helps to Give an Accurate Assessment of Cartilage Condition, by Providing More Clues to the Diagnosis, Severity, and Prognosis of the Condition

Arthroscopic assessment of cartilage condition is very important to the diagnosis and prediction of disability and disease progression. Cartilage condition was found to have stronger association with physical disability, damage progression, and clinical outcomes than bony erosion in rheumatoid arthritis [35, 36]. In rheumatoid arthritis, there are two major components of joint destruction. They are cartilage degradation and bony destruction, which are elicited by two different mechanisms. Bony destruction is mediated by synovial osteoclasts and direct invasion of the pannus into the adjacent bone [37, 38], whereas cartilage damage is mostly due to the action of metalloproteinases secreted into the synovial fluid by synovial fibroblasts and macrophages or produced locally by activated chondrocytes, activated and regulated by pro-inflammatory cytokines [39, 40]. These two mechanisms do not necessarily happen simultaneously. The severity of cartilage degradation and bony destruction is therefore not proportional to each other, especially in early disease or in certain patients with atypical presentation. Cartilage degradation is reflected radiologically by joint space narrowing and bony destruction by erosions. Radiographic erosive change is regarded more characteristic of rheumatoid arthritis, whereas joint space narrowing is less and can be interpreted as degenerative joint disease or other arthritic conditions when the erosive change is not apparent. Moreover, the degree of joint space narrowing in the wrist joint may not be easily determined and appreciated radiologically. In order to identify cartilage degradation while all the radiological features are not prominent, arthroscopy plays an important role to visualize the cartilage directly and differentiate degradation from degeneration or other inflammatory arthritis. In gouty arthritis, tophaceous material would invade and deposit on the cartilage (Fig. 14.4a). In primary or secondary osteoarthritis, there is softening, fissuring, fragmentation, or even exposure of subchondral bone, depending on the severity of the degeneration (Fig. 14.4b, c). In rheumatological diseases, cartilage appears thin, soft, easily wiped off on palpation (Fig. 14.4d), eroded (Fig. 14.4e, f), and honeycomb (Fig. 14.4f) and sometimes may be covered by a thin layer of inflamed synovium (Fig. 14.4g). Arthroscopy is helpful to assess the severity of cartilage destruction and gives the prediction of disability and disease progression.

Besides the diagnostic role of arthroscopy in rheumatoid wrist, it serves both the prophylactic and therapeutic role. The prophylactic role is to remove inflamed synovial tissue in an attempt to prevent articular damage, whereas the therapeutic role is to improve function and relieve pain in situations in which joint destruction is already present, such as arthroscopic wrist fusion or reconstruction surgeries that will be discussed later in this chapter.

Arthroscopy Allows for Synovectomy, Which Showed Favorable Results and Is Helpful in Controlling Joint Destruction

Over recent years, evidence has emerged linking rheumatoid arthritis with antibodies such as anti-citrullinated protein/peptide antibodies; pro-inflammatory cytokines such as TNFa, IL-1, IL-6, and IL-17; and platelet microparticles. They are shown to contribute prominently to the progression of the disease by attaching to, invading, and degrading cartilage [17]. They are found to be synthesized locally from the ectopic lymphoid structures [41], naive and memory B-cell and T-cell aggregates, monocytes, macrophages, macrophage-like synoviocytes [42], platelets, and fibroblast-like synoviocytes in the synovial tissues [43]. The removal of the diseased synovium is theoretically helpful in controlling destruction to the synovial joints through the autoimmune and inflammatory mechanisms. Moreover, study showed that sensory denervation explained the positive effects of synovectomy leading to pain reduction and improved mobility [44]. And in fact, throughout the years, favorable clinical results after open surgical synovectomy were reported in many joints [3–7]. It is also particularly helpful in patients who are resistant to the DMARDs and biologics [45, 46]. Arthroscopic synovectomy gains further advantages by providing a minimally invasive approach with low morbidity and an early return to daily activities [47–49]. Successful results with predictable pain relief, better grip strength, improved range of motion, and functional improvement were also reported in the wrists [9–15].

Arthroscopic Synovectomy Not Only Helps to Control Joint Destruction But May Also Retard Spread and Systemic Amplification of the Disease

Rheumatoid arthritis often presents as mono-/oligoarticular disease before becoming polyarticular. Study showed that fibroblast-like synoviocytes migrate via vasculature to the previously unaffected joints and cause spread and amplification of the disease [8]. Literatures have also suggested

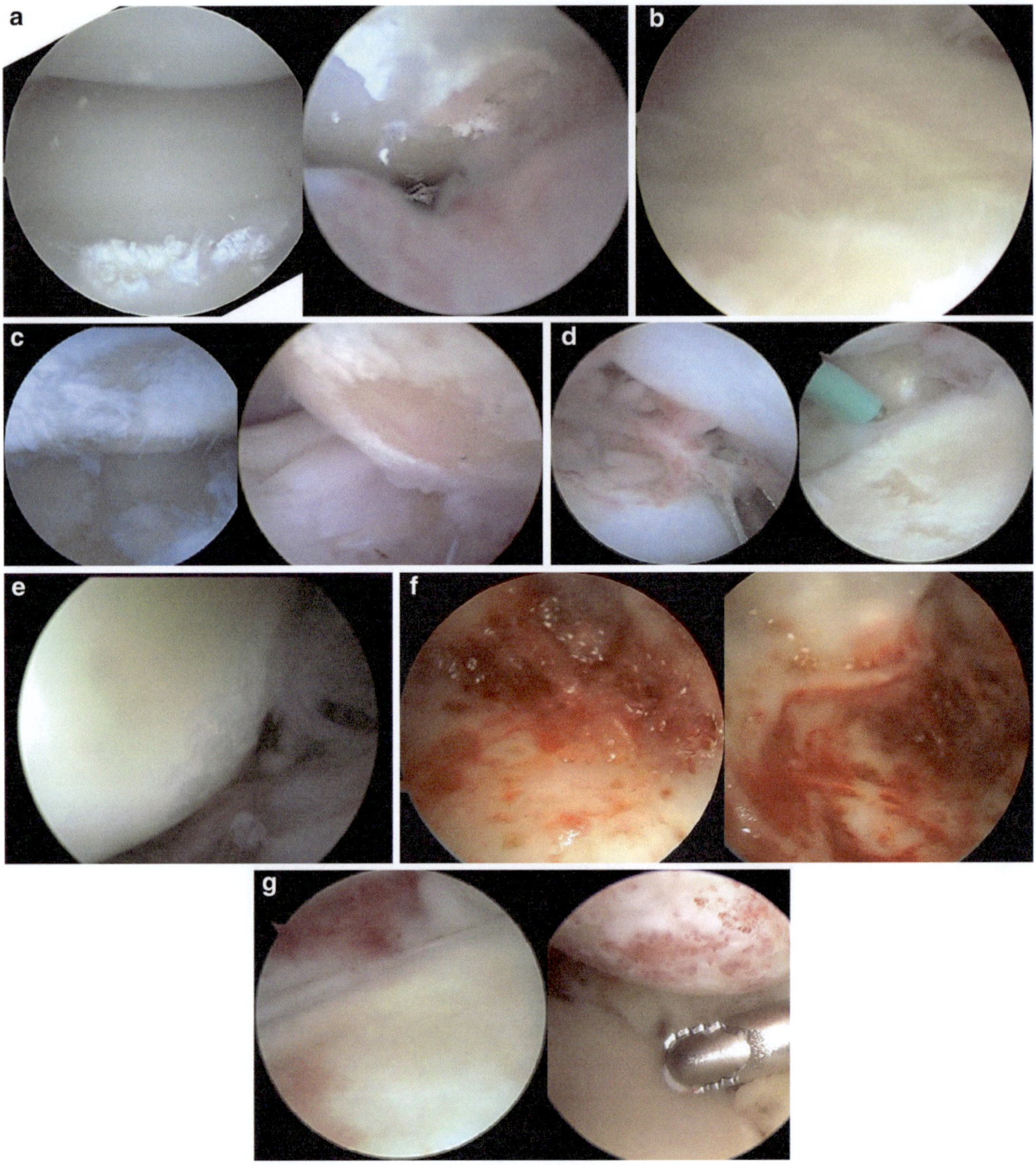

Fig. 14.4 Appearance of the cartilage in the arthroscopic view of the radiocarpal joint. (**a**) The cartilage was invaded by the tophaceous deposits in gouty arthritis. (**b**) There were softening and fissuring in the early stage of primary or secondary osteoarthritis. (**c**) There were fissuring, fragmentation, and exposure of subchondral bone in moderate to severe stage of primary or secondary osteoarthritis. (**d**) A 40-year-old man with rheumatoid arthritis; the cartilage appeared thin and soft and was easily wiped away by light palpation. (**e**) Patchy erosive changes in a rheumatoid patient whose disease is at a quiescent stage. (**f**) The cartilage had a honeycomb and erosive appearance. (**g**) The appearance of the cartilage at the active inflammatory phase. A layer of inflamed synovium on the cartilage eroding the cartilage

that synovectomy can decrease systemic level of inflammatory mediators [50–54]. Synovectomy should therefore be helpful in ameliorating the overall disease condition and arrest or slow progression, though recurrence is still possible.

Arthroscopic Synovectomy May Help to Prevent Ligament and Tendon Damage

Synovectomy of the wrist joint has another role that is not present in the lower limb weight-bearing joints. Distension of the wrist joint by the synovium and the collagenases, cytokines, and metalloproteinases released from the synovium leads to attenuation and ruptures of the wrist joint ligaments, instability, and deformity [55]. The extracapsular extrusion of the diseased synovium also contributes to tendon rupture [56]. Synovectomy, even if recurrence may still happen, protects the joint from instability and deformity and the tendon from rupture.

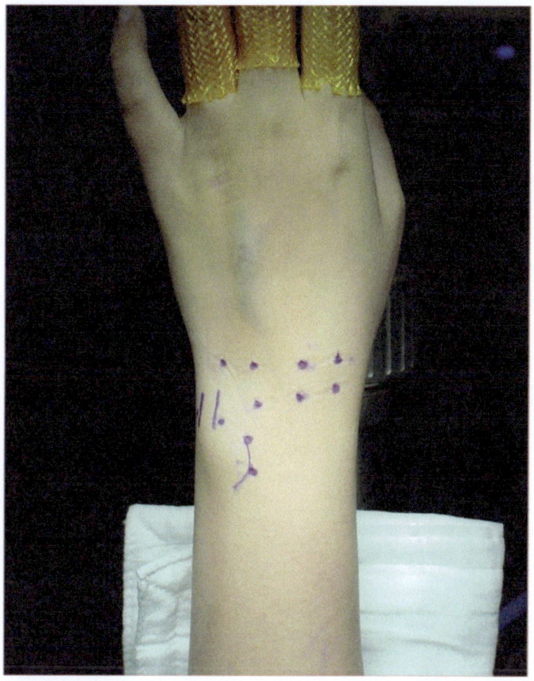

Fig. 14.5 All the routine arthroscopic portals are marked on skin with the wrist under traction prior to the surgical procedure

Surgical Techniques

Patient is put in supine position while the operated arm is supported on a hand table. An arm tourniquet is applied loosely but does not need to be inflated routinely. A tight application of a tourniquet without exsanguination leads to venous engorgement and can induce more troublesome bleeding. Most of the procedures can be done without the use of a tourniquet. Vertical traction of 4–6 kg force is applied through plastic finger trap devices to the middle three fingers for joint distraction via a wrist traction tower (Fig. 14.5). Metallic traction device is discouraged especially in patients with fragile skin. The wrist joint is continuously irrigated and distended by suspending a bag of 3 % of normal saline at 1–1.5 m above the operating table and instilling with the aid of gravity to maintain a clear arthroscopic view. Infusion pump is not necessary and is potentially harmful in causing fluid extravasation. In wrist arthroscopy, it is mainly the distraction device that keeps the joint opened, not the fluid irrigation as in shoulder arthroscopy. Essential arthroscopic instruments include motorized full-radius shaver of 2 mm and 2.9 mm diameter, arthroscopic bur of 2.9 mm, small angled curette, 2.5 mm suction punch, and radiofrequency thermal ablation system.

The operation can be performed under local or regional anesthesia. PSLA without a tourniquet is the preferred mode of anesthesia and is enough to complete the whole procedure [16]. Xylocaine 2 % with adrenaline 1:200,000 is injected to the portal site skin and capsule to reduce bleeding related to the incision and dissection. Intra-articular Xylocaine with adrenaline injection is used when extensive synovitis is encountered and can reduce bleeding associated with shaving and punching. Local anesthetic drug can also be injected through the arthroscopic portal to the volar joint capsule whenever necessary. Sterile tourniquet can be applied to the proximal forearm and the surgery then proceeds under forearm intravenous regional anesthesia (FIRA) (Fig. 14.6) or intravenous local anesthesia (IVLA), when patients encounter pain during the procedure.

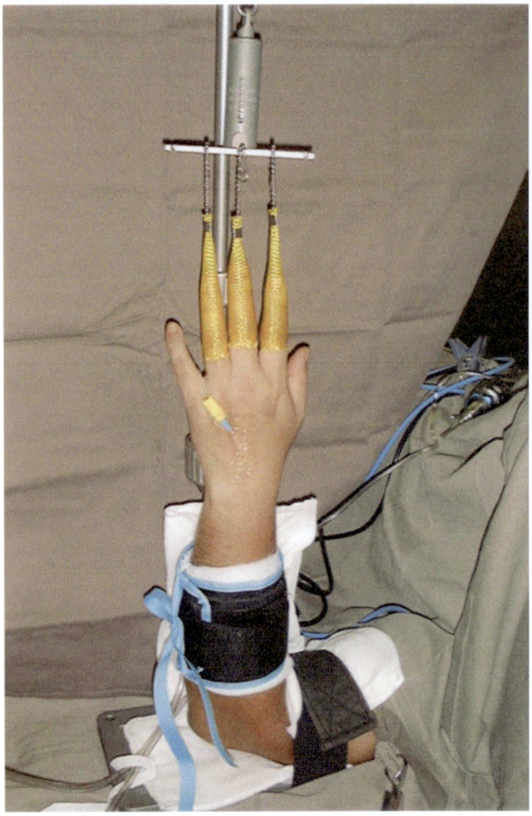

Fig. 14.6 Usually the operation can be completed under PSLA. A sterile tourniquet put at the forearm and FIRA can be used if patients encounter pain during the operation

Standard wrist arthroscopic techniques are employed. We perform routine inspection of the radiocarpal joint through 3/4 portal using 1.9 or 2.7 mm video arthroscope. The 4/5 portal is used for instrumentation. For cases with florid synovitis, additional access such as 1/2 and 6R portals need to be employed to allow more thorough and extensive synovectomy. Outflow portal is established at 6U portal just volar to the extensor carpi ulnaris tendon using 18G needle. The midcarpal joint is approached through the midcarpal radial (MCR) portal. Instruments are introduced through the midcarpal ulnar (MCU) portal. Accessory portals including scaphoid-trapezium-trapezoid STT and triquetral-hamate TH portals can be used for outflow and instrumentation.

Distal radioulnar joint (DRUJ) is also examined if there are clinical symptoms and signs of DRUJ pathology. Usually the triangular fibrocartilage complex (TFCC) has been perforated and the DRUJ can be accessed from the radiocarpal joint. A 1.9 mm arthroscope is used if separate portals for DRUJ are required (Fig. 14.7).

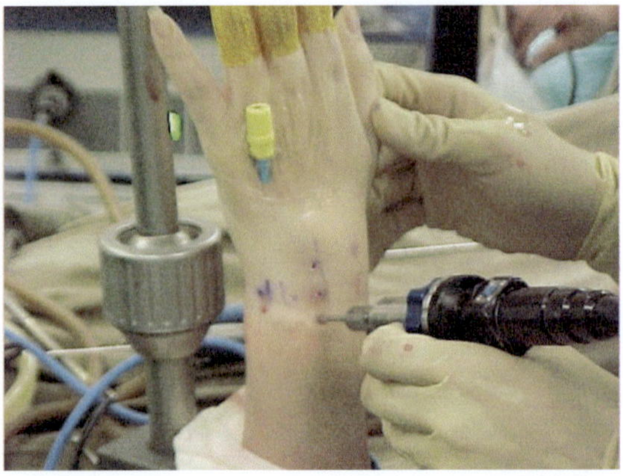

Fig. 14.7 The arthroscope is inserted to the DRUJ via the distal DRUJ portal

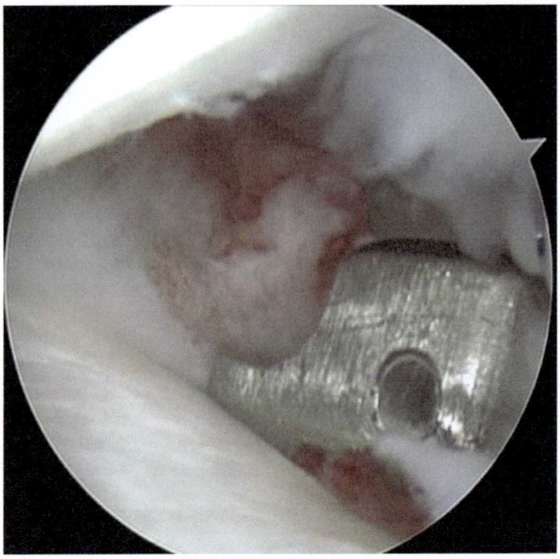

Fig. 14.8 A suction punch used to clear the synovitis and get the specimen for histo-microbiological diagnosis

Distribution of synovitis and cartilage damage is documented during initial assessment of the wrist joint. Synovectomy is then performed using punch forceps, motorized shaver system with suction, and radio-frequency probe (Fig. 14.8). All the extrinsic ligaments are carefully preserved. Radio-frequency energy is applied in short bursting mode to avoid accumulation of local heat which may damage ligaments and adjacent tendons, especially the extensor tendons. Torn TFCC is debrided of frayed tissue while the peripheral rim is preserved as far as possible. If bleeding is profuse, the instilling saline bag can be elevated higher to increase the hydrostatic pressure. Coagulation mode of the radio-frequency apparatus can also be used.

The portal sites are closed with sterile strips. Skin suture is usually not necessary. Light soft bandage is worn postoperatively, and active wrist mobilization exercise is started as soon as pain is tolerated.

Our Experience and Results

From 1997 to 2002, we did 39-wrist arthroscopic synovectomy in 30 patients with rheumatoid arthritis. They were diagnosed to have rheumatoid arthritis by rheumatologists. The average age of the patients was 39 (range 17–80). Five patients were male and 25 were female. Twenty-one right wrists and 18 left wrists were operated, and 18 dominant wrists were involved. Patients with evidence of tenosynovitis, weakened extensor tendon, or previous wrist open or arthroscopic surgery were excluded from this study group. Twenty patients were given DMARDs or biologics, whereas ten were not. They either had intolerable wrist pain and swelling despite the medications or they could not tolerate the side effects of the medications and refused them. Seven patients were diagnosed to have monoarthritis at the time of operation, whereas two of these progressed to have oligoarthritis during the follow-up period. Nine had oligoarthritis with arthritis of four or fewer joints. Fourteen had polyarthritis. The wrists were the most affected and symptomatic joints. The average duration of symptoms was 40 months (range 12–108 months). In these 30 patients, 2 patients had the wrist arthroscopic synovectomy on both wrists at the same time and operation setting

All patients received clinical and radiological assessment before and after the procedure. They were also referred to the occupational therapist for a formal wrist function assessment (Fig. 14.9). This was both an objective and subjective assessment of the activities of daily living (ADL) performance specifically designed for patients with wrist problems. We used this assessment protocol routinely in wrist pain patients since 1997 when we interviewed and studied on a group of Chinese patients having different kinds of wrist pain problems. Ten most problematic ADL tasks were identified. We found this assessment protocol was valid and reliable.

The assessment protocol consists of five elements (Fig. 14.9):

1. The ability to perform the ten ADL tasks. This is rated in five scores as shown in Table 14.1, with the higher score representing the better performance. The full score of each task is 4. The added scores for all the ten tasks is the "wrist total performance score," in which the full score is 40.

   The ten ADL tasks are listed in Table 14.2.
2. The pain perceived in performing the ten tasks. The full score is 20.
   (a) Score 2: moderate to severe pain.
   (b) Score 1: mild to moderate pain.
   (c) Score 0: no pain.

   The added score for all the ten tasks is the "total pain score," in which the full score is 20.
3. The wrist active range of motion, in flexion, extension, radial deviation, ulnar deviation, forearm supination, and forearm pronation.
4. The visual analog scale (VAS) of pain in maximum exertion, from 0 to 10, in which ten is the most severe pain.
5. The grip strength.

   Patient's overall satisfaction level after surgery was also documented.

Standard wrist X-rays were taken and arthritic changes were staged according to the five radiological grades described by Larsen-Dale-Eek (LDE) [57] (Table 14.3). The preoperative radiological staging is shown in Table 14.4.

All arthroscopic synovectomy were performed under regional or local anesthesia except three early cases which were operated under general

Prince of Wales Hospital
Occupational Therapy Department
Assessment of ADL Performance for Wrist Injury

Date					
Post-op (weeks)					
ADL Tasks by Affected Side		Performance	Pain	Performance	Pain
Wash back	(F,N,S,Rd,Ud,Pi)				
Pull out drawer 7lbs	(N,S,Gr)				
Pour out water from full pot	(N,F,Ud)				
Turn door knob/ turn key	(N,P,S)				
Open gate	(E,S)				
Lift weight 5lbs	(N,E,Ud,Gr)				
Write name	(E,Ud,Pi)				
Wring towel dry	(P,S,Gr,Ud,Rd,E,F)				
Hold a wok	(E,Ud,Gr,S)				
Open jar lid	(N,Ud,Rd,Gr)				
Total Performance Score		/40		/40	
Total Pain Score		/20		/20	
Remarks					
Overall Comment					
Wrist range		L	R	L	R
Extension					
Flexion					
Radial Deviation					
Ulnar Deviation					
Pronation					
Supination					
VAS Pain on Exertion					
Power Grip (kg)					
Lateral Pinch (kg)					

Performance
4: can do without difficulty and pain free
3: can do with minimum difficulty or pain, but with satisfactory outcome
2: can do with some modification of activities, with awkward and pain
1: pain affect the performance and the quality is poor, would stop doing it most of the time
0: cannot do at all

Pain
2: pain free in doing
1: tolerated pain in doing
0: intolerable pain in doing

Wrist/ forearm position
E Extension
F Flexion
S Supination
P Pronation
Ud Ulnar deviation
Rd Radial deviation
Gr Gripping action
Pi Pinching action
N Neutral wrist

Fig. 14.9 The wrist function assessment data sheet to be completed by occupational therapist. It consists of five elements, which are performance evaluation, pain evaluation, wrist range of motion, visual analog pain score, and grip and pinch strength

Table 14.1 Scoring system in performing the ten ADL tasks in wrist function assessment

Score 4	Can do the task without difficulty and is pain-free
Score 3	Can do with a minimum of difficulty or pain and with satisfactory outcome
Score 2	Can do with some modification of the activity; it is awkward and painful
Score 1	Pain affects the performance and the quality if poor; would stop doing it most of the time
Score 0	Cannot do the task at all

Table 14.2 The ten ADL tasks in wrist function assessment

1. Wash back
2. Pull out a drawer of 7 lbs
3. Pour out water from a full pot
4. Turn door knob/turn key
5. Open a door gate
6. Lift weight of 5 lbs
7. Write a name
8. Wring out a wet towel
9. Hold a wok
10. Open a jar lid

Table 14.3 Radiographic grading of rheumatoid arthritis according to Larsen-Dale-Eek [57]

Stage	Definition
0	No arthritic change (changes not related to arthritis may be present)
I	Slight changes: presence of one or more of the following: – Periarticular soft tissue swelling – Osteoporosis – Slight joint space narrowing
II	Definite early changes: one or several small erosions + joint space narrowing
III	Medium destructive changes: marked erosions + joint space narrowing
IV	Severe destructive changes: marked erosions + joint space narrowing + bone deformation
V	Mutilating changes: gross bone deformation + original articular surfaces disappeared

Dislocation and bony ankylosis are not considered in the grading system

Table 14.4 Preoperative and postoperative radiological staging of the wrist joint arthritis and number of grade progressed at the final follow-up

Preoperative X-ray arthritic changes (Larsen-Dale-Eek grading)	Number of wrists (% of cases)	Postoperative X-ray arthritic changes (Larsen-Dale-Eek grading)	Number of wrists (% of cases)	Number of grade progressed at the final follow-up	Number of wrists (% of cases)
I	5 (12.8)	I	3 (7.7)	0	10 (25.6)
II	10 (25.6)	II	3 (7.7)	1	19 (48.7)
III	21 (53.8)	III	8 (20.5)	2	7 (17.9)
IV	3 (7.7)	IV	16 (41.0)	3	2 (5.1)
V	0 (0)	V	9 (23.1)	4	1 (2.6)

anesthesia to allow familiarization with arthroscopic techniques. All subsequent cases were successfully completed under PSLA or regional anesthesia (IVLA/FIRA). The average operation duration was 86 min (range 60–135 min). Radiocarpal and midcarpal joints could be assessed arthroscopically in all cases even in Larsen grade III and IV arthritis. The DRUJ was explored in 26 wrists. Nine wrists required separate portals for DRUJ because of the relatively well-preserved TFCC. In the remaining 17 cases, working portals for DRUJ could be gained through 4/5 or 6R of radiocarpal joint via perforated TFCC.

Distribution and key areas of significant synovitis and cartilage damage were shown in Table 14.5 and Fig. 14.10.

Arthroscopic ulnar head ablation was performed in two cases. They had the clinical features of ulnar impaction syndrome. One case underwent arthroscopic wafer procedure, whereas the other underwent arthroscopic ulnar head hemiresection.

Table 14.5 Preoperative radiological staging of the wrist joint arthritis

Joint with synovitis and cartilage damage	% of cases
Midcarpal joint	56.8
Radiocarpal joint	86.5
Distal radioulnar joint	18.9

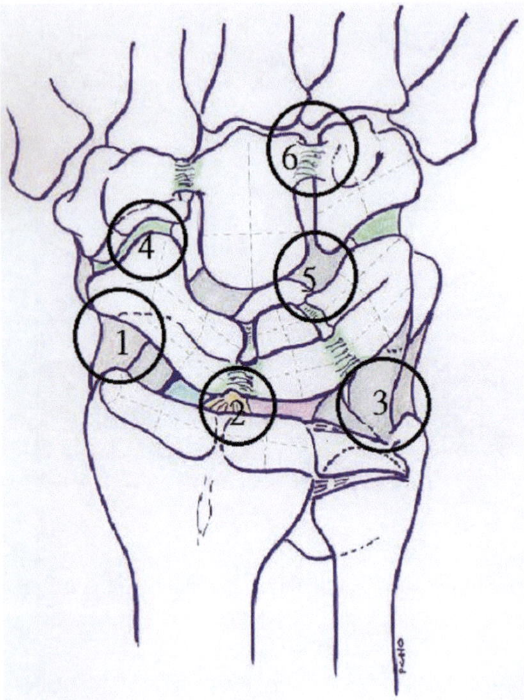

Fig. 14.10 Key areas of arthritis involvement: (1) radiostyloid region, (2) scapholunate region, (3) ulnostyloid region, (4) triscaphe region, (5) four-corner region (capitohamate and triquetrolunate), and (6) dorsal capitohamate close to carpometacarpal joint

All patients were followed up regularly for clinical, radiological, and occupational therapy assessment. Any complications and disease recurrence were noted. The average follow-up duration was 13 years (6–17.5 years). Statistical analysis was performed using Student's *t*-test and Pearson's correlation test to compare the preoperative and postoperative data and the correlations of each parameter.

All patients had significant resolution of synovial swelling within 2–3 weeks after the surgery (Fig. 14.11). VAS, total pain score, wrist total performance score, and grip strength were significantly better after the operation (Table 14.6). Only one patient experienced pain deterioration after the operation. Wrist range of motion was similar as shown in Table 14.7. There was no neurovascular or wound complication. Patient's overall satisfaction score was 7.6 over 10 (range 4–10) with ten being the most satisfied. Seven patients stopped the DMARDs at an average of 4.7 years (1–8 years) after the synovectomy because of symptomatic improvement. Seven requested the same operation on the contralateral wrists after arthroscopic synovectomy on one side. Comparing early stage (LDE grade I and II) and late stage (LDE grade III and IV) diseases, there was no statistical significant difference in the degree of improvement in VAS, total pain score, wrist total performance score, and grip strength. Seven wrists had a second arthroscopic synovectomy for recurrence of synovitis at an average of 4.3 years after the first operation (range 1–15 years) (Table 14.8). Two had open synovectomy because of the need of concurrent tenosynovectomy. Two had Sauve-Kapandji procedure, two had wrist fusion, and two had total wrist replacement. A total of 15 wrists need reoperation for recurrence of symptoms in which all seven wrists are having symptomatic and functional improvement after a second wrist arthroscopic synovectomy.

For the radiological progression (Table 14.6), preoperatively, there were 38.5 % LDE grade I and II, 61.5 % grade III and IV, and 0 % grade V. At the final follow-up, there were 15.4 % grade I and II, 61.5 % grade III and IV, and 23.1 % grade V. Ten wrists (25.6 % of all cases) did not have radiological progression at the average follow-up duration of 13 years (6–17.5 years) (Fig. 14.12), in which three wrists were of grade I and four wrists of grade III. Most of the cases (19 wrists, 48.7 %) progressed to one LDE grade, seven wrists (17.9 %) progressed to two grades, two (5.1 %) progressed to three grades, and one (2.6 %) progressed to one grade. The severity of the radiographic progression, recurrence of symptoms, and need of subsequent operations showed no correlation with the radiographic grading at the time of operation. In the 29 wrists having radiological progression, 21 wrists developed radiocarpal or midcarpal ankylosis (Figs. 14.13, 14.14, and 14.15) at

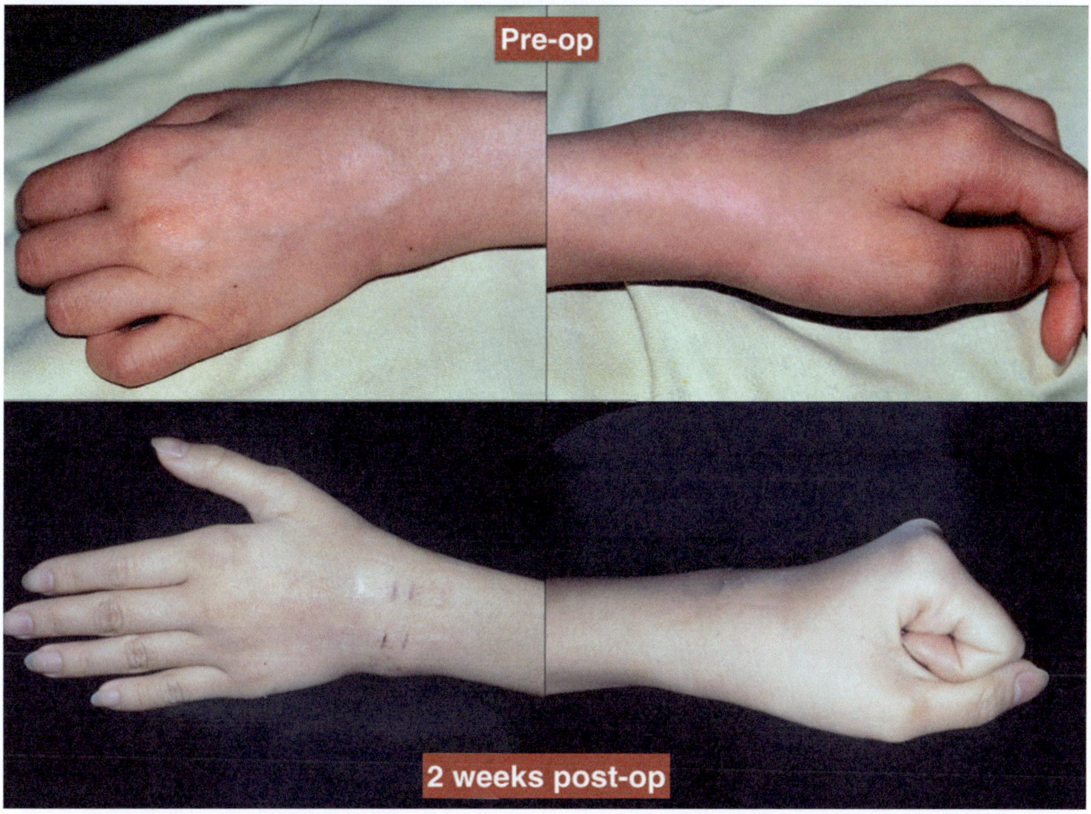

Fig. 14.11 Significant resolution of wrist synovial swelling 2 weeks after arthroscopic synovectomy in a rheumatoid patient

Table 14.6 The VAS, total pain score, wrist total performance score, and grip strength before the operation and at the final follow-up

	Preoperative value	Latest follow-up value	*p*-Value
VAS	6.1 ± 2.2	1.5 ± 2.3	0.005
Total pain score ± SD	12.9 ± 3.5	3.9 ± 6.6	0.005
Wrist total performance score ± SD	20.9 ± 8.6	31.3 ± 12.3	0.01
Grip strength (kg ± SD)	12.7 ± 8.0	23.7 ± 4.0	0.03

Table 14.7 The wrist range of motion before the operation and at the final follow-up

Range of motion (degree ± SD)	Preoperative value	Latest follow-up value	*p*-Value
Extension	42.5 ± 14.6	38.5 ± 10.1	0.03
Flexion	37.1 ± 13.3	25.3 ± 15.7	0.17
Radial deviation	10.2 ± 6.4	7.1 ± 7.0	0.18
Ulnar deviation	24.3 ± 9.5	23.2 ± 13.0	0.13
Pronation	72.3 ± 11.4	66.4 ± 15.3	0.05
Supination	72.4 ± 22.1	77.7 ± 12.5	0.08

Table 14.8 Reoperations were done for recurrence or progression of the disease as shown here

Nature of further surgery	Number of cases
Arthroscopic synovectomy	7
Open synovectomy + tenosynovectomy	2
Sauve-Kapandji procedure	2
Total wrist fusion	1
Limited wrist fusion	1
Total wrist replacement	2

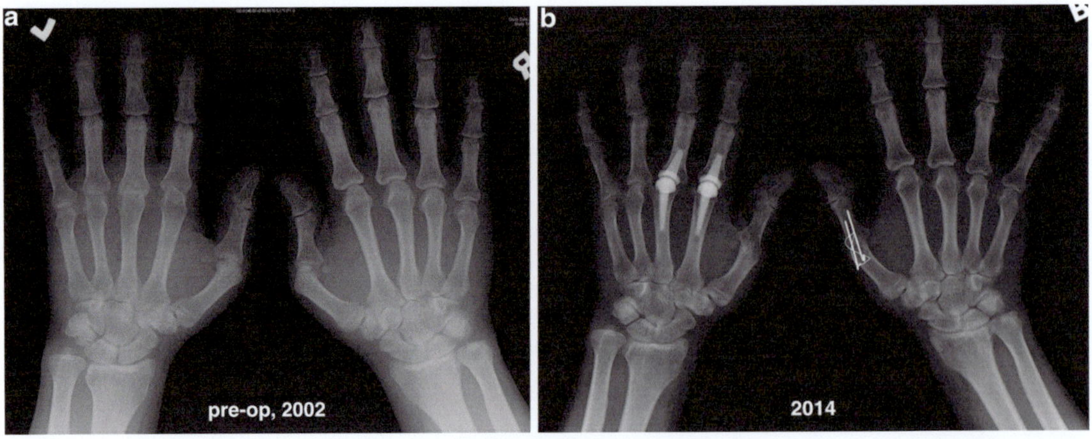

Fig. 14.12 (**a** and **b**) A 40-year-old man having bilateral wrist arthroscopic synovectomy done in 2002. There was no radiological progression 12 years after the operation. There was no wrist pain or swelling since the operation

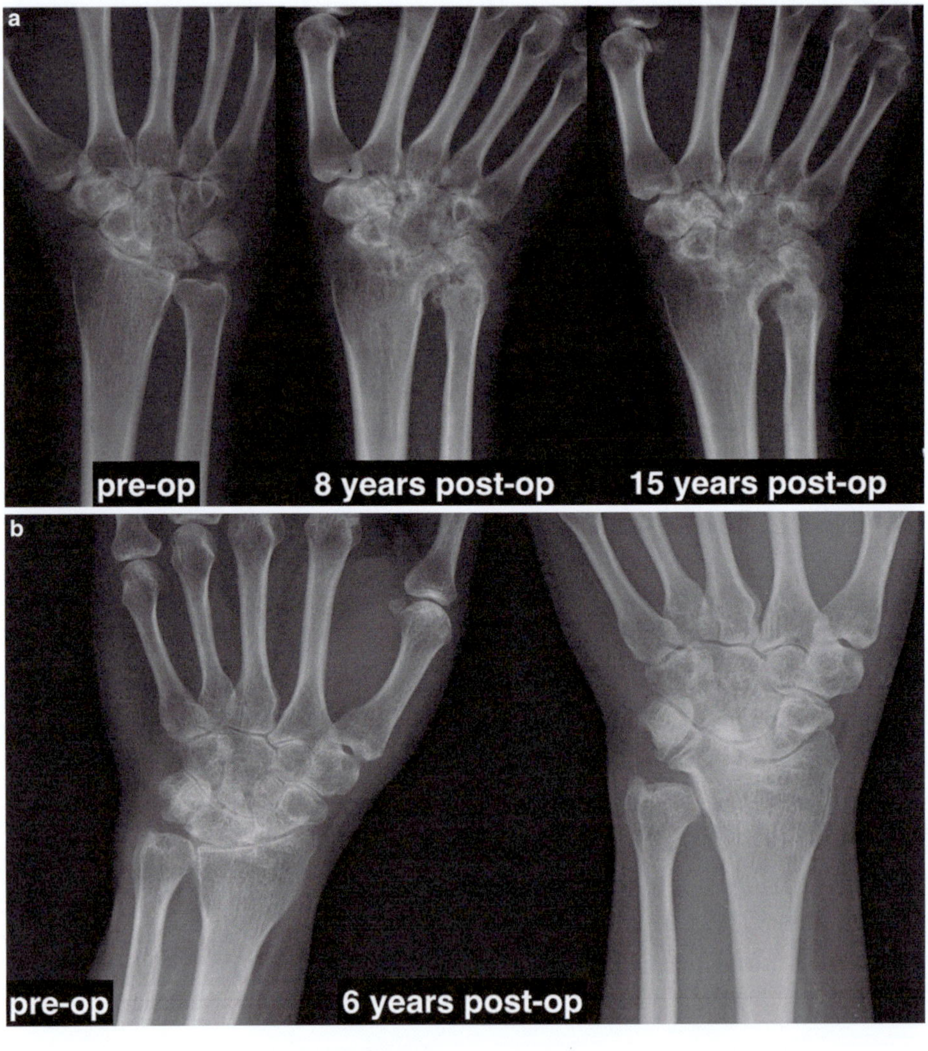

Fig. 14.13 (**a**) Solid spontaneous radioscapholunate arthrodesis was found 8 years after the arthroscopic wrist synovectomy. (**b**) Solid spontaneous radiolunate arthrodesis in a 42-year-old lady with rheumatoid arthritis 6 years after the arthroscopic wrist synovectomy

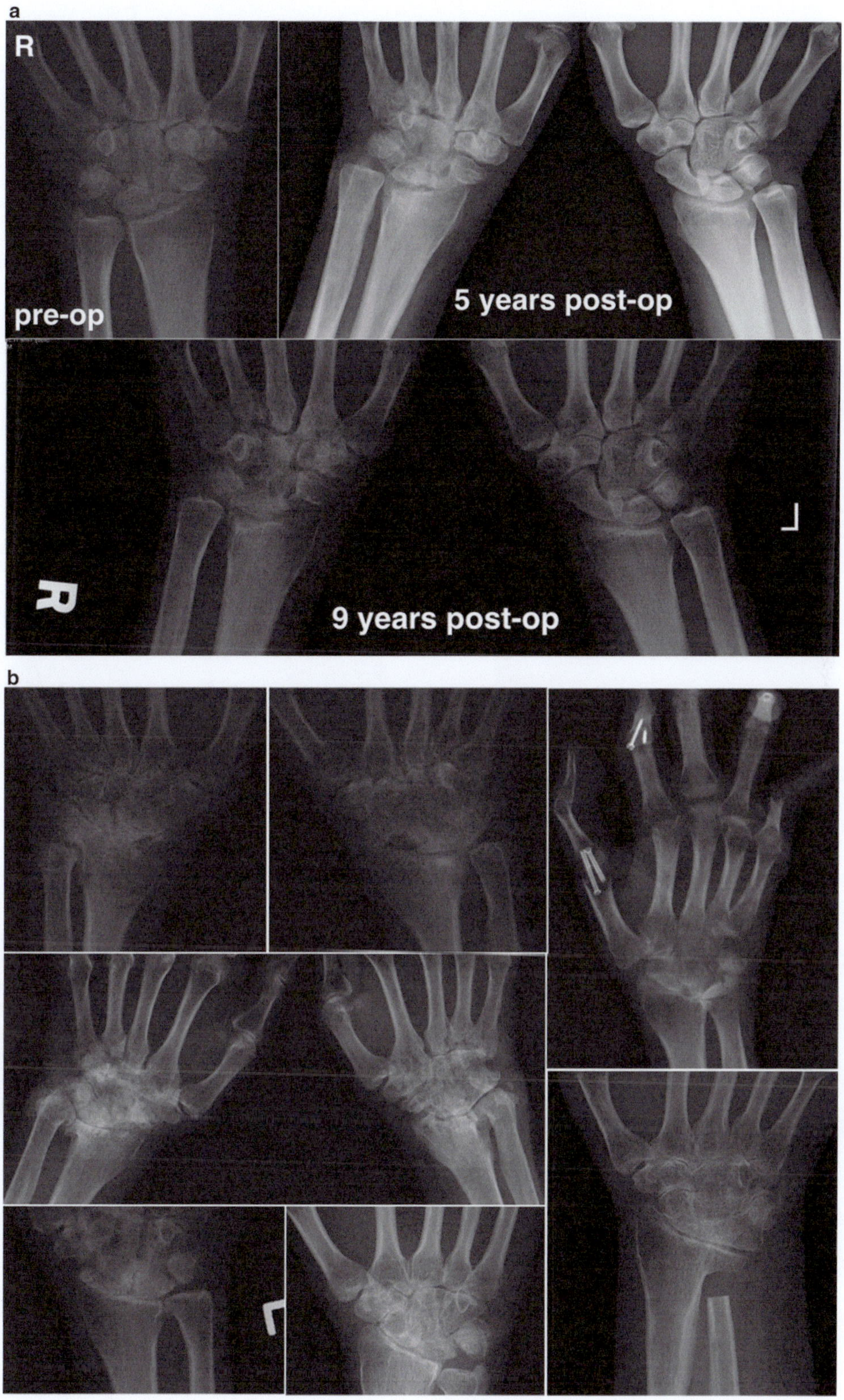

Fig. 14.14 (**a**) A 40-year-old lady with seropositive rheumatoid monoarthritis. Progressive capitolunohamate arthrodesis was observed. (**b**) Different kinds of midcarpal joint arthrodesis in our patients after arthroscopic wrist synovectomy

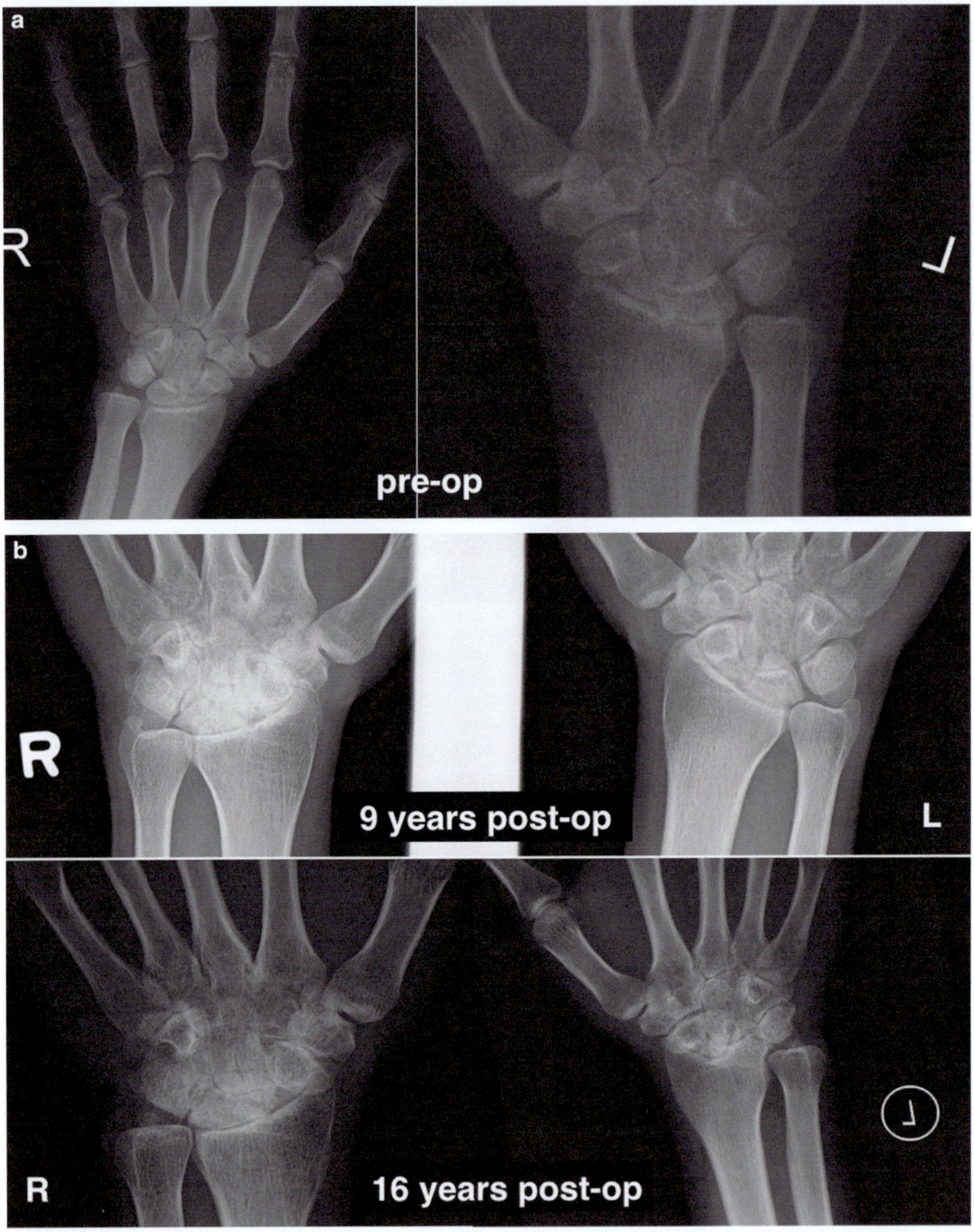

Fig. 14.15 (**a** and **b**) A 17-year-old boy who had juvenile rheumatoid arthritis affecting bilateral knees, bilateral ankles, feet, and wrists. He had bilateral arthroscopic wrist synovectomy done in 1997. He stopped the DMARDs after the operation. Definite radiological progression was seen. There was spontaneous right wrist midcarpal arthrodesis at around 6 years post-op and left radiolunate arthrodesis at 11 years post-op. He did not have any wrist pain now. His wrist total performance score was full

Table 14.9 Comparing the group (21 wrists) with midcarpal or radiocarpal joint ankylosis and the group (18 wrists) without; the group with ankylosis showed better VAS, grip strength, and wrist total performance score

	Wrists with ankylosis (21 wrists)	Wrists without ankylosis (18 wrists)	*p*-Value
VAS	0.8	2.8	0.02
Grip strength (kg)	19	10.1	0.004
Wrist total performance score	39.3	27.4	0.03

an average of 5.6 years (6 months to 11 years) after the synovectomy. When stratifying the group with ankylosis and the other with no ankylosis at the final follow-up, the group having ankylosis had significant better VAS and grip strength (Table 14.9). The wrist total performance score also improved though it was not statistically significant (Table 14.9).

Analysis on Our Results

We Had Good Outcomes After Arthroscopic Wrist Synovectomy

This is the long-term clinical results of wrist arthroscopic synovectomy for rheumatoid arthritis with an average follow-up period of 13 years (6–17.5 years) after the publications by Adolfsson et al. (1993) (6 months of follow-up) [9], Adolfsson et al. (1997) (3.8 years of follow-up) [11], Park et al. (2003) (2.4 years of follow-up) [13], Kim et al. (2006) (5.8 years of follow-up) [14], and Lee et al. (2014) (7.9 years of follow-up) [15]. We reported similar good results as them. VAS, wrist total performance score, and grip strength were significantly improved except one patient who did not have pain improvement. High patient satisfaction was gained. Seven patients requested the same operation for the other wrists, and seven stopped the DMARDs after the relief of their symptoms. There was no radiologic progression in ten wrists after the operations, in which two of them had all along no DMARDs, whereas three of them stopped the medications after the operation.

Clinical and Radiological Outcomes Were Not Associated with the Radiological Grading Preoperatively and We Had Good Outcomes in Both Early and Late Arthritis

It is well known that the best results of synovectomy are seen in the early stages of rheumatoid arthritis [11, 58, 59]. In the knee joint, many reports of long-term successful results from synovectomy were limited to chronically painful and swollen joints with early radiographic changes [60–62]. For the open wrist synovectomy, however, Chalmers reported that pain scores or need for subsequent arthroplasty did not correlate with the preoperative radiographic findings and joint changes [63]. Thirupathi also found that there was no significant relationship between radiological progression, in terms of carpal translocation or collapse, and the preoperative stage of disease [54]. The wrist is not a weight-bearing joint as opposed to the joints of the lower limb; therefore, it can cope well with applied loads during activities. The benefits of synovectomy therefore could be extended to patients with wrists of advanced grading. Nevertheless, for arthroscopic wrist synovectomy, Adolfsson et al. recruited 18 wrists in 16 patients, with radiographic changes more severe than LDE grade III excluded, and reported the arthroscopic results in 1993 [9]. In 1997, he concluded that the progression of arthritis was significantly less common in patients with no or very early changes at the time of surgery in his 24 wrists in 19 patients [11]. Until 2001, Park et al. studied the results of arthroscopic synovectomy in 19 wrists in 18 patients [13]. Though there was only one patient in LDE grade III disease and one in grade IV disease in his study, he suggested that the stage of radiological change before surgery did not correlate significantly with the clinical results. In 2006, Kim et al. studied the results of arthroscopic wrist synovectomy in advanced rheumatoid arthritis [14]. He noticed that patients with advanced radiographic changes and joint space narrowing had satisfactory surgical and clinical results after synovectomy. Though the 18 patients (19 wrists) he recruited were only limited to LDE grade III or less, he found that radiographic stage was not related to clinical outcomes. In the latest publication in 2014 by Lee et al., he analyzed his results with arthroscopic wrist synovectomy done in an average of 7.9 years of follow-up that an earlier radiologic stage did not indicate better clinical outcomes or less recurrence [15]. Although advanced arthritis with deformity LDE grade IV or V was excluded in the final 56 wrists in 49 patients, he advocated arthroscopic surgery even in wrists with advanced radiographic changes.

In our study, we had more than half of the patients with LDE grade III disease (21 wrists, 53.8 %) and three wrists with grade IV disease (7.5 %). Satisfactory results were demonstrated in both the early and late arthritis (LDE grade I and II versus grade III and IV). Clinical or radiological disease progression also did not show any correlation with the radiographic grading at the time of operation. Although the outcomes in advanced disease are not consistent in the literatures so far, our favorable results encouraged us operating on them. Given the less predictable disease course in patients with advanced diseases following arthroscopic synovectomy, restricting the procedure only to early disease would unfairly deny patients with advanced disease the pain and function improvement they could obtain, which we have shown to be not inferior to that obtained by patients with early disease. This is more so given the excellent risk-benefit ratio of the minimal invasive procedure compared with the existing options for advanced disease as there was no complication noted and most of the patients were satisfied with this operation.

Arthroscopic Wrist Synovectomy Could Be Done Under Local or Regional Anesthesia That Made Operation Safer for Rheumatoid Patients

Under the PSLA or combined FIRA/IVLA, patients could tolerate the procedure for an average operation time of 86 min. One case was even performed totally under PSLA without a tourniquet for 135 min. These techniques made arthroscopic synovectomy feasible under regional anesthesia and especially beneficial for rheumatoid patients with cervical spine instability and general anesthesia can be avoided.

Technically, Arthroscopic Wrist Synovectomy Was Easy for Even Advanced Arthritis

The procedure was technically possible even in advanced disease with extremely narrowed joint spaces shown in the radiographs. Capsular laxity conferred by the disease process enabled sufficient joint distension upon digital traction and saline irrigation. Feasibility for arthroscopy could also be predicted preoperatively by assessing the joint space under manual traction with an image intensifier (Fig. 14.1).

Technically, Arthroscopic Work in DRUJ Was Easy and Feasible and Gave Good Success

The portals for DRUJ were easier to be developed in rheumatoid patients. The process of synovitis distended the DRUJ and gave a spacious environment for the arthroscopic instruments to work. However, separate portals for DRUJ were not always required as the TFCC was usually perforated in late stage arthritis. Working portals for DRUJ could be gained through portals for the radiocarpal joint via perforated TFCC. Early results in our series were encouraging with good relief of DRUJ symptoms. Moreover, arthroscopic ulnar head ablation could be performed at the same time if patients experienced features of ulnar impaction syndrome. The two patients showed good forearm rotation without symptomatic DRUJ instability or ulnar impingement at the final follow-up.

Midcarpal Joints Were Not Spared and Were Commonly Involved in Our Series

In contrast to the usual findings of relatively spared and protected from destructive changes in midcarpal joint in rheumatoid arthritis [11, 64, 65], 56.8 % of our cases showed midcarpal joint involvement. This contradicted the hypothesis that midcarpal joint disease was spread from radiocarpal joint via triquetrolunate joint [66]. We showed that the key areas of midcarpal joint involvement were the triscaphe region, four-corner region (capitohamate and triquetrolunate junction), and finally dorsal aspect of the capitohamate junction near the carpometacarpal joint. The last area had not been mentioned in the literature and it did contribute partly to dorsal wrist swelling detected clinically.

There Was Radiological Progression and Clinical Recurrence in Our Series: Radiological Progression Was Not Correlated with the Clinical Outcomes and MidCarpal or Radiocarpal Joint Ankylosis Was Present in the Majority of Cases with Radiological Progression and Showed Better Clinical Outcomes

Basic sciences demonstrated the local and systemic destructive nature of the diseased synovium in rheumatoid arthritis as mentioned previously. Synovectomy theoretically helps to arrest or slow progression and sometimes allows erosive lesions to heal. Improvement in radiological appearance, with disappearance of the erosive lesions and restoration of joint space, had been reported after synovectomy since 1965 by Wilkinson et al. [7]. He believed that following synovectomy for rheumatoid arthritis, new synovial tissue was formed, capable of dialysis of synovial fluid. Nutrition of cartilage was restored and the removal of necrotic tissue favored revascularization, which explained the postoperative better radiological appearance in his cases. However, in our series, 29 wrists (74.4 %) had radiological progression and 13 wrists (33.3 %) had clinical recurrence of synovitis, which corresponded to previous studies showing that disease progression and recurrence were always possible after synovectomy [9–15]. Nevertheless, it is interesting to notice that in the 29 wrists having radiological progression, only seven (24.1 %) of them had recurrence of symptoms of pain and swelling. Statistical analysis showed that radiological progression to a higher grade was not associated with poor clinical outcomes. This echoed the finding by Kim et al. that nine patients had progression of their arthritis to a higher radiographic grade even though clinical symptoms improved [14]. More interestingly, in these 29 wrists, 21 (72.4 %) of them developed midcarpal or radiocarpal ankylosis at an average of 5.6 years (6 months to 11 years) after the synovectomy (Figs. 14.13, 14.14, and 14.15). Our follow-up duration was long enough to let us observe this phenomenon. That means 54 % of all the 39 wrists were found to have spontaneous arthrodesis of the midcarpal or radiocarpal joints in our series. This differs greatly from the data presented by Lee KH in the 68th Annual Meeting of the ASSH in 2013 that there were a total of 24.8 % of the 213 wrists in 164 patients having spontaneous midcarpal (18.3 %) or radiocarpal (6.5 %) arthrodesis [67]. Statistical analysis revealed that the group with ankylosis had significant better VAS and grip strength and improved wrist total performance score. Removing the diseased synovium helped to retard the erosion of the articular surface and surrounding joint ligaments. This conferred stability of the wrist joint lets the bare bone surfaces get in touch with each other and might therefore result in ankylosis. Mechanical pain from bone-to-bone articulation and stretching of the ligaments could then be eliminated after ankylosis, which might explain the better performance in this group of patients. Although ankylosis created a stiff joint, a significant deterioration of range of motion was not found. Probably, wrist pain had already limited their preoperative wrist range of motion. This ankylosis phenomenon may demonstrate one indirect mechanism arthroscopic wrist synovectomy offers to relieve symptoms and improve function.

There Were Many Monoarthritis Cases in Our Series and Rheumatoid Monoarthritis May be Especially Benefited from Arthroscopic Wrist Synovectomy

Monoarthritis due to rheumatoid arthritis is quite rare [68]. It may represent an early stage of the systemic disease and progress to oligoarthritis or polyarthritis with time. In our series, there were relatively a large proportion of patients (Fig. 14.14a), seven patients (23.3 %) having monoarthritis, in which only one patient was put on an antirheumatic drug, two stopped it after the operation, and four had never received any disease-modifying agent. Only two of them progressed to oligoarthritis during the 16 years of follow-up. We were unable to determine the reason for the relatively higher percentage of monoarthritis in our series. It could be that they were identified and operated early, and the spread to other joints was retarded by the systemic effect of synovectomy as mentioned previously [8]. Nevertheless, rheumatoid patients having monoarthritis may especially benefit from wrist arthroscopic synovectomy, which may help to retard the amplification of the disease locally at that joint, provide early relief of symptoms and improvement in function, give more diagnostic clue to guide treatment early, and exempt them from disease-modifying antirheumatic drugs if local disease is well controlled.

Arthroscopic Wrist Synovectomy Shared the Same Advantages of a Minimal Invasive Surgery

The findings in our series indicated that arthroscopic synovectomy for rheumatoid arthritis is effective in providing long-term pain relief, functional improvement, and grip strength even in advanced condition. It is well known that open procedures are relatively major trauma with consequent discomfort for the patient, longer rehabilitation, longer hospital stay, and risk of postoperative joint stiffness [53, 69–71]. Our patients having arthroscopic procedures had smaller incision, wrist joint capsulo-ligamentous structures preserved, minimal postoperative pain, no postoperative stiffness, no need for hospital stay or formal rehabilitation, and high patient satisfaction.

Other Applications

Besides synovectomy, with the advancement of arthroscopic techniques, the surgical application is extended to the reconstructive procedures in rheumatoid wrist. The following are the examples.

Arthroscopic Wafer Procedure

Patients with rheumatoid arthritis usually have ulnar wrist pain. It can be caused by ulnocarpal synovitis, DRUJ arthritis, and ulnocarpal impaction syndrome. Ulnocarpal impaction happens not only in those with preexisting ulnar plus variance but also in rheumatoid wrists having ulnar translation or bony deformity resulted in decreasing distance between ulnar head and the ulnar-sided carpal bones. TFCC is usually perforated and arthroscopic wafer procedure can be performed by passing a motorized bur through the radiocarpal joint (4/5 portal or 6R portal) via the perforated TFCC while viewing through the 3/4 portal. Perforated TFCC is first debrided, smoothened, and enlarged. The ulnar head is beveled with care to preserve the part articulating with the sigmoid notch. DRUJ synovitis is debrided. Pronation-supination movements are made to ensure even resection of the anterior and posterior parts of the ulnar head while respecting the DRUJ.

Arthroscopic Hemiresection of Ulnar Head

DRUJ is most commonly affected of the three articulations of the wrist, with 78 % of patients having evidence of rheumatoid arthritis in DRUJ at the late radiographic follow-up [72]. Progressive synovitis disrupts and attenuates the ulnocarpal and radioulnar ligaments, and TFCC results in DRUJ instability and subsequently caput ulna syndrome and extensor tendon ruptures. Bony erosions at the DRUJ result in ulnar impingement syndrome and radiographic appearance of scallop sign of sigmoid notch erosion. Early DRUJ synovectomy and soft tissue balancing procedures help to avoid the above sequelae. For established DRUJ erosive changes, osseous procedures are targeted to treat the pain and stiffness at forearm rotation, by clearing the bony contact between the radius and ulna. This can be done by complete (Darrach procedure) or partial resection of the distal ulna (hemiresection interposition arthroplasty, matched distal ulna hemiresection), fusing the joint (Sauve-Kapandji procedure), or replacing the distal ulna. In 1912, Darrach first performed a resection of the distal ulna for an unreduced dislocation of the distal ulna [73]. Several soft tissue procedures, using free tendon grafts, extensor carpi ulnaris (ECU), flexor carpi ulnaris, joint capsule, or pronator quadratus, have also been described to stabilize the ulnar stump. However, ulnar stump instability, impingement, pain, and snapping were still reported [74, 75]. Removal of the distal ulna also predisposes the carpus to ulnar-sided translation [76], acceleration of carpal supination deformity [77], ECU rupture [78], and grip weakness [79, 80]. Kingman determined that the only factor that correlated with better results was preserving more distal ulna bone [81]. Ulnar styloid tends to be retained to preserve the adjacent ligaments and TFCC insertion. In 1936, Sauve and Kapandji described arthrodesis of the DRUJ and distal ulnar pseudoarthrosis, which preserved the whole ulnar head [82]. It provides a buttress to prevent carpal translation and maintain normal load sharing between the ulna and carpus while enabling forearm rotation. However, problems of nonunion or delayed union of the arthrodesis, fibrous or osseous union at the pseudoarthrosis, painful instability of the proximal ulna stump, and painful wrist motion and stiffness were not uncommonly reported [83]. In 1985, Bowers described the modification of ulnar head resection, hemiresection interposition arthroplasty, in which only a portion of the distal ulna was removed, leaving intact the radioulnar and ulnar carpal ligaments as well as the TFCC in an effort to preserve the stability of the remaining ulna [75]. He also described interposing tendon, muscle, or dorsal capsule in the resected area. In 1992, Watson and Gabuzda described a further modification of distal ulnar resection, matched distal ulnar hemiresection [84]. Although the ulnar styloid and most of the head of the ulna are removed, ulnar length is preserved to the level of the radial articular surface, and the distal ulnar shaft is tapered to avoid impingement on the radius or ulnar carpus while exposing maximal cancellous bone so that the ulnocarpal ligaments can reattach to the ulnar remnant. Favorable long-term results were reported in various series when more ulnar head bone was preserved [75, 81, 84–89].

Arthroscopic hemiresection of the ulnar head serves the purpose of clearing the painful bony contact between the radius and ulna while meticulously preserving more ulnar head bone and surrounding stabilizing soft tissues and therefore minimizing the above complications. Because it can be performed under local anesthesia, any catching or uneven surface can be smoothened to make sure that there is no radioulnar impingement at both active and passive wrist and forearm movement. With the soft tissue structures preserved in the arthroscopic approach, interposition procedure is obviated (Fig. 14.16) (Video 14.1).

Arthroscopic TFCC Reconstruction

The synovitis process destroys and invades TFCC and radioulnar ligaments, resulting in destabilization of the DRUJ. Instability of DRUJ produces painful forearm rotation, ruptures extensor tendons, and exacerbates bony erosions at the DRUJ. Early synovectomy and DRUJ stabilization procedures help to avoid the above sequelae.

Arthroscopic TFCC reconstruction is advocated for the chronic DRUJ instability with the absence of DRUJ erosion [90]. TFCC is the most important stabilizer of DRUJ but the other secondary stabilizers also contribute significantly. Arthroscopic technique gives minimal surgical dissection while preserving the anatomical integrity and vascular supply of the delicate structures around the DRUJ. This is especially important to the rheumatoid patients when the postoperative pain is less and rehabilitation is faster.

The operation is performed under general anesthesia or brachial plexus block. Standard arthroscopic setup, small joint arthroscopic graspers of 2–3 mm, cannulated drills, and a fluoroscopic image intensifier are required. There are seven surgical steps:

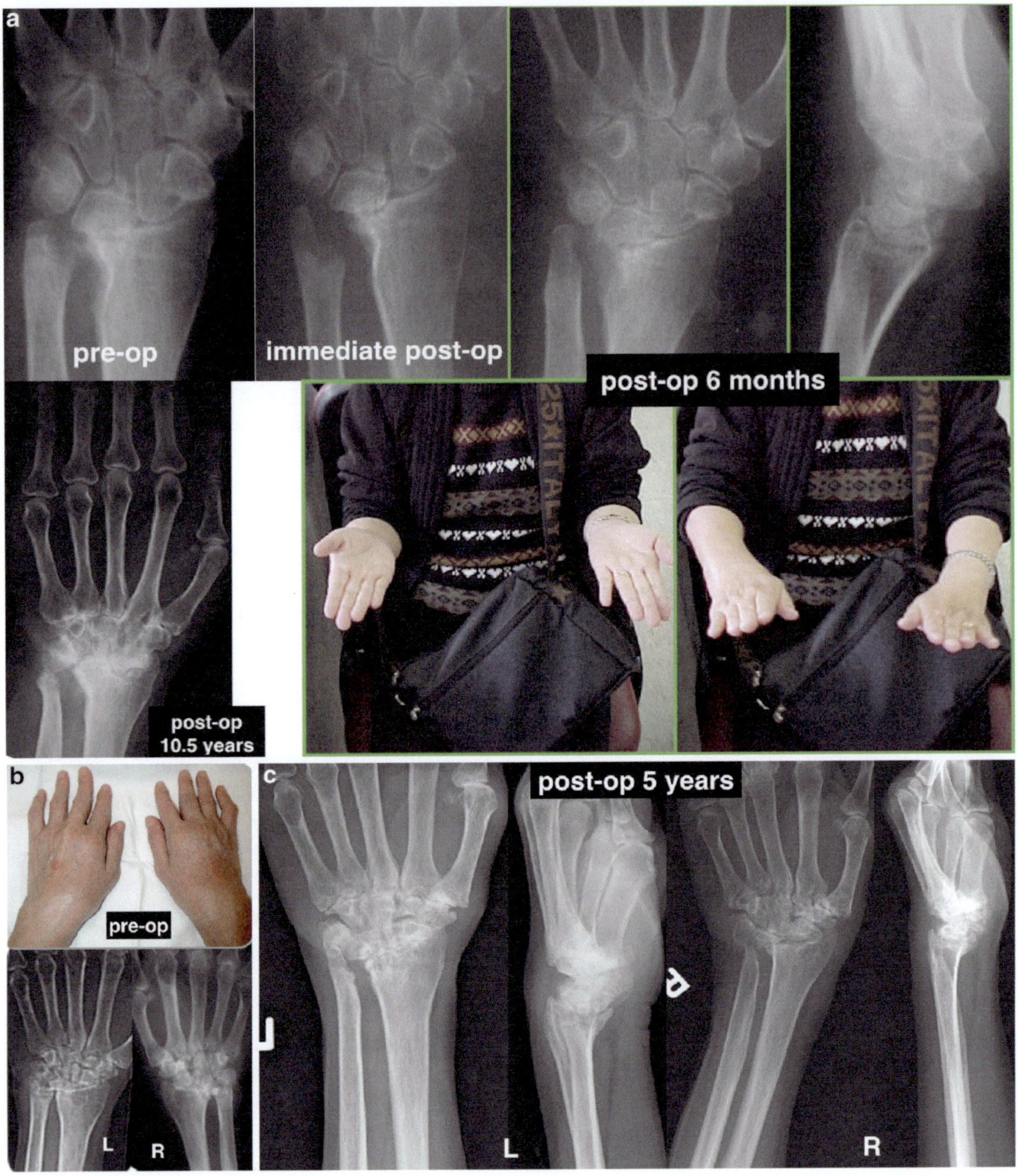

Fig. 14.16 (**a**) A 62-year-old lady with rheumatoid arthritis and significant right DRUJ pain and swelling and forearm stiffness. Arthroscopic hemiresection of ulnar head was done. The DRUJ symptoms were resolved for long and forearm range of motion was satisfactory. She had DMARDs stopped 1 year after the operation as they impaired liver function (Video 14.1). (**b** and **c**) A 54-year-old lady with rheumatoid arthritis and bilateral wrist swelling and painful wrist and forearm motion, which were not well controlled with medications. Bilateral arthroscopic synovectomy and hemiresection ulnar head excision were done. She had the right side operated first and requested the same operation for the left wrist (Video 14.2)

1. Arthroscopic synovectomy + TFCC central hole preparation (Fig. 14.17a)
2. Harvesting palmaris longus (PL) graft
3. Radial (sigmoid notch) tunnel preparation with passage of the PL graft through the radial tunnel (Fig. 14.17b)
4. Ulnar tunnel preparation (Fig. 14.17c)
5. Volar graft limb returning to the joint and exteriorizing through ulna head and tunnel (Fig. 14.17d)
6. Dorsal graft limb returning to the joint and exteriorizing through the ulnar head and tunnel (Fig. 14.17e)
7. Tensioning of the PL graft and tying around ulnar neck (Fig. 14.17f, g)

For surgical details, please refer to Tse et al. [90].

Arthroscopic Limited Wrist Fusion/ Total Wrist Fusion

Limited and total wrist fusions are two well-known treatment options for uncontrollable, painful, unstable, and deformed rheumatoid wrists. Progressive wrist joint destruction results in shortening and joint instability which cause pain, a significant loss of strength, and disability. Both wrist stability and mobility are indispensable for good hand function. However, in this scenario, priority has to be given to a painless and stable wrist to restore the function. Partial wrist fusion is indicated to the wrists in which only part of the articulating system is particularly affected and is not controlled with synovectomy,

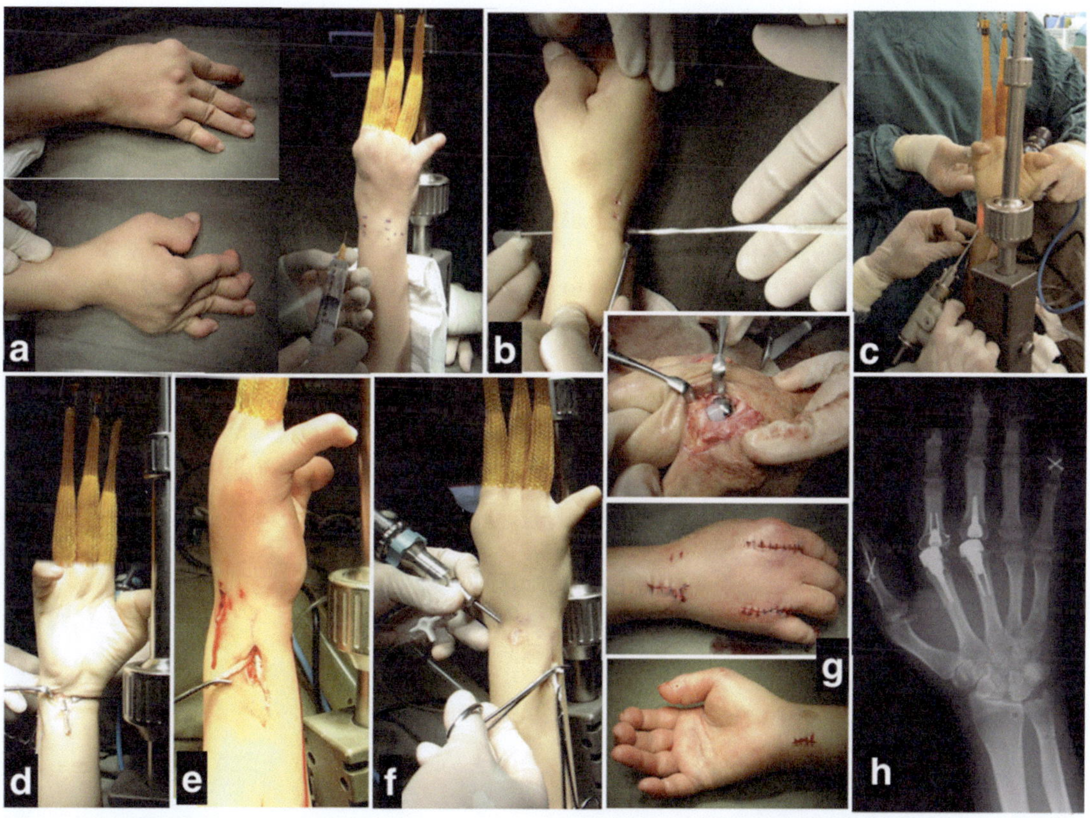

Fig. 14.17 (**a**) TFCC reconstruction in a rheumatoid wrist with DRUJ instability. The wrist joint was inspected under PSLA. (**b**) PL tendon graft was passed through the radial tunnel. (**c**) Ulnar tunnel was prepared. (**d**) Volar limb of the PL tendon graft returned to the ulnocarpal joint. (**e**) Both dorsal and volar limbs of the tendon graft had passed through the ulnar tunnel. (**f**) Tensioning and tightening of the 2 limbs and confirmed with arthroscope. (**g**) She also had joint replacement and reconstruction at the same operation setting. (**h**) Pos-operative X-ray showing the bone tunnels of the radius and ulna where the tendon graft passed

while the rheumatoid disease progression should also be optimally controlled by DMARDs and should not be at an active proliferative phase before the operation. Study showed that wrist arthrodesis in patients with low disease activity of rheumatoid arthritis yielded better results than previously reported for the union rate, postoperative flexion and extension arc, and radiological LDE grade [91]. The use of DMARDs and biologicals also helps to limit the use and reduce the dosage of steroid which has an adverse effect on bone quality and bone union [92, 93]. The wrist is composed of multiple bony linkages from the forearm to the metacarpus via the carpal bones. This anatomical peculiarity offers an opportunity to allow fusion of the painful diseased segments of the wrist while preserving motion in the other unaffected segments. The partial wrist fusion also helps to halt any predictable mechanical collapse of the carpal column and maintain carpal height in the presence of ligament or bony destructions (Fig. 14.18). In fact, the concept of partial wrist fusion in the rheumatoid wrist was first described by Chamay [94], a radiolunate fusion. It is an effective procedure to obtain reduction of the lunate, correct carpal malalignment, relieve pain, and retain some flexion and extension. In case of excessive damage to the radiocarpal joint, then radiolunate fusion is expanded to radioscapholunate fusion. When the bony resorption is so extensive that the lunate is gone, total wrist fusion is advocated.

Arthroscopic version of wrist fusion is a particular good option for rheumatoid patients who would have less postoperative pain, faster recovery, higher union rate, and low complications [95]. Union of arthrodesis should not be a problem in rheumatoid patients. High union rate of wrist arthrodesis by means of rods or pins was reported [96, 97]. In rheumatoid arthritis, poor bone quality and cortical thinning due to endosteal resorption are not conducive to the insertion of plates and screws. They also have thin and fragile skin that prominent plates may need to be removed [97]. A potential for fracture through screw holes following plate removal has also been noted [98]. Complications at the carpometacarpal joint and extensor tendon synovitis due to prominent implant material have been described [99]. Arthroscopic techniques using embedded percutaneous K-wire or screw fixation eliminate the above problems while giving the least surgical trauma and dissection and promoting vascularity and bony union.

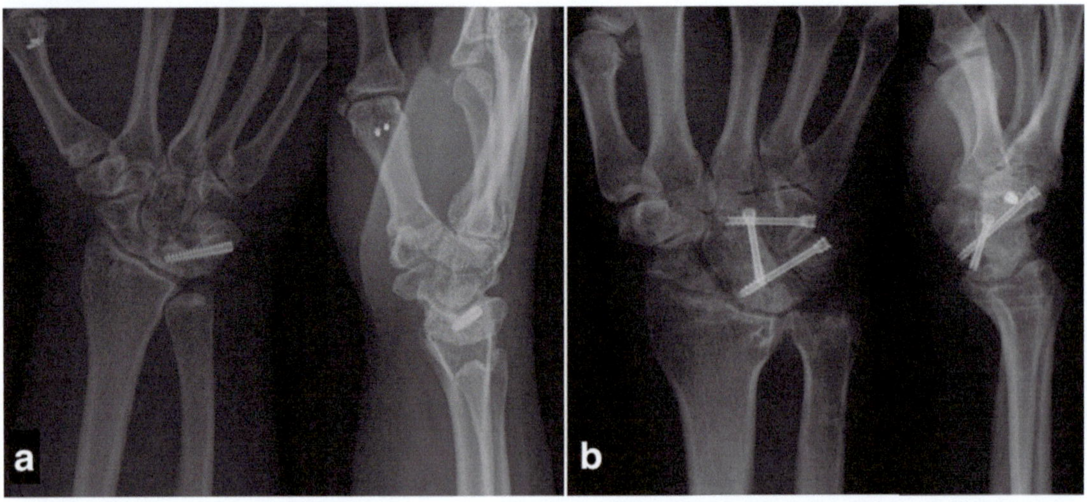

Fig. 14.18 (**a**) A rheumatoid patient having wrist synovitis particularly affecting the lunotriquetral joint with lunotriquetral instability and pain. Arthroscopic lunotriquetral fusion was done. (**b**) Another rheumatoid patient having wrist synovitis mainly affecting the midcarpal joint and chronic DRUJ instability. Arthroscopic four-corner fusion was done in addition to the TFCC reconstruction

The operation is performed under general anesthesia or plexus anesthesia, if no autologous bone grafting from the iliac crest is necessary. Fluoroscopy should be available. The list of essential instruments includes standard arthroscopy set, a motorized full-radius shaver and bur system of diameters ranging from 2.0 mm to 3.5 mm, small angled and ring curettes, 2.5 mm suction punch, radio-frequency thermal ablation system, and small cannulated screw system or K-wires. Foley catheter is sometimes necessary to block spillage of bone graft away from the fusion site. A tourniquet is applied but not inflated routinely and most of the procedures can be done without the use of a tourniquet. The surgical steps in arthroscopic wrist fusion include the following (Figs. 14.19 and 14.20):

1. Arthroscopic surveillance.
   - Assessment of both the radiocarpal and midcarpal joints to evaluate the status of the interosseous ligaments, synovitis, and articular cartilage of the joints intended to be fused.
2. Arthroscopic synovectomy.
3. Residual cartilage denudation and contouring of the opposing bone surfaces at the fusion site.
   - The extent and depth of cartilage denudation should be precisely controlled using 2.9 mm arthroscopic bur. There should be maximal preservation of the subchondral bone so as to maintain the carpal height. Burring is completed when the subchondral cancellous bone with healthy punctate bleeding is reached. This phenomenon is easily observed if the tourniquet is not inflated. Usually the bleeding is not profuse and can be well controlled with the hydrostatic pressure maintained through the irrigation system.
4. Correct carpal deformity.
   - Carpal malalignment is closely reduced and held with percutaneous K-wire. The tract should be carefully dissected bluntly to avoid iatrogenic injury or tethering of the extensor tendons during the introduction of K-wire through the skin, especially in rheumatoid patients with weak extensor tendons.
5. Provisional fixation at the fusion site.
   - The wrist is released from the traction tower and K-wires are inserted across the fusion site. The K-wires can be used as definitive fixation device or used as a guide pin for subsequent conversion to percutaneous cannulated screw fixation. The K-wires are then withdrawn from the fusion site but still left in the carpus or distal radius.
6. Augmentation of the fusion site with bone graft or bone substitute.
   - Autologous bone graft or artificial bone substitute is frequently required to fill up the voids between the opposing bone surfaces. If the vascularity and the bone quality of the fusing bone are adequate, autologous cancellous bone graft is not essential and there is an increasing role of using bone substitute to reduce the potential donor site morbidity with similar outcomes. In order to prevent spillage of the graft inside the joint to undesirable compartments, a French 6 Foley catheter can be inserted and the inflated balloon helps to block the flow of the bone graft. The wrist is put up to the traction tower again. Bone graft can then be passed through an arthroscopic cannula introduced through a working portal. The bone graft is impacted with the trocar until satisfactory amount of graft is achieved.
7. Definitive fixation.
   - The wrist is taken off from the traction tower. Definitive fixation is done by driving the provisional K-wires forwards across the fusion site. If cannulated screws are used, the K-wires serve as the guide pins. Percutaneous K-wires should then be cut short and buried underneath the skin. They are removed under local anesthesia when the bone healing is complete.

The incision wounds are opposed with Steri-Strips or simple sutures. Comfortable compression dressing and short arm slab are applied.

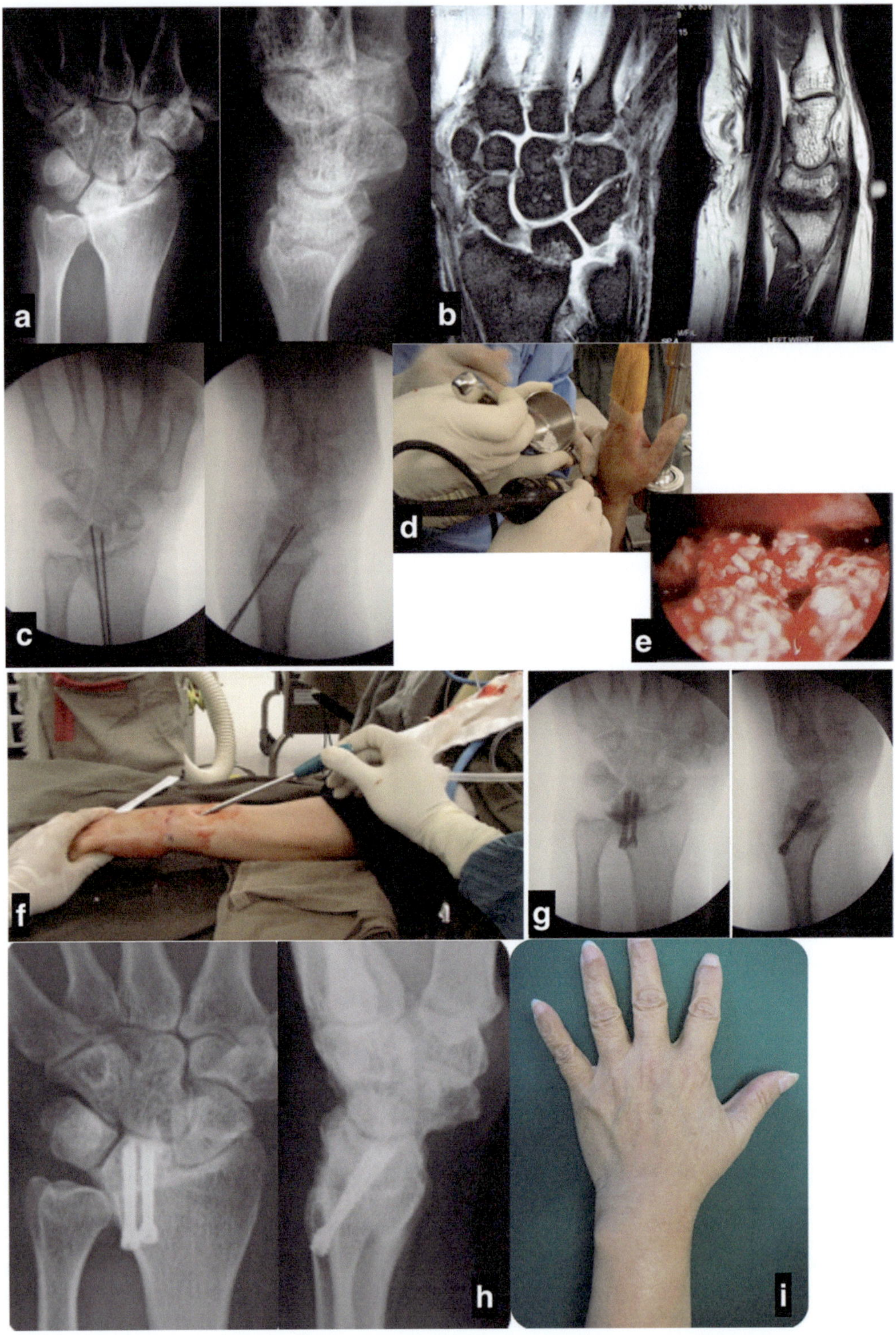

Fig. 14.19 A 53-year-old rheumatoid patient with left wrist pain and stiffness for 5 years. X-ray and MRI showed that the radiolunate joint was particularly affected. Arthroscopic radiolunate joint fusion with percutaneous cannulated screws and bone substitute was done (Videos 14.3 and 14.4). (**a**) Preoperative X-rays. (**b**) Preoperative MRI. (**c**) After arthroscopic synovectomy and burring of the fusion site, preliminary K-wires were inserted across the fusion site. (**d**) Artificial bone graft was inserted along an arthroscopic trocar cannula to the fusion site. (**e**) Appearance of the bone graft at the fusion site. (**f**) Percutaneous cannulated screw was inserted. (**g**) Immediate postoperative X-rays. (**h**) X-rays at 9 months post-op. (**i**) Inconspicuous scar and minimal wrist swelling

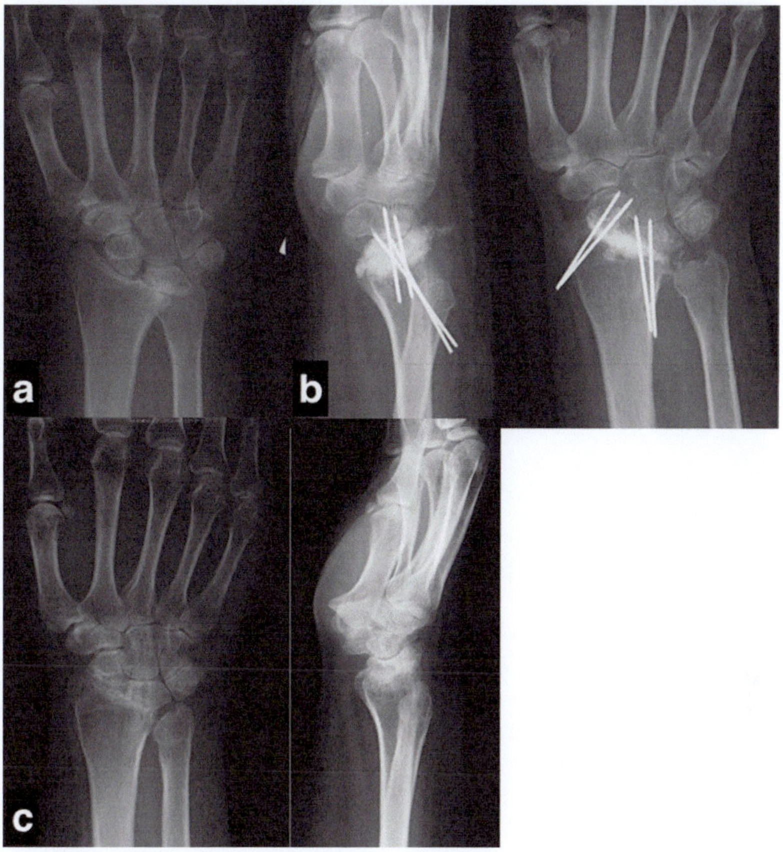

Fig. 14.20 A 58-year-old lady with rheumatoid wrist having painful wrist motion and forearm rotation. There was mild volar subluxation and ulnar translation of the lunate. Arthroscopic wafer procedure in addition to arthroscopic radioscapholunate fusion with the use of K-wires and artificial bone substitutes was done (Videos 14.5 and 14.6). (**a**) Preoperative X-ray. (**b**) Early postoperative X-rays. (**c**) Postoperative X-rays at 4 months showed good union at arthrodesis site

It is changed to a removable wrist splint at 1–2 weeks. In fusion across the radiocarpal joint and for K-wire fixation cases, active mobilization of the wrist is initiated after the fusion is united. For compression screw fixation cases, gentle active wrist mobilization out of splint can be started at 2 weeks. In fusion within the midcarpal joint, active mobilization can be initiated early out of splint 1–2 weeks after the operation.

For detailed surgical techniques and rehabilitation, please refer to Ho [95].

Complications

Arthroscopic procedures are overall safe and reliable. However, we still have to take special precaution in the use of arthroscopic bur and radio-frequency probe. Throughout the years, we encountered one case of superficial second-degree skin burn due to the use of a high-speed bur without a good protective sheath during arthroscopic wrist fusion. There were two cases of delayed extensor tendon ruptures after the use of radio frequency (Fig. 14.21). Radio-frequency probe should be avoided in the dorsal wrist, especially in rheumatoid patients with thin or incompetent dorsal wrist capsule where the extensor tendons are directly overlying. A lower temperature and shorter duration of use are also recommended.

Conclusion

Arthroscopic approach in diagnosing and treating the rheumatoid wrist may be a breakthrough in providing a higher standard of care to rheumatoid patients. The inherent ligamentous laxity in the rheumatoid wrist gives an easier visualization and working environment for the arthroscope. Arthroscopy improves the operative exposure,

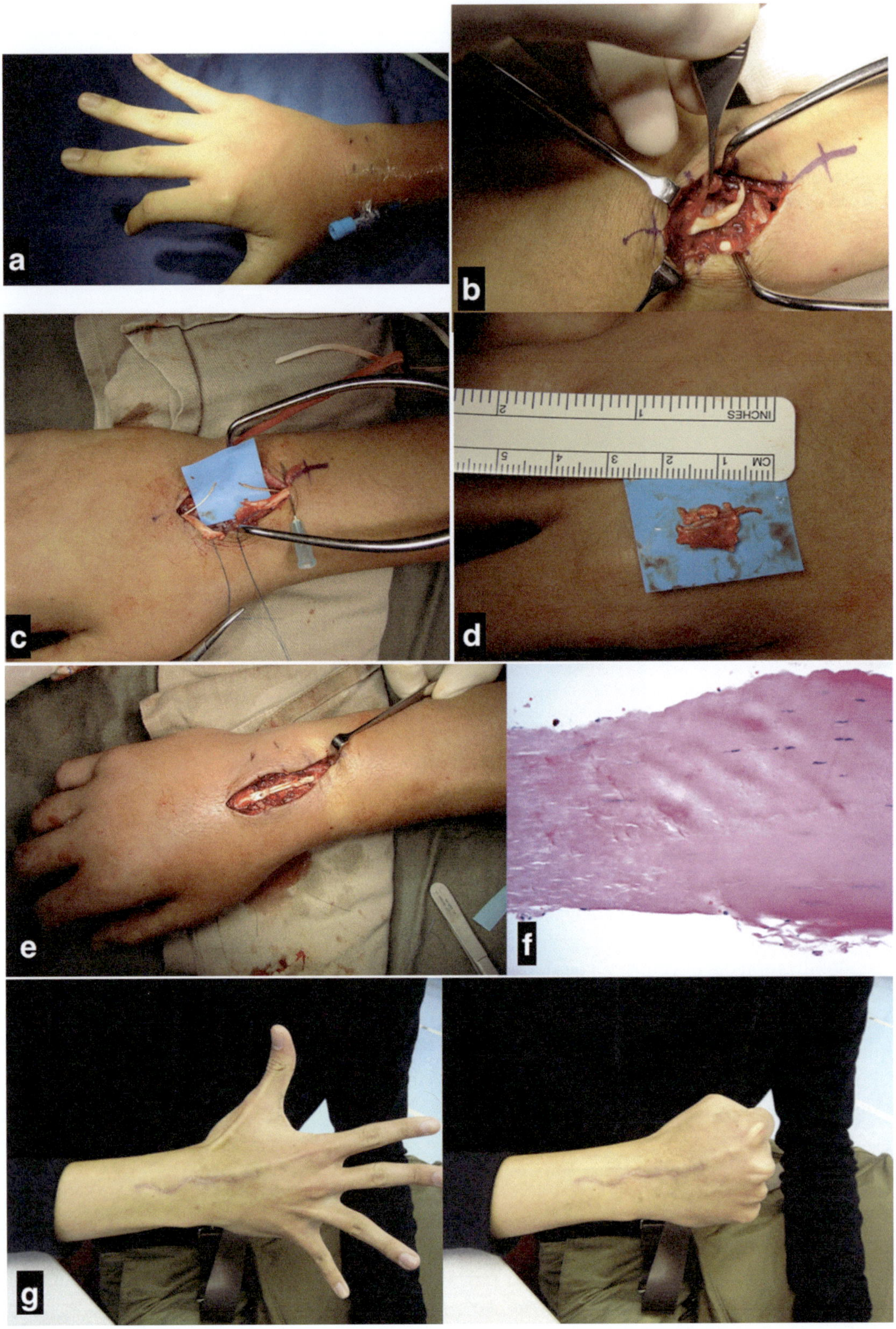

Fig. 14.21 (**a**) Failure of right index finger extension after arthroscopic wrist synovectomy. (**b**) Open exploration showed complete rupture of the extensor tendon. (**c**) Flimsy rupture ends of the extensor tendon. (**d**) Unhealthy part of the tendon was excised and sent for histopathology. (**e**) Direct repair of the extensor tendon to the index finger. (**f**) Histological features of thermal injury to the tendon. (**g**) Full finger range of motion was demonstrated after healing

gives a global assessment of wrist pathology for comprehensive surgical planning, gives minimal ligament disturbance and minimal scar and postoperative pain, has low anesthetic risk, accurately tackles mechanical symptoms, and hastens recovery and rehabilitation.

Rheumatoid arthritis is a systemic disease. A multidisciplinary approach with rheumatologists, hand surgeons, physiotherapists, and occupational therapists is of paramount importance to give high-quality care to the patients. Evidences also revealed that surgical intervention when the disease under pharmacological control gives the best outcomes [91–93, 100, 101]. However, less than 20 % of hand surgeons and rheumatologists treat rheumatoid patients in a multidisciplinary setting [102]. Rheumatologists may be skeptical of the role, efficacy, and benefits of prophylactic and therapeutic surgeries for rheumatoid arthritis. Hopefully, our promising results and experiences of the use of arthroscopy in the treatment of rheumatoid wrist can gain trust and confidence of more people; the success of the minimal invasiveness of the procedures can eliminate the worries of the patients and rheumatologists and gain popularity by hand surgeons. With the rapid progression of the disease in rheumatoid wrists [2], early diagnosis, early intervention, and good communications and consensus among the health-care providers are the keys to help and treat more patients.

References

1. Gibofsky A. Epidemiology, pathophysiology, and diagnosis of rheumatoid arthritis: a synopsis. Am J Manag Care. 2014;20:S128–135.
2. Rizzo M, Cooney III WP. Current concepts and treatment for the rheumatoid wrist. Hand Clin. 2011;27(1):57–72.
3. Rombouts JJ. Indications de la synovectomie chirurgicale dans le traitement de la polyarthrite rhumatoide. Louvain Med. 1978;97:151–8.
4. Thompson M, Douglas G, Davison EP. Evaluation of synovectomy in rheumatoid arthritis. Proc R Soc Med. 1973;66:197.
5. Gschwend N, Kentsch A. Late results of synovectomy of wrist, metacarpophalangeal and proximal interphalangeal joints. Multicenter study. Clin Rheumatol. 1985;4:23–5.
6. Brattsrom H. Long-term results of knee synovectomy in early cases of rheumatoid arthritis. A multicenter retrospective study. Clin Rheumatol. 1985; 4:19–22.
7. Wilkinson MC, Lowry JH. Synovectomy for rheumatoid arthritis. J Bone Joint Surg Br. 1965;47(3): 482–8.
8. Lefevre S, Knedla A, Tennie C, et al. Synovial fibroblasts spread rheumatoid arthritis to unaffected joints. Nat Med. 2009;15:1414–20.
9. Adolfsson L, Nylander G. Arthroscopic synovectomy of the rheumatoid wrist. J Hand Surg Br. 1993;18(1):92–6.
10. Adolfsson L. Arthroscopic synovectomy of the wrist. Hand Clin. 2011;27(3):395–9.
11. Adolfsson L, Frisen M. Arthroscopic synovectomy of the rheumatoid wrist: a 3.8 year follow-up. J Hand Surg Br. 1997;22(6):711–3.
12. Wei N, Delauter SK, Beard S, Erlichman MS, Henry D. Office-based arthroscopic synovectomy of the wrist in rheumatoid arthritis. Arthroscopy. 2001; 17(8):884–7.
13. Park MJ, Ahn JH, Kang JS. Arthroscopic synovectomy of the wrist in rheumatoid arthritis. J Bone Joint Surg Br. 2003;85(7):1011–5.
14. Kim SJ, Jung KA, Kim JM, Kwun JD, Kang HJ. Arthroscopic synovectomy in wrists with advanced rheumatoid arthritis. Clin Orthop Relat Res. 2006;449:262–6.
15. Lee HI, Lee KH, Koh KH, Park MJ. Long-term results of arthroscopic wrist synovectomy in rheumatoid arthritis. J Hand Surg Am. 2014;39(7): 1295–300.
16. Ong TYM, Ho PC, Wong WYC, Cheng HSS, Tse WL. Wrist Arthroscopy under Portal Site Local Anesthesia (PSLA) without Tourniquet. J Wrist Surg. 2012;1(2):149–52.
17. Firestein GS. Evolving concepts of rheumatoid arthritis. Nature. 2003;423:356–61.
18. Smolen JS, Aletaha D, Koeller M, Weisman M, Emery P. New therapies for the treatment of rheumatoid arthritis. Lancet. 2007;370:1861–74.
19. Van der Heide A, Jacobs JW, Bijlsma JW, Heurkens AH, van Booma-Frankfort C, van der Veen MJ, et al. The effectiveness of early treatment with "second-line" antirheumatic drugs: a randomized, controlled trial. Ann Intern Med. 1996;124:699–707.
20. Bukhari MA, Wiles NJ, Lunt M, Harrison BJ, Scott DG, Symmons DP, et al. Influence of disease-modifying therapy on radiographic outcome in inflammatory polyarthritis at five years: results from a large observational inception study. Arthritis Rheum. 2003;48:46–53.
21. Van Dongen H, van Aken J, Lard LR, Visser K, Ronday HK, Hulsmans HM, et al. Efficacy of methotrexate treatment in patients with probable rheumatoid arthritis: a double-blind, randomized, placebo-controlled trial. Arthritis Rheum. 2007;56: 1424–32.

22. Aletaha D, Neogi T, Silman AJ, et al. Rheumatoid arthritis classification criteria: an American College of Rheumatology/European League against Rheumatism collaborative initiative. Ann Rheum Dis. 2010;69:1580–8.
23. Bohndorf K, Schalm J. Diagnostic radiography in rheumatoid arthritis: benefits and limitations. Baillieres Clin Rheumatol. 1996;10:399–407.
24. Van der Heijde DM. Joint erosions and patients with early rheumatoid arthritis. Br J Rheumatol. 1995;34 Suppl 2:74–8.
25. Plant MJ, Jones PW, Saklatvala J, Ollier WE, Dawes PT. Patterns of radiological progression in rheumatoid arthritis: results of an 8 year prospective study. J Rheumatol. 1998;25:417–26.
26. Wolfe F, Sharp JT. Radiographic outcome of recent-onset rheumatoid arthritis: a 19-year study of radiographic progression. Arthritis Rheum. 1998;41: 1571–82.
27. Machold KP, Stamm TA, Eberl GJ, Nell VK, Dunky A, Uffmann M, et al. Very recent onset arthritis: clinical, laboratory, and radiological findings during the first year of disease. J Rheumatol. 2002;29: 2278–87.
28. Fillipucci E, da Luz KR, Di Geso L, Salaffi F, Tardella M, Carotti M, et al. Interobserver reliability of ultrasonography in the assessment of cartilage damage in rheumatoid arthritis. Ann Rheum Dis. 2010;69(10):1845–8.
29. Hariri A, Lebailly F, Zemirline A, Hendriks S, Facca S, Liverneaux P. Contribution of arthroscopy in case of septic appearance arthritis of the wrist: a nine cases series. Chir Main. 2013;32:240–4.
30. Kouri VP, Olkkonen J, Ainola M, Li TF, Bjorkman L, Konttinen YT, et al. Neutrophils produce interleukin-17B in rheumatoid synovial tissue. Rheumatology. 2014;53(1):39–47.
31. Kobayashi I, Ziff M. Electronic microscopic studies of the cartilage-pannus junction in rheumatoid arthritis. Arthritis Rheum. 1975;18(5):475–83.
32. Van de Sande MGH, Gerlag DM, Lodde BM, van Baarsen LGM, Alivernini S, Codullo V, et al. Evaluating antirheumatic treatments using synovial biopsy: a recommendation for standardisation to be used in clinical trials. Ann Rheum Dis. 2011;70(3):423–7.
33. Baeten D, Kruithof E, Rycke LD, Vandooren B, Wyns B, Boullart L, et al. Diagnostic classification of spondyloarthropathy and rheumatoid arthritis by synovial histopathology. Arthritis Rheum. 2004;50(9):2931–41.
34. Kiener H, Niederreiter B, Lee DM, Jimenez-Boj E, Smolen J, Brenner MB. Cadherin 11 promotes invasive behavior of fibroblast-like synoviocytes. Arthritis Rheum. 2009;60(5):1305–10.
35. Aletaha D, Funovits J, Smolen JS. Physical disability in rheumatoid arthritis is associated with cartilage damage rather than bone destruction. Ann Rheum Dis. 2011;70:733–9.
36. Mcqueen F, Mchaffie A, Clarke A, Lee A, Reeves Q, Curteis B, et al. The progression of cartilage damage in rheumatoid arthritis: a three year prospective 3T-magnetic resonance imaging study examining predictive factors. Arthritis Rheum. 2013; 65(Suppl10):S832–3.
37. Gravallese EM, Harada Y, Wang JT, Gorn AH, Thornhill TS, Goldring SR. Identification of cell types responsible for bone resorption in rheumatoid arthritis and juvenile rheumatoid arthritis. Am J Pathol. 1998;152:943–51.
38. Redlich K, Hayer S, Ricci R, David JP, Tohidast-Akrad M, Kollias G, et al. Osteoclasts are essential for TNF-alpha-mediated joint destruction. J Clin Invest. 2002;110:1419–27.
39. Goldring SR. Pathogenesis of bone and cartilage destruction in rheumatoid arthritis. Rheumatology (Oxford). 2003;42 Suppl 2:ii11–16.
40. Milner JM, Cawston TE. Matrix metalloproteinase knockout studies and the potential use of matrix metalloproteinase inhibitors in the rheumatic diseases. Curr Drug Targets Inflamm Allergy. 2005;4:363–75.
41. Humby F, Bombardieri M, Manzo A, et al. Ectopic lymphoid structures support ongoing production of class-switched autoantibodies in rheumatoid synovium. PLoS Med. 2009;6, e1.
42. Okada T, Tsukano H, Endo M, et al. Synoviocyte-derived angiopoietin-like protein 2 contributes to synovial chronic inflammation in rheumatoid arthritis. Am J Pathol. 2010;176:2309–19.
43. Wong C, Chen D, Tam L, et al. Effects of inflammatory cytokine IL-27 on the activation of fibroblast-like synoviocytes in rheumatoid arthritis. Arthritis Res Ther. 2010;12:R129.
44. Ossyssek B, Anders S, Grifka J, Straub RH. Surgical synovectomy decreases density of sensory nerve fibers in synovial tissue of non-inflamed controls and rheumatoid arthritis patients. J Orthop Res. 2011;29:297–302.
45. Lie E, van Der Heijde D, Uhlig T, Mikkelsen K, Kalstad S, Kaufmann C, et al. Treatment strategies in patients with rheumatoid arthritis for whom methotrexate mono therapy has failed: data from the NOR-DMARD register. Ann Rheum Dis. 2011;70(12):2103–10.
46. Ghattas L, Mascella F, Pomponio G. Hand surgery in rheumatoid arthritis: state of the art and suggestions for research. Rheumatology (Oxford). 2005;44(7): 834–45.
47. Choi WJ, Choi GW, Lee JW. Arthroscopic synovectomy of the ankle in rheumatoid arthritis. Arthroscopy. 2013;29(1):133–40.
48. Kang HJ, Park MJ, Ahn JH, Lee SH. Arthroscopic synovectomy for the rheumatoid elbow. Arthroscopy. 2010;26(9):1195–202.
49. Pan X, Zhang X, Liu Z, Wen H, Mao X. Treatment for chronic synovitis of knee: arthroscopic or open synovectomy. Rheumatol Int. 2012;32:1733–6.

50. McEwen C. Multicenter evaluation of synovectomy in the treatment of rheumatoid arthritis: report of results at the end of five years. J Rheumatol. 1988; 15:765–9.
51. Nicolle FV, Holt PJL, Calnan JS. Prophylactic synovectomy of the joints of the rheumatoid hand. Ann Rheum Dis. 1971;30:476–80.
52. Wilde AH. Synovectomy of the proximal interphalangeal joint of the finger in rheumatoid arthritis. J Bone Joint Surg Am. 1974;56:71–8.
53. Nakamura H, Nagashima M, Ishigami S, et al. The anti-rheumatic effect of multiple synovectomy in patients with refractory rheumatoid arthritis. Int Orthop. 2000;24:242–5.
54. Thirupathi RG, Ferlic DC, Clayton ML. Dorsal wrist synovectomy in rheumatoid arthritis—a long-term study. J Hand Surg Am. 1983;8:848–56.
55. Rombouts JJ, Rombouts-Lindemans C. L'atteinte de la main au cours de la polyarthrite rhumatoide: Essai de synthese. Louvain Med. 1980;99:693–704.
56. Nalebuff EA, Potter TA. Rheumatoid involvement of tendon and tendon sheaths in the hand. Clin Orthop Relat Res. 1968;59:147–59.
57. Larsen A, Dale K, Eek M. Radiographic evaluation of rheumatoid arthritis and related conditions by standard reference films. Acta Radiol Diagn. 1977;18:481–91.
58. Aschan W, Moberg E. A long-term study on the effect of early synovectomy in rheumatoid arthritis. Bull Hosp J Dis Orthop Inst. 1984;44:106–21.
59. Ishikawa H, Hanyu T, Tajima T. Rheumatoid wrists treated with synovectomy of the extensor tendons and the wrist joint combined with a Darrach procedure. J Hand Surg Am. 1992;17(6):1109–17.
60. Ishikawa H, Ohno O, Hirohata K. Long-term effects of synovectomy in rheumatoid patients. J Bone Joint Surg Am. 1986;68:198–205.
61. Laurin CA, Desmarchais J, Daziano L, Gariepy R, Derome A. Long term results of synovectomy of the knee in rheumatoid patients. J Bone Joint Surg Am. 1974;56:521–31.
62. Shibata T, Shiraoka K, Takubo N. Comparison between arthroscopic and open synovectomy for the knee in rheumatoid arthritis. Arch Orthop Trauma Surg. 1986;105:257–62.
63. Chalmers PN, Sherman S, Raphael BS, Su EP. Rheumatoid synovectomy: does the surgical approach matter? Clin Orthop Relat Res. 2011; 469(7):2062–71.
64. Ferlic DC, Cooney WP. Wrist in inflammatory arthritis. In: Metcalf PG, editor. Operative arthroscopy. New York: Raven; 1991. p. 641–46.
65. Hindley CJ, Stanley JK. The rheumatoid wrist: patterns of disease progression. A review of 50 wrists. J Hand Surg Br. 1991;16(3):275–9.
66. Feldon P, Millender L, Nalebuff EA. Rheumatoid arthritis in hand and wrist. In: Green DP, editor. Operative hand surgery. 3rd ed. New York: Churchill Livingstone; 1993. p. 1587–690.
67. Lee KH, Lee CH, Park HS, Sung IH, Choi WS. Longitudinal radiographic analysis of rheumatoid wrist: minimum 7 year follow-up. Poster presentation. 68th Annual Meeting of the ASSH. 2013;AM E-poster 15.
68. Douraiswami B, Thanigai S. Monoarticular rheumatoid arthritis of the wrist: a rare entity. OA Case Reports. 2013;2(8):80.
69. Matsui N, Taneda Y, Ohta H, Itoh T, Tsuboguchis S. Arthroscopic versus open synovectomy in rheumatoid knee. Int Orthop. 1989;13:17–20.
70. Kvien TK, Pahle JA, Høyeraal HM, Sandstad B. Comparison of synovectomy and no synovectomy in patients with juvenile rheumatoid arthritis. Scand J Rheumatol. 1987;16:81–91.
71. Vahvanen V, Pätiälä H. Synovectomy of the wrist in rheumatoid arthritis and related diseases. Arch Orthop Trauma Surg. 1984;102(4):230–7.
72. Leak RS, Rayan GM, Arthur RE. Longitudinal radiographic analysis of rheumatoid arthritis in the hand and wrist. J Hand Surg Am. 2003;28(3): 427–34.
73. Darrach W. Forward dislocation at the inferior radioulnar joint, with fracture of the lower third of the shaft of the radius. Ann Surg. 1912;56:801–2.
74. Bell MJ, Hill RJ, McMurtry RY. Ulnar impingement syndrome. J Bone Joint Surg Br. 1985;67:126–9.
75. Bower WH. Distal radioulnar joint arthroplasty: the hemiresection-interposition technique. J Hand Surg Am. 1985;10:169–78.
76. Rana NA, Diao E, Peimer CA, Sherwin FS. Comparative results of resection of the distal ulna in rheumatoid arthritis and post-traumatic conditions. J Hand Surg Br. 1999;24(6):667–70.
77. Blank JE, Cassidy C. The distal radioulnar joint in rheumatoid arthritis. Hand Clin. 1996;12(3): 499–513.
78. Newmeyer WL, Green DP. Rupture of digital extensor tendons following distal ulnar resection. J Bone Joint Surg Am. 1982;64(2):178–82.
79. Bieber EJ, Hinschied RL, Dobyns JH, Beckenbaugh RD. Failed distal ulna resections. J Hand Surg Am. 1988;13(2):193–200.
80. Tulipan DJ, Eaton RG, Eberhart RE. The Darrach procedure defended: technique redefined and long-term follow-up. J Hand Surg Am. 1991;16(3): 438–44.
81. Dingman PVC. Resection of the distal end of the ulna (Darrach operation): an end-result study of twenty-four cases. J Bone Joint Surg Am. 1952; 34:893–900.
82. Sauve L, Kapandji M. A novel surgical technique for the treatment of subluxations of the distal forearm. J Chir (Paris). 1936;47:589–94.
83. Lluch A. The Sauve-Kapandji procedure. J Wirst Surg. 2013;2:33–40.
84. Watson HK, Gabuzda GM. Matched distal ulna resection for post-traumatic disorders of the distal radioulnar joint. J Hand Surg Am. 1992;17:724–30.

85. Bain GI, Pugh DM, MacDermid JC, Roth JH. Matched hemiresection interposition arthroplasty of the distal radioulnar joint. J Hand Surg Am. 1995;20:944–50.
86. Faithful DK, Kwa S. A review of distal ulnar hemiresection arthroplasty. J Hand Surg Br. 1992;17:408–10.
87. Glowacki KA. Hemiresection arthroplasty of the distal radioulnar joint. Hand Clin. 2005;21:591–601.
88. Imbriglia JE, Matthews D. The treatment of chronic traumatic subluxation of the distal ulna by hemiresection interposition arthroplasty. Hand Clin. 1991; 7:329–34.
89. Minami A, Kaneda K, Itoga H. Hemiresection-interposition arthroplasty of the distal radioulnar joint associated with repair of triangular fibrocartilage complex lesions. J Hand Surg Am. 1991;16:1120–5.
90. Tse WL, Lau SW, Wong WY, Cheng HS, Chow CS, Ho PC, et al. Arthroscopic reconstruction of triangular fibrocartilage Complex (TFCC) with tendon graft for chronic DRUJ instability. Injury. 2013;44:386–90.
91. Motomiya M, Iwasaki N, Minami A, Matsui Y, Urita A, Funakoshi T. Clinical and radiological results of radiolunate arthrodesis for rheumatoid arthritis: 22 wrists followed for an average of 7 years. J Hand Surg Am. 2013;38:1484–91.
92. Solomon DH, Katz JN, Cabral D, Patrick AR, Bukowski JF, Coblyn JS. Osteoporosis management in patients with rheumatoid arthritis: evidence for improvement. Arthritis Rheum. 2006;55(6):873–7.
93. Lee SG, Park YE, Park SH, Kim TK, Choi HJ, Lee SJ, et al. Increased frequency of osteoporosis and BMD below the expected range for age among South Korean women with rheumatoid arthritis. Int J Rheum Dis. 2012;15(3):289–96.
94. Chamay A, Della Santa D, Vilaseca A. Radiolunate arthrodesis. Factors of stability for the rheumatoid wrist. Ann Chir Main. 1983;2(1):5–17.
95. Ho PC. Arthroscopic partial wrist fusion. Tech Hand Up Extrem Surg. 2008;12(4):242–65.
96. Clayton ML. Surgical treatment at the wrist in rheumatoid arthritis: a review of thirty-seven patients. J Bone Joint Surg Am. 1965;47(4):741–50.
97. Lee DH, Carroll RE. Wrist arthrodesis: a combined intramedullary pin and autogenous iliac crest bone graft technique. J Hand Surg Am. 1994;19(5):733–40.
98. Deluca PA, Lindsey RW, Ruwe PA. Refracture of bones of the forearm after the removal of compression plates. J Bone Joint Surg Am. 1988;70(9):1372–6.
99. Nagy L, Buchler U. AO-wrist arthrodesis: with and without arthrodesis of the third carpometacarpal joint. J Hand Surg Am. 2002;27(6):940–7.
100. Momohara S, Inoue E, Ikari K, Yano K, Tokita A, Suzuki T, et al. Efficacy of total joint arthroplasty in patients with established rheumatoid arthritis: improved longitudinal effects on disease activity but not on health-related quality of life. Mod Rheumatol. 2011;21(5):476–81.
101. Yano K, Ikari K, Inoue E, Tokita A, Sakuma Y, Hiroshima R, et al. Effect of total knee arthroplasty on disease activity in patients with established rheumatoid arthritis: 3-year follow-up results of combined medical therapy and surgical intervention. Mod Rheumatol. 2010;20(5):452–7.
102. Alderman AK, Chung KC, Kim HM, Fox DA, Ubel PA. Effectiveness of rheumatoid hand surgery: contrasting perceptions of hand surgeons and rheumatologists. J Hand Surg Am. 2003;28(1):3–11.

Case-Based Discussion of the Management of the Rheumatoid Wrist

15

Daniel Herren

Introduction

The aim of this chapter is to highlight current thinking on the surgical treatment of rheumatoid wrists. The cases illustrate the concepts of different indications and surgical performance. The cases presented are not intended to give only one possible treatment option but rather to stimulate thought and discussion.

Case 1 (Fig. 15.1)

Case 1: A 72-year-old man with rheumatoid arthritis (RA) for more than 20 years. At the present time, his condition is stable on infliximab (Remicade®) and methotrexate (MTX), with no major side effects. He has a painful nondominant left wrist: the pain on a VAS scores six on loading and two at rest. The fingers are functioning reasonably well, without any significant synovitis. Motion on flexion/extension of the wrist is 25°/0°/30°, with pain in the end positions. Pro-/supination accounts for 60°/0°/65°, with painful grinding of the distal radioulnar joint (DRUJ).

D. Herren, MD, MHA (✉)
Hand Surgery, Schulthess Klinik,
Lengghalde 2, Zurich 8008, Switzerland
e-mail: Daniel.Herren@kws.ch

The dominant hand is currently free from pain (maximum VAS of two on loading) with a functional range of motion.

The following points need to be addressed:

1. Which anatomical parts are responsible for the pain?
2. Is surgery indicated and, if so, which parts of the wrist require intervention?
3. What are the treatment options for the distal radioulnar joint?
4. What are the possibilities for treating the wrist?
5. How should we handle the current medication during surgical treatment?

Discussion

1. Which anatomical parts are responsible for the pain?

   The X-ray shows an AP view of a wrist with considerable destruction of the radiocarpal and midcarpal joints, as well as of the DRUJ. Cystic bone lesions indicate residual inflammatory activity in all parts of the wrist, including the capitate. The DRUJ shows protrusion into the radius, with sclerotic changes within the bone. There is no significant ulnar drift and good coverage of the lunate on the radius. The carpal height is well preserved

K.C. Chung (ed.), *Clinical Management of the Rheumatoid Hand, Wrist, and Elbow*,
DOI 10.1007/978-3-319-26660-2_15

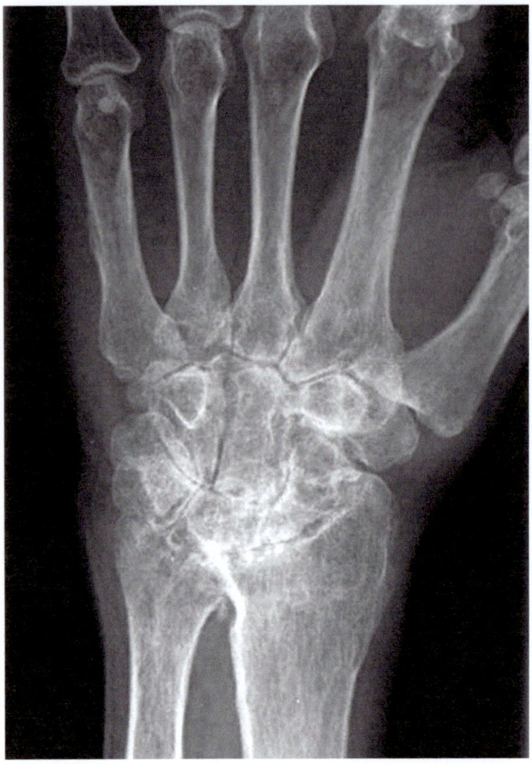

Fig. 15.1 AP radiograph of the wrist showing severe destruction in all wrist compartments including the distal radioulnar joint. There is little ulnar drift and it seems that the lunate starts to fuse with the radius

and the overall bone quality seems reasonable, despite the cystic lesions. In the Schulthess classification of RA wrists, this represents a type II wrist, with a stable bone situation similar to that seen in wrist joints undergoing osteoarthritic degeneration. In summary, there is destruction of all the compartments in the wrist, with the midcarpal joint probably the best preserved.

2. Is surgery indicated and, if so, which parts of the wrist require intervention?

   The medication seems to be working reasonably well, with the wrist on the other side being almost pain-free and little or no evidence of soft tissue synovitis. There is no need to change the medication, because the patient is not suffering from significant side effects. With such clear destruction of all compartments of the wrist, including the DRUJ, surgery is probably the best option for this patient. As all the components are painful, a "full service" should be considered; that is to say, we should treat the wrist as well as the DRUJ. Surgery on the DRUJ also has the potential to prevent problems with the extensor tendons in the future.

3. What are the treatment options for the distal radioulnar joint?

   The classic intervention in the DRUJ of patients with RA is resection of the ulnar head (Darrach procedure). Its main disadvantages include instability of the residual ulna with a loss of grip strength, possible destabilization of the radiocarpal joint, and an unsatisfactory aesthetic appearance of the wrist. Possible alternatives include a Sauvé-Kapandji procedure and a DRUJ prosthetic replacement. The choice of procedure depends on three factors: (1) the procedure planned for other parts of the wrist, (2) the patient's requirements, and (3) the expected future development.

   Classic ulnar head resection was first described by Darrach for post-traumatic destruction of the DRUJ. Instability of the DRUJ in RA, combined with wrist deformity, leads to the "caput ulnae syndrome." This syndrome includes dorsal subluxation of the ulna head (or more accurately, volar decent of the radius because the ulna is the fixed unit of the forearm and does not subluxate) which, together with bone spurs and local synovitis, can lead to extensor tendon attrition. The disadvantages of ulna head resection include some destabilization of the radiocarpal joint, possible instability of the ulna shaft, and a loss of grip strength due to the lack of support from the DRUJ. The Sauvé-Kapandji procedure may be considered as an alternative. It includes fusion of the ulna head with the radius and resection of a segment of the distal ulna. As a result, the DRUJ center of rotation is moved proximally. Compared with ulna head resection, it provides more residual stability for the radiocarpal joint, leaving support at the ulnar edge of the joint. In addition, maintaining the ulnar profile gives the wrist a more natural appearance. Possible residual ulna instability remains a problem in the same way as with ulnar head resection. It has never been proven that the Sauvé-Kapandji procedure provides better grip strength than ulnar head resection alone.

The ulna head prosthesis was developed primarily for post-traumatic destruction of the DRUJ. It is rarely used in RA patients and then only if disease activity is well controlled and the basic architecture of the joint is preserved. There can be no substantial subluxation or loss of stability if distal radioulnar joint replacement is to be considered.

4. What are the possibilities for treating the wrist?

   Figure 15.2 summarizes the possible surgical indications. In general, a Schulthess type II wrist is the ideal indication for either wrist arthroplasty or partial wrist fusion. The latter requires at least a partially intact midcarpal joint in order to perform radioscapholunate (RSL) fusion. In this patient, the capitate head has no cartilage and shows significant cystic lesions. As an alternative to RSL fusion alone, a combination of capitate resurfacing with an implant (e.g., pyrocarbon) and RSL fusion is theoretically an option. However, because the midcarpal joint shows significant changes the implant would come up against destroyed bone surface, making it a less than ideal solution. Wrist arthroplasty is, however, a valid option for a wrist in this condition. The tendons are preserved, the bone quality seems adequate, and, most importantly, the wrist is well centered. Wrist replacement can be expected to provide a range of motion similar to what the patient has at the moment, i.e., about 60° total ROM.

   The alternative to wrist arthroplasty is wrist fusion. Because it is the patient's nondominant hand, reasonable strength and a stable wrist would be acceptable. The optimal position for wrist fusion in this situation is about 30° of extension. This gives an ideal flexor tendon moment arm, with maximal grip force. Fusion is typically carried out with a wrist fusion plate, either extended up to the third metacarpal or with an implant that does not cross the CMC III joint and simply fuses the radiocarpal and midcarpal joints. The longer plate is more effective in neutralizing the forces of the long lever arm in the wrist but has the potential to cause problems at the CMC III joint, which is not usually fused in a panarthrodesis. This joint may subsequently become a source of persistent pain, and its residual motion may lead to distal plate loosening.

   To summarize, the most meaningful option for this wrist would be either total wrist fusion or arthroplasty, combined with a procedure to include the distal radioulnar joint (preferably ulnar head resection or the Sauvé-Kapandji procedure).

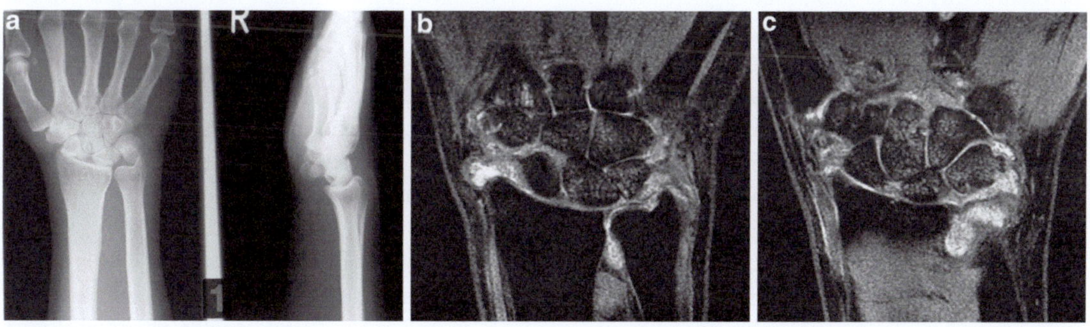

Fig. 15.2 (**a**) AP radiograph of the wrist showing a scapholunate dissociation with flexion of the scaphoid. There are no significant signs of inflammation in this wrist. (**b** and **c**) T2-weighted MRI of the wrist including gadolinium enhancement. There is synovial tissue especially in the radio-scaphoid joint compartment as well as in the distal radioulnar joint. The cartilage is thinned but preserved around the ulnar head and in the radiocarpal joint. The midcarpal joint shows significant cartilage thinning. There are few signs of inflammation within the bones

After intensive discussion with the patient, we decided to perform wrist fusion with a plate and ulnar head resection.

5. How should we handle the current medication during surgical treatment?

   Because both possible solutions, arthroplasty and fusion, are major procedures with operating times of about 2 h and include implants with significant surface areas, it would be advisable to stop the biologic medications prior to surgery. The medication should be stopped in line with its half-life and 1–2 cycles omitted until wound healing is guaranteed (typically about 2–3 weeks postoperatively). There is some evidence in the literature that the infection rate in such interventions might be higher on biologics. Methotrexate can be continued with an appropriate dose adjustment or combined with glucocorticosteroids in the perioperative phase, in order to prevent a flare-up of disease. Good communication with the treating rheumatologist is not only advisable but absolutely essential.

Case 2 (Fig. 15.2)

Case 2: A 32-year-old man with a slightly swollen wrist. RA factor is positive with scapholunate dissociation in standard X-ray views, diminished carpal height, and well-preserved midcarpal joint. The distal radioulnar joint seems unchanged in the plain X-ray but erosions and significant synovitis can be seen on MRI. A lesser degree of synovitis is present in the radial compartment of the radiocarpal joint.

The patient has painful forearm rotation, especially under loading (VAS: max. 4–5), but no pain at rest. Flexion/extension is possible in a range of 50°/0°/60°. There is no synovial swelling around the tendons. The patient is currently on medication with a TNF-alpha blocker and methotrexate.

The following points need to be addressed:

1. Is surgery indicated and, if so, which parts of the wrist require intervention?
2. What are the treatment options for the distal radioulnar joint?
3. What are the possibilities for treating the wrist?
4. How should we handle the current medication during surgical treatment?
5. How urgently is intervention needed?

Discussion

1. Is surgery indicated and, if so, which parts of the wrist require intervention?

   The patient's symptoms are arising mainly from the synovial process in the distal radioulnar joint. The DRUJ cartilage seems intact and it is the inflammatory process that needs to be controlled. Because the rest of the wrist and, in particular, the soft tissue structures are responding well to the current medication, DRUJ surgery is a viable option. The X-ray shows scapholunate dissociation due to the inflammatory process; although it does not seem active at the moment, structural damage is present and the carpus is starting to destabilize. It has been shown that early intervention with scapholunate fusion to stabilize the wrist can prevent further deterioration. It seems likely in this patient that the deformity of the wrist will continue. Scapholunate dissociation is often the first sign of ongoing carpal collapse. Surgical intervention at the wrist might therefore be beneficial, given the probable progression of the disease. On the other hand, we have a patient with little to no pain in the radiocarpal joint. From his point of view, there is no obvious immediate gain from surgery of any type at that level. On the contrary, radiocarpal surgery carries the risk of reduced mobility in flexion/extension.

   Another aspect to consider is the conservative medical treatment. Although the patient is on a modern treatment regimen, there would appear to be some residual disease activity. It is necessary to talk to the rheumatologist in order to optimize the pharmaceutical treatment.

   Taken overall, surgery is indicated if (a) the burden of the pain is sufficiently heavy and (b) the clinical progression and the course of the disability are obvious. If the patient is unsure about having surgery, a repeat MRI in 3–4 months' time might be an option for monitoring disease activity and judging the effects of a change in medication.

2. What are the treatment options for the distal radioulnar joint?

   When considering a surgical procedure, the following points need to be clarified:

   - Is the structural defect such that a salvage procedure is needed for the DRUJ?
   - If only a soft tissue intervention (synovectomy) is indicated, should it be performed by open or arthroscopic surgery?

   From what we can see on the plain X-ray and especially in the MRI, the cartilage is well preserved in all parts of the distal radioulnar joint. A salvage procedure for the DRUJ should be avoided at any cost in this young active patient. The only meaningful intervention is therefore synovectomy of the DRUJ. The tendons are not clinically affected, nor does the MRI show any signs of their involvement, so the choice of an open versus an arthroscopic procedure can be discussed.

   The open procedure has been the standard for a long time, but new possibilities have opened up with the evolution of arthroscopic techniques. Both techniques have advantages, disadvantages, and limitations. The open procedure provides the possibility of inspecting and, if necessary, treating the extensor tendons. MRI sometimes underestimates the synovial changes in the tendons. Direct demonstration of the radioulnar joint and complete synovectomy requires a generous open surgical approach, with the danger of scarring around the DRUJ and subsequently limited range of motion for pro- and supination. The arthroscopic procedure, on the other hand, has the advantage of being less invasive and causing less internal scarring. Arthroscopic assessment of the DRUJ is technically demanding, however, and requires skill and experience. The decision on the correct procedure depends on the surgeon's experience and technical skills. So far, there is no evidence in the literature as to which of these procedures gives the better results, especially in the long term.

3. What are the possibilities for treating the wrist?

   The symptoms and clinical examination do not demand surgical intervention. The extent of both the radiocarpal and midcarpal synovial changes is minor. The indication for surgical intervention, including synovectomy, must be evaluated critically. Open removal of the inflamed synovial tissue often leads to stiffness in this joint. Whether or not it helps to stabilize the wrist in the long term is debatable. Arthroscopic synovectomy seems to have less morbidity and the potential to preserve mobility. During arthroscopy of the wrist for treatment of the distal radioulnar joint, the radiocarpal joint can also be inspected and treated if necessary.

   The radiographic picture, however, shows scapholunate dissociation, which indicates instability of this joint. Conversely, there is no sign of instability in another plain X-ray of the wrist and, in particular, no ulnar drift. As the patient has little in the way of complaints, the only reason to perform surgery would be to stabilize the wrist for the future, in order to prevent further carpal collapse. The theoretical possibilities for achieving this goal are scapholunate ligament reconstruction and some sort of midcarpal fusion. The latter is accompanied by a significant loss in the range of motion. In addition, it has to be remembered that the midcarpal joint stays intact for a long time in most forms of inflammatory wrist disease and is often the last part of the wrist to remain mobile. So the price to pay for intervention seems rather high.

   With respect to SL ligament reconstruction in rheumatoid arthritis, there is no indication for such a procedure. Firstly, the patterns of carpal instability in rheumatoid wrists seem to be more complex, involving combined laxity of the intrinsic and extrinsic carpal ligaments. Secondly, some cartilage involvement in the radiocarpal joint is often observed in rheumatoid arthritis, even in the early stages. Scapholunate ligament reconstruction may increase the pressure in the radiocarpal joint, which may in turn produce more symptoms, and limit the range of motion due to scarring.

Overall, the indication for radiocarpal joint surgery must be evaluated critically. When carrying out arthroscopic treatment of the distal radioulnar joint, it makes sense to inspect the radiocarpal and midcarpal joints and perform synovectomy in these compartments as well, if appropriate.

4. How should we handle the current medication during surgical treatment?

   If an open or arthroscopic synovectomy is performed, the current medication can be continued. There is some evidence in the literature that the risk of infection in minor procedures is not significantly elevated on treatment with biologics. Routine antibiotic cover is indicated for these procedures.

5. How urgently is intervention needed?

   The timing of an intervention always depends on different factors. In this wrist, there is obviously some residual inflammatory disease activity. In situations like this, it is important to communicate with the rheumatologist: are there any plans to look for pharmaceutical alternatives or is the disease generally well controlled, even though residual inflammation in the wrist is in need of special attention?

   The inflammatory process in the wrist, especially in the mechanically heavily loaded distal radioulnar joint, has great potential for further destruction of both the cartilage and the surrounding soft tissues. We therefore advised that surgery should be performed within the next few months, with the aim of diminishing the mass of inflammatory tissue [1–14].

References

1. Adolfsson L. Arthroscopic synovectomy of the wrist. Hand Clin. 2011;27(3):395–9.
2. Chantelot C et al. Radiographic course of 39 rheumatoid wrists after synovectomy and stabilization. Chir Main. 1998;17(3):236–44.
3. Chung KC, Pushman AG. Current concepts in the management of the rheumatoid hand. J Hand Surg Am. 2011;36(4):736–47. quiz 747.
4. De Smet L. The distal radioulnar joint in rheumatoid arthritis. Acta Orthop Belg. 2006;72(4):381–6.
5. Ito J et al. Radiologic evaluation of the rheumatoid hand after synovectomy and extensor carpi radialis longus transfer to extensor carpi ulnaris. J Hand Surg Am. 2003;28(4):585–90.
6. Kozlow JH, Chung KC. Current concepts in the surgical management of rheumatoid and osteoarthritic hands and wrists. Hand Clin. 2011;27(1):31–41.
7. Lee HI et al. Long-term results of arthroscopic wrist synovectomy in rheumatoid arthritis. J Hand Surg Am. 2014;39(7):1295–300.
8. Murray PM. Current concepts in the treatment of rheumatoid arthritis of the distal radioulnar joint. Hand Clin. 2011;27(1):49–55.
9. Cavaliere CM, Chung KC. Total wrist arthroplasty and total wrist arthrodesis in rheumatoid arthritis: a decision analysis from the hand surgeons' perspective. J Hand Surg Am. 2008;33(10):1744–55. 1755 e1–2.
10. Kluge S et al. The modified Clayton-Mannerfelt arthrodesis of the wrist in rheumatoid arthritis: operative technique and report on 93 cases. J Hand Surg Am. 2013;38(5):999–1005.
11. Motomiya M et al. Clinical and radiological results of radiolunate arthrodesis for rheumatoid arthritis: 22 wrists followed for an average of 7 years. J Hand Surg Am. 2013;38(8):1484–91.
12. Ogunro S, Ahmed I, Tan V. Current indications and outcomes of total wrist arthroplasty. Orthop Clin North Am. 2013;44(3):371–9. ix.
13. Raven EE, Ottink KD, Doets KC. Radiolunate and radioscapholunate arthrodeses as treatments for rheumatoid and psoriatic arthritis: long-term follow-up. J Hand Surg Am. 2012;37(1):55–62.
14. Rizzo M, Cooney 3rd WP. Current concepts and treatment for the rheumatoid wrist. Hand Clin. 2011; 27(1):57–72.

Part III

Rheumatoid Hand

The Rheumatoid Finger: Treatment Concepts and Indications for Surgery

16

Philippe Kopylov and Magnus Tägil

Introduction

In rheumatoid arthritis, all mesenchymal tissues are involved and not only the joints. The disease most often starts as a synovitis, which is the initiating factor for the subsequent deformities and the main factor to be treated. The synovial proliferation primarily causes a capsular distension. Secondarily bone erosions and destruction of tendon and ligament will follow. The severity of the disease, as well as the distribution of the bone, tendon, and ligament pathology, may differ, and a large variety of deformities may be encountered. The goal of the treatment, besides pain relief, is the restoration of finger and hand function, in combination with an improved appearance. The modern drugs introduced in recent years may have changed at least partially the evolution of the disease with less frequent typical finger deformities but may not have a lasting effect on the development of synovitis in small joints in all patients. It must be stated that with the new drugs, there is no place for just surgical treatment. Instead a combination of medical and surgical treatment has become the standard, together with well-conducted rehabilitation and physiotherapy including splints in a true rheumatoid team effort. It should be borne in mind that full restoration of a normal anatomy and normal function is not a realistic goal.

Finger Anatomy

Functionally, the finger can be described as two joints, the proximal interphalangeal (PIP) joint and the distal interphalangeal (DIP) joint, with an extensor complex tendon dorsally and two flexor tendons volarly. The finger is attached to the hand at the level of the metacarpophalangeal (MCP) joint. The tendons have origins proximally in the hand, and/or the finger deformity is seldom isolated but part of a deformity of the whole hand and wrist. Deviations in one direction are compensated by other deformities proximally or distally to the affected joint.

The PIP Joint

The PIP joint is a bicondylar joint that moves from zero degrees in full extension to approximately 100° in full flexion. The two concave facets of the middle phalanx are connected by a

P. Kopylov, MD, PhD (✉)
Department of Orthopedics, Central Hospital Kristianstad, Kristianstad, Sweden
e-mail: philippe.kopylov@med.lu.se

M. Tägil, MD, PhD
Department of Orthopedics, Lund University Hospital, Lund, Sweden
e-mail: magnus.tagil@med.lu.se

K.C. Chung (ed.), *Clinical Management of the Rheumatoid Hand, Wrist, and Elbow*,
DOI 10.1007/978-3-319-26660-2_16

marked bony ridge, which fits the depression between the two condyles of the base phalanx, by providing a perfect congruency of the joint. These, together with the collateral ligaments, create the prerequisites for a solid lateral and volar/dorsal stability. On the volar side, the volar plate forms a strong and competent structure in preventing the joint to hyperextend. In contrast, the lax dorsal capsule can easily be stretched by the condyles in flexion [1].

The extensor mechanism intimately follows the dorsum of the bony structures and is divided into three parts at the dorsum of the proximal phalanx—the central band and the two lateral bands (Fig. 16.1). The central band contains a fibrocartilage thickening, the dorsal plate, at its insertion at the base of the middle phalanx by contributing to the stability of both the joint and the extensor mechanism. The dorsal plate has a similar function as the patella in the knee and is histologically similar to the volar plate with a fibrocartilaginous structure. The two lateral bands run laterally and conjoin at the level of the middle phalanx to insert onto the distal phalanx proximally/dorsally. The three bands, two lateral and one central, are interconnected by a thin connective tissue, which gives freedom in motion in relation to each other. The lateral bands can move from a dorsal position and an extending function to a lateral position that allows flexion of both the PIP and the DIP joints simultaneously but only if the lateral bands remain dorsal to the PIP joint in the flexion/extension axis (Fig. 16.2). The relatively loose and thin transverse retinacular ligaments of Landsmeer control this physiologic displacement of the lateral bands. If the central band extends the PIP joint only, the lateral band participates to the extension of both the PIP and DIP joints.

The flexor tendons run in a tendon sheath volar to the three phalanges, forming a loose structure, which easily distends with the expanding synovitis. At the joint levels, the tendon sheath is equipped with pulleys, strong fibrous reinforcements that usually do not distend.

Both the extensor mechanism as well as the flexor tendons are arranged to be able to flex and extend the PIP joint separately, allowing a simultaneous extension or flexion of the DIP. The two

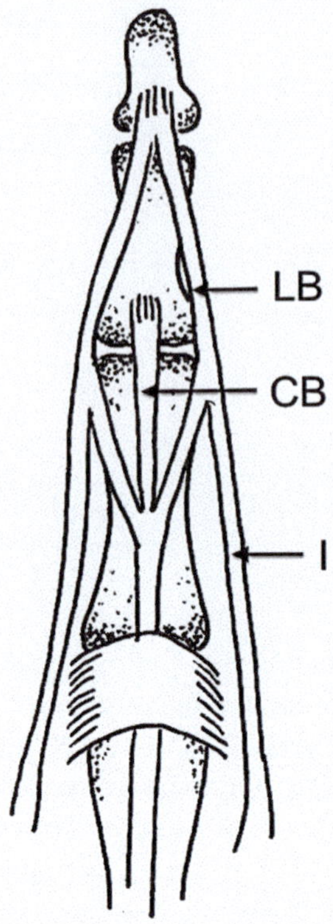

Fig. 16.1 A dorsal view of the finger extensor mechanism shows the relation between the central band (CB) acting on the PIP joint and the lateral bands (LB) acting on both PIP and DIP joints

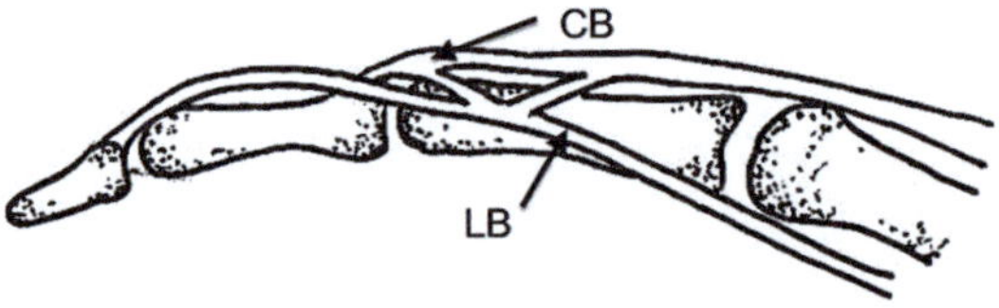

Fig. 16.2 A lateral view of the finger shows the dorsal position of the extensor mechanism including central band (CB) and lateral band (LB) in relation to the PIP axis of flexion/extension

flexor tendons insert at both sides of the DIP joint. The superficial tendon (FDS) inserts at the middle phalanx and the profundus tendon (FDP) at the volar side of the distal phalanx. In a similar fashion, the central band inserts at the base of the middle phalanx and the conjoined lateral bands at the distal phalanx (Fig. 16.3).

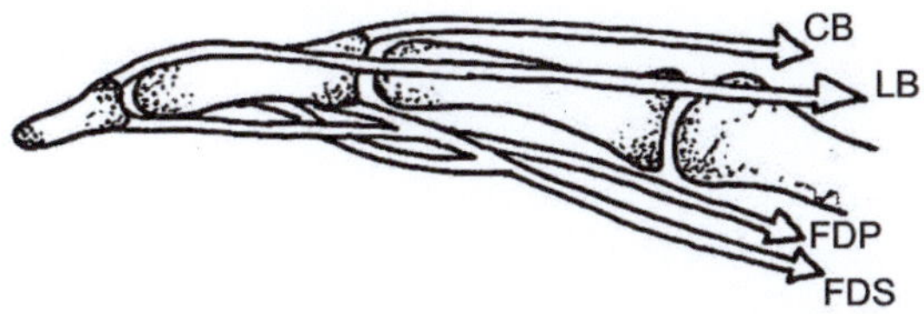

Fig. 16.3 The balance between the extensor and flexor mechanisms. The FDP tendon and the lateral bands (LB) act on both joints with the FDS tendon and the central band (CB) acting on the PIP joint only

Effect of the Disease on Finger Anatomy and Finger Function

The cause of the finger deformities in rheumatoid arthritis is the synovial inflammation in both the joints and in the flexor tendon sheaths [2]. The volume of the synovium increases and the joint capsules and the tendon sheath bulge with a gradual distension of the weak structures. In time, the synovitis in the joints will cause bone erosions, primarily around the ligament insertions, and destroy the stabilizing ligaments. The synovitis of the tendon sheath causes tendon degeneration in a similar way. Owing to the mechanical load when using the fingers and the distribution of the bone, ligament, and tendon derangements, a variety of deformities may evolve.

Unlike the flexors, the extensor tendons are not covered by a synovial lining and are therefore not subject to the destructive effects of the synovitis. The extensor tendon lesions are therefore only secondary to the joint synovitis. At the PIP level, the distension of the joint capsule will secondarily distend the loose connective tissue between the lateral and central band. This initiates an elongation of the central band, and the lateral bands are dislocated volarly, causing a lack of PIP extension. Indirectly, the volar displacement of the lateral bands will have consequences more distally and the DIP joint may hyperextend. Though rarely occurring, laterally directed deformation of the PIP joint is, however, not related to the PIP synovitis but secondary to an MCP involvement [3, 4].

Although the flexor tendon synovitis occurs along the two tendons, disease manifestations are mainly found where the synovial tendon sheath is present. Proximally, the tendons passing through the carpal tunnel may be involved, and distally, the tendons in the tendon sheath are affected from the MCP level to the DIP. The synovitis initially develops close to the vascularizing structures of the tendons and mobility is primarily affected in flexion. The PIP is affected early with a restriction of the active flexion. In time, the intrinsic muscles are progressively reduced in their relative length, leading to an intrinsic tightness that compensates this lack of flexion.

Ruptures of the flexor tendons within the flexor sheath today are rare, due to the success of modern medication. FDP rupture is readily noticed by the patient himself or herself, in contrast to the FDS rupture, which usually is diagnosed as an imbalance between the extensor and flexor tendons at the PIP level. A change in the length of the tendons, by distention, rupture, or simply an inability to glide, will provoke an imbalance leading to the boutonnière or swan-neck deformity. Although the synovitis initiates the deformity by causing the imbalance between structures, a successful treatment of the synovitis does not always guarantee the regress of the deformity. Once the imbalance is established, it may progress by itself even without any signs of active synovitis.

Modern medication has been successful and boutonnière and swan-neck deformities today do not normally fully develop. However, the deformity of the fingers in rheumatoid arthritis still follow the patterns of these two typical deformities, and the knowledge of the biological and mechanical pathologic pathways makes the treatment more logical and easier.

The Boutonnière Deformity

Boutonniere is the French word for the buttonhole deformity (Fig. 16.4). A rupture of the central band, with a lateral or even volar dislocation

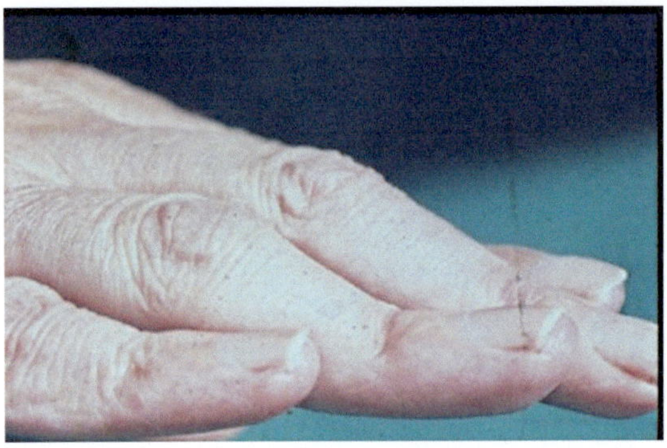

Fig. 16.4 A mild boutonnière of the middle finger and a more advanced deformity in the ring finger

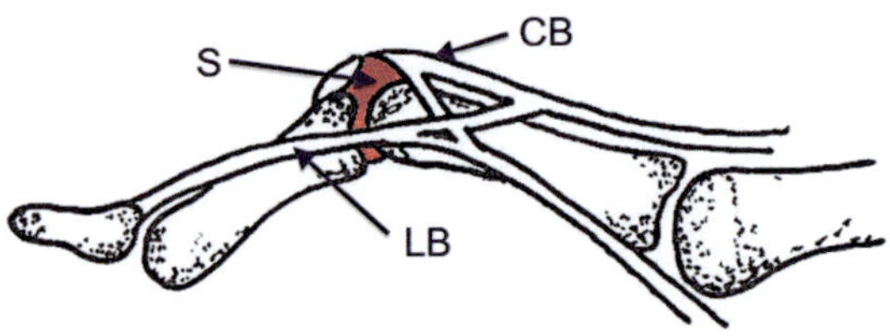

Fig. 16.5 A boutonnière deformity provoked by the synovitis (S) and the distention and rupture of the central band (CB). As a consequence, the lateral bands (LB) displace volarly and become PIP joint flexors and at the same time participate in the hyperextension of the DIP joint

of the lateral bands, mimics the buttonhole of a shirt. The PIP joint protrudes dorsally through the extensor mechanism, which then poses the equivalent to the button itself. The boutonniere deformity is the result of a *joint* synovitis and not a *tendon* synovitis (Fig. 16.5). The boutonniere deformity is a joint and not a tendon lesion. However, once the deformity is established, it will cause a disturbance of the entire extensor mechanism, which has to be treated. Treating only the joint synovitis is not enough. To determine the proper treatment, the boutonniere deformity is divided into two stages, depending on whether the PIP extension defect and the DIP flexion defect are possible to passively correct. The extent of the active PIP extension deficit, per se, appears less important. In early correctable deformities, the DIP joint can be flexed by extending the PIP joint, and a dorsal mobilization of the lateral bands is still possible. In late cases, the deformity is fixed [3, 4]. In end cases, the

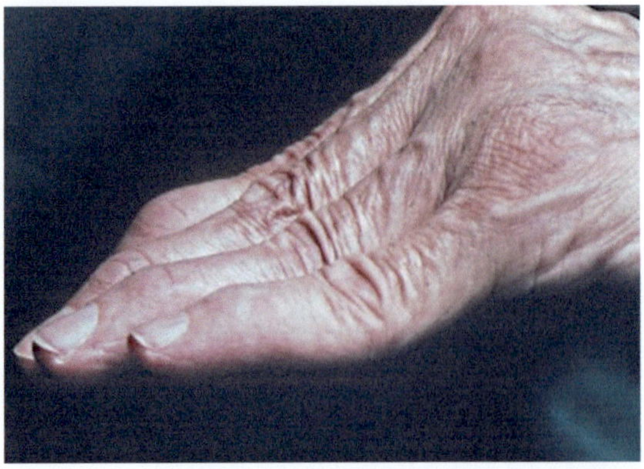

Fig. 16.6 Four fingers with swan-neck deformities and MCP extension deficits

subchondral bone and the joint cartilage have been destroyed by the synovitis and the mechanical load and soft tissue procedures cannot fully address the deformity. Prosthetic replacement combined with rebalancing may be the choice, or even arthrodesis.

The Swan-Neck Deformity

Also the swan-neck deformity has its French eponym, "la déformation en col de cygne" (Fig. 16.6). The swan-neck deformity is in one way the opposite of the boutonnière deformity in presenting with a hyperextension of the PIP joint and a flexion of the DIP joint. If the pathogenesis of the boutonnière deformity is quite clear, the swan-neck deformity has a multifactorial origin. If the boutonniere deformity is caused by an extensor insufficiency, the swan-neck deformity is caused by an imbalance in PIP by a disturbed flexor mechanism [5, 6]. The reduced PIP flexion can be secondary to a volar dislocation of the basal phalanx in the MCP joint, due to MCP joint synovitis, or an excessive tension of the intrinsic muscles. The synovitis of the flexor tendons again is the primary cause of the deformity, with a reduction of the active finger joint flexion (Fig. 16.7). The intact intrinsic muscles flex the MCP and extend the PIP joints. In PIP joint synovitis, a distension or even rupture of the volar structures of the PIP joint increases the extension. In the swan-neck deformity, the concomitant

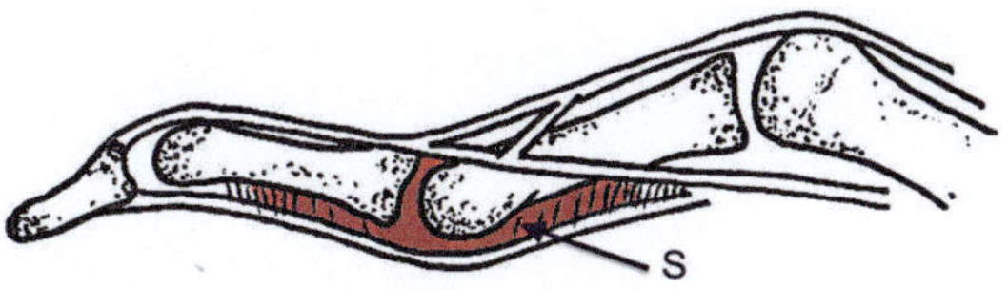

Fig. 16.7 Swan-neck deformity initiated by volar flexor tenosynovitis (S), distension of the PIP volar plate, and compensatory flexion of the MCP joint. A secondary intrinsic tightness may accentuate the deformity even after the regress of the synovitis

presence of an imbalance between the flexor and extensor mechanism, together with a weakness of the volar capsule of the PIP joint, is the primary cause. It is important to note that swan-neck deformities in RA almost always are associated with a lack of MCP extension and that the extent of the swan-neck deformity relates to the extent of the limitation of the PIP passive flexion, especially in relation with the MCP position.

Intrinsic Tightness

Intrinsic tightness is caused by a contracture of the intrinsic muscles inserting into the extensor tendon. In MCP flexion, the length of the intrinsic muscles is sufficient to allow extension of the PIP joint. In MCP extension, in contrast, the intrinsic muscles are too short to allow extension of the PIP joint. Intrinsic tightness has to be recognized as an important factor aggravating a nascent or mild finger deformity in RA (Fig. 16.8). Normally, the shortening is equal in both the radial and ulnar intrinsic muscles, but in ulnar or radial deviation of the MCP joints, one of the intrinsic muscles will be tighter than the other with some possible consequence such as a lateral deviation of the PIP joint. The intrinsic tightness is evaluated by examining the ability of the patient to flex the PIP actively or passively when the MCP joint is extended. When the structures are tight, shortened intrinsic muscles reduce the flexion of the PIP [7].

Joint Deformities

A long-standing active synovitis in joints will not only distend and elongate the surrounding tissues but will also destroy ligament insertions and

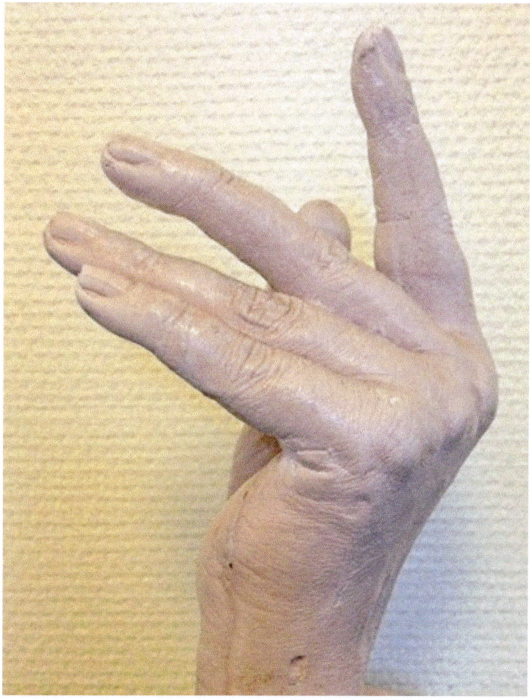

Fig. 16.8 A three-dimensional reconstruction of the right hand of a 31-year-old woman before surgery (plaster of Paris model from 1972). The fingers present with different grades of swan-neck deformities and advanced flexion contractures in MCP and intrinsic tightness. The treatment should start with MCP surgery in order to evaluate the need of future treatment for the fingers

cartilage leading to instability, lateral deviation, and joint collapse. All kinds of malpositions can follow the joint destructions, depending on the evolving malposition, the deformation of adjacent joints, as well as the patient activity. A joint instability or destruction, especially in the PIP joint, limits the therapeutic and reconstruction possibilities, which motivates an early treatment before established deformity (Fig. 16.9).

Rheumatoid Nodule

Subcutaneous nodules are relatively frequent in RA and consist histologically of a fibrinoid necrosis surrounded by fibrous tissue. The nodules are often located over bony prominences like the MCP or PIP joints but may also appear on the palmar side of the hand, especially in the finger pulp. The nodules are cosmetically embarrassing for the patient but may also disturb the

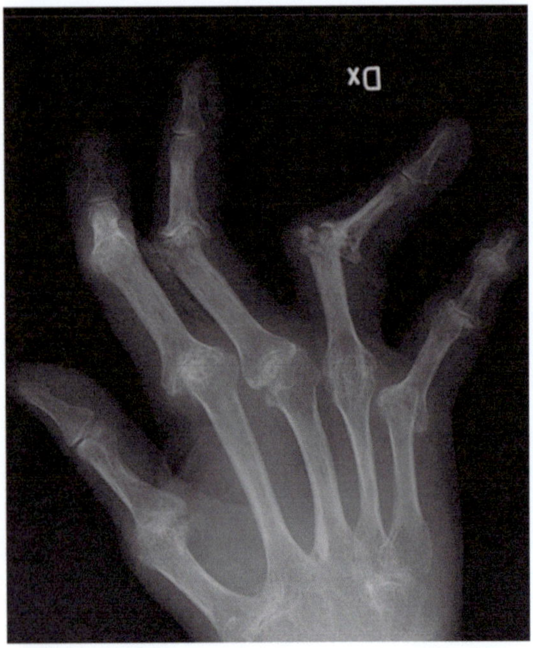

Fig. 16.9 Different finger deformities can be seen on this radiograph of a patient with juvenile rheumatoid arthritis: an advanced boutonnière deformity of the index finger and PIP joint destruction with ulnar deviation of the long and ring fingers. Note also the different deformations of the MCP joints

grip function when located in the pulp and be painful when located laterally by interfering with other fingers (Fig. 16.10).

Treatment Options

Before contemplating surgical intervention, the reduction or rather the eradication of the synovitis is mandatory to eliminate the cause of the finger deformity. The modern medical approach with potent drugs has reduced the indications for a surgical joint or tendon synovectomy, which was so common not too long ago. Early medical treatment is logical. The use of splints and physiotherapy is relatively safe, but prophylactic surgery always comes with a risk of deteriorating the function in a patient with more or less absent subjective deficits. Still, the surgical treatment preferably should be considered before the deformities become fixed [8–10]. When surgical procedures are initiated, the results always depend

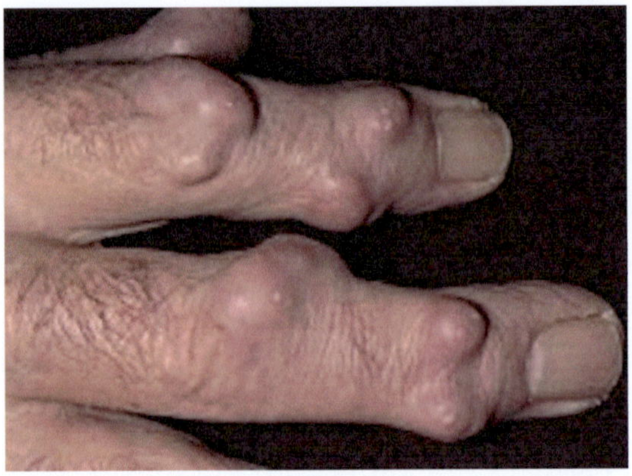

Fig. 16.10 Rheumatoid nodules

on competent physiotherapy, preferably in specialized rheumatoid centers, including the use of postoperative splints to allow the tissues to adapt to as near physiologic motion arcs as possible. The patient has to be meticulously informed of the importance of the rehabilitation and be aware of the length of time of the postsurgical treatment. The deformities have rarely reached the same stage and often different deformities are found in the same hand. Three adjacent fingers may present differently, with a boutonnière in one, a swan neck in the other, and a lateral deformity in the third finger. Therefore, the treatment of the finger deformities should be individualized for each finger, but with the whole hand, carpus, or upper extremity in mind [11]. A surgical plan is to be proposed to the patient, preferably as a single session but sometimes as staged procedures. Often stabilization of the carpus is necessary before treating the finger deformity itself, with reduction of the radial deviation, reduction of an ulnarly deviated MCP joint, recentralization of the tendons at the MCP level, and reduction of an often volarly dislocated proximal phalanx. Before deciding or even suggesting treatment of the rheumatoid finger, the hand function and the deformity patterns should be evaluated with an analysis of the needs of the individual fingers. The precise and complete examination of the finger deformities and the analysis of the radiographs help in the choice of possible treatment but are never in themselves an indication for treatment. The patient instead has to try to define the difficulties for which he or she seeks surgical remedy and what function or tasks are to be improved or recovered [12].

The sequence of surgery is still a matter of debate but it may appear logical to start proximally. It is important to consider what is possible to achieve in one operative session, not only for technical and time reasons but maybe more for the postoperative rehabilitation. For these reasons, often surgery on the volar/flexor side of the hand precedes surgery on the dorsal/extensor side of the hand [13, 14]. It is rarely possible to recover full range of motion in the MCP, PIP, and DIP joints, and these three joints should be considered as a unique functional entity with the capacity of one joint to compensate for the lack of motion or deformity in another. The disabilities and patient complaints are most often associated with lack of MCP extension and/or a lack of flexion in PIP and/or DIP malposition (hyperextension or hyperflexion). In advanced cases, in which the finger deformity is not isolated, the following sequence can be proposed:

1. Volar synovectomy of fingers with complete tenosynovectomy, including nerve decompression. Intraoperatively, the freedom of the joints to move can be evaluated by pulling both the FDS and FDP at the different anatomical levels.
2. Dorsal tenosynovectomy, combined if necessary with recentralization of the extensor tendons at the MCP level by soft tissue plasty, or implants together with a carpal recentralization and stabilization by radio-lunate fusion.
3. Reduction of the volar luxation of the proximal phalanx in the MCP joint and treatment of the intrinsic tightness.
4. Treatment of the finger deformity itself.

The goal in the treatment of the boutonnière deformity is to reduce the PIP extension defect but also the hyperextension of the DIP joint. Before surgery, the elasticity of the soft tissue and the possibility to reduce the deformity is evaluated. Preoperative physiotherapy includes splints to reduce the passive deformity. If the deformity can be reduced, the reinsertion of the central band and a relocation of the lateral band, dorsal to the PIP center of rotation, have to be performed. Although technically demanding, a trans-osseous central band reinsertion with careful adaptation of the length will normally reposition the lateral bands. If not, a careful dissection and mobilization of the lateral bands and a suture of the structures in a dorsal position can be done. Suture anchors or other devices that may interfere with implants in future surgery are best avoided. A plethora of techniques for lateral band transfer and sutures has been proposed to secure the relocation but are almost all sources of secondary stiffness.

A fixed DIP joint extension deformity is often identified by the patient as the main disturbing factor of the boutonnière deformity and has to be addressed in all cases. A simple division of the extensor tendon proximal to the DIP joint normally gives good results without secondary flexion deformity. None of the different described tenotomy techniques have shown to be superior. In late cases of boutonnière deformity, with a fixed PIP in flexion, a PIP fusion can be proposed. The shortening associated with the procedure may in some cases make the tenotomy at DIP level unnecessary.

The swan-neck deformity is often identified by the patient as a severe impairment of hand and finger function. Here, the goal of treatment is the recovery of a smooth PIP flexion. If a moderate lack of extension after treatment is acceptable to the patient, the surgical treatment offers a relatively good end result. If the tenosynovectomy on the volar side cannot solve the recurrent PIP joint hyperextension, some type of tendon transfer has to be suggested. One lateral band is mobilized and detached proximally, keeping only its distal attachment. The tendon slip is rerouted volarly to the Cleland transverse ligament before sutured to the A2 pulley. The rerouted lateral band is maintained in adequate tension in order to gently flex the PIP. To avoid the recurrence, an extension block is used as a postoperative splint, and the goal should not be to recover full extension but rather a PIP extension of maybe 10–20°. A free tendon graft or other rerouting or suture procedures can be used but have not shown to be superior. In case of a decreased passive flexion of the PIP joint, the joint may be surgically released, but the results are often disappointing in spite of a long and demanding rehabilitation period. In these cases, in our view, a joint fusion in a slight flexed position is preferable. The DIP flexion deformity is often reduced spontaneously by restoring the normal PIP joint mobility, but the DIP joint sometimes needs to be fused also in order to position the finger pulp in a functional position.

The use of an implant by itself is not sufficient to treat a boutonnière or swan-neck deformity. In stiff fingers with large bone erosions, the mobility of the PIP joint may be recovered but the rebalancing of the extensor mechanism is difficult. A proper positioning of the implant in relation to the center of rotation must be respected and a special technique approaching the joint has to be used in order to shorten or elongate the soft tissue. The results with an implant are far better when treating a swan neck than a boutonnière.

Technical Tips

Approach and Incision

RA is a chronic disease and patient treatment may need several surgical procedures over time. For this reason, it is important at the primary surgery to use an approach and incision that can be reused for subsequent surgeries in order to avoid multiple scars with an increased risk of healing problems or even skin necrosis.

Rheumatoid Nodule

Despite the relative high risk of recurrence, surgical excision may be proposed for cosmetic and functional reasons. Laser excision can be used but does not reduce the level of recurrence. Excision can be difficult due to the close adherence to the skin and the neurovascular bundles.

Joint Fusion

Small and noninvasive fixation material has to be used in RA patient because of the quality of the skin and the soft tissues. The position of the fused joint has to be purposeful with proper orientation of the finger pulp, taking into account the adjacent joint deformities or decreased mobility. For the same reason, a minimal shortening of the finger permits optimal thumb or hand grip. The position of the pins securing the arthrodesis has to be carefully chosen to avoid interfering with hand function during rehabilitation [15].

Central Band Suture

The central band is mobilized distally after dissection and resutured or reinserted into its original insertion. The flexion capacity has to be tested during surgery, and a good PIP flexion is the priority by accepting some degrees of residual extension lack. In our opinion, complicated tendon transfer or free tendon graft is to be avoided due to a high risk of secondary stiffness [16, 17].

Lateral Band Relocation in Boutonnière

If quite extensive surgery and dissection can be done to mobilize the lateral band back in place dorsally to the PIP axis of rotation, the suture repair should not restrict motion.

Lateral Band Rerouting in Swan Neck

One lateral band is mobilized and detached proximally, keeping only its distal attachment. The tendon slip is rerouted volarly to the Cleland transverse ligament before sutured to the A2 pulley. The rerouted lateral band is maintained in adequate tension to gently flex the PIP. To avoid the recurrence, an extension block is used as a postoperative splint, and the goal should not be full extension but rather a PIP extension of maybe 10–20° (Fig. 16.11).

Tenotomy at DIP Level

A tenotomy may be the procedure of choice for a DIP hyperextension deformity. A simple incision of the extensor tendon proximal to PIP is

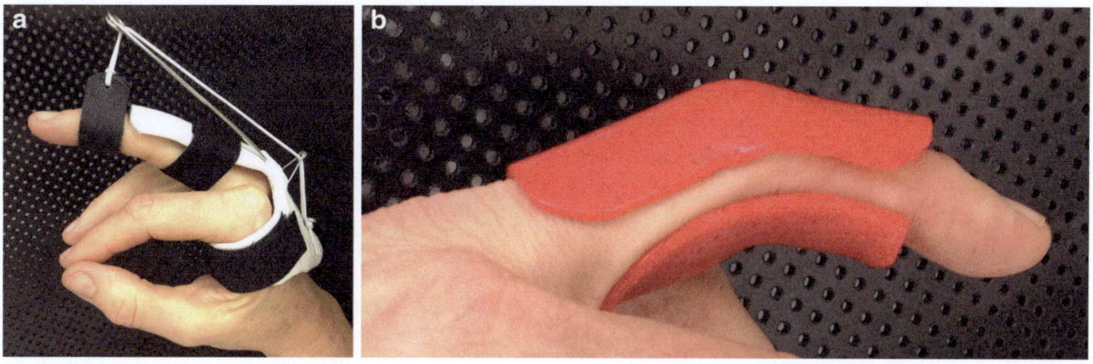

Fig. 16.11 An example of splint that allows early motion of PIP after tendon transfer for swan-neck deformity or implant surgery. Note the block with an extension defect of 10–20° (**a**). A night splint has to be used for a period of almost 3 months after surgery (**b**)

made percutaneously associated with a gentle mobilization of the DIP in flexion. We avoid pin fixation by giving priority to an early active mobilization.

Implants

Implants are part of the treatment of finger deformities in RA but should be used with care. The proper positioning of the implant in relation to the axis of rotation in the PIP joint in combination with the imbalance of tendons makes the procedure very demanding. In our hands, only a dorsal approach provides the possibility to adjust the tendon length. The silicone PIP implants in our hands have been associated with instability and lateral deviation and are only used in rare cases in the central fingers. Bicondylar implants and non-constrained implants like the pyrocarbon implants have been used with good results especially in young patients. The size of the implants remains a problem in these often very small fingers. In a few cases, we have used only the proximal part of the implant as a hemiarthroplasty. Implants in DIP are not used today [18, 19] (Fig. 16.12).

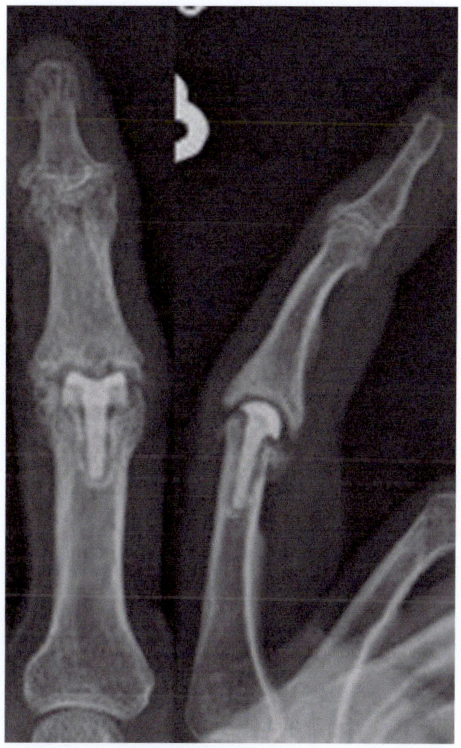

Fig. 16.12 A proximal pyrocarbon hemiarthroplasty in order to correct a boutonniere deformity. An approach according to Chamay was used to correct the elongation of the central band

Conclusion

The consequences of slowly evolving finger deformities in RA may cause a deteriorating hand function, and even in the era of the modern drug-based rheumatoid treatment, hand and finger involvement has to be followed carefully from the beginning of the disease. The patient preferably should be in contact with a hand surgeon long before surgery is considered necessary. The treatments of the established deformities are often difficult and the results may be disappointing for the patient. Thus, all efforts are to be considered to avoid the development into fixed joint deformities. Ergonomic advice and the use of splints may help but it should be kept in mind that the main factor to be treated is the synovitis. In some cases, prophylactic surgical synovectomy has to be proposed if medical treatment is insufficient. A set goal for the treatment has to be defined in collaboration with the patient, combining the need and wishes of the patient but also the activity of the disease and the associated deformation and joint involvements in both hands. The possibilities of surgery have to be presented to the patient with full disclosures of the possible problems and drawbacks. It is better for the patient to have more use of a good joint fusion than a bad arthroplasty. In all cases, the surgery has to be as simple as possible, by avoiding complicated tendon transfer and extensive surgery, bearing in mind that the results have to be predictable and persisting over time.

References

1. Carrera A, Forcada P, Garcia-Elias M, Lusa Pérez M. Hand and finger anatomy. In: Llusa Pérez A, editor. Atlas de Disseccion Anatomiquirurgica de la Muneca y de la Mano. Barcelona: Elsevier Masson; 2007. p. 122–44.
2. Allieu Y. Deformities of the hand in rheumatoid arthritis. Etio-pathogenesis and pathological anatomy. Therapeutical deductions. Rev Rheum Mal Osteoartic. 1973;40(3):203–5.
3. Lluch A. Surgical management of the rheumatoid hand. In: Bentley G, editor. European Surgical Orthopedics and Traumatology. The EFORT textbook, vol. 3. London: Springer; 2014. p. 2051–83.
4. Lluch A. The treatment of finger joint deformities in rheumatoid arthritis. In: Allieu Y, editor. The Rheumatoid Hand and Wrist. Surgical treatment. Paris: Expansion Scientifique Publications; 1988. p. 85–104.
5. Horner G, Terrano A. Soft tissues procedures for the rheumatoid swan-neck finger deformity. Tech Hand Up Extrem Surg. 2000;4:22–9.
6. Nalebuff EA. The rheumatoid swan-neck deformity. Hand Clin. 1989;5:203–14.
7. Chetta M, Burns PB, Kim HM, Burke FD, Wilgis EF, Fox DA, Chung KC. The effect of swan neck and boutonnière deformities on the outcome of silicone metacarpophalangeal joint arthroplasty in rheumatoid arthritis. Plast Reconstr Surg. 2013; 132(3):597–603.
8. Dahl E, et al. Flexor tendon synovectomy of the hand in rheumatoid arthritis. A follow up study of 201 operated hand. Scand J Rheumatol. 1976;5:103–7.
9. Duché R, Canovas F, Thaury MN, Bouges S, Allieu Y. Tenosynovectomy of the flexor in rheumatoid polyarthritis. Analytic study of short term and long term mobility of the fingers. Ann Chir Main Memb Super. 1993;12(2):85–92.
10. Tolat AR, Stanley JK, Evans RA. Flexor tenosynovectomy and tenolysis in longstanding rheumatoid arthritis. J Hand Surg. 1996;21-B:538–43.
11. Sebastin SJ, Chung KC. Reconstruction of digital deformities in rheumatoid arthritis. Hand Clin. 2011;27(1):87–104.
12. Malcus Johnsson P, Sandqvist G, Sturesson AL, Gulfe A, Kopylov P, Tägil M, Geborek P. Individualized outcomes measures of daily activities are sensitive tools for evaluating hand surgery in rheumatic diseases. Rheumatology (Oxford). 2012;51(12): 2246–51.
13. Stanley D, Norris SH. The pathogenesis and treatment of rheumatoid wrist and hand deformities. Br J Hosp Med. 1988;39(2):156–60.
14. Fowler JR, Baratz ME. Distal interphalangeal joint arthrodesis. J Hand Surg Am. 2014;39(1):126–8.
15. Nalebuff EA, Millender LH. Surgical treatment of the boutonnière deformity in rheumatoid arthritis. Orthop Clin North Am. 1975;6(3):753–63.
16. Williams K, Terrono AL. Treatment of boutonnière finger deformity in rheumatoid arthritis. J Hand Surg Am. 2011;36(8):1388–93.
17. Boyer MI, Gelberman RH. Operative correction of swan-neck and boutonniere deformities in the rheumatoid hand. J Am Acad Orthop Surg. 1999; 7(2):92–100.
18. Rizzo M, Beckenbaugh RD. Proximal interphalangeal joint arthroplasty. J Am Acad Orthop Surg. 2007; 15(3):189–97.
19. Tägil M, Geijer M, Abramo A, Kopylov P. Ten years' experience with a pyrocarbon prosthesis replacing the proximal interphalangeal joint. A prospective clinical and radiographical follow-up. J Hand Surg Eur Vol. 2013;39(6):587–95.

Biomechanics of Rheumatoid Finger Deformities

17

Nathan T. Morrell and Arnold-Peter C. Weiss

Introduction

The human finger is an amazing mechanical structure. The complex anatomy of the digit imparts stability to an otherwise unstable mechanical setup, allowing the finger to perform an incredible variety of precise mechanical functions. Rheumatoid arthritis is a chronic, progressive, systemic, autoimmune, inflammatory disorder that affects numerous organ systems and frequently involves the musculoskeletal system in the hand [1]. The synovial hypertrophy, collagenous destruction, and bony resorption that are typical of rheumatoid arthritis lead to a disruption of normal anatomy and hence a disruption of the normal biomechanics of the digit. In order to fully appreciate the biomechanical changes that are frequently present in the rheumatoid finger, one must understand the intricate workings of the non-pathologic finger. In this chapter we review normal finger anatomy and biomechanics and then discuss the biomechanical changes of common rheumatoid finger deformities.

N.T. Morrell, MD (✉)
Department of Orthopaedics & Rehabilitation, University of Vermont, Burlington, VT, USA
e-mail: nathan.morrell@uvmhealth.org

A.-P. C. Weiss, MD (✉)
Department of Orthopaedics, Brown University/ Rhode Island Hospital, Providence, RI, USA
e-mail: apcweiss@brown.edu

Normal Anatomy and Mechanics

Joint Anatomy

In the normal human finger, there are two types of joints: the metacarpophalangeal (MCP) joint is an ellipsoidal joint, while the interphalangeal joints are hinge joints. Ellipsoidal joints have reciprocal, elliptical convex (metacarpal head) and concave (proximal phalangeal base) surfaces that allow both flexion-extension and abduction-adduction movements (two degrees of freedom). Hinge joints are conceptually simpler, allowing only flexion-extension around a fixed axis of rotation (one degree of freedom) [2, 3].

The metacarpal head is asymmetric in both the sagittal and coronal planes. The volar aspect of the metacarpal head is longer and broader than the dorsal aspect; this allows the center of rotation to move volarly with flexion and also creates a cam effect that causes the proper collateral ligaments to tighten in flexion. Additionally, the radial condyle is larger than the ulnar condyle, causing the metacarpal head to slope ulnarly and proximally in the coronal plane; this is especially true in the second and third metacarpals [2, 4]. This becomes readily apparent when one considers the common volar and ulnar deformity seen at the MCP joint in

K.C. Chung (ed.), *Clinical Management of the Rheumatoid Hand, Wrist, and Elbow*,
DOI 10.1007/978-3-319-26660-2_17

rheumatoid arthritis. The interphalangeal joints have more congruent anatomy. At each joint, there is a trochlea on the proximal aspect that is perpendicular to the axis of rotation. This provides medial, lateral, and rotational stability. The trochlea matches reciprocally with an intercondylar groove on the opposite side of the joint.

Extensor Anatomy

The extensor apparatus is composed of extrinsic tendon contributions, intrinsic tendon contributions, and intrinsic ligament contributions. The extensor digitorum communis tendon (and proprius) merges with an extensor hood at the level of the MCP joint. Sagittal bands arising from the volar plate and intermetacarpal ligaments centralize the extrinsic extensor tendon(s) at the MCP joint. The anatomy gets even more complicated at the level of the proximal interphalangeal (PIP) joint. Here, tendinous contributions from the intrinsic muscles merge with an extension of the extrinsic tendon to form the central slip which has a bony attachment at the base of the middle phalanx. Additionally, contributions from both the extrinsic and intrinsic muscles merge to form the lateral bands on both the radial and ulnar aspects of the digit. The lateral bands are maintained in relation to the central slip by the transverse retinacular ligament, which has both dorsal and lateral components and arises from the volar plate. The lateral bands on either side of the digit merge distally on the dorsal surface of the middle phalanx with the triangular ligament and eventually insert at the base of the distal phalanx as the terminal extensor tendon. Also merging with the terminal extensor tendon is the oblique retinacular ligament which arises from the volar plate and flexor tendon sheath at the level of the PIP joint.

Basic Mechanical Concepts

A few basic mechanical concepts are worth reviewing. A *moment* is a vector quantity. A *moment arm* (or lever arm) is the perpendicular distance from a joint's axis of rotation to the force (e.g., tendon) that acts upon it. The *moment about the axis* is the cross product of a force and its moment arm about an axis: M (moment) $= F$ (force) $\times L$ (moment arm). *Torque* is also the product of force and moment arm, though is a scalar quantity (rather than a vector quantity like a moment). *Mechanical advantage* relates to the efficiency of a moment (lever) arm; the larger the moment arm, the smaller the force needed to achieve the same torque [2].

The normal anatomy of the flexor tendon sheath with its numerous pulleys serves to provide a mechanical advantage to the extrinsic finger flexor tendons. By maintaining the tendons close to the joints that they act upon, less excursion (or force) is needed to create a given angular change. This is expressed as: θ (angle) $= s$ (tendon excursion) $\div r$ (moment arm). On average, the flexor digitorum profundus tendon passes 5 mm from the axis of rotation of the DIP joint, 7.5 mm from that of the PIP joint, and 10 mm from that of the MCP joint; the flexor digitorum superficialis tendon passes 7 mm from the axis of rotation of the PIP joint and 13 mm from that of the MCP joint [2].

Rheumatoid Pathoanatomy and Mechanics

Sagittal Plane Deformities

From a mechanical standpoint, three bodies articulating in series, as the phalanges do in the fingers, are inherently unstable [2]. The normal extrinsic and intrinsic anatomy of the fingers stabilizes the digits, creating a biomechanical equilibrium that allows fine and intricate control. In rheumatoid arthritis, the disease process leads to a disruption of this inherent stability, causing a variety of deformities. Characteristic deformities are seen in the sagittal plane, videlicet, boutonniere and swan-neck deformities, of course variations and combination deformities can also occur [5]. The prevalence of these deformities in patients with established rheumatoid arthritis is 36 % and 14 %, respectively [6]. Much is due to disruptions of the extensor mechanism, which, because of its complex anatomy, can cause significant biomechanical changes. As Littler wrote many years ago, “Unlike the flexor mechanism, useful extensor function is readily jeopardized by the alteration of even a few millimeters’ excursion in the conjoined central and lateral tendon length relationship” [7].

Boutonniere Deformity

A boutonniere deformity is flexion at the proximal interphalangeal (PIP) joint and hyperextension at the distal interphalangeal (DIP) joint; it is invariably due to a loss of tendon balance at the PIP joint. “Boutonniere” is literally the French word for “buttonhole”; this makes sense when considering the pathogenesis of the deformity. In rheumatoid arthritis, synovial proliferation distends the PIP joint capsule and surrounding extensor apparatus. The central slip is attenuated and often ruptures; the dorsal aspect of the transverse retinacular ligament between the central slip and lateral bands is also stretched [5]. This dorsal attenuation allows the PIP joint to “buttonhole” through the extensor apparatus.

The pathologic changes in anatomy at the PIP joint have an adverse effect on the normal biomechanics of the digit. At the PIP joint itself, the attenuation of the central slip leads to a decreased extensor moment at that joint. Additionally, as the buttonholing progresses, the lateral bands migrate in a palmar direction, ultimately coursing volar to the axis of rotation and becoming flexors of the PIP joint, rather than extensors. As such, there is a strong flexion moment at the PIP joint. The volar position of the lateral bands increases their effectiveness as extensors of the DIP joint; thus, a flexion deformity at the PIP joint reciprocally causes an extension deformity at the DIP joint [5] (Fig. 17.1).

The treatment of boutonniere deformities in rheumatoid arthritis depends on the severity of the disease and deformity, existing joint motion (passive and active), and the condition or the articular surface [8]. Nalebuff and Millender provided a three-staged classification [9]. In stage 1, there is a mild (10–15°) active extensor lag at the PIP joint that is passively correctable. Additionally, there is little, if any, active DIP flexion when the PIP joint is held in extension. Most of the disability experienced by patients at this early stage is related to the lack of DIP flexion [5]. In stage 2, there is a moderate (typically 30–40°) flexion deformity at the PIP joint; this stage is subdivided based on the passive correctability of the PIP joint and the degree of the contracture. At this stage, most of the disability is due to the deformity at the PIP joint. In stage 3, there is articular destruction on radiographs and the typically severe PIP contracture is fixed. As the PIP deformity progresses, there is frequently

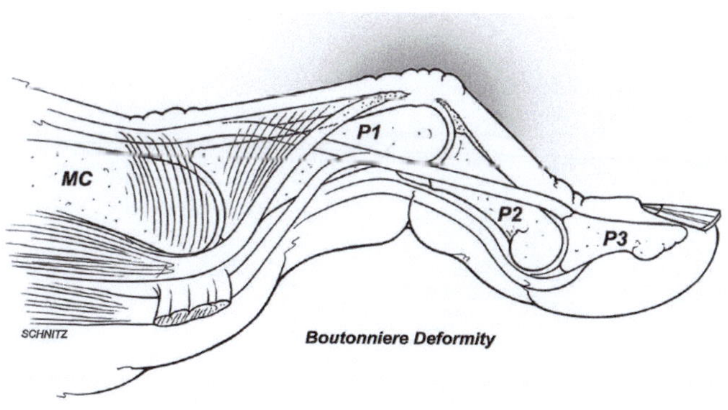

Fig. 17.1 Disruption of the central extensor tendon slips occurs at the dorsal PIP joint secondary to erosive synovitis. The extensor tendon, released from its insertional tether, retracts proximally. The lateral bands slide off the dorsal aspect of the PIP joint and migrate volar to the axis of rotation, causing a PIP flexion moment arm. Since the lateral bands connect to the extensor mechanism, they are pulled proximally and result in DIP hyperextension. From Gonzalez MH, Mohan V, Elhassan B, Amirouche F. Biomechanics of the Digit. J Am Soc Surg Hand. 2005;5(1):48–59. Reprinted with permission from the Journal of the American Society for Surgery of the Hand

a compensatory hyperextension at the metacarpophalangeal (MCP) joint to allow continued use of the digit.

Swan-Neck Deformity

A swan-neck deformity is hyperextension at the PIP joint and flexion at the DIP joint. Whereas a boutonniere deformity is classically due to biomechanical changes originating at the PIP joint, a swan-neck deformity may be due to the sequelae of biomechanical alterations originating at any of the three digital joints (the MCP, PIP, or DIP joints) [5]. The most common is when hypertrophied rheumatoid synovium infiltrates the volar plate, collateral ligaments, and flexor digitorum superficialis insertion about the PIP joint allowing the extensor mechanism to pull the PIP joint into hyperextension. Synovitis-induced attenuation of the lateral portion of the transverse retinaculum allows the lateral bands to migrate dorsally, increasing their distance from the PIP joint axis of rotation and thus increasing their moment arm as extenders of this joint. Synovitis at the DIP joint can lead to attenuation or disruption of the terminal extensor tendon. This leads to a relative flexor over-pull at the DIP joint causing the mallet deformity classically seen in swan-neck deformity. Additionally, the loss of the terminal extensor function actually enhances the extensor forces at the PIP joint, causing or contributing to a swan-neck deformity. The extensor moment at the PIP joint can be accentuated by alterations at the MCP joint as well, such as intrinsic tightness, volar MCP subluxation, and extensor digitorum communis tendon subluxation [2, 10].

The MCP joint is actually the most commonly affected joint in the rheumatoid hand [4]. In general, there is a volar and ulnar subluxation of the proximal phalanx, relative to the metacarpal head, as the disease progresses. This is in part due to the normal geometry of the MCP joint, as well as the pathologic changes brought by rheumatoid arthritis. Synovial proliferation leads to destruction of adjacent soft tissues. Attenuation of the accessory collateral ligaments and volar plate allows for volar displacement of the flexor sheath; this increases the flexion moment (and volar subluxation force) of the flexor tendons at the MCP joint [2, 4]. Increasing subluxation of the extensor tendons potentiates this volar moment, as does interosseous muscle contracture [4] (Fig. 17.2).

Just as with boutonniere deformities, the treatment of swan-neck deformities in rheumatoid arthritis depends on the severity of the disease and deformity, existing joint motion (passive and active), and the condition or the articular surfaces. Nalebuff and Millender described four types of increasing severity: Type I is characterized by a flexible hyperextension deformity of the PIP joint; Type II is characterized by intrinsic

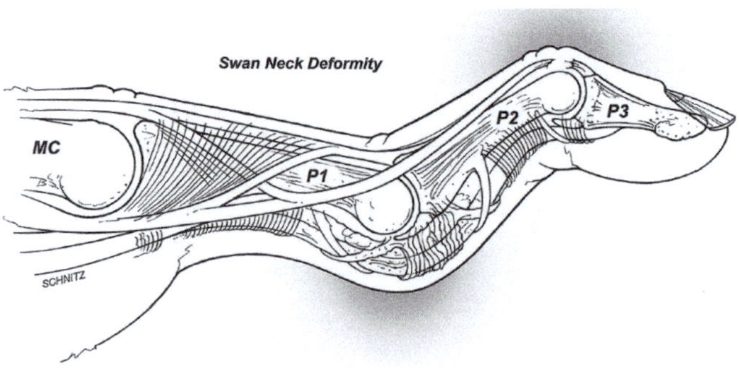

Fig. 17.2 Synovitis at the DIP joint erodes the terminal extensor tendon insertion causing rupture. The entire extensor mechanism, now untethered, migrates proximally, causing an extra proximal pull on the central slip resulting in PIP hyperextension. Since the terminal tendon ruptures, the DIP joint falls into flexion. From Gonzalez MH, Mohan V, Elhassan B, Amirouche F. Biomechanics of the Digit. J Am Soc Surg Hand. 2005;5(1):48–59. Reprinted with permission from the Journal of the American Society for Surgery of the Hand

muscle tightness that limits PIP joint flexion when the MCP joint is maintained in extension; Type III is characterized by limited PIP joint flexion, regardless of MCP joint position, due to the inability of the lateral bands to translate volar to the axis of rotation of the PIP joint; and Type IV is characterized by articular surface destruction of the PIP joint [10, 11].

Coronal Plane Deformity

While boutonniere and swan-neck deformities are frequent sagittal plane deformities, a common coronal plane deformity occurs in the rheumatoid finger with ulnar drift at the metacarpophalangeal joint. Previous studies have found that ulnar drift is present in 29–45 % of patients with established rheumatoid arthritis [12]. This coronal plane deformity is multifactorial, though intimately related to the wrist. While the interrelationships of wrist deformity and finger deformity in rheumatoid arthritis have been well documented [4, 12], it is not the intent of this chapter to discuss in detail the anatomical and biomechanical changes observed at the wrist in rheumatoid arthritis. Briefly though, a zigzag deformity exists: as radial deviation of the wrist progresses, so typically does ulnar deviation of the fingers.

From a biomechanical standpoint, there is a relatively large ulnarly directed moment (torque) at the finger MCP joints due to the pathologic changes seen in rheumatoid arthritis. Flexor tenosynovitis thins the flexor tendon sheath, and synovitis within the MCP joint attenuates the extensor hood, both allowing the extrinsic tendons that course across the MCP joint to subluxate in an ulnar direction. The radial deviation at the wrist changes the line of pull of the extrinsic flexor and extensor tendons, increasing their ulnar moment arm at the MCP joint and leading to ulnar subluxation. Additionally, destructive changes at the metacarpal head and contracture of the ulnar-sided intrinsics (shortened already by the ulnar drift of the digit) further contribute to the progression of ulnar drift [12].

MCP Arthroplasty

As the MCP joint is the most commonly affected hand joint in rheumatoid arthritis, MCP arthroplasties are commonly performed in rheumatoid arthritis patients. Indications for implant arthroplasty include severe flexion contractures fixing the digit in a poor functional position; an arc of motion ≤40°; MCP joint pain with advanced radiographic destruction (Larsen grades III–V); and severe ulnar drift (>30°) [4]. MCP arthroplasties are designed to balance the flexor and extensor forces and reestablish the center of rotation as close to that of the native joint as possible. Anatomically neutral (30° pre-bend) block-hinge silicone-based implant arthroplasties approximate normal joint kinematics more closely than straight (zero degree bend) implants [13].

Functional Disability

While clinical experience reveals that some patients with deformed hands are able to adapt and perform a wide range of hand functions, certainly many experience disability. It has been estimated that 80–90 % of patients with rheumatoid arthritis have reduced hand function [14]. A recent study found that maximum finger flexion and extension forces were considerably lower in rheumatoid patients than in healthy controls [14]. This is likely due to the loss of biomechanical equilibrium related to rheumatoid finger deformities.

Conclusion

The human finger is an amazing mechanical structure. Complex anatomy creates a biomechanical equilibrium that allows precise and intricate function. Rheumatoid arthritis, via a myriad of mechanisms, disrupts the normal anatomy and hence the normal biomechanics of the digit. Boutonniere, swan-neck, and MCP ulnar drift are common deformities seen in the rheumatoid hand. In this chapter we have reviewed normal finger anatomy and biomechanics and discussed the biomechanical changes of these common rheumatoid finger deformities.

References

1. McInnes IB, Schett G. The pathogenesis of rheumatoid arthritis. N Engl J Med. 2011;365(23):2205–19.
2. Gonzalez MH, Mohan V, Elhassan B, Amirouche F. Biomechanics of the Digit. J Am Soc Surg Hand. 2005;5(1):48–59.
3. Rath S. Hand kinematics: Application in clinical practice. Indian J Plast Surg. 2011;44(2):178–85.
4. Abboud JA, Beredjiklian PK, Bozentka DJ. Metacarpophalangeal joint arthroplasty in rheumatoid arthritis. J Am Acad Orthop Surg. 2003;11(3):184–91.
5. Rizio L, Belsky MR. Finger deformities in rheumatoid arthritis. Hand Clin. 1996;12(3):531–40.
6. Eberhardt K, Johnson PM, Rydgren L. The occurrence and significance of hand deformities in early rheumatoid arthritis. Br J Rheumatol. 1991;30(3):211–3.
7. Littler JW. The digital extensor-flexor system. In: Converse J, editor. Reconstructive plastic surgery. 6. 2nd ed. Philadelphia: W.B. Saunders Company; 1977. p. 3166–214.
8. Williams K, Terrono AL. Treatment of boutonniere finger deformity in rheumatoid arthritis. J Hand Surg Am. 2011;36(8):1388–93.
9. Nalebuff EA, Millender LH. Surgical treatment of the boutonniere deformity in rheumatoid arthritis. Orthop Clin North Am. 1975;6(3):753–63.
10. Boyer MI, Gelberman RH. Operative correction of swan-neck and boutonniere deformities in the rheumatoid hand. J Am Acad Orthop Surg. 1999;7(2):92–100.
11. Nalebuff EA, Millender LH. Surgical treatment of the swan-neck deformity in rheumatoid arthritis. Orthop Clin North Am. 1975;6(3):733–52.
12. Oster LH, Blair WF, Steyers CM, Flatt AE. Crossed intrinsic transfer. J Hand Surg Am. 1989;14(6):963–71.
13. Weiss AP, Moore DC, Infantolino C, Crisco JJ, Akelman E, McGovern RD. Metacarpophalangeal joint mechanics after 3 different silicone arthroplasties. J Hand Surg Am. 2004;29(5):796–803.
14. Brorsson S, Nilsdotter A, Pedersen E, Bremander A, Thorstensson C. Relationship between finger flexion and extension force in healthy women and women with rheumatoid arthritis. J Rehabil Med. 2012;44(7):605–8.

Treatment of MCP Joints in the Rheumatoid Hand

18

Alberto Lluch

Functional Anatomy and Pathomechanics of the Deformities

The finger extensor tendons do not insert at the base of the proximal phalanx, as they need to glide proximally and distally to provide extension of the interphalangeal joints (IPJ). The extensor tendons are stabilized at the dorsum of the metacarpal heads by two aponeurotic expansions, the sagittal bands (SB), which insert at both sides of the volar plate of the metacarpophalangeal joints (MPJ). The SB are responsible for maintaining the extensor tendon at the dorsum of the joint during radial and ulnar inclination of the fingers, as well as allowing the tendon to glide proximally and distally during extension and flexion of the finger joints. If the intrinsic muscles are paralyzed, as seen after median and ulnar nerve lesions, the extensor tendon will only extend the MPJ, causing a claw deformity of the fingers. In these circumstances, if the MPJ are passively held in flexion, because the extensor tendon does not insert into the proximal phalanx (PP), it will be capable of extending the IP joints.

The flexion forces at the MPJ, provided by the extrinsic flexors and the intrinsic musculature, are far greater than the extension force provided by the extensor tendon. The collateral ligaments (CL) originate on the dorsum of the metacarpals and insert at the most anterior part of the base of the proximal phalanx, for the purpose of preventing the PP from displacing anteriorly. Anterior displacement of the PP is also prevented by the ball and socket joint morphology, as well as the constraint of the SB, which insert at both sides of the volar plate and should be considered as a proximal extension of the PP.

Synovitis of the MPJ will attenuate the collateral ligaments (CL) and the SB, allowing the PP to displace volarly from the pull of the extrinsic and intrinsic flexor muscles. The intensity and characteristics of the joint synovitis, as seen in cases of lupus, may rapidly destroy the CL and both SB, causing a complete anterior dislocation of the PP. When the dorsal stabilizers are not completely disrupted, the PP will partially sublux causing a scalloping deformity from wear of the dorsal part at its base.

Another common deformity is an ulnar inclination of the fingers, known as ulnar drift. There is no single cause for the ulnar drift deformity, but rather a combination of several factors and the relative importance of each of them are difficult to determine. The following causes have been described as contributing to ulnar drift of the fingers in the rheumatoid hand: gravity, thumb

A. Lluch, MD, PhD (✉)
Department of Orthopaedic Surgery, Surgery of the Hand and Upper Extremity, Institut Kaplan, Paseo Bonanova, 9, Barcelona, Spain
e-mail: alluch@telefonica.net

K.C. Chung (ed.), *Clinical Management of the Rheumatoid Hand, Wrist, and Elbow*,
DOI 10.1007/978-3-319-26660-2_18

pressure, morphology of the metacarpal heads, length of the collateral ligaments, radial inclination of the wrist, traction from the flexor tendons, intrinsic muscle spasticity or retraction, and dislocation of the extensor tendons [1, 2]. There is no space in this chapter to analyze each of the aforementioned factors. Radial inclination of the wrist has classically been described as the main cause of ulnar inclination of the fingers at the MPJ level [3, 4]. However, when only the wrist is involved, it always inclines toward the ulnar side. From our clinical and radiological studies, we have concluded that the radial inclination of the metacarpals is a volitional deformity done by the patient in order to align the fingers with the long axis of the forearm, for aesthetic and functional purposes [5].

Due to an imbalance of forces toward the ulnar side, mainly caused by the pull of the extensor tendons when flexing the carpometacarpal joints of the little and ring fingers, the radial SB will progressively elongate, allowing the extensor tendon to displace toward the ulnar side of the metacarpal head [6]. When this occurs, the pull of the extensor tendons through their intertendinous connections will bring the fingers into ulnar inclination, starting with the small finger and then progressively with the most radial fingers. The volar plate of the MPJ is attached to the PP, and all volar plates are attached to each other by the intervolar plate ligament (IVPL) (Fig. 18.1). This structure should not be called "deep intermetacarpal ligament," as it does not insert into the metacarpals. As the PP of the little finger displaces volarly and ulnarly, the rest of the fingers will displace in the same direction from the pull of the IVPL. Progressive ulnar displacement of the extensor tendons will cause loss of active extension and increased ulnar inclination of the finger upon muscle contraction. When the radial sagittal band is fully attenuated, the extensor tendons will dislocate below the axis of rotation of the MPJ, and they will become flexors of the MPJ. In long-standing deformities, the intrinsic muscles will be remodeled in a shortened position, mainly the ulnar intrinsics, and the test for intrinsic tightness will be positive. Intrinsic muscle retraction should not be considered as muscle pathology but rather muscle physiology: if the muscle origin and insertion approximate, its sarcomere will remodel in a shortened position.

The dislocated extensor tendons will also cause flexion of the carpometacarpal (CMC)

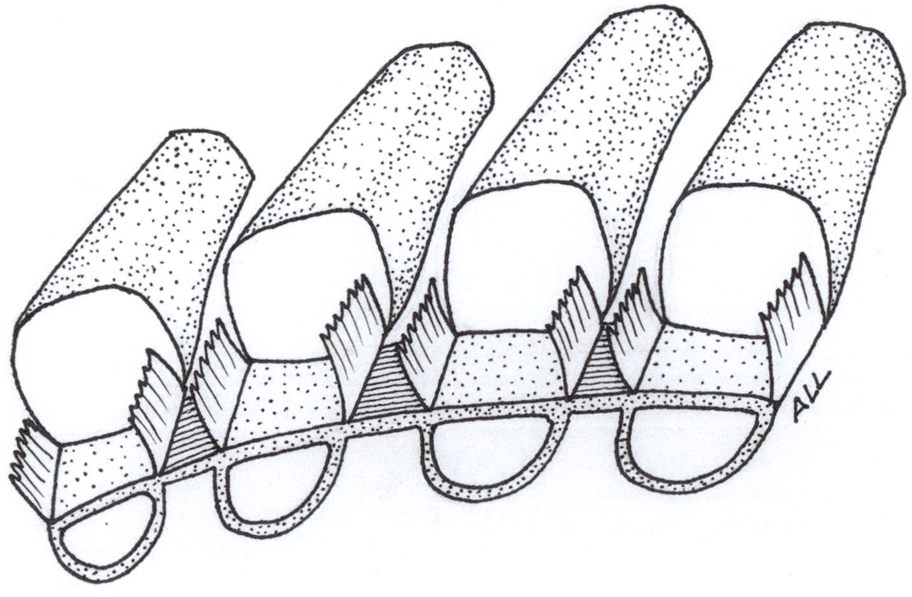

Fig. 18.1 The volar plate of the metacarpophalangeal joint attaches distally to the base of the proximal phalanx. The sagittal bands, holding the extensor tendon at the dorsum of the joint, insert at both sides of the volar plate. All volar plates are united to each other by the intervolar plate ligament, also known as deep intermetacarpal ligament

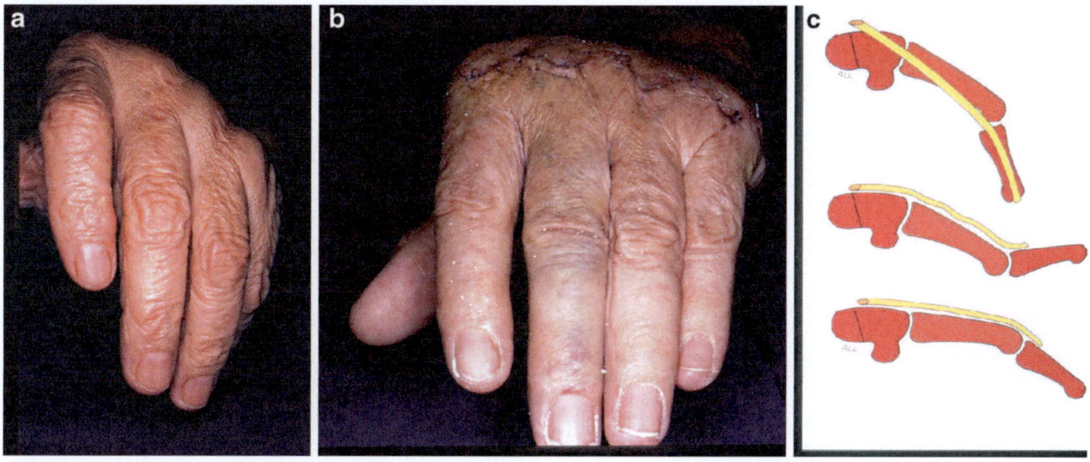

Fig. 18.2 (**a**) Increased "metacarpal descent" in a rheumatoid hand with ulnar dislocation of the extensor tendons. (**b**) The "metacarpal descent" has corrected after having relocated the extensor tendons at the dorsum of the metacarpophalangeal joints. (**c**) On the top drawing, we can see how the ulnarly dislocated extensor tendon causes flexion of the carpometacarpal joint and supination of the little finger. After relocating the extensor tendon, flexion of the carpometacarpal joint and supination of the little finger are corrected

joints of the ring and little fingers, along with some finger rotation into supination. In normal hands, flexion of about 33° of the CMC joints is possible due to muscle contraction [7]. An increased "metacarpal descent" and supination of the fingers is frequently observed in rheumatoid hands secondary to CMC joint laxity and can be confused with a supination deformity of the carpus (Fig. 18.2).

Surgical Treatment

When the joint cartilage has not yet been destroyed, joint synovectomy can be done as an isolated procedure in those cases of persistent MPJ synovitis not responding to rest and pharmacological treatment. Soft tissue rebalancing is very important, such as dorsal relocation of the extensor tendons and ulnar intrinsic muscle release if present. MP joint arthroplasty is only indicated in cases of cartilage and bone destruction.

A transverse zigzag skin incision allows for the best exposure. The proximal flaps of the zigzag, forming a 90° angle, should be placed over the metacarpal heads, disregarding the position of the fingers, which may be markedly displaced volarly and ulnarly (Fig. 18.3). By doing so, the skin flaps will provide the best coverage of the underling joint implants. Zigzag incisions will facilitate a better exposure as opposed to linear incisions, without the need for excessive skin retraction, and provide a far better aesthetic result (Fig. 18.4). By blunt longitudinal dissection, the dorsal veins and nerves located within fat pads in the interdigital spaces are freed from the sides of the extensor hood covering the metacarpal heads. With the veins retracted on both sides of the metacarpal heads, the loose connective tissue underneath the skin is bluntly dissected with small curved scissors until the extensor system is exposed from the distal third of the metacarpal up to the middle of the PP. The skin of the dorsum of the hand is very mobile, allowing for a close inspection of the extensor tendons and its intertendinous connections on the back of the hand, the sagittal bands at both sides of the MP joint, and the extensor hood around the proximal phalanx.

We can gain access to the MPJ by a longitudinal division of the extensor tendon or by dividing either one of the SB. If the tendon remains located dorsally over the metacarpal head, the best approach is by longitudinal division of the tendon, as it will facilitate a better and more symmetrical exposure of the metacarpal heads, as

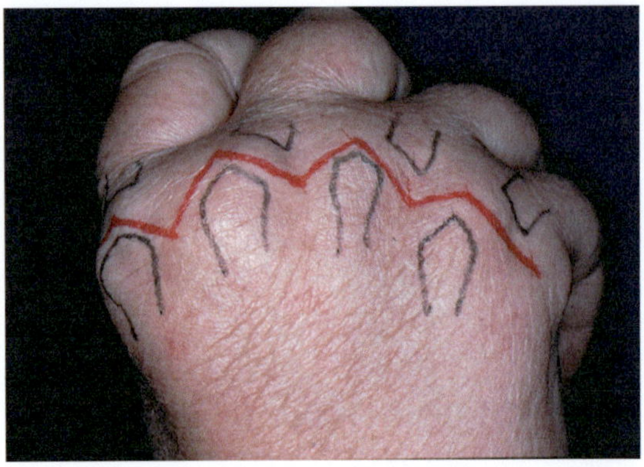

Fig. 18.3 A zigzag skin incision should be made over each of the metacarpal heads, disregarding a possible deformity of the fingers. The incision is extended slightly toward the ulnar side for adequate visualization of the ulnar sagittal band and the tendon of the abductor digiti minimi. From Lluch A. Swanson silicone metacarpo-phalangeal arthroplasty in the rheumatoid hand. In: Arthropaties des metacarpo-phalangiennes et inter-phalangiennes de la main. Allieu Y, Roux JL, Meyer zu Reckendorf G (eds). Montpellier-Paris: Sauramps Medical, 2008: 201–210. Reprinted with permission from Sauramps Medical

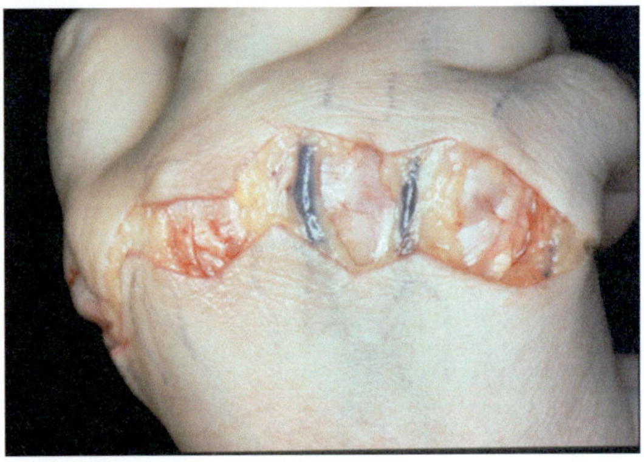

Fig. 18.4 A dorsal zigzag incision provides the best exposure of the extensor apparatus

well as allowing for a stronger surgical repair. However, in most patients the extensor tendons are displaced toward the ulnar side of the metacarpal heads. In such cases, we longitudinally divide the ulnar SB, as it is usually remodeled in a shortened position, making the dorsal relocation of the tendon very difficult if this is not released [5, 8] (Fig. 18.5). In the presence of a long-standing and marked ulnar drift, the ulnar intrinsic muscles will be remodeled in a shorter position. In these circumstances, the entire insertion of the intrinsic muscle into the extensor hood should also be divided, as well as the tendon of the abductor digiti quinti muscle (Fig. 18.6). The tendon of the short flexor of the small finger should not be cut if possible. If this is done, the patient will lose flexion force, and this will result in a postoperative stiffness in extension of the MPJ. After the proximal phalanx of the small finger has been axially aligned with its corresponding metacarpal head, its extensor tendons are displaced toward the radial side, exposing the MPJ. The soft tissue release should begin with the little finger, followed by the ring, middle, and index fingers [5]. If the correction is started on the index finger, an extensive soft tissue release will be necessary to correct the finger displacement, as all fingers are anchored to each other by the intertendinous connections dorsally and by the deep intermetacarpal ligament volarly. Excessive release of the extensor hood and intrinsic musculature will result in a postoperative extension lag and a loss of grip strength of the fingers.

After the soft tissue release is performed and the extensor tendons are displaced toward the radial side of the metacarpal heads, the synovium is first detached from the base of the proximal phalanx and then from the neck of the metacarpal until the metacarpal head is clearly seen. The head can be transected with either a narrow surgical saw or a bone cutting forceps. The amount of head to be removed depends on the amount of the volar and proximal displacement of the proximal phalanges, although the osteotomy is generally done at the level of or just proximal to the origin of the CL (Fig. 18.7). The origin of the collateral ligaments is usually destroyed by the synovial tissue, otherwise volar subluxation of the proximal phalanges would not be possible. Based on the above figure, we usually divide whatever is left of the collateral ligaments at its origin on the metacarpal head. This allows for a more thorough synovectomy and facilitates removal of the metacarpal head (Fig. 18.8). Division of the CL will not cause an anterior subluxation of the

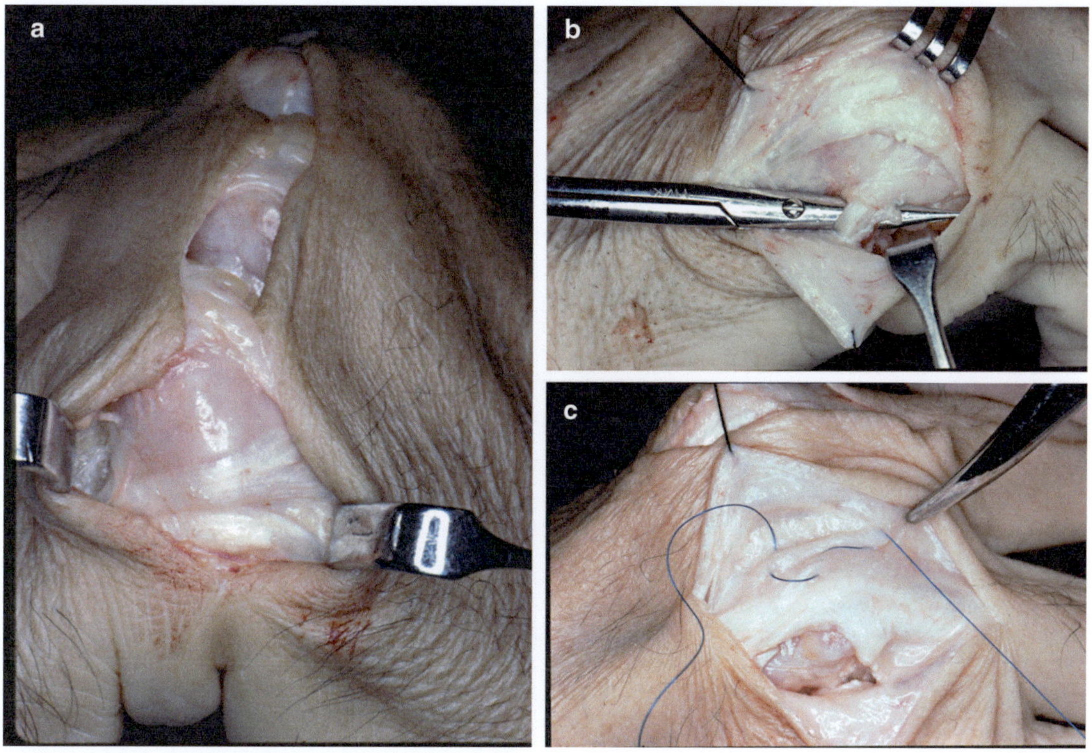

Fig. 18.5 (**a**) Ulnar dislocation of the communis and proprius extensor tendons of the little finger, secondary to the elongation of the radial sagittal band. (**b**) The ulnar sagittal band has been longitudinally divided and the extensor tendons relocated at the dorsum of the metacarpal head. The tendon of the abductor digiti minimi should also be transected. (**c**) The extensor tendons are maintained at the dorsum of the metacarpal head by transverse and longitudinal plication of the radial sagittal band. The defect on the retracted and divided ulnar sagittal band can be clearly seen. From Lluch A. Swanson silicone metacarpophalangeal arthroplasty in the rheumatoid hand. In: Arthropaties des metacarpo-phalangiennes et interphalangiennes de la main. Allieu Y, Roux JL, Meyer zu Reckendorf G (eds). Montpellier-Paris: Sauramps Medical, 2008: 201–210. Reprinted with permission from Sauramps Medical

proximal phalanx, as this never occurs when they are transected for the release of an MPJ contracture in extension. Kirschenbaum et al. did not reconstruct the radial collateral ligament in 144 arthroplasties and did not observe any deleterious effects on the functional results [9].

With the base of the proximal phalanx placed opposite to the metacarpal, a reasonable space should be created, so as to be able to insert the implant with the joint in full extension. If there is not enough space, soft tissue detachment from the volar aspect of the metacarpal should be done, avoiding division of the intrinsic musculature into the proximal phalanx to prevent loss of postoperative grip strength. We should then direct our attention to the shape of the base of the proximal phalanx, as its possible deformity is difficult to ascertain in most preoperative radiographic examinations. If the base is not deformed, we should only remove the remains of joint cartilage and the subchondral bone, to prevent splitting of the base during reaming of the endomedullary canal (Fig. 18.9). If the base of the proximal phalanx has a dorsal scalloping, we should carefully remove part of its volar edge, so as not to completely detach the insertion of the intrinsic muscles, the volar plate, and the flexor tendon sheath. In the presence of a greatly deformed proximal phalanx, with scalloping of its dorsal aspect, we should be careful not to direct the reamer perpendicular to its articular surface, as we could perforate the volar cortex of the phalanx. It is always

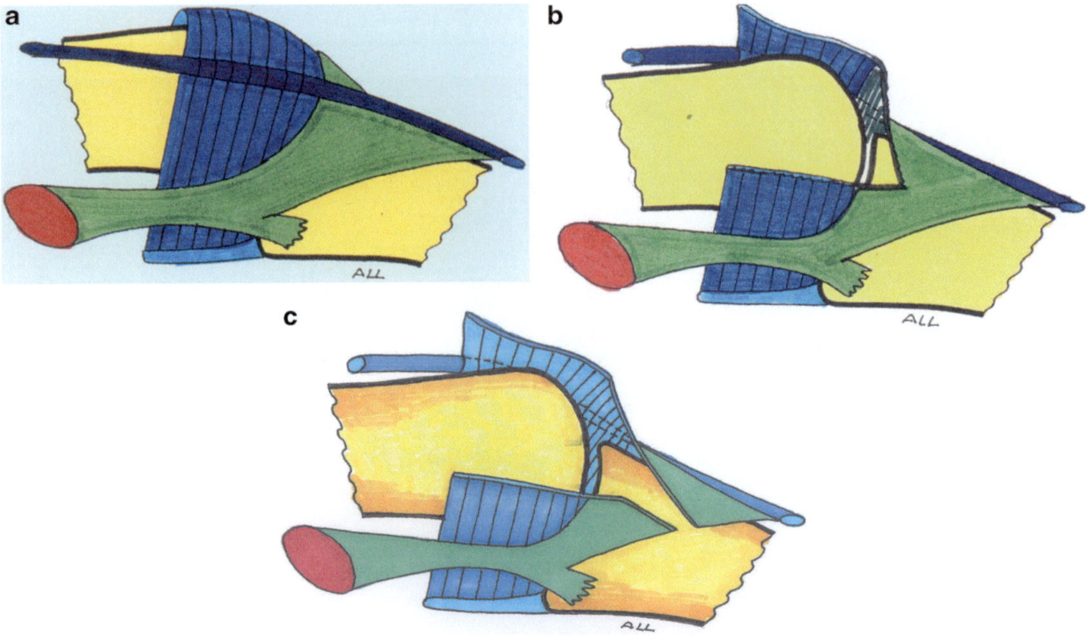

Fig. 18.6 (**a**) Schematic drawing of the metacarpophalangeal joint of the little finger as seen from the ulnar side. The extensor tendon is dislocated, and the proximal part of the extensor hood is rotated into supination from the pull of the tendon and the abductor digiti minimi muscle. (**b**) Longitudinal division of the ulnar sagittal band and proximal part of the extensor hood used to gain access to the metacarpophalangeal joint and relocate the extensor to the dorsum. (**c**) In cases of severe ulnar drift of the finger, the entire extensor hood should be transected

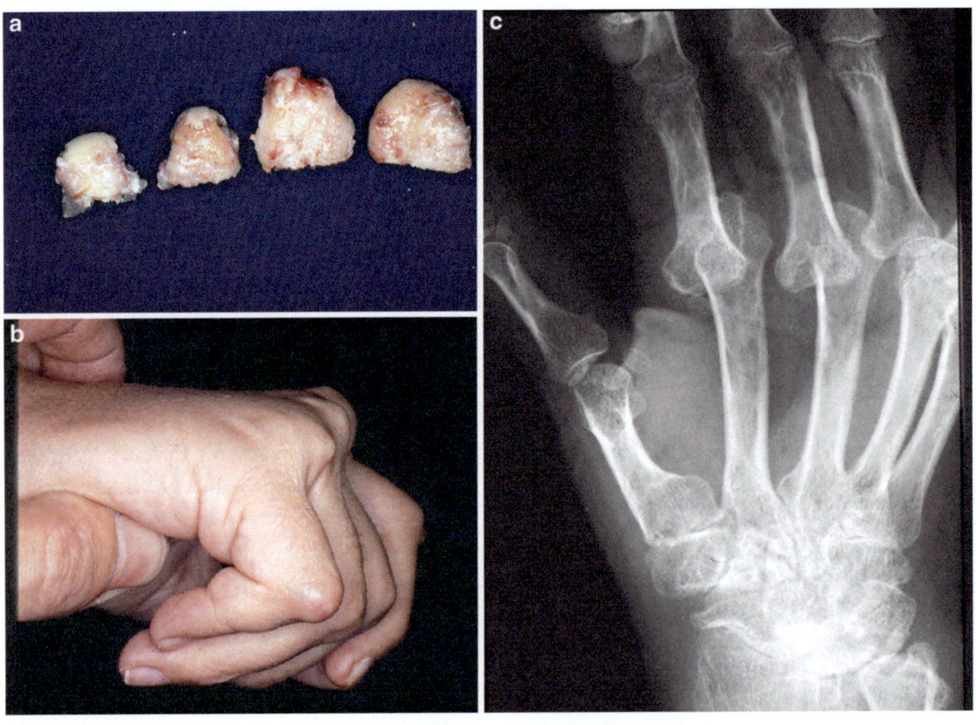

Fig. 18.7 (**a**) In severe deformities, the metacarpal heads should be excised proximal to the insertion of the collateral ligaments. (**b**) The proximal phalanx of the fingers is dislocated and displaced proximally underneath the metacarpal heads. (**c**) Radiograph showing a marked dislocation of the metacarpophalangeal joints

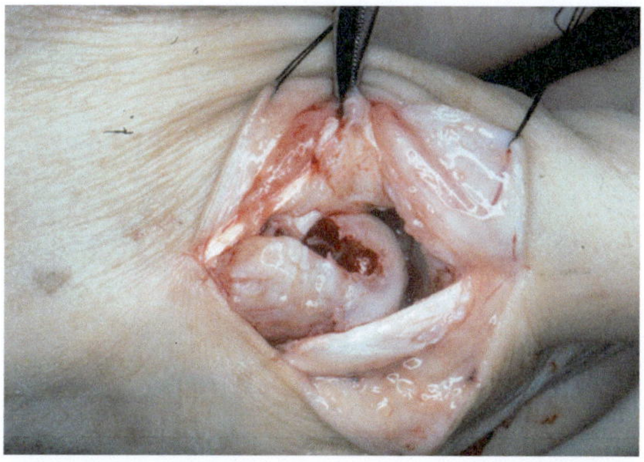

Fig. 18.8 Division of the collateral ligament will facilitate a more complete joint synovectomy. The thumb forceps holds the synovial tissue invading and destroying the metacarpal head

safer to direct the reamer toward the thicker dorsal cortex or to check the direction of the medullary cavity with a straight instrument, such as a straight clamp. We should then proceed with power tools or even better with the appropriate manual reamers. The use of manual reamers has the advantage of impacting the bone rather than removing it, as well as providing direct information about the size of the implant to be used. We should use the largest implant that will fit inside the bone. The medullary cavities of the metacarpals, particularly the ring finger, are usually narrower than those of the PP, and therefore we should begin first with reaming the metacarpals. This will provide information about the maximum size reamer we should use for the proximal phalanx. After the bone ends have been prepared, the volar pouch of the joint is inspected, and bone debris and any remaining synovium are removed until the volar plate is clearly seen. If flexor tendon synovitis or tendon adhesions have been diagnosed or suspected preoperatively, the volar plate is longitudinally divided while applying longitudinal traction to the finger. Through this incision, the flexor tendons can be pulled out with a hook or other curved instrument until independent gliding of both tendons is obtained. If necessary, a partial tendon synovectomy can also be performed (Fig. 18.10).

The trial implants should then be introduced and tested for proper fitting and placement (Fig. 18.11). Flexible silicone implants are first placed inside the medullary cavity of the metacarpal, keeping the proximal stem in place while holding their transverse part with a smooth forceps. The distal stem is then flexed with another forceps until it is driven inside the proximal phalanx while applying some traction and flexion to the finger. Once the distal stem has been introduced inside the medullary cavity of the proximal phalanx, the finger is brought into extension and maintained in this position until the end of the procedure. When using rigid two-component implants, the distal stem should be inserted first. Implant stability can be checked by flexing and extending the joint. The trial implants are removed and the wound irrigated. Bone preparation will differ slightly according to the type of implant to be used. The manufacturer's instructions should be followed carefully.

The radial sagittal band should be plicated with several fine caliber sutures, such as 5-0 USP, size 1 metric, using reabsorbable and colorless material. After the plication of the radial sagittal band, the extensor tendon should be relocated over the implant, checking that it does not dislocate toward the ulnar side while flexing the finger at the MPJ level. If there is still some tendon subluxation, further distal plication of the extensor hood on the radial side should be done. Extensor tendon stability is best determined by flexing the MPJ with the IP joints completely flexed. In those cases in which extensor tendon excursion is limited, simultaneous flexion of MP and IP joints will be difficult. It is better that the extensor tendon be slightly displaced toward the radial side of the MP joint (Fig. 18.12).

Implant Designs

Hinged Metallic Prosthesis

The earliest MP joint implants were hinged metallic prostheses with the main advantage of providing stability, allowing early mobilization and an initial good range of motion [10, 11]. These implants have been discontinued because of their high complication rate due to loosening and fracture [12].

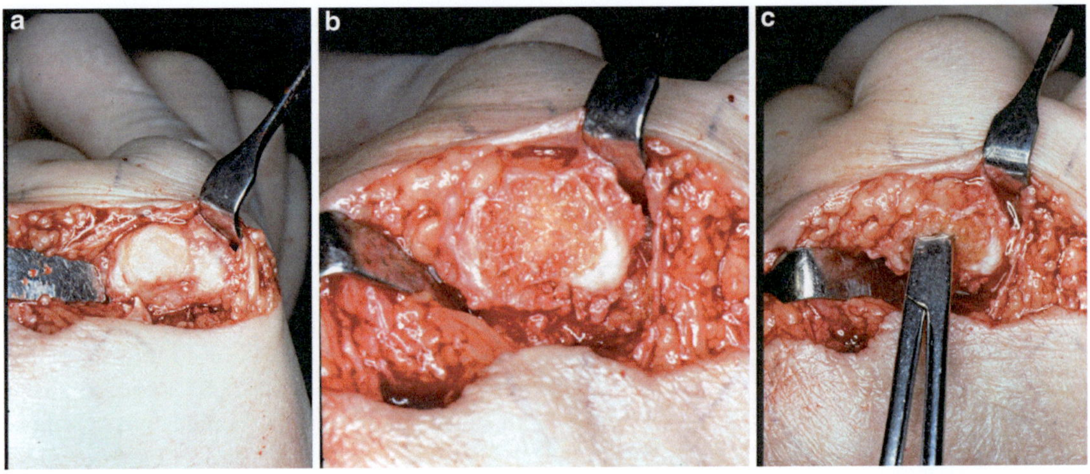

Fig. 18.9 (**a**) After release of the ulnar sagittal band and extensor hood and removal of the metacarpal head, the base of the proximal phalanx should be easily displaced over the plane of the metacarpal. (**b**) Only the cartilage and subchondral bone should be removed. This will prevent splitting of the bone during reaming, as well as preserving the insertion of the intrinsic tendons and the volar plate. (**c**) Prior to reaming, the direction of the endomedullary canal should be identified with a blunt instrument, such as a straight clamp. Care should be taken not to perforate the anterior cortex in cases of dorsal "scalloping" of the proximal phalanx

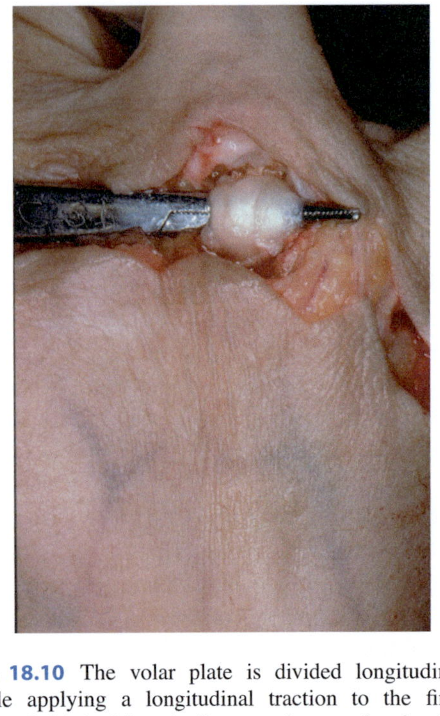

Fig. 18.10 The volar plate is divided longitudinally while applying a longitudinal traction to the finger. Through this incision, the flexor tendons can be visualized in order to perform a tenolysis and limited synovectomy

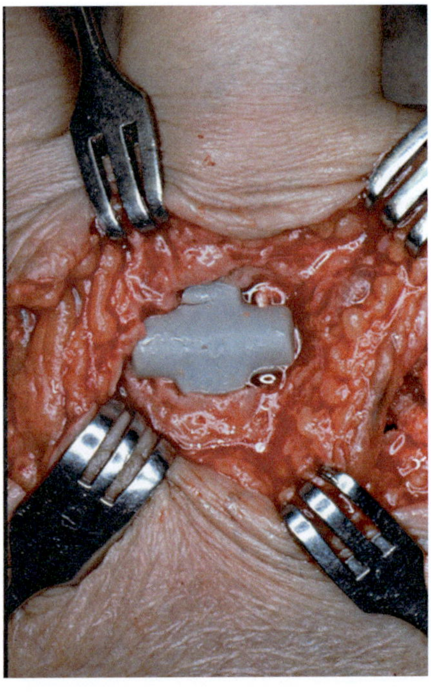

Fig. 18.11 A flexible silicone trial implant is placed and tested for proper fitting

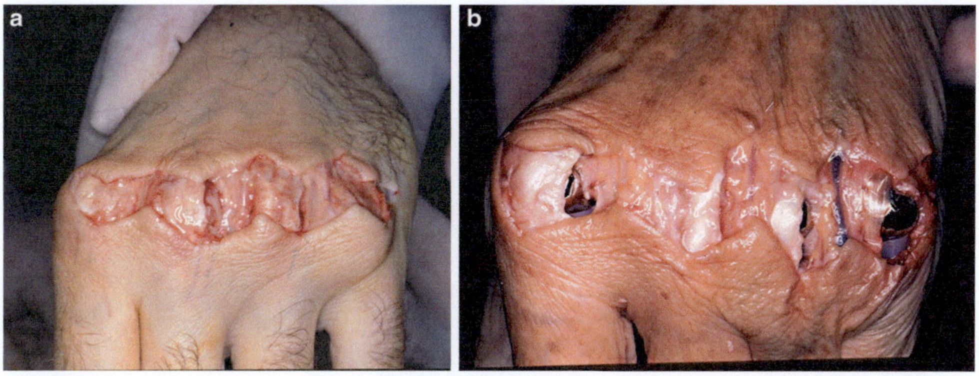

Fig. 18.12 (**a**) After release of the ulnar sagittal bands and plication of the radial sagittal bands, the extensor tendons should remain at the dorsum of the metacarpal heads after full metacarpophalangeal joint flexion. (**b**) The extensor tendons should remain at the dorsum or slightly radial to the metacarpophalangeal joint implants after full metacarpophalangeal joint flexion

Flexible Silicone Implants

Flexible silicone implants for the MPJ were designed by Swanson in 1964 [13]. Implant breakage was common at the base of the distal stem. In 1986, the implants were manufactured using a silicone more resistant to rupture called *Silastic HP 100®*. In 1992, titanium grommets were introduced. The use of grommets is recommended, as they protect the Swanson silicone implants from breakage and wear against the cortical bone. The placement and stability of the grommets are easily accomplished at the metacarpals but may pose some difficulties at the level of the proximal phalanges, particularly in those cases with a dorsal bone defect known as "scalloping." In these cases, they may not sit flush against the anterior part of the proximal phalanx because the volar plate or the collateral ligaments may be interposed.

In the late 1960s, several flexible silicone implants were available, such as those of *Calnan-Nicolle* [14, 15], *Niebauer* [16], and *Kessler* [17], but their manufacturing has been discontinued.

Flexible silicone implants are relatively inexpensive and placement is an easy procedure to perform. Subsequently, other silicone implants have also been designed, such as the *Sutter*™ [18] and the *NewFlex*™ [19, 20]. Clinical results are similar with the use of the different flexible implants [21–23], although there is a lower breakage rate for the Swanson implants [24].

Semiconstrained Rigid Two-Component Implants

The third generation of prosthesis is semiconstrained with two components: metal for the metacarpal component and HMWPE for the distal component [12, 25, 26]. Other implants are made of ceramic or graphite covered with a thin layer of pyrocarbon [27].

Associated Procedures

Cross Intrinsic Transfer (CIT)

This procedure was first described by Straub [28] and later popularized by Flatt and others [29, 30], for the purpose of preventing a recurrence of the ulnar deviation of the fingers. The ulnar intrinsic tendons of the ring, middle, and index fingers are divided and later sutured to the radial extensor hood of the adjacent ulnar finger. In order to prevent a possible postoperative limitation of PIP joint flexion or even a swan-neck deformity, it has been proposed to insert the transfer to the radial collateral ligament at the proximal phalanx [31]. Ellison et al. performed some biomechanical studies in freshly amputated fingers comparing four insertion sites of the transferred intrinsic tendon: dorsum of middle of proximal phalanx, anterior

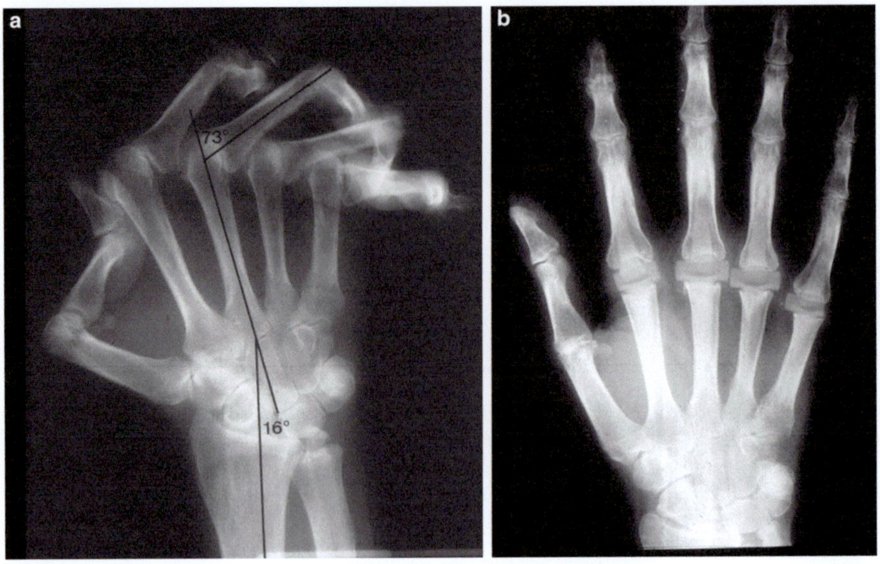

Fig. 18.13 (**a**) Posteroanterior radiograph of a hand with a severe ulnar drift of the fingers. The metacarpals show a compensatory radial inclination. (**b**) After correction of the ulnar drift, the radial inclination of the wrist has corrected spontaneously. From Lluch A. Swanson silicone metacarpo-phalangeal arthroplasty in the rheumatoid hand. In: Arthropaties des metacarpo-phalangiennes et inter-phalangiennes de la main. Allieu Y, Roux JL, Meyer zu Reckendorf G (eds). Montpellier-Paris: Sauramps Medical, 2008: 201–210. Reprinted with permission from Sauramps Medical

part of middle of proximal phalanx, extensor hood at mid-shaft of proximal phalanx, and insertion of the radial CL [29]. They observed that attachment of the intrinsic muscle to the distal end of the CL was less likely to cause an intrinsic contracture or a swan-neck deformity, as occurred in 12 of the 25 patients initially reported.

We do not routinely perform a CIT transfer as this would increase the time and difficulties of the surgical procedure. Published studies on the results of CIT seem to demonstrate a decreased incidence of recurrent postoperative ulnar drift of the fingers. However, from an academic point of view, this technique does not follow the principles of a successful tendon transfer, which are an adequate postoperative immobilization period and use of a muscle that has good contractility and has not already been shortened [8]. According to Wood et al., the ulnar intrinsic muscle to be transferred should stretch 4 mm or more with gentle traction [32].

Rebalancing of Forces at the Wrist

We do not simultaneously perform a rebalancing of forces at the wrist, by means of tendon transfers or transpositions, to correct a preoperative radial deviation of the metacarpals, as we have observed that the radial deviation of the wrist is always secondary to the ulnar deviation of the fingers. After the finger deformity is corrected, the wrist tends to correct itself (Fig. 18.13). If the radial inclination cannot be passively corrected and there is an ulnar translocation of the carpus, we prefer to perform a radio-lunate or radio-scapho-lunate arthrodesis after correction of the carpal deformity [33] (Fig. 18.14).

Postoperative Care

The wrist is immobilized in a neutral position or moderate extension correcting a possible preoperative radial inclination. The MPJ are immobilized in full extension with the correction of any

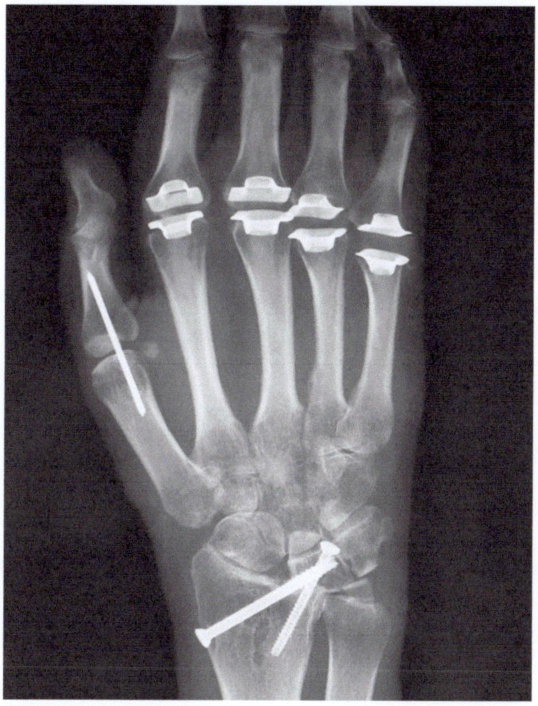

Fig. 18.14 A radio-lunate arthrodesis is performed to correct a radial inclination of the wrist and ulnar translocation of the carpus

preoperative ulnar inclination. The interphalangeal joints are left free in most cases.

The precise details of the postoperative program are not defined in most publications except for that of Madden et al. [34]. The entire dressing is removed 5–7 days after the procedure and a dynamic splint is applied. The fingers are kept in extension and aligned with the metacarpals with an outrigger and rubber bands (Fig. 18.15). The rubber bands should be removed a few times during the day in order to make it easier for the patient to flex the fingers at the level of the arthroplasties. Patients should be encouraged to actively flex the MP joints as much as possible, with the only precaution being that this should not be accomplished at the expense of an active extension loss or ulnar inclination of the fingers. For most grasping activities, it is more important for the ring and little fingers to regain flexion rather than extension. To accomplish this, it may be necessary to remove the rubber bands from these fingers earlier and for longer periods of time than for the index or middle fingers [34, 35].

Patients with good proximal interphalangeal joints will tend to flex the fingers at this level, and there is the risk for the MPJ to become stiff in extension (Fig. 18.16). This can be prevented by external immobilization with dorsal aluminum splints on each finger or better yet with an internal immobilization with Kirschner wires done at the time of surgery (Fig. 18.17). Dynamic splints are usually replaced by static splints 6 weeks after the procedure, used mainly at nighttime.

Although dynamic splintage is the most widely used postoperative regime, many variations are in common use. There is no study that has evaluated the efficiency or suitability of any one in particular [36]. Burr et al. reported that that a static splintage regime provided similar results as a dynamic outrigger [37]. Static splintage is recommended for patients suffering from lupus arthritis because of their inherent joint instability and decreased scar formation [38].

Patients with good proximal interphalangeal (PIP) joints will tend to flex the fingers at this level, and therefore there is the risk for the MP joints to become stiff in extension. This can be prevented by external immobilization with dorsal aluminum splints on each finger or better yet with an internal immobilization of the interphalangeal joints with axial Kirschner wires.

Results

MP joint arthroplasty provides pain relief, correction of deformities, and increased flexion force. The degree of joint mobility will vary, with the final arch of motion usually being displaced to one of increased extension. Up to 60° of motion can be obtained following an adequate rehabilitation program, but frequently the range of active movement is less (Fig. 18.18). Madden et al. reported the best postoperative results, probably due to prolonged supervision and splinting [34]. They reviewed 238 MPJ arthroplasties using a Swanson-designed silicone implant. Preoperative active mobility was from 42.5 to

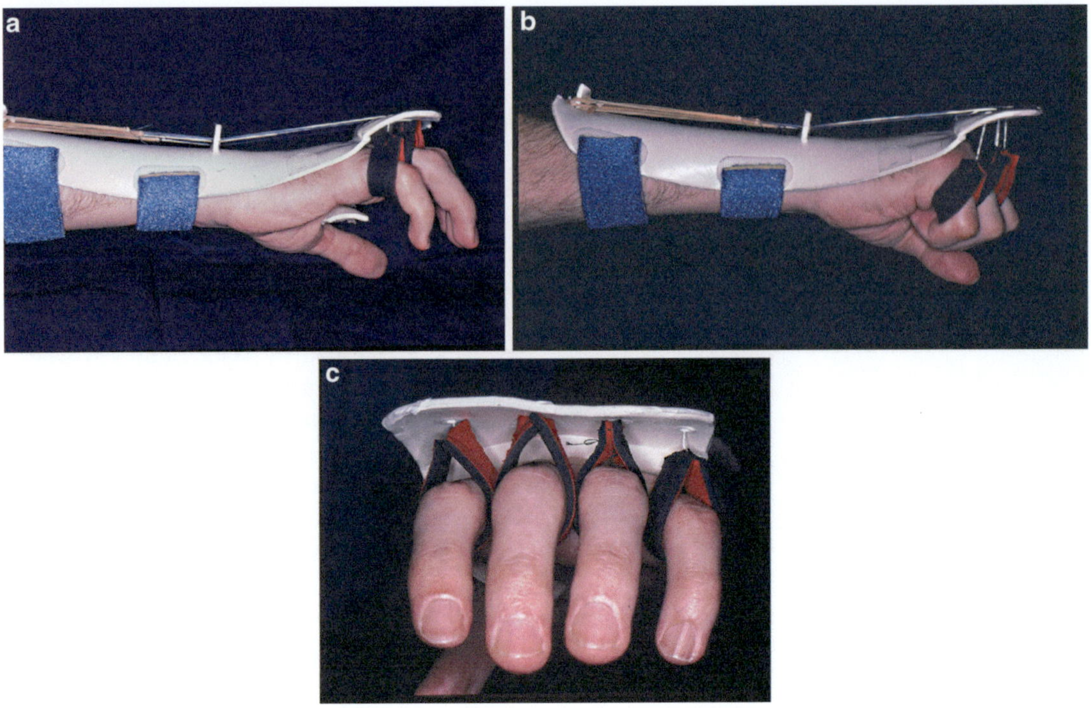

Fig. 18.15 (**a**) Dynamic splint to keep the metacarpophalangeal joints in extension. (**b**) The proximal phalanges are aligned with the longitudinal axis of the metacarpals by means of outriggers. (**c**) The rubber bands of the outriggers should be long enough to allow for active flexion of the metacarpophalangeal joints. (**c**) From Lluch A. Swanson silicone metacarpo-phalangeal arthroplasty in the rheumatoid hand. In: Arthropaties des metacarpophalangiennes et inter-phalangiennes de la main. Allieu Y, Roux JL, Meyer zu Reckendorf G (eds). Montpellier-Paris: Sauramps Medical, 2008: 201–210. Reprinted with permission from Sauramps Medical

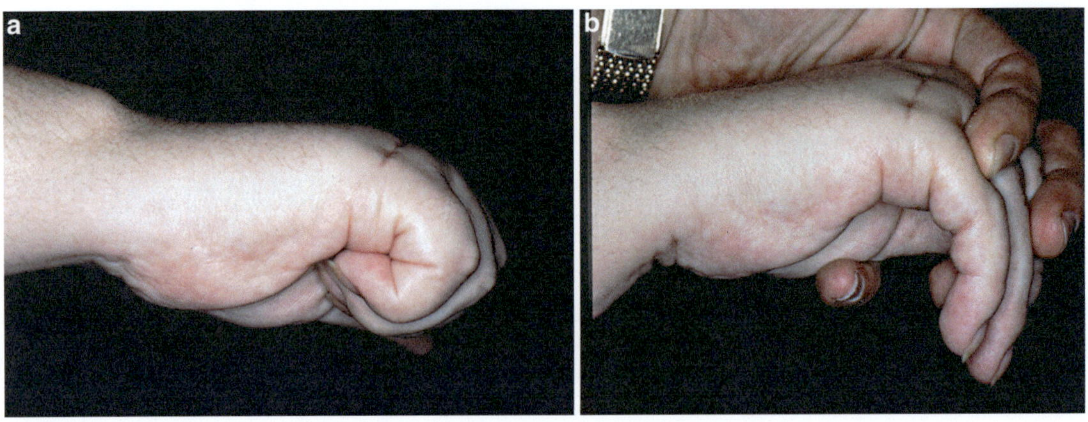

Fig. 18.16 (**a**) Patients with good interphalangeal joints show a tendency to decreased flexion of the metacarpophalangeal joints during the postoperative period. (**b**) In these cases, passive flexion of the arthroplasties is greater than active flexion

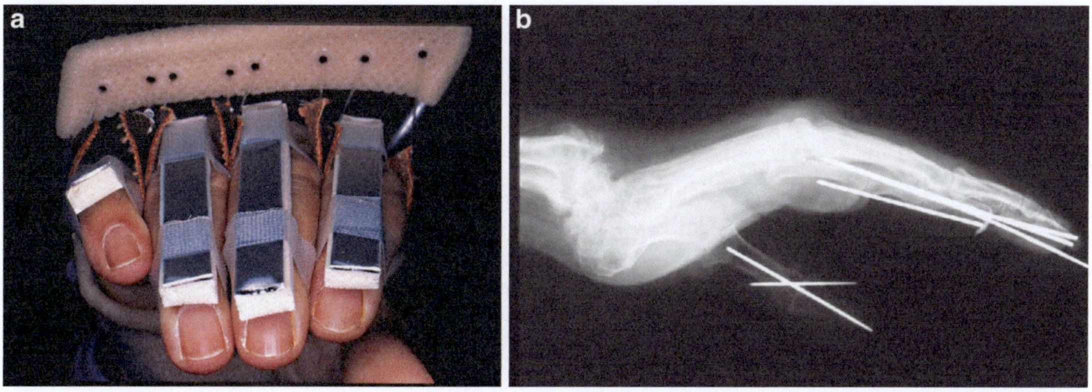

Fig. 18.17 (**a**) Flexion of the interphalangeal joints can be prevented by immobilization with dorsal aluminum splints. (**b**) Immobilization of the interphalangeal joints in extension can also be achieved with axial Kirschner wires placed at the time of surgery. This method of immobilization is preferred in those patients who live alone and have difficulties in placing the aluminum splints by themselves due to severe deformities in the opposite hand as well

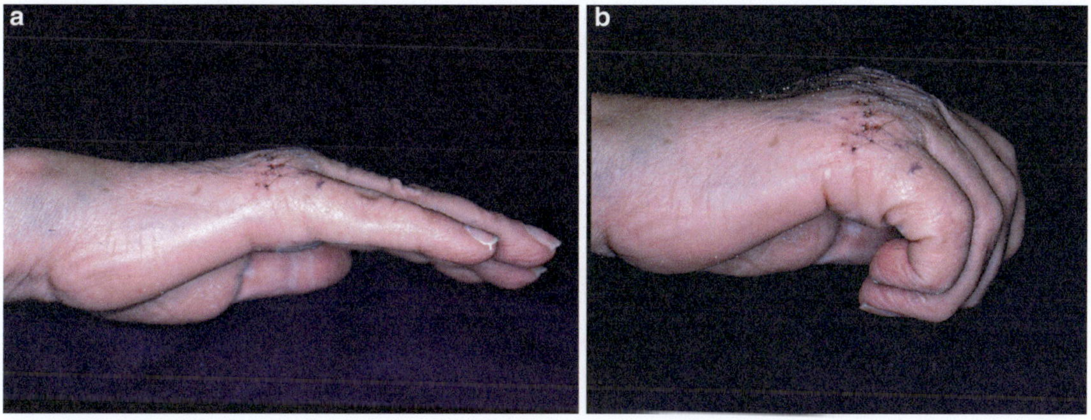

Fig. 18.18 (**a**) Ulnar drift correction and average active extension lag during the early postoperative period. (**b**) Active metacarpophalangeal flexion in the patient of the previous figure

85.7° of flexion (total of 43.2°) and postoperatively from 9.2 to 66.8° of flexion (total of 57.6°). Swanson also reported 3–65° of flexion (total of 62°), although this was passive mobility [39]. Most authors report an average active mobility of 36° on average, going from 10 to 46° of flexion [40–45]. In a meta-analysis of 1.661 implants postoperative average active ROM was 36.7° [33]. However, most of the gain is in the correction of ulnar drift. Hume et al. studied the functional ROM for the MPJ, during 11 activities of daily living, and reported to be from 33 to 73° of flexion, with an average of 61° [46].

Few reports have been published comparing the results with and without CIT, and most of them report a decreased recurrence of ulnar drift after CIT [47–55]. In some of the above studies, the group of patients undergoing both techniques were not homogeneous, and the length of follow-up varied within the groups. Other authors claim that CIT does not significantly affect the outcome [56]. After reading all the above reports, one becomes aware of how difficult it is to draw conclusions in relation to effectiveness of CIT, as ulnar deviation of the fingers is difficult to measure. Roentgenograms in the posteroanterior projection should be made with some elevation of the palm above the X-ray film to ensure that the fingers are in a relaxed position and not corrected by the technician placing them resting over the cassette. Ideally, ulnar drift should be clinically measured individually for each finger [9, 42, 57]. The results will vary depending on the preoperative status of the MP and PIP joints, the duration of the postoperative treatment by dynamic splinting, the length of the follow-up period, and, what it is more important, the details of the surgical technique, in particular the tension of the transferred muscle and its place of insertion.

Extension lag and mainly the ulnar drift deteriorate with time [51, 58–60]. We have the impression, confirmed after reoperation, that the deformities are due to a recurrence of subluxations of the extensor tendons as consequence of a physiological imbalance of forces toward the ulnar side. Recurrence of ulnar drift is greater than extension lag, because there is less scar tissue on the radial side of the MPJ.

Silicone implant breakages have been reported from 0 % to 26 %, with less than 5 % in most reports [58, 61]. The reason why a fracture rate of 26 % was reported can be explained because implants manufactured with the original silicone, available before 1973, were used. *Sutter*™ silicone implants showed a higher incidence of breakage than *Swanson* implants [24]. However, there are no clinical significant differences between the results using *NeuFlex*™, *Sutter*™, or *Swanson* implants [18, 21–24].

The incidence of foreign body reaction to silicone microparticles, usually referred to as siliconitis or silicone synovitis, is negligible in flexible implants, as compared to scaphoid or lunate implants, which are subjected to wear from friction against the distal radius [60, 62–64].

In summary, patients treated with a silicone metacarpophalangeal arthroplasty are pleased with the results, mainly because the finger deformity has been corrected, particularly the ulnar drift [65]. The arc of joint mobility may not increase much, but it is placed in more extension, which makes it more functional and improves the aesthetic appearance of the hand [35, 43] (Figs. 18.19 and 18.20). Objective functional outcomes and patient satisfaction using the Michigan Hand Outcome Questionnaire demonstrated that patients were satisfied with only modest gains in grip and pinch strength [65–67]. Although patients rated function as the most important motivator for surgery, appearance was highly ranked postoperatively [68]. It is possible that patients are reluctant to admit that they are seeking hand surgery mainly to improve the appearance of their hands [69].

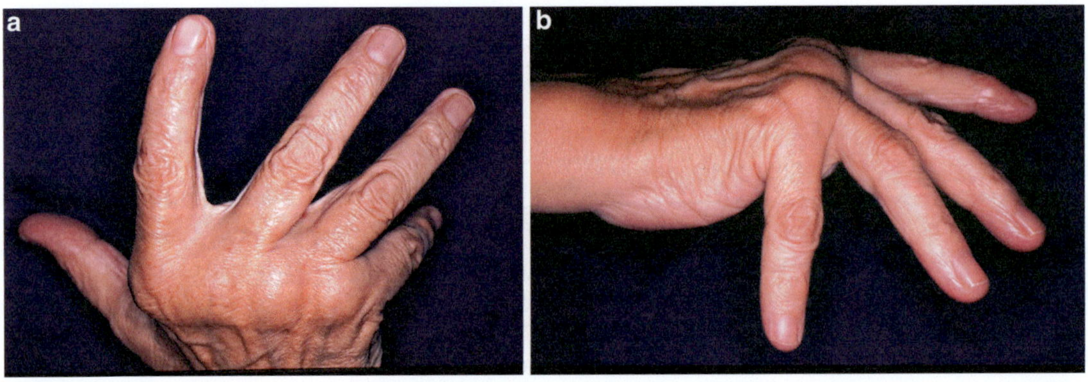

Fig. 18.19 (**a**) The aesthetic appearance of the hand is affected by the ulnar inclination of the fingers. (**b**) Severe extension lag causes hand disability, as the patient will not be able to grasp large objects. Note also an almost 90° rotation into supination of the little finger

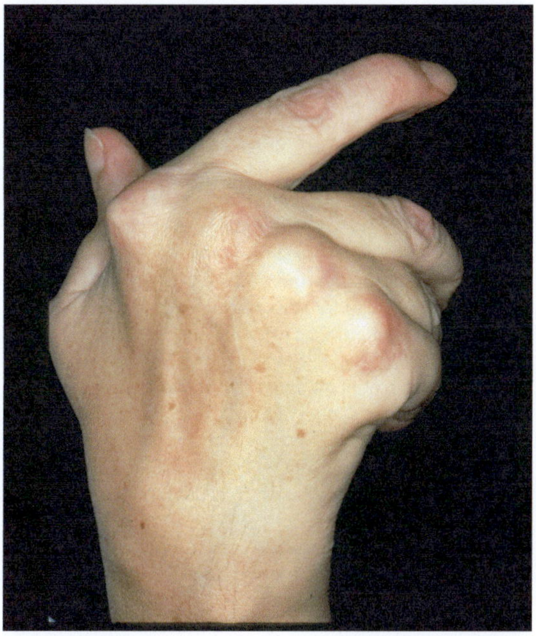

Fig. 18.20 A rheumatoid hand with great functional loss and an unpleasant aesthetic appearance, secondary to dislocation of the extensor tendons toward the ulnar side of the metacarpophalangeal joints. Only the index finger showed some active extension

References

1. Smith RJ, Kaplan E. Rheumatoid deformities at the metacarpophalangeal joints of the fingers. J Bone J Surg. 1967;49-A:31–47.
2. Wise KS. The anatomy of the metacarpophalangeal joints, with observations of the aetiology of ulnar drift. J Bone J Surg. 1975;57-B:485–90.
3. Shapiro JS. A new factor in the etiology of ulnar drift. Clin Orthop. 1970;68:32–43.
4. Shapiro JS, Heijna W, Nasatir S, Ray RD. The relationship of wrist motion to ulnar phalangeal drift in the rheumatoid patient. Hand. 1971;3:68–75.
5. Lluch A. Swanson silicone metacarpophalangeal arthroplasty in the rheumatoid hand. In: Allieu Y, Roux JL, Meyer zu Reckendorf G, editors. Arthropaties des metacarpo-phalangiennes et interphalangiennes de la main. Montpellier-Paris: Suramps Medical; 2008. p. 201–10.
6. Zancolli E. Structural and dynamic bases of hand surgery. Philadelphia: J.B. Lippincott Company; 1968. p. 54–63.
7. Tucker SC, Titley OG. Metacarpal descent, definition and normal range. J Hand Surg. 2002;27B:289–92.
8. Lluch A. Metacarpophalangeal joint arthroplasties. In: Duparc J, editor. Surgical techniques in orthopaedics and traumatology. Paris: Elsevier; 2000. 55-320-C10: 1–5.
9. Kirschenbaum D, Schneider LH, Adams DC, Cody RP. Arthroplasty of the metacarpophalangeal joints with use of silicone-rubber implants in patients who have rheumatoid arthritis. Long term results. J Bone Joint Surg. 1993;75-A:3–12.
10. Brannon EW, Klein G. Experiences with a finger-joint prosthesis. J Bone Joint Surg. 1959;41A:87–102.
11. Flatt AE. Restoration of rheumatoid finger-joint function. Interim report on trial prosthetic replacement. J Bone Joint Surg. 1961;43A:753–74.
12. Beevers DJ, Seedhom BB. Metacarpophalangeal joint prosthesis. A review of the clinical results of past and current designs. J Hand Surg. 1995;20B:125–36.
13. Swanson AB. Silicone rubber implants for replacement of destroyed joints in the hand. Surg Clin. 1968;48:1113–27.
14. Calnan JA, Reis ND. Artificial finger joints in rheumatoid arthritis development and experiment assessment. Ann Rheum Dis. 1968;27:207–17.
15. Nicolle FV, Calnan JS. A new design of the finger joint prosthesis for the rheumatoid hand. J Hand Surg. 1972;4:135–46.
16. Niebauer JJ, Shaw JL, Doran WW. Silicone-Dacron hinge prosthesis: design, evaluation and application. Ann Rheum Dis. 1969;28:56–8.
17. Kessler I. A new silicone implant for replacement of destroyed metacarpal heads. Hand. 1974;6:308–10.
18. McArthur PA, Nilner RH. A prospective randomized comparison of Sutter and Swanson silastic spacers. J Hand Surg. 1998;23B:574–7.
19. Weiss A-PC. NeuFlex prostheses. In: Simmen BR, Allieu Y, Lluch A, Stanley J, editors. Hand arthroplasties. London: Martin Dunitz; 2000. p. 315–22.
20. Schindele S, Herren D, Flury M, Simmen BR. Early results of NeuFlex silastic implant in MCP arthroplasty. Handchir Mikrochir Plast Chir. 2005;37:13–7.
21. Delaney R, Trail IA, Nuttal D. A comparative study of outcome between the Neuflex and Swanson metacarpophalangeal joint replacements. J Hand Surg. 2005;30B:3–7.
22. Möller K, Sollerman C, Geijer M, Kopylov P, Tägil M. Avanta versus Swanson silicone implants in the MCP joint – a prospective, randomized comparison of 30 patients followed for 2 years. J Hand Surg. 2005; 30B:8–13.
23. Parkkila T, Belt EA, Hakala M, Kautiainen H, Leppilahti J. Comparison of Swanson and Sutter metacarpophalangeal arthroplasties in patients with rheumatoid arthritis: a prospective and randomized trial. J Hand Surg. 2005;30A:1276–81.
24. Bass RL, Stern PJ, Nairus JG. High implant fracture incidence with Sutter silicone metacarpophalangeal joint arthroplasty. J Hand Surg. 1996;21A:813–8.
25. Linscheid RL. Implant arthroplasty of the hand: Retrospective and prospective considerations. J Hand Surg. 2000;25A:796–816.
26. Steefe A, Beckenbaugh R, Linscheid RL. The development, technique and early results of total replacement for the metacarpophalangeal joint of the fingers. Orthopedics. 1981;4:175–80.

27. Cook SD, Beckenbaugh RD, Redondo J, Popich BS, Klawitter JJ, Linscheid RL. Long-term follow-up of pyrolytic carbon metacarpophalangeal implants. J Bone Joint Surg. 1999;81A:635–48.
28. Straub LR. The intrinsic muscles in disease with particular reference to the rheumatoid hand. In: Dixième Congrès de la Société Internationale de Chirurgie Orthopedique et de Traumatologie, Paris 1966. Bruxelles: Acta medica Belgica, 1967; p. 863–72.
29. Ellison MR, Flatt AE, Kelly KJ. Ulnar drift of the fingers in rheumatoid disease. J Bone Joint Surg. 1971;53A:1061–82.
30. Flatt AE. The care of the arthritic hand. 5th ed. St. Louis, MO: Quality Medical Publishing; 1995. p. 370–3.
31. Oster LH, Blair WF, Steyers CM, Flatt AE. Crossed intrinsic transfer. J Hand Surg. 1989;14A:963–71.
32. Wood VE, Ichtertz DR, Yahiku H. Soft tissue metacarpophalangeal reconstruction for treatment of rheumatoid hand deformity. J Hand Surg. 1989; 14-A:163–74.
33. Goldfarb CA, Dovan TT. Rheumatoid arthritis: Silicone metacarpophalangeal joint arthroplasty. Indications, technique and outcomes. Hand Clin. 2006;22:177–82.
34. Madden JW, DeVore G, Arem AJ. A rational postoperative management program for metacarpophalangeal joint arthroplasty. J Hand Surg. 1977;2:358–66.
35. Stirrat CR. Metacarpophalangeal joints in rheumatoid arthritis of the hand. Hand Clin. 1996;12:515–29.
36. Massy-Westroop N, Johnston RV, Hill C. Postoperative therapy for metacarpophalangeal arthroplasty. Cochrane Database Syst Rev 2008: CD003522.
37. Burr N, Pratt AL, Smith PJ. An alternative splinting and rehabilitation protocol for metacarpophalangeal joint arthroplasty in patients with rheumatoid arthritis. J Hand Ther. 2002;15:41–7.
38. Nalebuff EA. Surgery of systemic lupus erythematosus arthritis of the hand. Hand Clin. 1996;12:591–602.
39. Swanson AB. Flexible implant arthroplasty for the arthritic finger joints: rationale, technique and results of treatment. J Bone Joint Surg. 1972;54-A: 435–55.
40. Millender LH, Nalebuff EA. Metacarpophalangeal joint arthroplasty utilizing the silicone rubber prosthesis. Orthop Clin. 1973;4:349–71.
41. Gschwend N, Zimmermann J. Analyse von 200 MCP Arthroplastiken. Handchirgie. 1974;6:7–15.
42. Mannerfelt L, Andersson K. Silastic arthroplasty of the metacarpophalangeal joints in rheumatoid arthritis. Long term results. J Bone Joint Surg. 1975; 57A:484–9.
43. Vahvanen V, Viljakka T. Silicone rubber implant arthroplasty of the metacarpophalangeal joint in rheumatoid arthritis: a follow-up study of 32 patients. J Hand Surg. 1986;11A:333–9.
44. Wilson RL, Carlblom ER. The rheumatoid metacarpophalangeal joint. Hand Clin. 1989;5:223–37.
45. Rothwell AG. Hand function following silastic arthroplasty of the metacarpophalangeal joins in the rheumatoid hand. J Hand Surg. 1997;22-B:90–3.
46. Hume MC, Gellman H, McKellop H, Brumfield Jr RH. Functional range of motion of the joints of the hand. J Hand Surg. 1990;15A:240–3.
47. Hellum C, Vainio K. Arthroplasty of the metacarpophalangeal joints in rheumatoid arthritis with transposition of the interosseous muscles. Scad J Plast Rec Surg. 1968;2:139–43.
48. Harrison DH, Harrison SH, Smith P. Re-alignment procedure for ulnar drift of the metacarpophalangeal joint in rheumatoid arthritis. Hand. 1979;11:163–8.
49. Blair WF, Shurr DG, Buckwalter JA. Metacarpophalangeal joint implant arthroplasty with a silastic spacer. J Bone Joint Surg. 1984;66A: 365–70.
50. Stothard J, Thompson AE, Sherris D. Correction of ulnar drift during silastic metacarpophalangeal joint arthroplasty. J Hand Surg. 1991;16B:61–5.
51. El-Gammal T, Blair WF. Motion after metacarpophalangeal joint reconstruction in rheumatoid disease. J Hand Surg. 1993;18A:504–11.
52. Blair WF, Jebson PJL. Crossed intrinsic transfers versus metacarpophalangeal joint arthroplasty in rheumatoid arthritis. In: Saffar P, Amadio PC, Foucher G, editors. Current practice in hand surgery. London: Martin Dunitz; 1997. p. 203–6.
53. Gellman H, Stetson W, Brumfield Jr RH, Costigan W, Kuschner SH. Silastic metacarpophalangeal joint arthroplasty in patients with rheumatoid arthritis. Clin Orthop. 1997;342:16–21.
54. Egloff DV. Flexible silicone implant arthroplasties. In: Simmen BR, Allieu Y, Lluch A, Stanley J, editors. Hand arthroplasties. London: Martin Dunitz; 2000. p. 295–300.
55. Clark DI, Delaney R, Stilwell JH, Trail IA, Stanley JK. The value of cross intrinsic transfer after metacarpophalangeal silastic arthroplasty: a comparative study. J Hand Surg. 2001;26B:565–77.
56. Pereira JA. A comparison of metacarpophalangeal joint silastic arthroplasty with or without crossed intrinsic transfer. J Hand Surg. 2001;26B:229–34.
57. Chung KC, Kotsis SV, Wilgis EF, Fox DA, Regan M, Kim HM, et al. Outcomes of silicone arthroplasty for rheumatoid metacarpophalangeal joints stratified by fingers. J Hand Surg. 2009;34A:1647–52.
58. Bieber EJ, Weiland AJ, Volenec-Dowling S. Silicone-rubber implant arthroplasty of the metacarpophalangeal joints for rheumatoid arthritis. J Bone Joint Surg. 1986;68A:206–9.
59. Goldfarb CA, Stern PJ. Metacarpophalangeal joint arthroplasty in rheumatoid arthritis. A long-term assessment. J Bone Joint Surg. 2003;85A:1869–78.
60. Wilson YG, Sykes PJ, Niranjan NS. Long-term follow-up of Swanson's silastic arthroplasty of the metacarpophalangeal joints in rheumatoid arthritis. J Hand Surg. 1993;18B:81–91.
61. Beckenbaugh RD, Dobyns JH, Linscheid RL, Bryan RS. Review and analysis of silicone-rubber metacar-

pophalangeal implants. J Bone Joint Surg. 1976;58-A: 483–7.
62. Foliart DE. Swanson silicone finger joint implants: a review of the literature regarding long-term complications. J Hand Surg. 1995;20A:445–9.
63. Trail IA et al. Seventeen-year survivorship analysis of silastic metacarpophalangeal joint replacement. J Bone Joint Surg. 2004;86-B:1002–6.
64. Trail IA. Silastic metacarpophalangeal joint arthroplasty. In: Trail I, Hayton M, editors. Surgery of the rheumatoid hand and wrist. Amsterdam: Elsevier; 2006. p. 129–43.
65. Chung KC et al. Patient outcomes following Swanson silastic metacarpophalangeal joint arthroplasty in the rheumatoid hand: systematic overview. J Rheumatol. 2000;27:1395–402.
66. Chung CK, Kotsis SV, Kim HM. A prospective outcomes study of Swanson metacarpophalangeal joint arthroplasty for the rheumatoid hand. J Hand Surg. 2004;29A:646–53.
67. Waljee JF, Chung KC. Objective Outcomes and patient satisfaction after silicone metacarpophalangeal arthroplasty for rheumatoid arthritis. J Hand Surg. 2012;37A:47–54.
68. Bogoch ER, Escott BG, Ronald K. Hand appearance as a motivation for surgery a determinant of satisfaction with metacarpophalangeal joint arthroplasty for rheumatoid arthritis. J Hand Surg. 2011;36A:1007–14.
69. Chung KC, Kotsis SV, Kim HM, Burke FD, Wilgis EF. Reasons why rheumatoid arthritis patients seek surgical treatment for hand deformities. J Hand Surg. 2006;31A:289–94.

Treatment of Boutonniere and Swan-Neck Deformities in Rheumatoid Fingers

19

Alfredo Olazábal and Alexandra L. Mathews

Swan-neck and boutonniere deformities are both found in patients with rheumatoid arthritis (RA) [1]. A careful evaluation of each deformity is essential to determine proper treatment [2]. Principles guiding operative correction focus on relief of pain, improvement of function, and elimination of the deformity [3]. A swan-neck deformity is characterized by hyperextension of the proximal interphalangeal (PIP) joint with flexion of the distal interphalangeal (DIP) joint. The boutonniere deformity is characterized by the inverse posture. Both deformities, which are not exclusively found in RA, are the result of the loss of balance between the different forces that act on the finger.

Swan-neck finger deformities are ultimately the result of hypertrophied rheumatoid synovium. Although the deformity is described as occurring at the PIP joint, it may be caused by the destructive effect of the synovitis at any of the three digital joints (MCP, PIP, or DIP joint). The abnormal posturing arises from an imbalance of what is normally a complex, delicately balanced, and dually innervated extrinsic and intrinsic tendon system. The extrinsic and intrinsic extensor contributions normally combine to form the central slip and lateral bands that, in concert, extend the PIP joint. The normal restraint to PIP hyperextension is partially static (volar plate and collateral ligaments) and partially dynamic (flexor superficialis). Through attenuation of the volar plate and collateral ligaments caused by synovitis or with rupture of the flexor digitorum superficialis (FDS), the extensor force is unopposed, causing hyperextension. With time, the lateral bands slide dorsally as the transverse retinacular ligaments stretch. As the hyperextension worsens, reciprocal flexion occurs at the DIP joint causing the swan-neck deformity. This is likely to occur for several reasons including lengthening of the extensor apparatus, tightening of the flexor profundus, or superimposed intrinsic contracture.

The swan-neck deformity can also result from synovitis at the DIP joint, MCP joint, or wrist joint. Synovitis of the DIP joint causes weakening and rupture of the terminal extensor tendon insertion. As the tendon insertion migrates proximally, the lateral bands become lax. The deformity at the DIP joint subsequently forces the PIP joint into hyperextension, resulting in a swan-neck deformity. A similar secondary effect occurs from synovitis at the MCP joint. The synovitis causes attenuation of the volar plate, resulting in a volar subluxation of the proximal phalanx at the

A. Olazábal, MD (✉)
Department of Orthopaedics, Hospital Aleman Buenos Aires, Pueyrredon 1640, M.T. de Alvear 2421, Buenos Aires 1122, Argentina
e-mail: alfredoeolazabal@gmail.com

A.L. Mathews, BS
Section of Plastic Surgery, Department of Surgery, The University of Michigan Health System, Ann Arbor, MI, USA

K.C. Chung (ed.), *Clinical Management of the Rheumatoid Hand, Wrist, and Elbow*,
DOI 10.1007/978-3-319-26660-2_19

MCP joint. This shortens the intrinsic extensors and the PIP joint becomes hyperextended. Finally, synovitis at the wrist can cause carpal collapse and proximal migration of the carpal-hand unit. An imbalance is created, resulting in an "extrinsic minus" phenomena and swan-neck finger deformity [3].

According to Nalebuff [1], the swan-neck deformity is classified into four types:

Type I: Flexible with complete range of motion
Type II: Flexible with restricted motion according to MCP joint position
Type III: Stiff with normal PIP joint articular surfaces
Type IV: Stiff with destruction of PIP joint articular surfaces

Type I

In type I cases (Figs. 19.1 and 19.2), patients retain complete mobility of the PIP joint. Conservative treatment options to prevent hyperextension at the PIP joint include the use of silver ring splints (Fig. 19.3); however, surgical treatment in some cases may be necessary. There are many surgical options available for treating type I deformities, which aim to limit PIP joint hyperextension. Options include dermadesis of the PIP joint, tenodesis of the FDS, and lateral band tenoplasty. Dermadesis is only helpful in mild cases and consists of a resection of palmar skin and immobilization of the finger in 45° of flexion for 3 weeks. Tenodesis of the FDS aims to create a slight flexion contracture of the PIP joint. This technique uses one slip of the tendon, which is divided proximally by keeping its distal insertion intact and is sutured to itself to make a loop on the A1 pulley. This loop will act to prevent PIP joint extension. Postoperatively, hyperextension is blocked for 6–8 weeks. When the swan-neck deformity begins at the DIP joint, laxity of the volar plate of the PIP joint allows hyperextension. If the deformity starts in the DIP joint, reconstruct by means of a tenoplasty or directly perform an arthrodesis, which usually yields a better result [4].

Additional approaches to correct type I deformities have been reported. For patients with RA in which soft tissue fixation may be unreliable, bone fixation techniques using modern suture anchors can be used to repair the volar plate. Littler's technique (retinacular ligament reconstruction) consists of detaching the ulnar lateral band of the extensor mechanism proximally, keeping its distal end attached. The lateral band is then passed volar to Cleland fibers and sutured to the fibrous sheath under tension to prevent PIP hyperextension. Zancolli's technique also uses the lateral band, fixing it in the flexor sheath [5]. Lateral band translocation involves

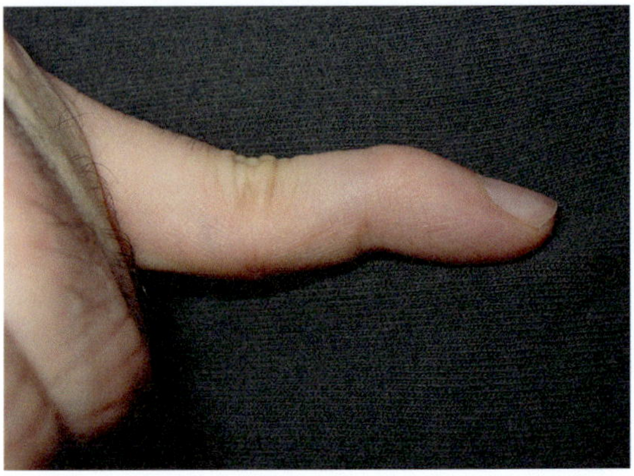

Fig. 19.1 Small finger type I swan-neck deformity showing PIP hyperextension and DIP flexion

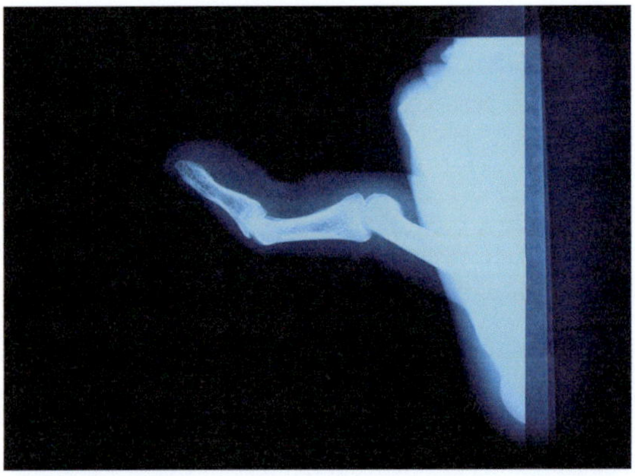

Fig. 19.2 Small finger type I swan-neck deformity X-ray with evidence of hyperextension at the PIP joint and flexion at the DIP joint

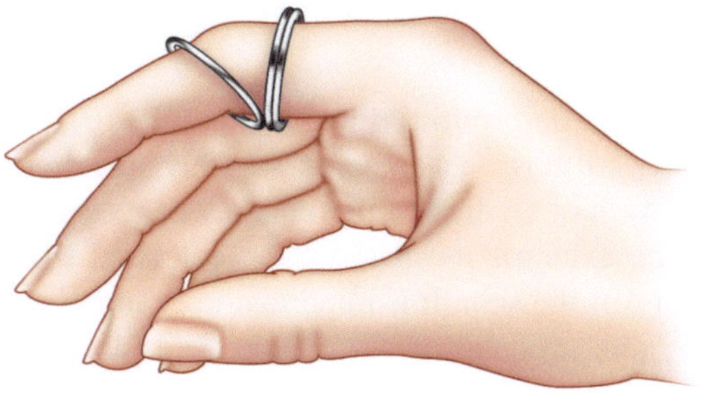

Fig. 19.3 A silver ring splint is used to conservatively treat mild to moderate hyperextension at the PIP joint

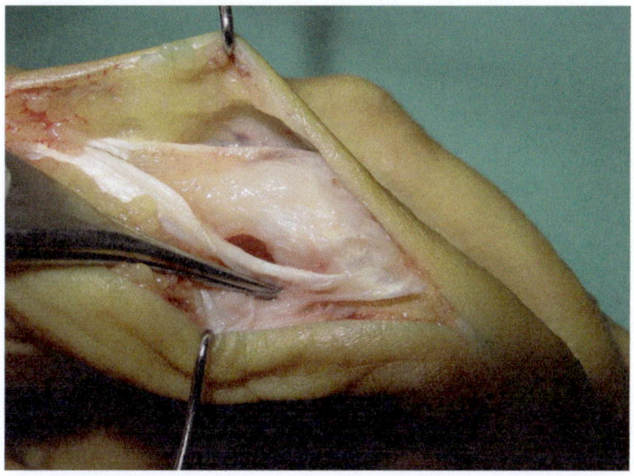

Fig. 19.4 Mobilization of the lateral bands using Zancolli's technique to treat a type II swan-neck deformity

transfer of the dorsally subluxed radial lateral band to the palmar aspect of the joint where it is maintained by a sling created between the flexor superficialis tendon and the palmar plate.

Zancolli's Surgical Procedure

A mid-lateral incision is made on the radial side of the finger. The lateral band of the extensor mechanism is mobilized from the midpoint of the proximal phalanx to the midpoint of the middle phalanx by separating the lateral band from the central tendon mechanism dorsally and by dividing the transverse retinaculum ligament of Landsmeer on the palmar aspect of the lateral band (Fig. 19.4). The accessory collateral ligament is divided at its insertion into the palmar plate to display the free lateral margin of that structure (Fig. 19.5). The insertion of the palmar plate into the base of the middle phalanx and its origin from the proximal phalanx remain intact. A synovectomy of the PIP joint may be done if indicated. The flexor tendon sheath is open between the A2 and A4 pulleys. The radial slip of the superficialis insertion is identified. The mobilized lateral band is translocated palmarly, below the PIP joint axis, and is retained in this position by creating a sling between the free margin of the palmar plate and the radial slip of the superficialis tendon. Two 4-O Tycron sutures are placed at the distal edge of the PIP joint between the palmar plate and the superficialis tendon to create the sling. The tension of the translocated tendon is checked so that the PIP joint does not extend beyond 5° of flexion when the finger is supported at the finger pulp alone. The tension may be adjusted by altering the position of the proximal point of dissection of the lateral band from the central tendon mechanism. Further proximal dissection loosens the tension. The lateral band may be resutured to the central slip to tighten the translocated band if necessary. A single suture at the point of proximal and distal separation prevents subsequent splitting of the translocated tendon from the central tendon. If an extension lag remains at the DIP joint, temporary Kirschner (K-) wire fixation maintains this joint in extension for 4 weeks. Alternatively, a DIP joint arthrodesis may be considered. After hemostasis is obtained, the skin alone is sutured [5].

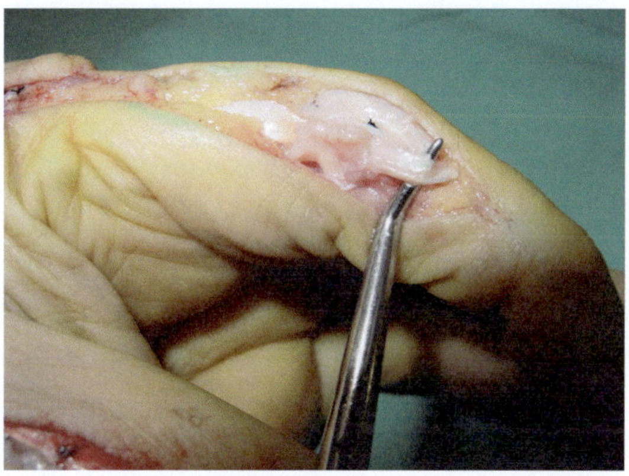

Fig. 19.5 Division of the accessory collateral ligament at its insertion into the palmar plate

Sirotakova et al. use a new lateral extensor band technique by combining Littler's and Zancolli's techniques. The lateral band on the ulnar side of the finger is dissected from the central slip and divided proximally just distal to the MCP joint level. The lateral band on the radial side is also dissected from the central slip to improve its lateral mobility during PIP flexion. A pulley is created as in Zancolli's technique and finally the ulnar lateral band is fixed to the proximal phalanx by a bone tag with the PIP joint in 30° [6].

Type II

In type II swan-neck deformities (Fig. 19.6), the intrinsic muscles are retracted and finger flexion is restricted in certain positions. For instance, when the MCP joint is placed in extension, the PIP joint cannot be passively flexed. A type II deformity may begin as subluxation of the MCP joint and secondarily cause the intrinsic muscles to retract. Correction of the subluxation using MCP joint arthroplasty plus intrinsic tenotomy may be required to fix the deformity. The intrinsic retraction is treated by resecting the triangular part of the extensor apparatus in the proximal phalanx. Postoperative results for the treatment of a type II deformity are shown in Figs. 19.7 and 19.8.

Type III

In type III deformities (Figs. 19.9 and 19.10), the ability to grasp an object is severely impaired. Passive motion of the PIP joint may be restricted by the extensor mechanism, the collateral ligaments, or the skin. It is important to examine the PIP joint articular cartilage before deciding the correct surgical treatment. If an X-ray shows that the joint is destroyed, arthrodesis is indicated. If the PIP joint is not affected, PIP joint manipulation can be performed. When performing this technique, the joint is flexed gently under anesthesia and fixed with a K-wire in 90° for 3–4 weeks. If the skin is under tension, a skin relaxing incision can be made just distal to the PIP

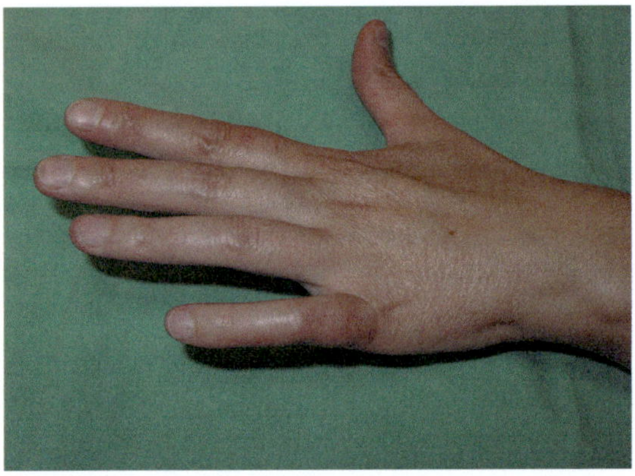

Fig. 19.7 Postoperative photograph of type II swan-neck deformity showing good finger posture

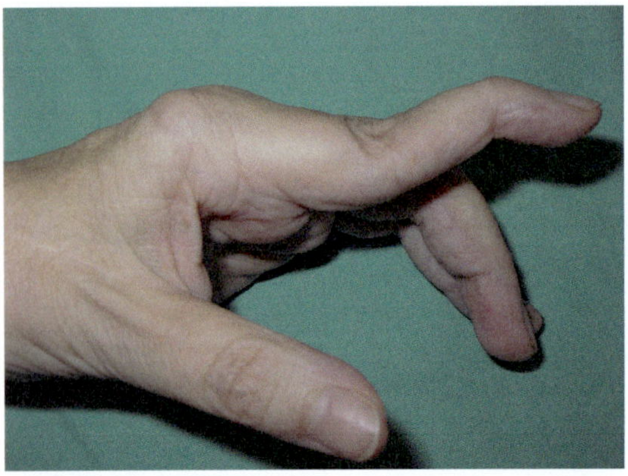

Fig. 19.6 Index finger type II swan-neck deformity. PIP joint flexion is limited in certain positions of the MCP joint

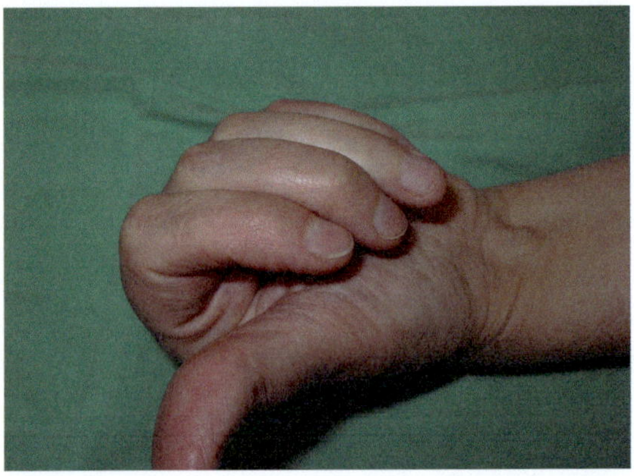

Fig. 19.8 Postoperative results of type II swan-neck deformity. Good flexion maintained after surgery

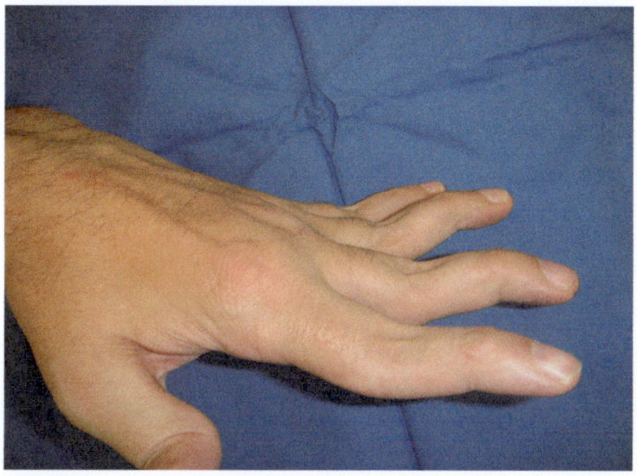

Fig. 19.9 Type III swan-neck deformity showing a partial lateral hand with significant PIP joint hyperextension in all fingers. PIP joint flexion is limited irrespective of MCP joint position

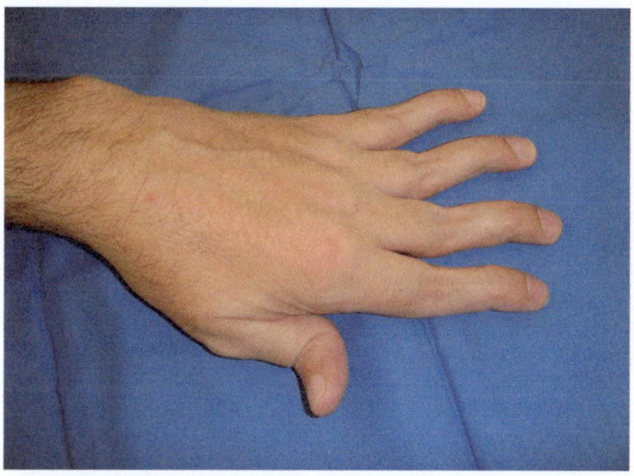

Fig. 19.10 Dorsal view of the same hand, showing type III swan-neck deformity

joint. The distal part of the incision is left open and does not require a skin graft. If the manipulation is difficult, lateral band mobilization is indicated.

Lateral Band Mobilization

A dorsal incision is made and the lateral bands are separated from the central part of the extensor apparatus (Fig. 19.11). The lateral bands are then moved palmarly so the PIP joint can be easily flexed (Figs. 19.12 and 19.13). The joint is splinted in 90° of flexion for 4–6 weeks. It is

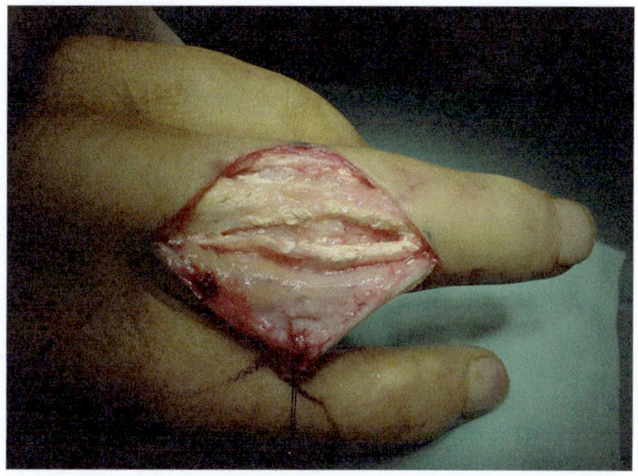

Fig. 19.11 Separation of lateral bands from the central part of the extensor apparatus

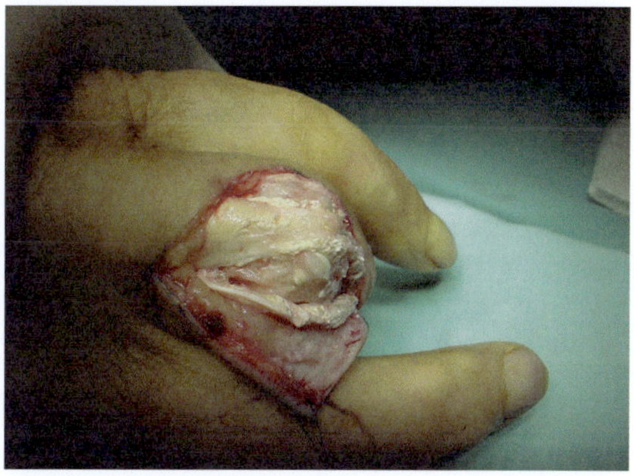

Fig. 19.12 Lateral bands are moved palmarly and the PIP joint is flexed easily

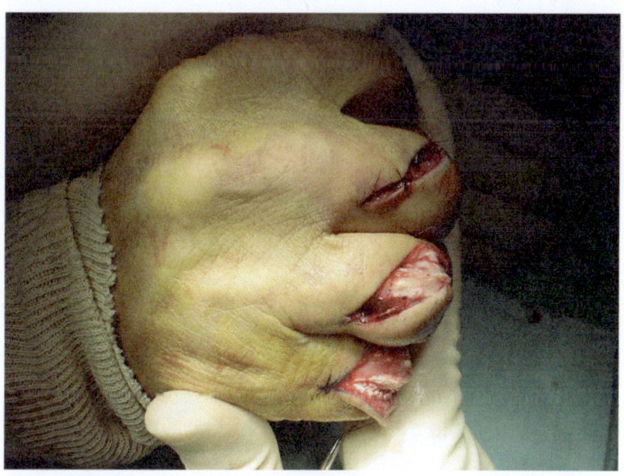

Fig. 19.13 Correction of type III swan-neck deformity

important to check the function of the flexor tendons in every case. If flexion is impaired, it can be corrected simultaneously, for example, performing a tenosynovectomy in case of "trigger finger" [7, 8]. Specialized physiotherapy is mandatory to obtain the best possible results.

Type IV

A type IV deformity is characterized by a fixed hyperextension deformity of the PIP joint resulting in a stiff joint and radiographic image that shows joint destruction (Figs. 19.14, 19.15, and 19.16). When the PIP joint is destroyed, either arthrodesis or arthroplasty can be performed. A careful evaluation of the whole hand is necessary to determine the best treatment option. In general, we prefer an arthrodesis in the index and middle finger and an arthroplasty in the ring and little finger. It is possible but it is not advisable to perform two arthroplasties in the same finger. If an MCP arthroplasty is performed in the same finger, we prefer to arthrodese the PIP joint. The PIP joint is fixed at 25° in the index finger and 30° in the middle finger. Postoperative results of PIP arthrodesis of the little finger are shown in Figs. 19.17 and 19.18. Sirotakova et al. corrected the swan-neck deformity using a new procedure that combines the distally based extensor lateral band technique described by Littler and the FDS-palmar plate pulley introduced by Zancolli [6].

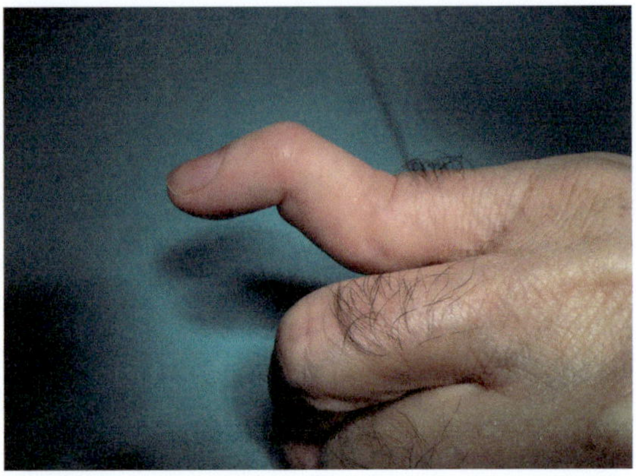

Fig. 19.15 Lateral view of the type IV swan-neck deformity at the little finger. The finger shows significant PIP joint hyperextension and DIP flexion

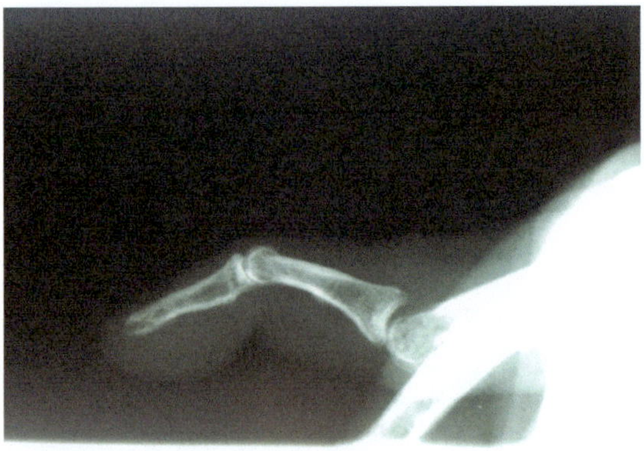

Fig. 19.16 Type IV swan-neck deformity X-ray demonstrating poor radiographic appearance at the PIP joint

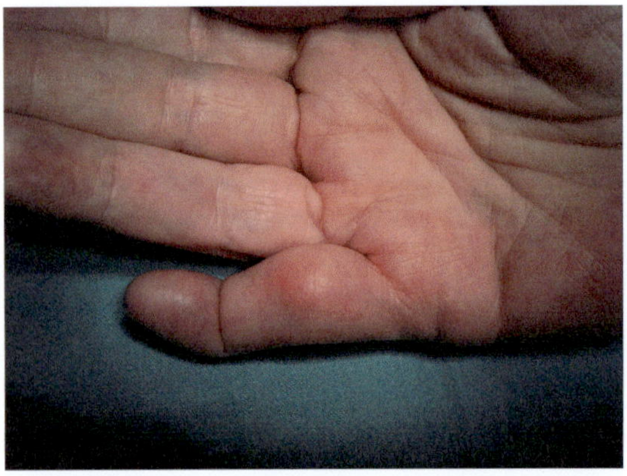

Fig. 19.14 Palmar view of a type IV swan-neck deformity at the little finger. The PIP joint is stiff

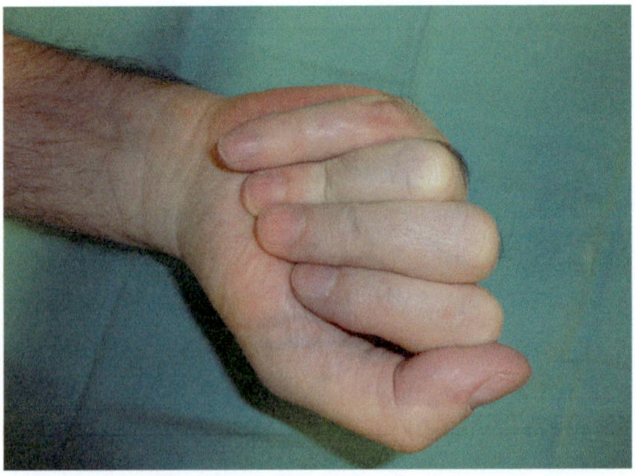

Fig. 19.17 Result after arthrodesis to treat a type IV swan-neck deformity in the little finger

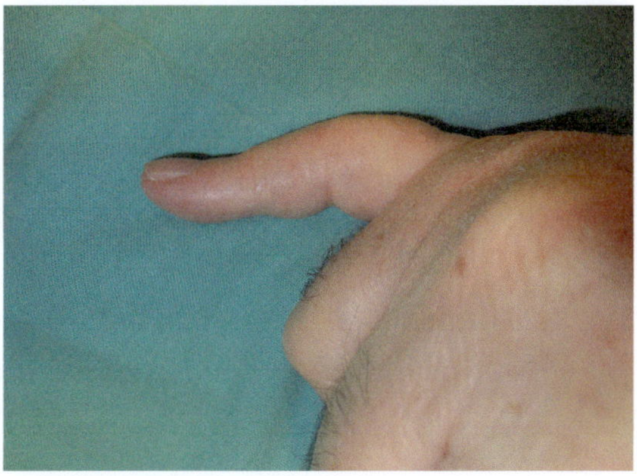

Fig. 19.18 Lateral view of the little finger after arthrodesis to treat a type IV swan-neck deformity

Personal Series [9]

Twenty-eight patients, mean age 50 (31–82), with 82 rheumatoid swan-neck digital deformities were selected: 26 belonged to type I, 30 to type II, 14 to type III, and 12 to type IV.

Results

All the patients were evaluated pre- and postoperatively at least 1 year after surgery.

PIP range of motion was recorded (Fig. 19.19).

Postoperative PIP range of motion: type II −15° to 67° and type III −12° to 65°. Type IV PIP joints were arthrodesed at 60° in the little finger, 50° in the ring finger, 40° in the middle finger, and 30° in the index finger.

Final Conclusion

Careful evaluation of each case is mandatory to determine the best treatment option. In our series, all swan-neck deformities were caused by RA, and surgical correction was usually accompanied by other surgical procedures in the wrist and MP joints. The classic sequence from proximal to distal was always the rule. In every case, we obtained a functional improvement due to better range of motion or better positioned arc of motion. We had three recurrences in type II deformity. Swan-neck deformity deserves our attention because we can help patients improve function either by a motion improvement or a better positioned arc of motion.

Boutonnière Deformity

A boutonnière deformity may be flexible or fixed and is characterized by flexion of the PIP joint and hyperextension of the DIP joint [1]. The pathology begins with synovitis of the PIP joint, which causes elongation of the central slip and triangular ligament. As this occurs, the central slip is unable to maintain full extension of the PIP joint and the lateral bands sublux below the axis of rotation. The retinacular ligaments contract and a stiff joint is the result [2]. The intrinsic-intrinsic plus test can be used to determine whether an oblique retinacular ligament retraction exists. A positive test is indicated when there is limited, passive DIP joint motion with the PIP joint placed in extension.

Nalebuff and Millender Classification [10]

The rheumatoid boutonnière deformity begins in the PIP joint, and any changes in the adjacent joints are secondary. As the PIP flexion deformity becomes more advanced, MCP joint hyperextension may occur as a result. Hand function is not limited significantly until the deformity becomes severe. Nalebuff and Millender classified three stages for boutonnière deformities:

Stage I: Mild deformity; there is only a slight extension lag at the PIP joint.
Stage II: Moderate deformity; the MCP joint is hyperextended.
Stage III: Severe deformity; the joints cannot be passively corrected.

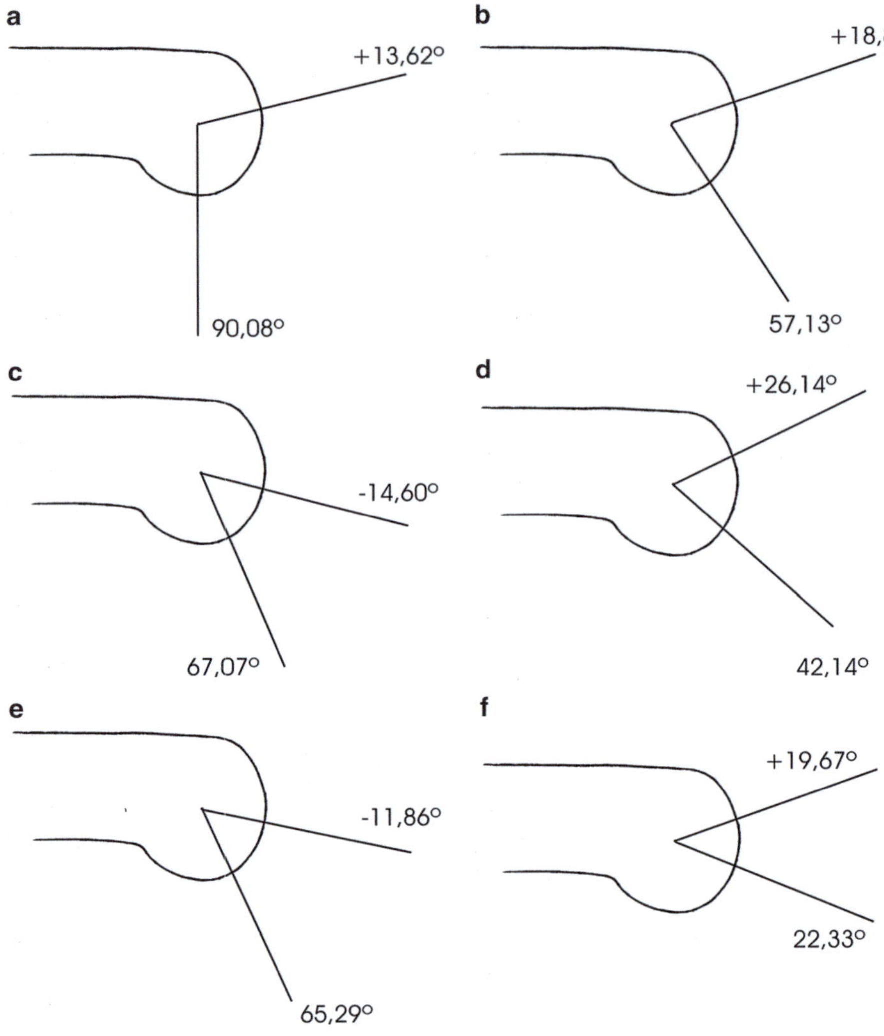

Fig. 19.19 (**a**) PIP range of motion: type I +14° to 90. (**b**) Preoperative: type II +19° to 57°. (**c**) Postoperative: type II −15° to 67°. (**d**) Preoperative: type III +26° to 42°. (**e**) Postoperative: type III −12° to 65°. (**f**) Preoperative: type IV +20° to 22°

Treatment

Fixed contractures may develop as the deformity becomes more severe. Surgical treatment options consist of synovectomy plus surgical reconstruction of the central slip to reposition the lateral bands and a distal tenotomy of the extensor mechanism to relieve the extension contracture of the DIP joint. Stage III deformities are most severe and result in a fixed flexion contracture at the PIP joint with joint space destruction evident on patient radiographs [11]. The complete deformity consists of three components: flexion of the PIP joint, hyperextension of the DIP joint, and hyperextension of the MCP joint. Surgical options to correct stage III deformities include either arthrodesis or arthroplasty. Arthrodesis is usually indicated and is the most reliable treatment option. The joint is fixed with a K-wire for 3–4 weeks at varying angles depending on which finger is being treated. For example, the PIP joint is fused at 25° in the index finger, 30° in the middle finger, 35° in the ring finger, and 40° in the little finger. Arthroplasty is very seldom performed in cases involving the ring and little fingers because we must simultaneously reconstruct the extensor mechanism and results are unreliable.

Reconstruction of the Extensor Mechanism [4]

Preoperative images are shown in Figs. 19.20 and 19.21. A dorsal curved incision is made over the PIP joint. The central slip is divided distally, leaving a cuff of tendon attached to the base or the middle phalanx. The central band is separated from the lateral bands, and after resecting a few millimeters, it is reattached to the base of the middle phalanx. The lateral bands are sutured to each other dorsally (Fig. 19.22). Postoperative results are shown in Figs. 19.23 and 19.24. If necessary, the extensor mechanism is divided at the middle phalanx to allow for flexion of the DIP joint. The reattachment of the central slip to the middle phalanx may also be achieved using a suture anchor [12]. This technique is indicated if the central slip is separated from its middle phalanx insertion or is too attenuated to hold sutures (Figs. 19.25, 19.26 and 19.27).

Postoperative Care

Following reconstruction of the extensor mechanism, the PIP joint is immobilized in full extension

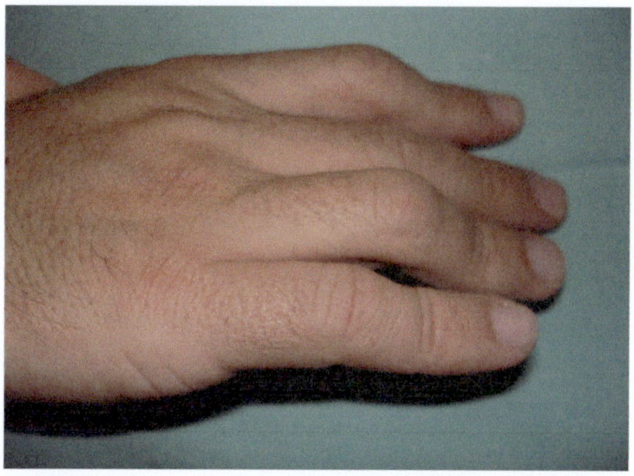

Fig. 19.21 Dorsal view of the ring finger boutonniere deformity

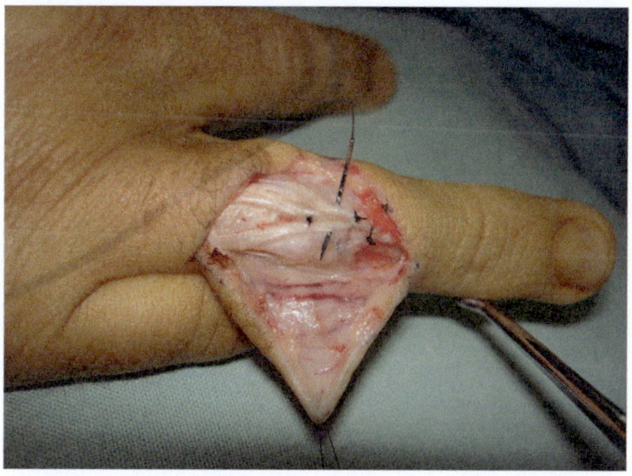

Fig. 19.22 Lateral bands sutured to each other dorsally

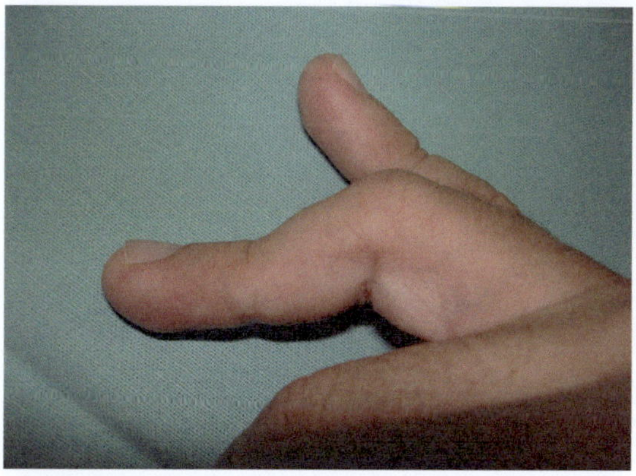

Fig. 19.20 Ring finger boutonniere deformity showing flexion at the PIP joint and hyperextension at the DIP joint

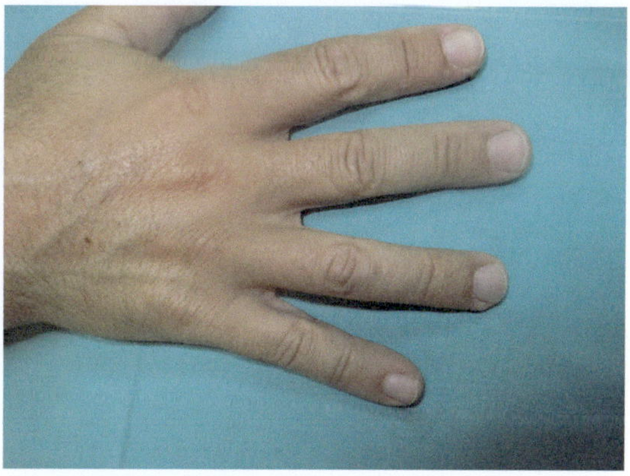

Fig. 19.23 Boutonniere Littler's technique post-op

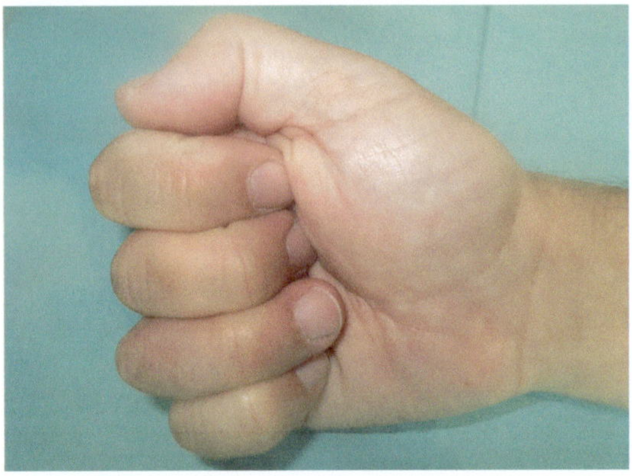

Fig. 19.24 Boutonniere Littler's technique post-op

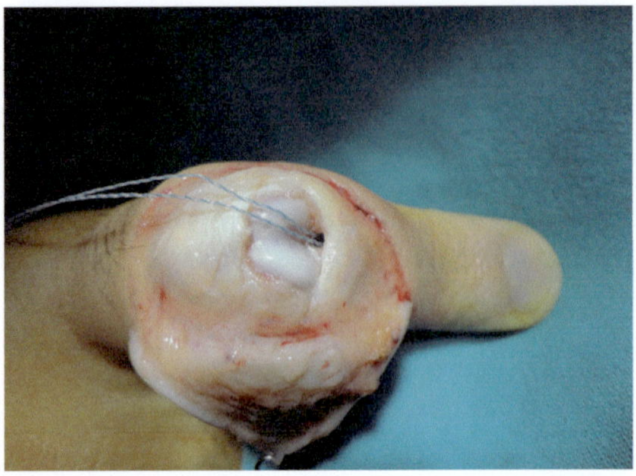

Fig. 19.26 Reattachment of central slip to the middle phalanx

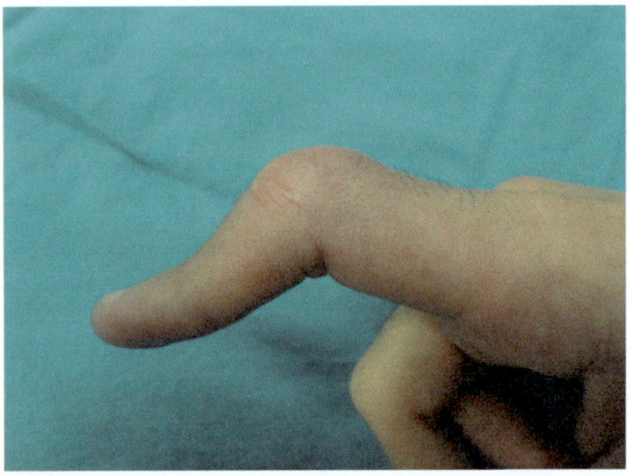

Fig. 19.25 Pre-op of index finger boutonniere deformity before surgical treatment with a bone anchor

using a K-wire or volar splint for 14 days. Patients may begin active flexion exercises of the DIP joint within 3 days of surgery. Active flexion exercises of the PIP joint are initiated after 14 days of immobilization is completed; however, active extension exercises should not be performed for several weeks.

Final Conclusion

Boutonniere deformities can severely affect the hand function of patients with RA. It is important to treat the deformity early to prevent secondary

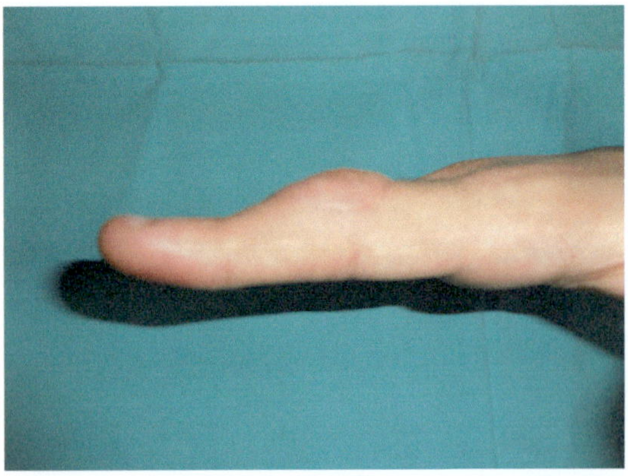

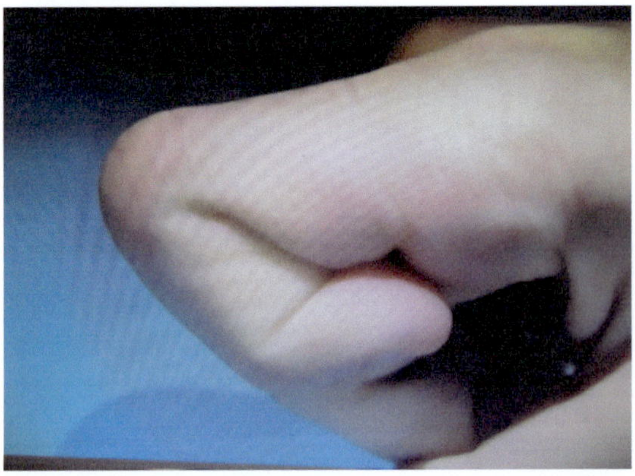

Fig. 19.27 Boutonniere post-op with bone anchor

effects to the MCP joint. Full passive correctability of the PIP joint should be achieved before surgery to allow for optimum results after reconstruction of the extensor mechanism [11]. Careful consideration of all other RA deformities is advised before deciding on the best treatment option.

References

1. Boyer MI, Gelberman RH. Operative correction of swan-neck and boutonniere deformities in the rheumatoid hand. J Am Acad Orthop Surg. 1999;7(2): 92–100.
2. Nalebuff EA. The rheumatoid swan-neck deformity. Hand Clin. 1989;5(2):203–14.
3. O'Brien ET. Surgical principles and planning for the rheumatoid hand and wrist. Clin Plast Surg. 1996;23(3):407–20.
4. Green DP. Operative hand surgery, vol. 2. 3rd ed. New York: Churchill Livingstone; 1993. p. 1654–70.
5. Tonkin MA, Hughes J, Smith KL. Lateral band translocation for swan-neck deformity. J Hand Surg Am. 1992;17(2):260–7.
6. Sirotakova M, Figus A, Jarrett P, Mishra A, Elliot D. Correction of swan neck deformity in rheumatoid arthritis using a new lateral extensor band technique. J Hand Surg Eur Vol. 2008;33(6):712–6.
7. Kiefhaber TR, Strickland JW. Soft tissue reconstruction for rheumatoid swan-neck and boutonniere deformities: long-term results. J Hand Surg Am. 1993;18(6):984–9.
8. Gainor BJ, Hummel GL. Correction of rheumatoid swan-neck deformity by lateral band mobilization. J Hand Surg Am. 1985;10(3):370–6.
9. Olazabal A. Surgery of the rheumatoid wrist and hand. J Bone Joint Surg Br. 2008;90(Supp 2):262.
10. Nalebuff EA, Millender LH. Surgical treatment of the boutonniere deformity in rheumatoid arthritis. Orthop Clin North Am. 1975;6(3):753–63.
11. Williams K, Terrono AL. Treatment of boutonniere finger deformity in rheumatoid arthritis. J Hand Surg Am. 2011;36(9):1388–93.
12. Slesarenko YA, Hurst LC, Mai K. Suture anchor technique for anatomic reconstruction in chronic boutonniere deformity. Tech Hand Up Extrem Surg. 2005; 9(3):172–4.

Concepts in Ulnar Drift Deformity

20

Shepard P. Johnson and Kevin C. Chung

Introduction

Ulnar drift occurs when there is a biomechanical imbalance of forces at the metacarpophalangeal (MCP) joint (Fig. 20.1). Ulnar drift deformity is distinct from ulnar deviation, the normal rotation of the proximal phalanx on the metacarpal that facilitates hand grip [1]. Classically seen in rheumatoid arthritis, the pathophysiology of ulnar drift is commonly attributed to MCP joint synovitis causing dorsoradial ligament damage and resultant extensor tendon ulnar subluxation [1–6]. More accurately, ulnar drift is a result of multiple factors including innate MCP anatomy, normal hand use, ulnar translation of the flexor tendons, and proximal joint disease (e.g., radial deviation of the wrist). Disruption of stabilizing ligaments at the MCP joint also leads to palmar subluxation of the proximal phalanx and permanent flexion deformities [1–4].

S.P. Johnson, MBBS
Department of Surgery, St. Joseph Mercy Ann Arbor, 5333 McAuley Drive, Suite 2111, Ann Arbor, MI 48197, USA

K.C. Chung, MD, MS (✉)
Comprehensive Hand Center, Section of Plastic Surgery, Department of Surgery, The University of Michigan Health System, 2130 Taubman Center, SPC 5340, 1500 E. Medical Center Drive, Ann Arbor, MI 48109-5340, USA
e-mail: kecchung@med.umich.edu

Ulnar drift can profoundly affect a patient's quality of life by impairing power grip and precision hand functions [1, 7]. Furthermore, pain and esthetic discomfort are common complaints by patients [8, 9]. When conservative management is exhausted, surgical interventions may be considered. Silicone metacarpophalangeal arthroplasty (SMPA) is the most proven intervention to correct ulnar drift deformity, relieve pain, and improve hand function [7, 10, 11]. Commonly, soft tissue reconstructive procedures are performed concomitantly to reestablish normal anatomical alignment at the MCP joint [6, 12, 13]. Long-term follow-up of a multicenter prospective outcomes study of SMPA in rheumatoid arthritis patients showed improvement in hand function and appearance when compared to nonsurgical controls [7, 14].

Metacarpophalangeal Joint Anatomy

To appreciate the pathological consequence of rheumatoid arthritis on the MCP joint, one needs an understanding of the joint anatomy. The metacarpal/proximal phalanx, periarticular connective tissues, extrinsic/intrinsic hand muscles, and extensor/flexor tendons function to stabilize and move the joint (Fig. 20.2). Knowledge of the anatomical relationships of these structures is critical to understanding the biomechanical properties of the MCP joint and how it contributes to hand

K.C. Chung (ed.), *Clinical Management of the Rheumatoid Hand, Wrist, and Elbow*,
DOI 10.1007/978-3-319-26660-2_20

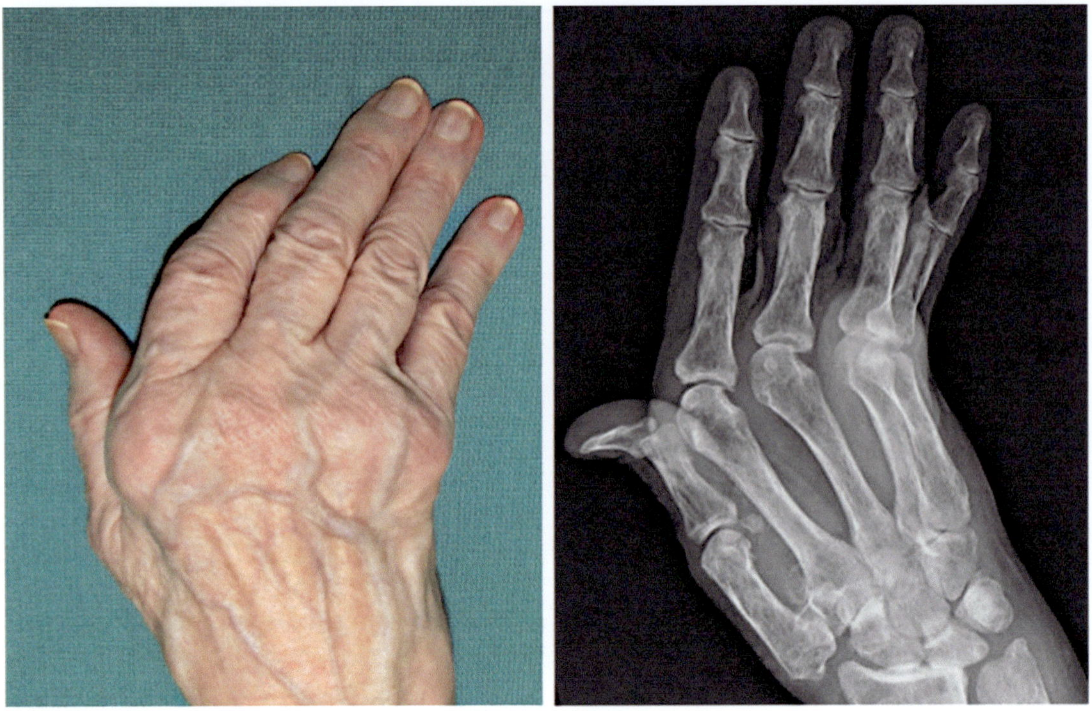

Fig. 20.1 Ulnar drift deformity in a patient with rheumatoid arthritis

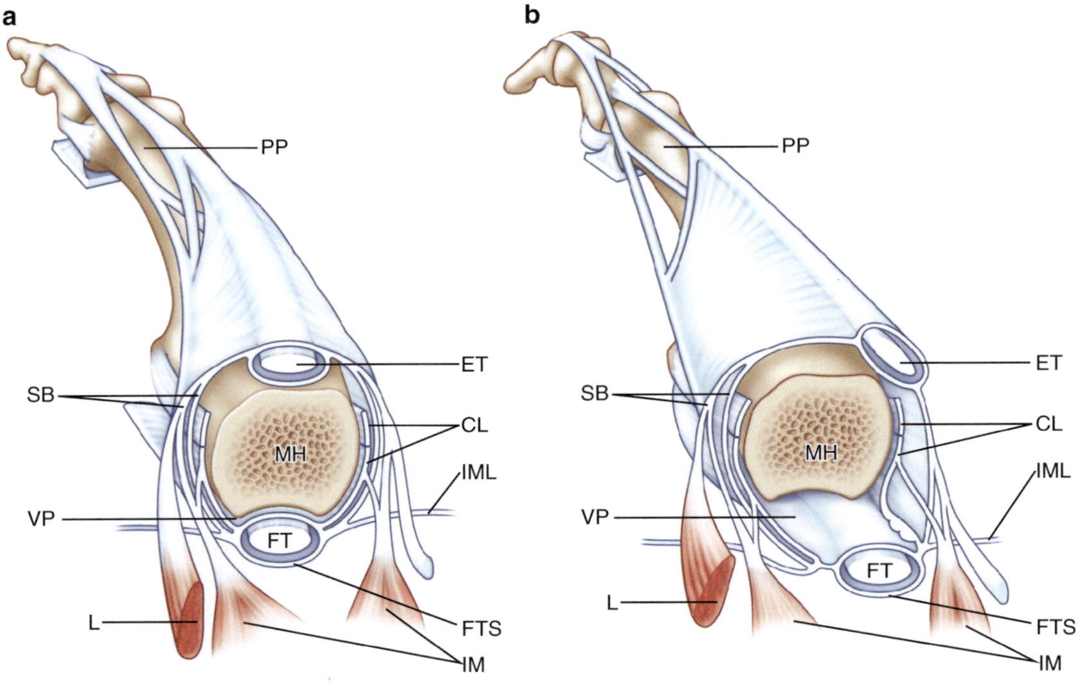

Fig. 20.2 (**a**) Metacarpophalangeal anatomy in normal alignment. (**b**) Soft tissue changes in ulnar drift deformity represented include radial sagittal band attenuation, ulnar subluxation of extensor and flexor tendons, and contracted intrinsic muscles [*CL* collateral ligament, *ET* extensor tendon, *FT* flexor tendon, *FTS* flexor tendon sheath, *IM* interosseous muscle, *IML* intermetacarpal ligament (deep transverse metacarpal ligament), *L* lumbrical, *MH* metacarpal head, *PP* proximal phalanx, *SB* sagittal band, *VP* volar plate]

Table 20.1 Anatomical causes of ulnar deviation in a normal metacarpophalangeal joint

Influences on natural ulnar deviation	Details
Metacarpophalangeal anatomic characteristics	
Asymmetrical metacarpal head	Small sloping ulnar condyle
Asymmetrical collateral ligaments	Radial collateral ligaments are more oblique, attenuated, and weaker than ulnar collateral ligaments
Transverse intermetacarpal ligament and volar plates	Transmits the ulnar pull of the abductor digiti minimi
Thin radial extensor triangle	Synovial swelling preferentially bulges into the thin, weak radial extensor triangle, leading to radial collateral ligament laxity
Intrinsic hand force system—intrinsic muscles	
Asymmetrical interossei muscles	Greater bulk and strength of ulnar sided interossei muscles
Influence of hypothenar muscle on little finger	Greater bulk and strength than the third radial volar interosseous muscle
Ulnar pull of the abductor digiti minimi (Zancolli's ulnar force)	Ulnar forces are translated across the metacarpal arch through the deep transverse metacarpal ligament
Intrinsic hand force system—extrinsic muscles	
Ulnar vector forces from flexor tendons	Flexor tendons of the index and long finger exert an ulnar force at the entrance of the flexor tunnel
Extrinsic hand force system	
Pinch grip	Pressure of thumb on radial side of digits exerts an ulnar force
Power grip	Lifting heavy objects is typically performed such that ulnar directed forces occur at the MCP joint
Gravitational pull	Accentuates proximal phalanx volar subluxation and ulnar deviating forces at the MCP joint

MCP metacarpophalangeal

functions, such as precision grip. Armed with knowledge of the normal function of the MCP joint, it becomes intuitive why ulnar drift deformity occurs as a consequence of joint destruction in rheumatoid arthritis (Table 20.1).

The MCP joint is formed by the condylar articulation between the larger convex metacarpal head and smaller concave base of the proximal phalanx [3, 15]. The metacarpal head is asymmetrical, having a larger radial condyle and a small, sloping ulnar condyle. This ulnar inclination, and the influence of asymmetrical radial and ulnar collateral ligaments, has important implication on normal hand grips [3, 4]. With active flexion, the proximal phalanx rotates and ulnar deviates. Therefore, ulnar deviation refers to the medial-lateral rotation of the proximal phalanx on the metacarpal, which brings the digits into opposed flexion onto the thenar eminence (Fig. 20.3) [1, 3, 4]. This is distinct from ulnar drift, which describes pathological ulnar translation of the proximal phalanx with respect to the metacarpal head (Fig. 20.4).

Enveloping the articulating bones of the MCP joint is a dense fibrous capsule lined by a synovial membrane, the target tissue of inflammatory changes in rheumatoid arthritis. The capsule provides joint stability by restricting passive movements and is reinforced by laterally orientated collateral ligaments and a volar (palmar) plate [15]. The collateral ligaments originate on the distal dorsal metacarpal, travel distally and volarly, and terminate on the base of the proximal phalanx [3, 4]. Landsmeer identified an important distinction (most prominently in the index and long fingers) between the radial and ulnar collateral ligaments [16]. The radial collateral ligament is thinner, wider, extends more dorsally, and takes a more oblique course than the ulnar collateral ligament [3, 16]. As a consequence, with proximal phalanx flexion rotation, the radial ligaments are more lax and offer less resistance to ulnar deviation of the digits. The more robust and tight ulnar ligaments prevent radial deviation.

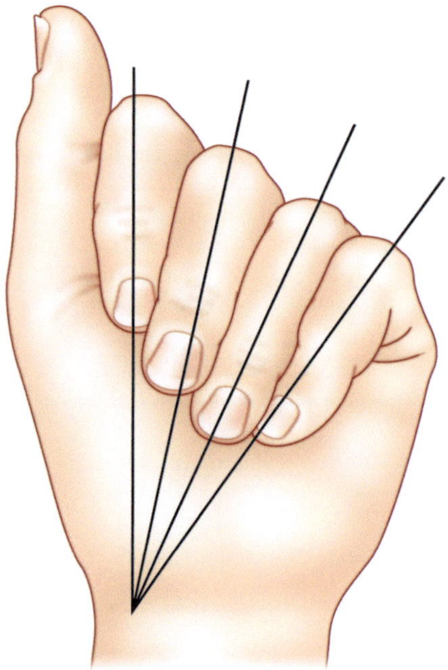

Fig. 20.3 Metacarpophalangeal joint flexion results in medial-lateral rotation and ulnar deviation of the proximal phalanx on the metacarpal (most pronounced in ulnar digits). This brings the digits into opposed flexion onto the thenar eminence

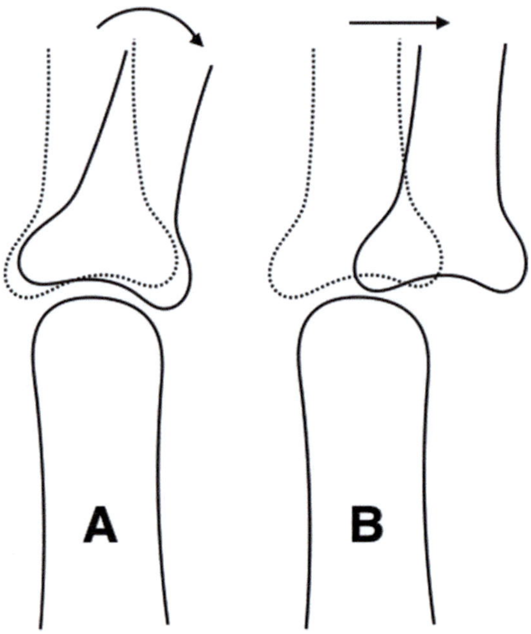

Fig. 20.4 (**a**) Ulnar deviation, present in normal digits, is the ulnar rotation of the phalanx in relation to the metacarpal. (**b**) Ulnar shift, a pathological finding, is ulnar translation of the phalanx in relation to the metacarpal. Ulnar drift is the consequence of deviation and shift

The fibrocartilaginous volar plate covers the palmar aspect of the MCP joint capsule and resists hyperextension. The volar plate consists of the proximal membranous portion adherent to the metacarpal and the distal, robust cartilaginous portion that adheres to the proximal phalanx [2]. The metacarpoglenoid (accessory collateral) ligament extends from the volar plate forming a sling that suspends the flexor digitorum profundus and flexor digitorum superficialis as they pass between the metacarpal tubercles and enter the flexor tendon sheath (Fig. 20.5) [15]. In 1966, Smith et al. proposed that the metacarpoglenoidal ligament acts as a pulley and prevents bowstringing of the flexor tendons during grasp or pinch grip. Figure 20.6 demonstrates the oblique course of the flexor tendons of the index and long finger as they enter the flexor tunnel and how the metacarpoglenoid ligament prevents flexor tendon bowstringing in both palmar and ulnar directions [2].

The deep transverse metacarpal ligament (intermetacarpal ligament) connects the volar plates of the second through fifth MCP joints [1, 15] (Fig. 20.7). This structure provides intercapsular stability, prevents fanning of the metacarpal heads, and distributes forces across the volar plates [15]. For example, the ulnar pull of the abductor digiti minimi on the small digit is translated across the metacarpal arch through the deep transverse metacarpal ligament. Zancolli described this as the ulnar force of the hand [17]. This force also influences a natural palmar descent on the metacarpals of the ring and small fingers, which facilitates tightening of the power grip (Fig. 20.8).

Covering the dorsum of the MCP joint capsule is the dorsal hood (extensor apparatus). This is an aponeurotic expansion of the extensor digitorum that covers the distal metacarpal and proximal phalanx and is the site of distal attachments for the intrinsic hand muscles [15, 18, 19]. Providing stability to the dorsal hood are the sagittal bands, tendinous attachments originating on the radial and ulnar side of the volar plate. This transversely orientated structure encircles the MCP joints and functions to centralize the extensor tendon over the metacarpal head (Fig. 20.2) [18, 19].

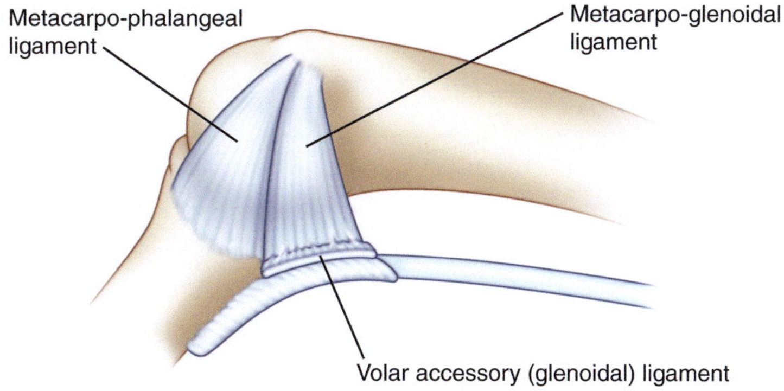

Fig. 20.5 The metacarpoglenoid (accessory collateral) ligament extends from the volar plate forming a sling that suspends the flexor tendons as they enter the flexor tendon sheath

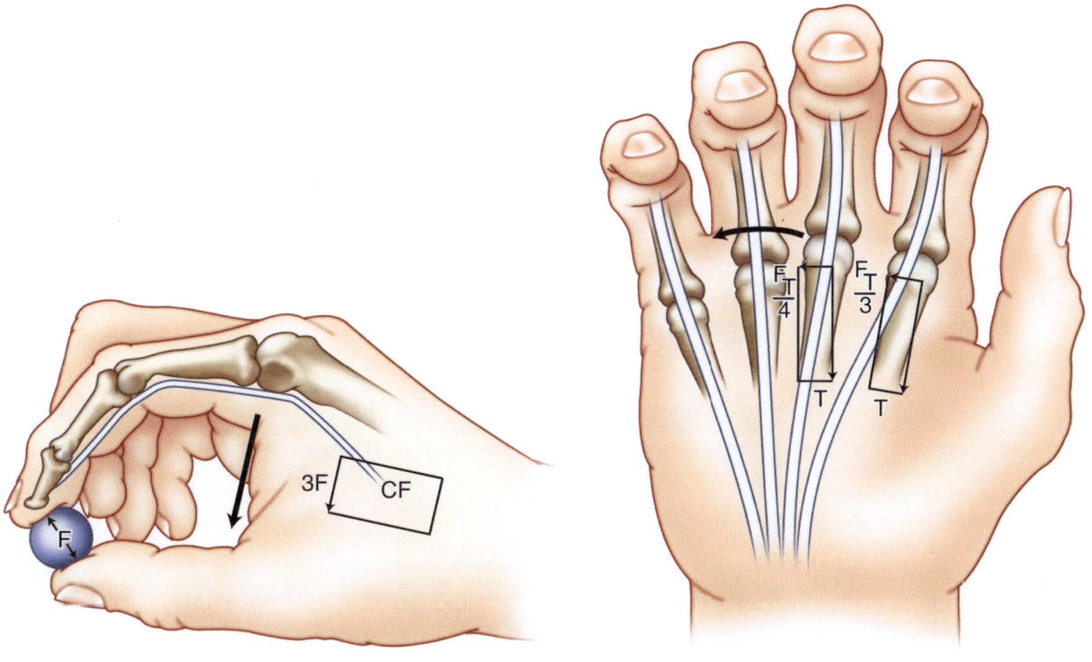

Fig. 20.6 Flexor tendons exert palmar forces (*left image*) and ulnar forces (*right image*) with pinch grip as they enter the flexor tunnel. Notice the oblique course of the tendons of the index and long finger (*blue line*). The metacarpoglenoid ligament helps prevent flexor tendon bowstringing in both palmar and ulnar directions (*black arrows*)

By adhering to the dorsal hood, the bands help limit hyperextension of the MCP joint.

The intrinsic muscles of the hand contributing to MCP joint movement are the four lumbricals and seven (three palmar and four dorsal) interossei [15]. The lumbricals cause MCP joint flexion, whereas the interossei muscles contribute to both flexion of the MCP joint and digit abduction and adduction. The lumbricals originate from the flexor digitorum profundus tendons, pass palmar to the MCP joints, and insert onto the radial aspect of the dorsal hood. The interossei arise from the metacarpals and insert onto the proximal phalanx and dorsal hood [18]. The tendons of the palmar and dorsal interosseous muscles on the ulnar side of the digit form the common intrinsic tendon [13]. On the radial side, the lumbrical tendon joins with the interossei muscles to form the common intrinsic tendon [13].

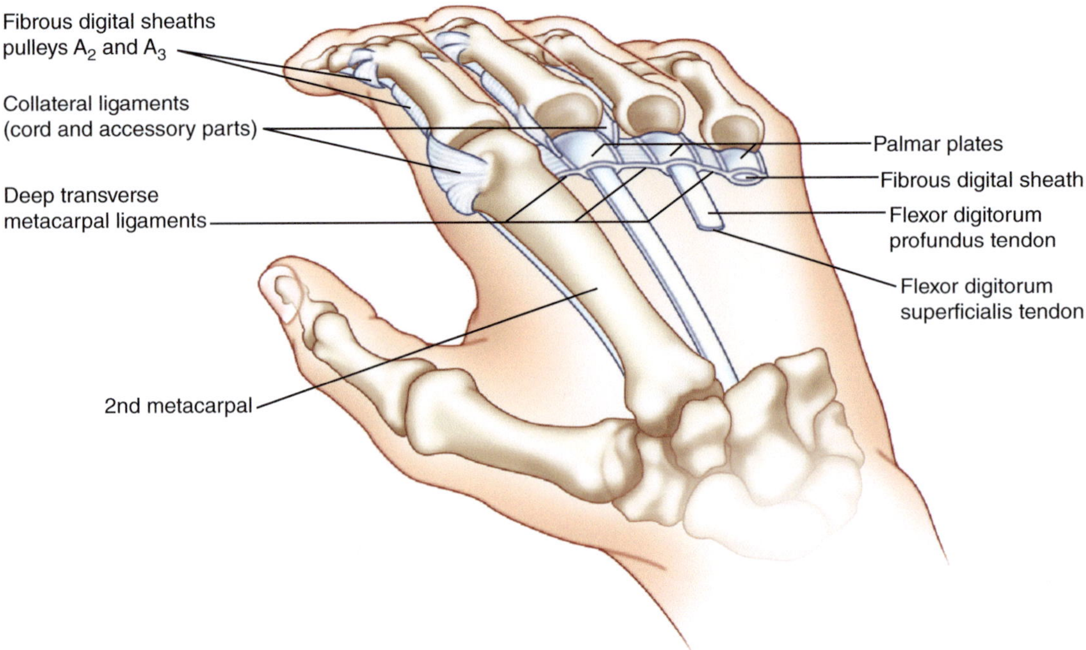

Fig. 20.7 The deep transverse metacarpal ligament (intermetacarpal ligament) connects the palmar (volar) plates and distributes forces across the metacarpophalangeal joints

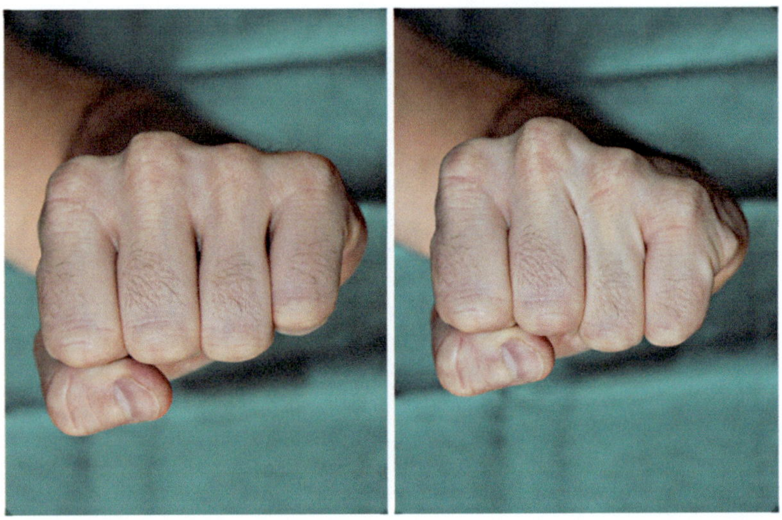

Fig. 20.8 Depicted is the natural palmar descent of the metacarpals of the ring and small finger, which facilitates tightening of the power grip (*right*, loose handgrip; *left*, tightened handgrip)

Intrinsic hand muscles exert forces that contribute to ulnar deviation [1, 3, 18]. Backhouse conceptually grouped the intrinsics into ulnar and radial muscle groups to simplify their influence on hand mechanics [3]. Mechanical studies have shown that the ulnar insertions of intrinsic muscles are broader, stronger, and more transverse than their radial counterpart and therefore work to a better mechanical advantage [1, 3, 18–20]. Because of the dominance of ulnar intrinsics, the already less-robust radial collateral ligaments are subjected to greater forces, and therefore, ulnar deviation occurs in normal MCP joint flexion.

Metacarpophalangeal Mechanics

The diarthrodial MCP joint permits motion through several axes; flexion, extension, abduction, adduction, distraction, and circumduction of the proximal phalanx on the metacarpal head [4]. The MCP joint is critical for hand function, as the arc of motion for hand grip is initiated through flexion at this joint [12]. Unlike interphalangeal joints, the MCP joint permits lateral mobility when in extension, which facilitates complex fine motor activity, such as typing on a keyboard. This is made possible by the stabilizing contributions of the intrinsic muscles, collateral ligaments, and volar plate at the MCP joint [15]. Consequently, the mechanical integrity of the MCP joint is dependent on these structures.

Precise control of MCP joint mobility is attained through a balance between active and counteractive forces. Active extension at the MCP joint is stabilized by passive tension within intrinsic muscles and the volar plate. Passive tension describes tension arising from the elastic properties of muscles not actively being contracted. Lateral stability of the MCP joint follows a similar principle. Active abduction of MCP joints is balanced by passive adduction of interosseous muscles and tension within lateral collateral ligaments. Therefore, in ulnar drift when the radial collateral ligaments are compromised, the interossei muscles remain the primary source of lateral stability [15].

Ulnar and radial collateral ligaments contribute to lateral stability during MCP joint flexion. The collateral ligaments run dorsal to the center of motion of the joint and therefore are stretched and tightened with proximal phalanx flexion [3, 4]. Additionally, they are stretched over the widened volar portion of the metacarpal head. As previously described, asymmetry of the collateral ligaments permits ulnar deviation during flexion. With MCP joint flexion, supination of the proximal phalanx (dorsal rotation) relaxes the radial collateral ligament, allowing it to take a less oblique course across the joint [3]. Unwinding of the radial ligament allows ulnar deviation.

The natural tendency of the MCP joint to rotate and ulnar deviate with flexion has important implications on both precision (pinch) grip and power grip (grasp) [21]. Precision grip describes pad-to-pad opposition of the thumb to finger (Fig. 20.9). With ulnar deviation, the tips of the thumb and opposing finger have greater surface area contact [3]. Likewise, the power grip takes advantage of flexion, rotation, and ulnar deviation at the MCP joint by placing the fingers in opposed flexion onto the thumb eminence [21]. Tightening of the power grip accentuates the palmar descent on the metacarpals of the ring and small finger [17].

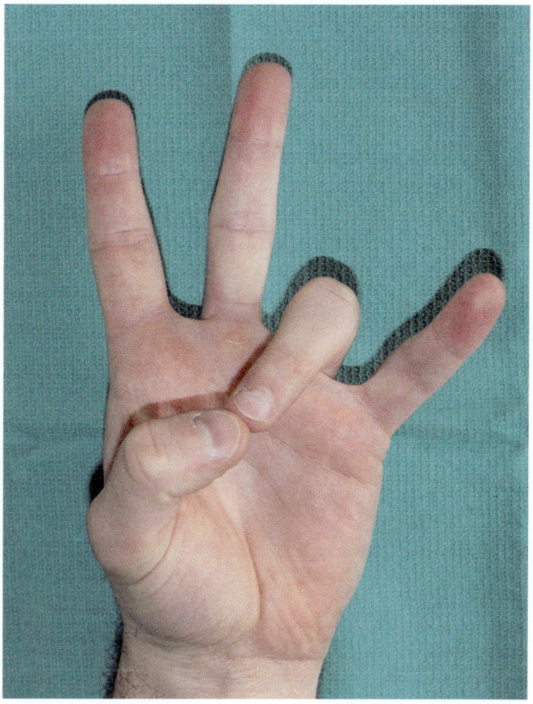

Fig. 20.9 Natural ulnar deviation facilitates opposition between the thumb and digits in precision grip

In 1966, Smith et al. provided insight on the mechanical influence of the flexor tendons on ulnar deviating forces acting at the MCP joint [2]. With pinch and grasp activities, the flexor tendons transmit large forces on the sling arrangement of the metacarpoglenoidal ligament and flexor tendon sheaths. Smith et al. geometrically demonstrated that the flexor tendon exerts a force at the metacarpoglenoidal ligament that is six times the pinch force exerted at the fingertip (Fig. 20.6) [2]. Furthermore, in the long and index finger, the tendons exert an ulnar force at the entrance of the flexor tendon sheath (Fig. 20.6). Therefore, the radial portion of the metacarpoglenoidal ligament is subjected to large ulnar bowstringing forces. Under significant strain, accessory collateral ligaments already stretched by inflammatory changes in rheumatoid arthritis may lead to flexor tendon palmar and ulnar subluxation.

Forces at the Metacarpophalangeal Joint

Flatt alluded two force systems exerting stress and influencing movement at the MCP joint [1]: the intrinsic forces, generated by action of the extrinsic and intrinsic muscles, and the extrinsic forces, created by usage. The ligamentous and retinacular tissues that surround the joint absorb these potentially deforming forces. Zancolli thought of these ligamentous structures as a closed circuit composed of functional units [17]. He referred to a "force nucleus" of each unit, to describe where the forces acting on the MCP joint are in balance [17]. Force nuclei exist on the radial and ulnar aspect of each MCP joint at the intersection of the volar plate, sagittal bands, flexor sheath, and deep transverse metacarpal ligament (Fig. 20.10).

Damage to any stabilizing structure will lead to an imbalance at the force nucleus and permanent deformity. Zancolli used this concept to describe the pathomechanical changes of rheumatoid arthritis at the MCP joint. For example, when the radial collateral ligament is disrupted by local synovitis, there is one less structure resisting ulnar forces. The remaining supportive tissues must compensate. Under greater stress, the radial sagittal band may weaken and stretch. Laxity of the sagittal band allows the extensor tendon to subluxate into the ulnar intermetacarpal sulcus (Fig. 20.10) [5]. In the subluxed position, the tendons exert aberrant ulnar and flexion

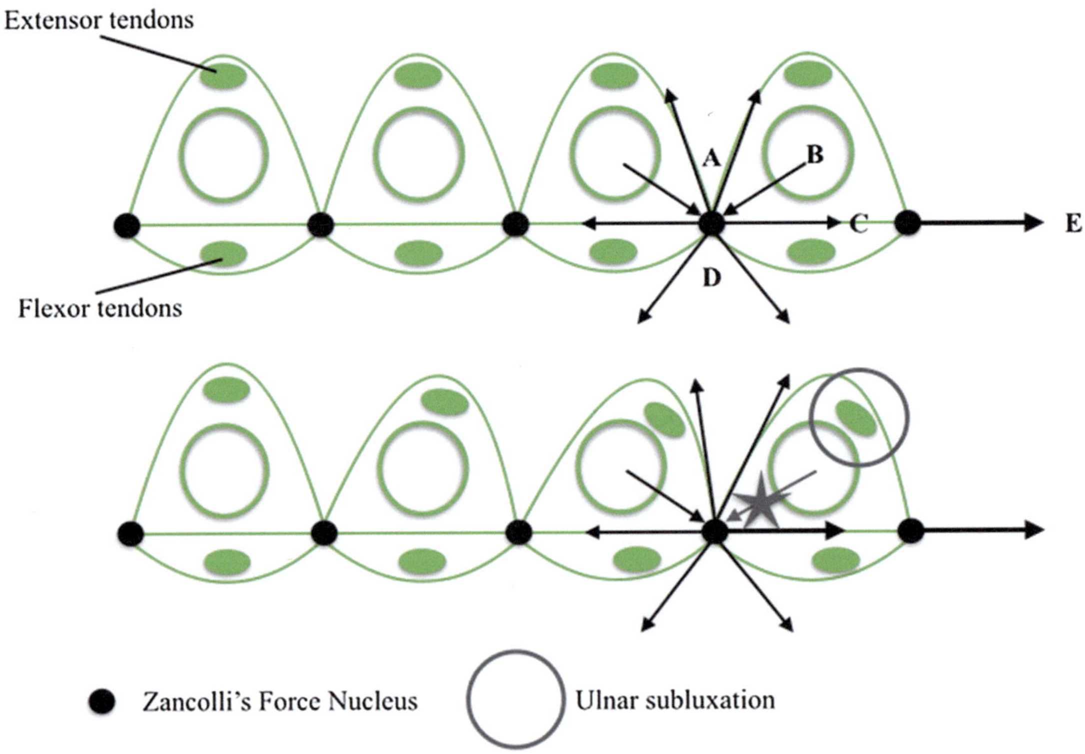

Fig. 20.10 Zancolli's force nucleus. *Star* represents damaged radial collateral ligament, which disrupts the force nucleus, weakens the radial sagittal band, and results in ulnar subluxation (*A* sagittal bands, *B* collateral ligaments, *C* volar plate and intermetacarpal ligament, *D* flexor tendon sheath, *E* ulnar force of the hand)

forces on the MCP joint. Therefore, disruption of the radial collateral ligament has led to an imbalance of the force nucleus, resulting in an ulnar drift deformity. The deep transverse metacarpal ligament connects all the force nuclei, and therefore, instability at one MCP joint leads to deforming forces in the remaining joints [1, 17].

Zancolli also described the ulnar force of the hand that originates from the fifth MCP (ulnar pull of the abductor digiti minimi) and exerts traction along the deep transverse metacarpal ligament and volar plates [17]. This force is accentuated by the natural palmar descent of the ring and small finger metacarpals. In rheumatoid ulnar drift, contracture of the hypothenar muscles, palmar subluxation of long flexor tendons, and ulnar subluxation of extensor tendons (imparting MCP flexion) results in permanent palmar descent [1, 17]. The ulnar force of the hand thus influences all the MCP joints.

Rheumatoid Arthritis at the Metacarpophalangeal Joint

Inflammatory change in rheumatoid arthritis is characterized by an autoimmune-driven synovial proliferation [22]. At the MCP joint, the inflamed synovium becomes edematous; distention of the joint capsule stretches the collateral ligaments and membranous portion of the volar plate [4]. Unclear is whether rheumatoid inflammation has a greater propensity to involve the radial side of MCP joint, leading to the pathognomonic ulnar drift deformity. Backhouse offered a sound hypothesis that synovial swelling preferentially bulges into the thin, weak radial extensor triangle, leading to radial collateral ligament and sagittal band laxity, setting the stage for ulnar subluxation of the extensor tendons [3].

Progressive inflammation leads to direct invasion and degeneration of collateral ligaments. Pannus, a membrane of fibrovascular tissue, develops at the site of synovial bony attachments and advances over the articular surface [4]. This highly vascularized tissue releases inflammatory cytokines, lysosomal enzymes, and free radicals that lead to degeneration of the hyaline cartilage [23]. Proliferation of pannus leads to erosion and softening of the metacarpal and proximal phalanx [4]. The result of inflammatory changes is a poorly articulating joint with stretched and attenuated supporting structures. Accompanying soft tissue changes seen in ulnar drift, including intrinsic muscle contracture and tendon lag, are secondary deformities rather than a direct consequence of rheumatoid inflammation.

Ulnar Drift Deformity

Ulnar drift deformity is a consequence of unbalanced forces at the MCP joint and proximal joints. As demonstrated, normal extrinsic and intrinsic force systems favor ulnar deviation, but the pathological condition of ulnar drift deformity only manifests with compromise to the major structural defenses in the MCP joint [1]. Literature has failed to identify a singular cause of ulnar drift deformity. Rather, it is a product of multiple influences including joint anatomy, rheumatoid tissue damage, and the pathomechanics of unbalanced forces. External forces have also been implicated in the development and progression of ulnar drift. Many activities exert an ulnar vector on the MCP joint, for example, wielding a hammer [12]. Table 20.2 summarizes rheumatologic changes that influence the formation of ulnar drift deformity.

At the MCP joint, synovitis leads to laxity and degradation of the radial collateral ligament, accessory collateral ligament, and sagittal band. Failure of these supportive ligaments permits extensor tendon subluxation into the ulnar intermetacarpal sulcus and ulnar deviating stress [1, 5, 15]. Weakening of the volar plate and rupture of the extensor tendon insertion on the proximal phalanx base results in palmar subluxation of the phalanx on the metacarpal head. On the palmar side, synovitis may cause laxity of the metacarpoglenoid ligament, allowing ulnar bowstringing of the flexor tendons [2]. Lengthening of the flexor and extensor tendons from carpal collapse allows unopposed MCP flexion from the relatively tighter intrinsic muscles. Prolonged flexion leads to intrinsic contractures.

Table 20.2 Biomechanical consequences of rheumatoid pathology at the metacarpophalangeal joint

Pathologic changes	Structural and biomechanical alterations
Metacarpophalangeal pathology	
Laxity and rupture of radial collateral ligaments	Loss of resistance to ulnar deviation
Laxity and rupture of extensor tendon insertion on base of proximal phalanx	Palmar subluxation of the proximal phalanx
Laxity and rupture of volar plate	Palmar subluxation of the proximal phalanx
Laxity and rupture of sagittal band	Extensor tendon ulnar subluxation into intermetacarpal sulcus
Laxity of metacarpoglenoidal ligaments	Flexor tendon ulnar subluxation into intermetacarpal sulcus
Intrinsic hand force system—intrinsic pathology	
Contracture deformities of intrinsic muscles	MCP flexion deformity and palmar subluxation of the proximal phalanx
Intrinsic hand force system—extrinsic pathology	
Extensor tendon ulnar subluxation into intermetacarpal sulcus	Ulnar drift
Flexor tendon ulnar subluxation into intermetacarpal sulcus	Ulnar drift and palmar subluxation of the proximal phalanx
Radial deviation at the wrist	Oblique forces along a multi-jointed system result in ulnar buckling (ulnar deviation) at the MCP joint

MCP metacarpophalangeal

Proximal joint malalignment contributes significantly to the development and progression of ulnar drift deformity [24]. In 1971, Shapiro et al. described the zigzag deformity, or *z*-collapse, of radial deviation at the wrist and ulnar deviation at the proximal phalanx [24]. Radial deviation at the wrist is a consequence of synovitis causing stretching of the extensor carpi ulnaris and disruption of the distal radioulnar joint, radiocarpal joint, and the triangular fibrocartilage complex. Unopposed extensor carpi radialis longus and brevis cause radial deviation of the metacarpals. This is compounded by carpal collapse and migration of the carpals along the ulnar aspect of the radius [6, 25]. Zigzag deformities can occur with collapse of any multibeam jointed system [1]. Joint buckling is a consequence of forces acting outside the linear plane of the system, and radial deviation of the wrist creates oblique forces that result in ulnar buckling at the metacarpals.

Surgical Management of Ulnar Drift Deformity

Surgical intervention to address ulnar drift deformity aims to improve patient-related outcomes including hand function, pain, and esthetics [26]. Patient-related outcomes reflect the patient's perspective on treatment benefits and are more important than objective measurements, such as range of motion, pinch strength, and degrees of residual ulnar drift [27]. Alleviating symptoms caused by ulnar drift is more complex than simply restoring anatomical alignment. Rheumatoid arthritis is a polyarticular disease, and often patients have multiple hand ailments (e.g., swan neck deformities) that inhibit their ability to carry out activities of daily living. Hand surgeons must individualize treatment plans based on coexisting conditions, the patient's expectations in context of their needs and occupation, and realistic surgical outcomes.

Unfortunately, there is a lack of robust evidence on the effectiveness of surgical interventions to address ulnar drift [23]. Furthermore, there are differing opinions between hand surgeons and rheumatologists regarding the appropriateness and timing of surgery [28–30]. Advancements in medical therapy have provided greater systemic control of rheumatoid arthritis, but have perpetuated the practice of rheumatologists referring patients to hand surgeons late in the disease process, when operative intervention is more challenging. Regardless, literature has demonstrated that patients with severe ulnar drift deformity benefit from surgical intervention [30].

Despite the absence of a consensus on how to surgically approach ulnar drift deformity, a few principles exist. First, before operative intervention is contemplated, conservative management should be optimized, including systemic immunosuppressants, physical and occupational therapy, splinting, and local intra-articular corticosteroid injections. Second, the treating surgeon must clearly outline the indications and expectations of the surgery, and that ulnar drift has a high propensity to recur. Lastly, the biomechanical stability of the MCP joint is dependent on the stability of proximal joints. In particular, radial wrist deviation may need partial or complete fusion to axially align the wrist before addressing the MCP joint. Correction of ulnar drift deformity will inevitably fail if deviating forces persist at the wrist.

Procedures to address ulnar drift deformity can be classified as prophylactic or reconstructive. Prophylactic procedures include synovectomy, tendon rebalancing, and ulnar intrinsic release [6, 13, 23]. Removing pathologic tissue and restoring the biomechanical balance of hand function offer the promise of pain relief and improved functionality. The effectiveness of these procedures is controversial, and with dramatic improvement in medical therapy, their use has declined. In general, 6 months of medical management is recommended before considering soft tissue procedures [13]. If joint destruction prohibits the indication of prophylactic procedures, hand surgeons may consider MCP arthroplasties, including resection arthroplasties, implant arthroplasty, and arthrodesis. SMPA remains the most widely used and investigated operation [6].

Soft Tissue Procedure: Synovectomy

MCP joint synovectomy removes the target tissue of intra-articular inflammation in rheumatoid arthritis. Indications for synovectomy include painful synovitis associated with restricted range of motion without significant joint deformity or radiographic changes [6, 13]. Ideally, this is performed before significant stretching and attenuation of the joint capsule, collateral ligaments, and volar plate have occurred. Despite this prophylactic approach, maintenance of capsule integrity and control of inflammation may not be sustaining. Synovial resection does little to ameliorate the disruption of mechanical balance in a rheumatoid hand with multiple diseased joints. Therefore, synovectomy does not improve ulnar drift deformities but may provide palliation of pain. Synovectomy alone is rarely performed, as recurrence of symptoms may be as high as 50 %, with symptoms returning in a few years [6, 9].

Soft Tissue Procedure: Tendon Rebalancing/Crossed Intrinsic Transfer

To improve the effectiveness of synovectomies, concomitant restoration of retinacular tissues can be performed, including sagittal band reefing, volar plate repair, ulnar intrinsic muscle release, and extensor tendon realignment. Clinically, if ulnar drift deformities are passively reducible, these procedures have theoretical benefit. Previous studies have demonstrated long-term anatomical alignment with a crossed intrinsic transfer [31]. Soft tissue procedures may be performed in conjunction with MCP joint arthroplasty, although evidence is conflicting regarding improved ulnar drift maintenance [32, 33].

Crossed intrinsic transfer is indicated in patients with ulnar subluxation of the extensor tendon at the MCP joint without arthritis or subluxation of the proximal phalanx [13]. This involves transferring the ulnar lateral bands of the second, third, or fourth finger to the extensor tendon of the ulnar adjacent digit (Fig. 20.11) [6, 23]. This has a twofold biomechanical benefit at the MCP joint. Releasing a contracted ulnar intrinsic tendon removes an ulnar deviating force (on the donor digit), and suturing the lateral band to the extensor tendon creates a radial deviating force on the ulnar adjacent digit. After the transfer, a double-breasted repair of the radial sagittal band can reinforce the transferred intrinsic tendon and centralize the extensor tendon over the MCP joint.

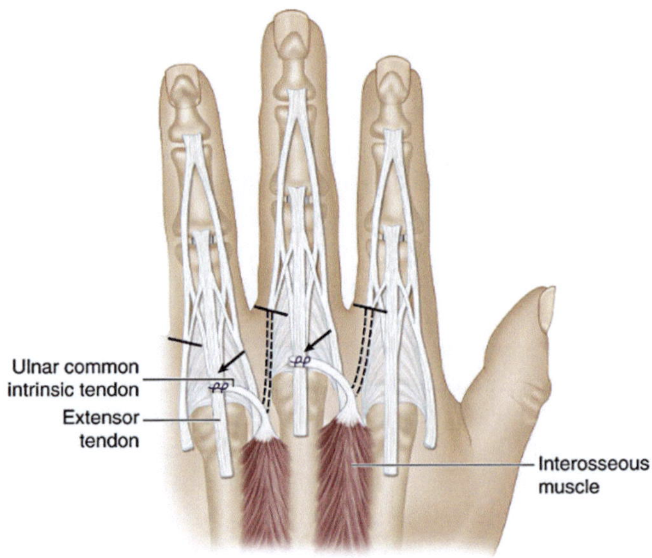

Fig. 20.11 Crossed intrinsic transfer. From Chung KC. Operative Techniques: Hand and Wrist Surgery. 2nd edition. Philadelphia, PA: Saunders; 2012:300–303. Reprinted with permission from Elsevier

Intrinsic transfers are not possible at the index finger, given the absence of an ulnar lateral band at the thumb. Addressing ulnar drift deformity at the index MCP joint is limited to tightening the radial sagittal band, reefing the radial collateral ligaments, and releasing a tightened intrinsic muscle. Intrinsic muscle contracture is clinically apparent when there is restricted flexion at the proximal interphalangeal joint while the MCP is passively held in extension. The abductor digiti minimi may be divided to remove the ulnar force on the small finger [23].

Arthroplasties: Metacarpophalangeal Joint Implant Arthroplasty

MCP joint arthroplasty is reserved for patients with ulnar drift deformity accompanied by MCP joint contracture or proximal phalangeal subluxation. These deformities indicate ligamentous damage and contractures not amenable to soft tissue reconstructive procedures [6, 13]. Despite clinical or radiographic evidence of major ulnar drift deformity, patients can maintain an unexpected degree of functionality [11]. In these patients, if pain is well controlled, arthroplasty procedures should not be pursued as they may decrease grip strength [6, 11, 23]. Several prosthetic designs have been used over the past 60 years, with silicone arthroplasty currently being the preferred implant given its safety profile, ease of placement and removal, durability, and effectiveness [6, 12, 27].

Indications for SMPA are clouded by a contentious debate between rheumatologists and hand surgeons. A national survey has highlighted the dichotomy of beliefs, which revealed that 34 % of rheumatologist and 83 % of hand surgeons had a positive view regarding outcomes of SMPA [28]. Rheumatologist favors delaying SMPA until severe deformity is present. Hand surgeons prefer to intervene early. Despite the trend of rheumatologist to refer patients late in their disease process, SMPA remains beneficial to patients with severe ulnar drift deformities [34].

Literature has shown SMPA to be effective in improving patient-related outcomes related to ulnar drift deformity [7, 10, 27, 34–36]. Long-term outcomes of SMPA have shown improvement in hand function and appearance [14]. A multicenter prospective study by Chung et al. comparing silicone arthroplasty in rheumatoid arthritis patients with medical treatment demonstrated improvement in mean overall Michigan Hand Outcomes Questionnaire scores in the surgical group but not in the medical group [7, 14]. Ulnar deviation, extensor lag, and arc of motion at the MCP joint also improved. Nevertheless, there is controversy over its value, as studies have failed to show improvement in grip strength, pinch strength, or mean Arthritis Impact Measurement Scales scores [7, 14, 37].

The silicone implant is considered an interpositional arthroplasty, or spacer, because the prosthesis is not wedded to the bone [38]. The success of silicone implants is based on Swanson's theory of joint encapsulation, where the implant is dependent on the formation of fibrotic tissue to provide joint stability [38]. Silicone elastomer implants are constructed of flexible material that bends at the "stem" (connection between central hinge and body) and at the central hinge [15]. The rubbery design allows pistoning of the implant within the medullary canal which permits added range of motion and distribution of forces along the implant-bone interface [38]. Although silicone implants have reported high fracture rates, ranging from 0 to 67 % [14], this is not an absolute indication for revision surgery, and patients often retain appropriate functionality.

Silicone implants are favored over early generation MCP arthroplasty designs. Metal-hinged prostheses, introduced by Brannon and Klein in 1953, have fallen out of favor given issues with bone resorption, digit shortening, loss of range of motion, and high failure rates [11, 15]. Modern designs, including articulating, nonconstrained pyrolytic carbon implants, utilize more sophisticated materials [15]. They are designed to recreate joint anatomy and have superior mechanical properties with low wear rates. Unfortunately, their use in rheumatoid arthritis is limited as they rely on stable periarticular soft tissue restraints, making them a more appropriate prosthesis for osteoarthritic joints [12].

Silicone metacarpophalangeal joint arthroplasty is carried out through a transverse or longitudinal skin excision over the joint. The extensor hood is exposed and an incision parallel to the extensor tendon is made through the ulnar sagittal band. The dorsal joint capsule is identified and a complete synovectomy is performed. The metacarpal head is excised. Adequate shortening of the bone is critical to allow correction of proximal phalanx subluxation and realignment of the joint [13]. This also decreases tension on the tendons and ligaments contributing to ulnar drift [6]. Releasing soft tissues, including the volar plate or ulnar intrinsic muscles, is sometimes necessary to allow alignment of the joint, although care is taken to maintain the radial attachments which inhibit ulnar drift [11, 13]. The medullary canals of the metacarpal and proximal phalanx are prepared with sequential awls, and the implant is sized and placed (Fig. 20.12). The radial collateral ligament is imbricated through predrilled holes through the radial side of the metacarpal. Tension in the ligament can be adjusted to place the digit in slight radial deviation. The extensor tendon is then centralized over the joint by reefing the radial sagittal band (and releasing the ulnar sagittal band).

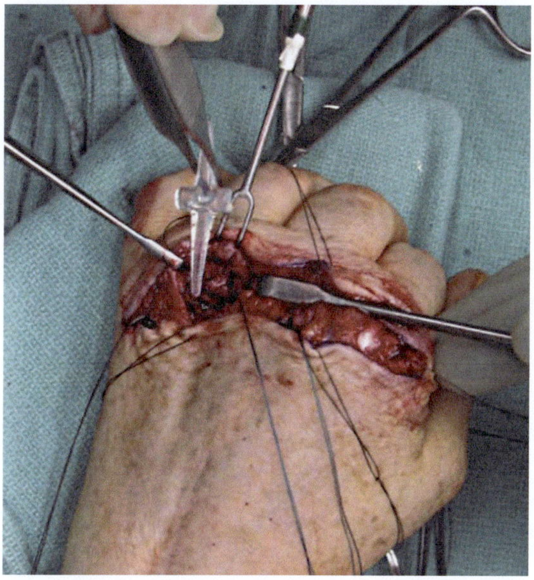

Fig. 20.12 Insertion of a silicone metacarpophalangeal arthroplasty implant. From Chung KC. Operative Techniques: Hand and Wrist Surgery. 2nd edition. Philadelphia, PA: Saunders; 2012:325–328. Reprinted with permission from Elsevier

In the surgical cohort of the multicenter prospective trial by Chung et al., patients reported clinically significant improvements from the Michigan Hand Outcomes Questionnaire in hand function, activities of daily living, esthetics, and satisfaction over time [7, 14]. There was also a 20° improvement in ulnar drift, 30° improvement in extensor slag, and 9° increase in arc of motion over 3 years, which are comparable values to previous investigations of SMPA [14]. Although this gain in range of motion may enable patients to form a grip, strength is not improved. The study was not randomized, and therefore patients who opted for surgical intervention may have been motivated by the prospective of relief from their debilitating symptoms. The cumulative results from publications support the use of silicone implants in selected patients. Even though literature may suggest conflicting evidence regarding the functional outcomes of silicone arthroplasty, the esthetic benefit of the surgery has been well documented [14, 26, 27].

References

1. Flatt AE. Ulnar drift. J Hand Ther. 1996;9:282–92.
2. Smith EM, Juvinall RC, Bender LF, Pearson R. Flexor forces and rheumatoid metacarpophalangeal deformity. JAMA. 1966;198(2):150–4.
3. Backhouse KM. The mechanics of normal digital control in the hand an analysis of the ulnar drift of rheumatoid arthritis. Ann R Coll Surg Engl. 1968; 43:154–73.
4. Smith R, Kaplan EB. Rheumatoid deformities at the metacarpophalangeal joints of the fingers. J Bone Joint Surg. 1967;49(A):31–47.
5. Snorrason E. The problem of ulnar deviation of the fingers in rheumatoid arthritis. Acta Med Scand. 1951;140:359–63.
6. Ono S, Entezami P, Chung KC. Reconstruction of the rheumatoid hand. Clin Plast Surg. 2011;38:713–27.
7. Chung KC, Burns PB, Wilgis S, Burke FD, et al. A multicenter clinical trial in rheumatoid arthritis comparing silicone metacarpophalangeal joint arthroplasty with medical treatment. J Hand Surg. 2009;34(A):815–23.
8. Alderman AK, Arora AS, Kuhn L, et al. An analysis of women's and men's surgical priorities and willingness to have rheumatoid hand surgery. J Hand Surg Am. 2006;31:147–1453.
9. Anderson RJ. Controversy in the surgical treatment of the rheumatoid hand. Hand Clin. 2011;27:21–5.
10. Chung KC, Kowalski CP, Kim HM, et al. Patient outcomes following Swanson silastic metacarpophalangeal joint arthroplasty in the rheumatoid hand: a systematic overview. J Rheumatol. 2000;27(6):1395–402.
11. Goldfarb CA, Stern PJ. Metacarpophalangeal joint arthroplasty in rheumatoid arthritis. J Bone Joint Surg Am. 2003;85:1869–78.
12. Burke FD. The rheumatoid metacarpophalangeal joint. Hand Clin. 2011;27:79–86.
13. Chung KC. Operative techniques: hand and wrist surgery. 2nd ed. Philadelphia, PA: Saunders; 2012.
14. Chung KC, Burns PB, Kim MH, et al. Long-term followup for rheumatoid arthritis patients in a multicenter outcomes study of silicone metacarpophalangeal joint arthroplasty. Arthritis Care Res. 2012;64(9): 1292–300.
15. Neligan PC. Plastic surgery. 3rd ed. Philadelphia, PA: Saunders; 2012.
16. Landsmeer JMF. Anatomical and functional investigations on the articulation of the human fingers. Acta Anat. 1955;25(24):5–69.
17. Zancolli E. Structural and dynamic bases of hand surgery. Philadelphia, PA: JP Lippincott; 1968.
18. Tubiana R, Valentin P. The anatomy of the extensor apparatus of the fingers. Surg Clin North Am. 1964; 44:897–906.
19. Tubiana R, Valentin P. The physiology of the extension of the fingers. Surg Clin North Am. 1964;44: 906–18.
20. Straub LR. The etiology of finger deformities in the hand affected by rheumatoid arthritis. Bull Hosp J Dis. 1960;21:322–9.
21. Napier JR. The prehensile movements of the human hand. J Bone J Surg. 1956;38B:902.
22. McFarland G, Sherman MS. The synovial reactions of rheumatoid arthritis. Clin Orthop. 1964;36:10–21.
23. Kozlow JH, Chung KC. Current concept in the surgical management of rheumatoid and osteoarthritic hands and wrists. Hand Clin. 2011;27:31–41.
24. Shapiro JS, Heijna W, Nasatir S, Ray RD. The relationship of wrist motion to ulnar phalangeal drift in the rheumatoid patient. Hand. 1971;3:68–75.
25. Papp SR, Athwal GS, Pichora DR. The rheumatoid wrist. J Am Acad Orthop Surg. 2006;14:65–77.
26. Chung KC, Kotsis SV, Kim HM, et al. Reasons why rheumatoid arthritis patients week surgical treatment for hand deformities. J Hand Surg Am. 2006;31: 289–94.
27. Chung KC, Kotsis SV, Kim HM. A prospective outcomes study of Swanson metacarpophalangeal joint arthroplasty for the rheumatoid hand. J Hand Surg. 2004;29(A):646–53.
28. Alderman AK, Chung KC, Kim HM, et al. Effectiveness of rheumatoid hand surgery: contrasting perceptions of hand surgeons and rheumatologists. J Hand Surg Am. 2006;28:3–11.
29. Alderman AK, Ubel PA, Kim HM, et al. Surgical management of the rheumatoid hand: consensus and controversy among rheumatologists and hand surgeons. J Rheumatol. 2003;30:1464–72.
30. Ghattas L, Mascella F, Pomponio G. Hand surgery in rheumatoid arthritis: state of the art and suggestions for research. Rheumatology. 2005;44:834–45.
31. Oster LH, Blair WF, Steyers CM, et al. Crossed intrinsic transfer. J Hand Surg Am. 1989;14:963–71.

32. Clark DI, Delaney R, Stilwell JH, et al. The value of crossed intrinsic transfer after metacarpophalangeal silastic arthroplasty: a comparative study. J Hand Surg [Br]. 2001;26:565–7.
33. Pereira JA, Belcher JH. A comparison of metacarpophalangeal joint silastic arthroplasty with or without crossed intrinsic transfer. J Hand Surg [Br]. 2001; 26:229–34.
34. Chung KC, Burke FD, Wilgis EFS, Regan M, et al. A prospective study comparing outcomes after reconstruction in rheumatoid arthritis patients with severe ulnar drift deformities. Plast Reconstr Surg. 2009;123: 1769–77.
35. Sollerman CJ, Geijer M. Polyurethane versus silicone for endoprosthetic replacement of the metacarpophalangeal joints in rheumatoid arthritis. Scand J Plast Reconstr Surg Hand Surg. 1996;30: 145–50.
36. Rothwell AG, Cragg KJ, O'Neill LB. Hand function following silastic arthroplasty of the metacarpophalangeal joints in the rheumatoid hand. J Hand Surg. 1997;22(B):90–3.
37. Blair WF, Shurr DG, Buckwalter JA. Metacarpophalangeal joint implant arthroplasty with silastic spacer. J Bone J Surg Am. 1984;66: 365–70.
38. Swanson AB. Flexible implant arthroplasty for arthritic finger joints: rationale, technique, and results of treatment. J Bone J Surg Am. 1972;54(3): 435–55.

The Rheumatoid Thumb

21

Michel E.H. Boeckstyns

Introduction

Rheumatoid arthritis tends to cause complex deformities in the thumb in contrast to osteoarthritis in which isolated destruction of the carpometacarpal joint of the thumb is more common. Nalebuff described three patterns of deformity but the original classification has since been extended to include six patterns, based on which joints are affected and in which direction instability develops (Table 21.1, Figs. 21.1, 21.2, 21.3, 21.4, 21.5, and 21.6) [1].

In addition, rupture of the tendons may occur, caused by tenosynovitis, attrition, or rarely corticosteroid injections. In the early phase of the disease, before the thumb is destabilized or when the deformities are still passively correctable, nonoperative treatment is indicated. Medical treatment should attempt to reduce synovial activity and hence decrease swelling of the joints and stretching of the capsule and ligaments. Besides the administration of antirheumatic drugs, intra-articular injections of corticosteroids are often effective. The use of a splint may be helpful to reduce pain, for example, in case of correctable boutonniere deformity [2]. Any treatment program must include joint protection measures with instruction to the patients and with the aid of devices when performing activities of daily living.

Surgical treatment must be considered if synovitis or pain cannot be controlled by nonoperative treatment or if there is significant functional impairment. Synovectomy may be performed when joints are chronically swollen and radiographic evaluation indicates well-maintained cartilage. In case of joint destruction, reconstructive procedures are indicated. The Nalebuff classification is helpful in understanding the surgical strategy for thumb reconstruction.

In type I boutonniere deformity, the key is to correct the flexion deformity of the metacarpophalangeal joint (MCP joint). If the deformity is passively correctable and the joint is well preserved, rerouting of the extensor pollicis longus (EPL) tendon is an option but if the deformity is fixed or the joint is destroyed, MCP fusion is recommendable. Arthroplasty is not used at the MCP joint because stability rather than motion is the goal to regain more confidence with grip and pinch. If hyperextension of the interphalangeal (IP) joint does not correct spontaneously when correction of the MCP joint is performed, transection of the EPL at the IP level may solve the problem, at least temporarily (Dolphin procedure). The preserved intrinsic muscles of the

M.E.H. Boeckstyns, MD (✉)
Clinic for Hand Surgery, Gentofte Hospital, University of Copenhagen, Niels Andersens Vej 65, 2900 Hellerup, Denmark
e-mail: mibo@dadlnet.dk

K.C. Chung (ed.), *Clinical Management of the Rheumatoid Hand, Wrist, and Elbow*,
DOI 10.1007/978-3-319-26660-2_21

Table 21.1 The extended Nalebuff classification

Type	CMC1 joint	MCP joint	IP joint
I (Boutonniere I)	Not involved	Flexed	Hyperextended
II (Boutonniere II)	Subluxed, flexed, and adducted	Flexed	Hyperextended
III (Swan neck)	Subluxed, flexed, and adducted	Hyperextended (palmar plate unstable)	Flexed
IV (Gamekeeper)	Flexed and adducted	Radially deviated (UCL unstable)	Not involved
V (Swan neck)	Usually not involved	Hyperextended (palmar plate unstable)	Not involved
VI (Mutilans)	Bony loss at any level		

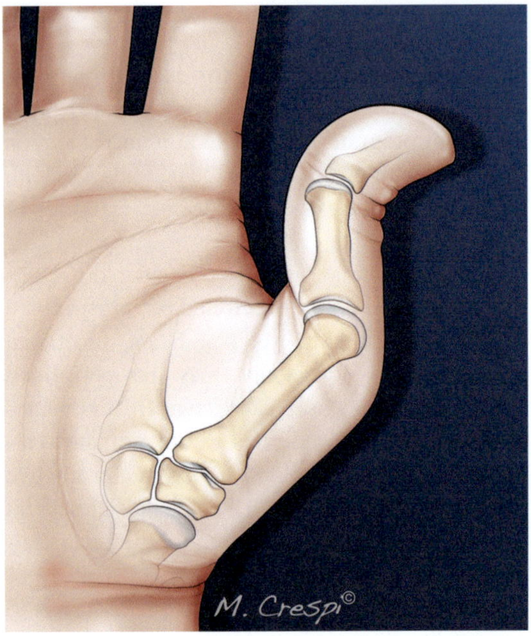

Fig. 21.1 Type I boutonniere deformity begins with synovitis at the MCP joint, which weakens the joint capsule and ligaments, stretches the extensor pollicis brevis (EPB), and causes the extensor pollicis longus (EPL) to sublux ulnarly. The IP joint becomes secondarily hyperextended as extensor power is concentrated distally. When pinch is attempted, the thumb collapses with hyperextension at the IP joint and abnormal flexion at the MP joint. The MCP and IP deformities are passively correctable in Type I and the CMC1 joint is not involved. When the IP joint is destroyed, radially deviation of the distal phalanx may occur

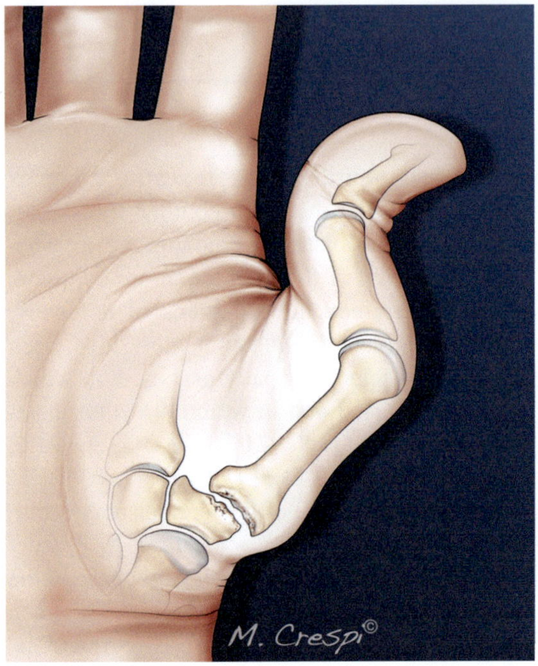

Fig. 21.2 In type II boutonniere deformity, the CMC1 joint is involved as well

thumb will then act to actively extend the distal joint. In case of flexor pollicis longus (FPL) tendon rupture, tendon repair is necessary. In case of IP joint destruction, fusion of this joint is performed.

In type II boutonniere, addressing the CMC joint is necessary in addition to the procedures described for Type I. Trapeziectomy with or without additional stabilizing procedures remains the method of choice, although joint replacement with silicone spacers or other implants have been used.

Type III—swan-neck deformity—usually requires correction of the CMC as well as the MCP joint in order to restore a proper balance in the thumb. The standard procedure to stabilize the MCP joint is fusion, but palmar capsulodesis or seamoidesis can be alternative procedures.

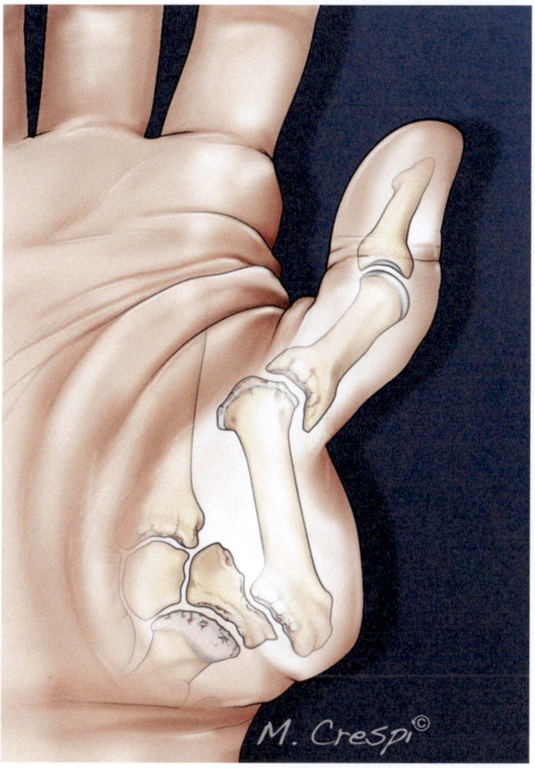

Fig. 21.3 Type III describes a swan-neck deformity beginning at the CMC1 joint [19]. Synovitis causes dorsal and radial subluxation, which adducts the distal end of the metacarpal. To compensate for the narrowing of the first web space, the thumb hyperextends at the MCP joint and the volar plate weakens. The resulting flexor-extensor imbalance causes the IP joint to go into flexion

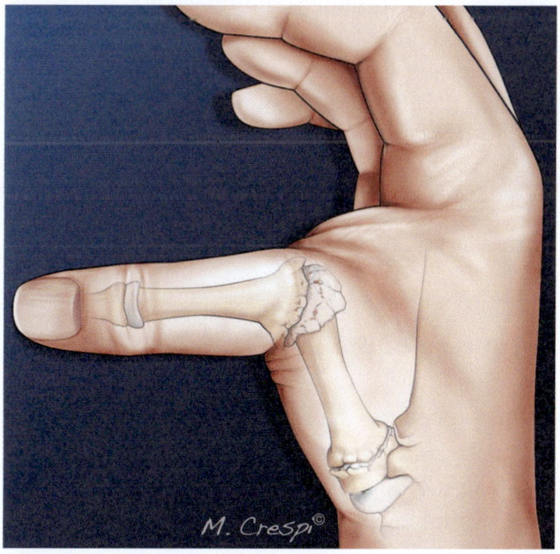

Fig. 21.4 In the relatively rare Type IV deformity, the ulnar collateral ligament of the MCP joint is ruptured, due to attrition

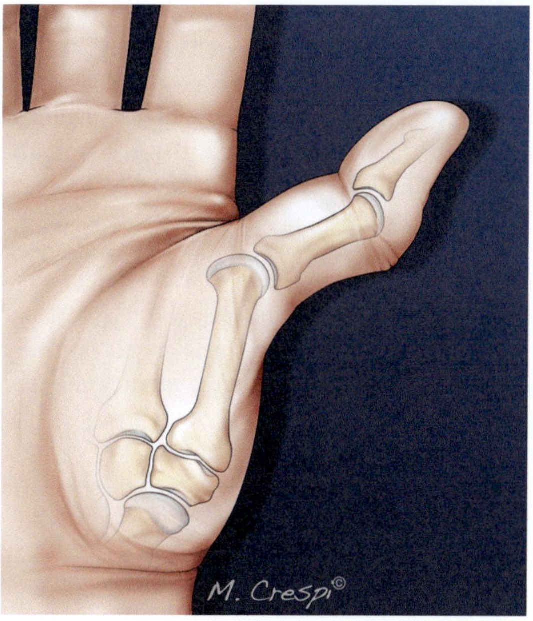

Fig. 21.5 Type V is a swan-neck deformity that has its origin in the MCP joint, in principle without CMC1 joint involvement

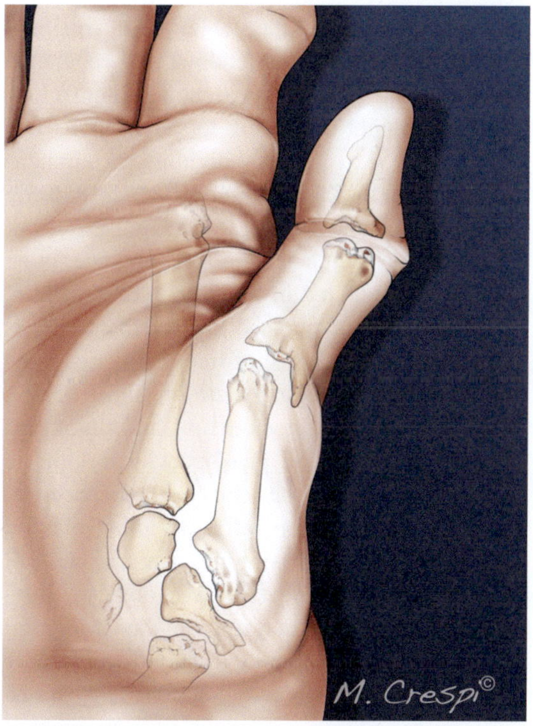

Fig. 21.6 Type VI results from aggressive and mutilating bone resorption, resulting in telescoped shortened digits and loss of the articulations

The uncommon type IV obviously requires ulnar stabilization of the MCP joint to restore pinch function. Again, fusing of the MCP achieves stability, but reconstruction of the ulnar collateral ligament is possible if the joint cartilage is well preserved. Treating the CMC joint is often necessary.

In the relatively rare type V—swan neck without CMC joint involvement—stabilizing the MCP joint is needed as described in Type III.

In case of arthritis mutilans (type VI), only fusion of the joints can arrest progression and restore stability.

Surgical Procedures

Fusion of the Thumb MCP Joint

MCP joint replacement has been used with success for the fingers [3–5], but MCP joint fusion for the thumb remains one of the winners in surgery of the rheumatoid hand and is the most reliable method to reconstruct stability and treat deformity in this joint. Fusion will also shorten the thumb a little, which will contribute to relaxing the extensor tendons and rebalance the thumb. The joint is approached through a longitudinal straight or curved dorsal incision. The joint capsule is exposed by dividing the aponeurosis between the EPL and the EPB. The capsule is opened and the collateral ligaments excised. Remaining cartilage is removed and the bone surfaces are prepared in a cup-and-cone fashion, which offers a larger contact surface than flat surfaces and offers a degree of freedom in positioning of the fusion. Usually, no or slight flexion (maximum 10°), slight abduction, and slight pronation of the proximal phalanx will provide an adequate position but this can be adapted according to the actual thumb deformity: more flexion may relieve the CMC joint in pinch grip but will reduce the ability to grasp large objects, especially if an adduction deformity in the CMC joint cannot be corrected. Stable fixation is preferable in order to allow early mobilization. This can be achieved by adding a cerclage wire to crossed K-wires, by a traditional tension band fixation, or by using plates or screws. The author's preferred method is fixation with a rotation controlling dorsal plate (Fig. 21.7). It acts as a tension band, as it applies tension to the dorsal cortex and compression to the fusion surfaces when activating the relatively stronger flexor forces. Unless the bone is very fragile, splinting is not necessary and early unloaded mobilization can be started. Regardless of the method of fixation, it is important that the IP joint is kept mobile to avoid adhesion of the EPL tendon to the fusion site. Fusion is reliable and can be expected to be solid after 6–8 weeks. Loaded usage of the thumb can be started at this time [6].

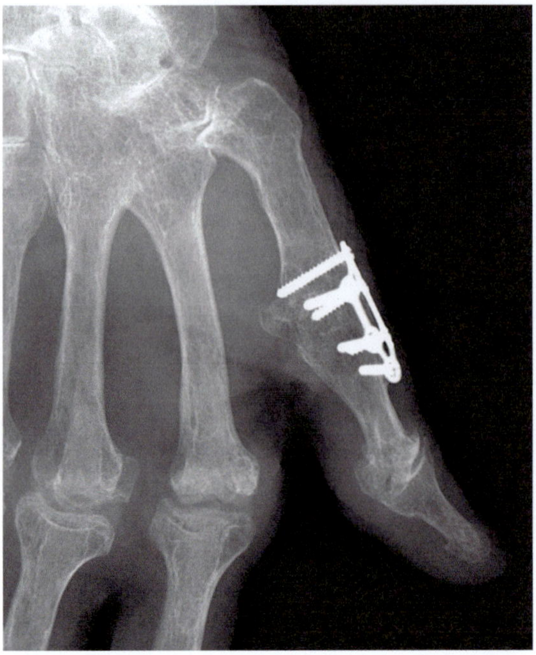

Fig. 21.7 Fusion of the MCP joint, fixated with a rotational stabilizing dorsal plate, allowing immediate mobilization

Rerouting of the EPL Tendon

In this procedure, the EPL is rerouted through the dorsal capsule or attached to the proximal phalanx to provide additional extensor force at this level. Simultaneously, the extensor force at the IP level is weakened but active extension of the IP joint will still be possible through the action of

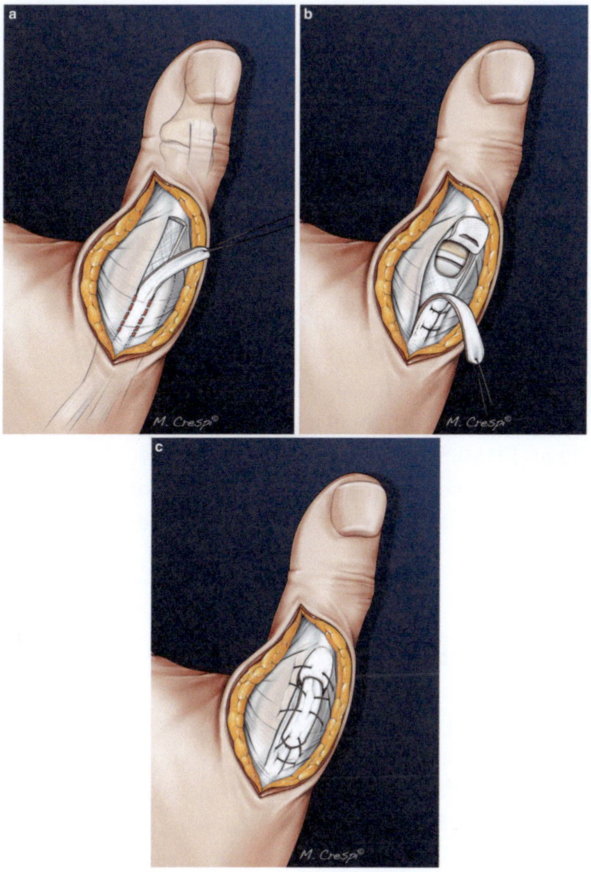

Fig. 21.8 (a–c) Rerouting of the EPL tendon for the correction of a supple boutonniere deformity

the intrinsic muscles. A curved longitudinal incision is made over the dorsal MP joint and proximal phalanx. The EPL tendon is freed from the EPB tendon; it is divided near to its distal insertion and detached from the extensor hood (Fig. 21.8). The joint capsule is opened through two small transverse incisions and synovectomy performed. The EPL tendon is then passed through the incisions and sutured back to itself with the MCP joint in extension. Alternatively, the tendon may be fixated to the proximal phalanx by means of an anchor. The EPB and EPL tendons are sutured together. The joint is transfixed with a K-wire and the thumb is protected by a splint. After 4 weeks, the K-wire is removed and unloaded mobilization is initiated. Between exercise sessions the thumb is protected by a splint during the first 2–4 weeks. Recurrence rate of the deformity is rather high, as much as 64 % at 6 years [3].

MCP Joint Sesamoidesis/ Capsulodesis

The radial sesamoid is exposed through a palmar Bruner-type incision. The radial digital nerve and artery are protected. Cartilage is removed from the sesamoid and corresponding area of the metacarpal head. The sesamoid is attached to the metacarpal head with a K-wire with the MCP joint in slight flexion. A supplementary protective K-wire may be passed through the MCP joint. The thumb is protected by a splint during 6 weeks.

An alternative procedure for hyperextension instability is to simply divide and reattach the palmar capsule on the metacarpal head [7].

Reconstruction of the Ulnar Collateral Ligament of the MCP Joint

In the relatively rare Nalebuff type IV, reconstruction of the ulnar collateral ligament can be considered. The author's preferred method is to use a tendon graft through bony tunnels, mimicking the normal triangular anatomy of the ligament. Fixation with an interference screw allows early mobilization [8]. Still, fusion will often be the most reliable procedure in the rheumatoid patient.

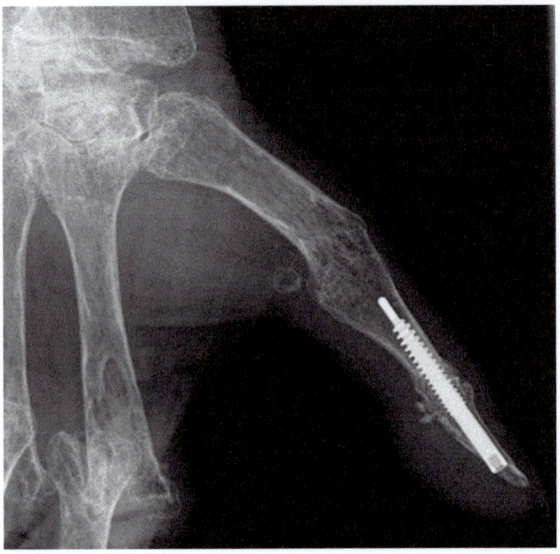

Fig. 21.9 Fusion of the IP joint, fixated with an Acutrak fusion screw

Fusion of the IP Joint

The IP joint is approached through a dorsal transverse incision that is angulated proximally and distally in each end (double Y-incision). The extensor apparatus is transected and the joint opened. The surfaces of the joint are fashioned in a similar way as described for MCP joint fusion. Fixation is secured by a screw inserted through a small incision at the tip of the finger, just beneath the edge of the nail (Fig. 21.9). The joint is positioned in neutral extension or slight flexion. This usually provides enough stability to permit immediate, careful mobilization of the thumb. K-wire fixation may be used as an alternative, and if supplemented with a cerclage wire, it will also permit early mobilization. Bone grafting is usually not necessary. Fusion of the IP joint may be done even when the MCP joint is fused but will result in a rigid thumb so for this reason, the indication must be very strict.

Procedures on the CMC Joint

In previous decades, replacement of the trapezium with silicone spacers was popular. The advantages of this procedure are claimed to be the restoration of the length of the thumb ray and a much shorter recovery time, compared to resection/suspension/interposition arthroplasty. Despite a relatively high complication rate, many papers report favorable clinical results and a high patient satisfaction [9, 10]. Although there is a general agreement on a rather high rate of subluxation or even dislocation, the importance of silicone synovitis is much more debatable [11], and the silicone implants are rarely if ever used today [12]. In more recent decades, an increasing number of implants have been designed for replacement of the CMC joint of the thumb. Total joint replacement does not reliably give better results than trapeziectomy and some have very high rates of failure [13, 14].

Fusion of the CMC joint of the thumb may be indicated in young patients with isolated degenerative osteoarthritis [15] but is usually not a good option in patients with rheumatoid arthritis, in whom the bone stock is of lesser quality and in whom soft-tissue procedures generally give good results.

Various types of resection and suspension/interposition arthroplasties have been described. Although well established, none have reliably been shown to give a better outcome than trapeziectomy [13, 16–18]. Trapeziectomy is performed through a radial-dorsal incision. The author's preferred incision extends from the radial styloid to the proximal part of the first metacarpal. The branches of the superficial radial nerve are identified and carefully protected. The first compartment may be released after subcutaneous exposure. The dissection continues between the tendon of the extensor pollicis brevis and the abductor pollicis longus. The radial artery is exposed and its branches off the dorsal joint capsule are electrocoagulated and divided. The capsule is incised in a U-shape, with the base at the attachment on the metacarpal and the proximal incision at the scapho-trapezial joint. This U-shaped flap is freed from the trapezium and lifted up. The remaining capsule is dissected off the trapezium and the bone itself removed in pieces with a rongeur. While an assistant is holding the metacarpal abducted, the dorsal capsule flap is interposed in the cavity between the metacarpal and the scaphoid, and the capsule is closed, taking care of the radial artery. Finally the wound is closed and dressings and a thumb spica cast are applied that allows full motion of the IP joint. The cast is removed after 3 weeks and unresisted exercises initiated. At 6 weeks the patient is encouraged to use the thumb for activities of daily living. Slips of the tendons of the abductor pollicis longus, flexor carpi radialis, and extensor carpi radialis longus all can be used, if a tendinous interposition or a ligament reconstruction between the first and second metacarpals is preferred.

Tendon Reconstruction

Flexor pollicis longus tendon ruptures are usually secondary to attrition around the scaphoid bone in the carpal tunnel and are referred to as a Mannerfelt lesion. Its presence may aggravate a boutonniere deformity and repair of a ruptured FPL tendon is necessary to obtain a well-balanced thumb. Likewise, a MCP joint fusion may be required to achieve a functional FPL repair. Direct suture is rarely possible, even when the patient presents with an acute rupture. Transfer of the flexor digitorum superficialis of the ring finger is the most used procedure. An interpositional tendon graft can be an alternative. In any case, it is important to debride any bony prominences that could cause re-rupture of the repaired tendon.

Rupture of the extensor pollicis longus most often occurs by attrition at Lister tubercle. To avoid this complication, the tendon is, whenever possible, placed superficially to the extensor retinaculum after surgery in the rheumatoid wrist. Usually, direct suture is not an option due to loss of tendon substance. The most commonly used repair involves transferring the extensor indicis proprius tendon to the ruptured EPL. The procedure and rehabilitation are rewarding. Alternatively, the extensor carpi radialis longus tendon can be used. In case of a severely destroyed IP joint, fusion of this joint can be an alternative to tendon repair.

References

1. Terrono AL. The rheumatoid thumb. J Am Soc Surg Hand. 2001;1(2):81–92.
2. Silva PG, Lombardi Jr I, Breitschwerdt C, Poli Araujo PM, Natour J. Functional thumb orthosis for type I and II boutonniere deformity on the dominant hand in patients with rheumatoid arthritis: a randomized controlled study. Clin Rehabil. 2008;22(8):684–9. PubMed.
3. Terrono A, Millender L, Nalebuff E. Boutonniere rheumatoid thumb deformity. J Hand Surg. 1990; 15(6):999–1003. PubMed.
4. Figgie MP, Inglis AE, Sobel M, Bohn WW, Fisher DA. Metacarpal-phalangeal joint arthroplasty of the rheumatoid thumb. J Hand Surg. 1990;15(2):210–6. PubMed.
5. Dyer GS, Simmons BP. Rheumatoid thumb. Hand Clin. 2011;27(1):73–7. PubMed.
6. Rasmussen C, Roos S, Boeckstyns M. Low-profile plate fixation in arthrodesis of the first metacarpophalangeal joint. J Hand Surg Eur Vol. 2011;36(6):509–13. PubMed.
7. Miller NJ, Davis TR. Palmar plate capsulodesis for thumb metacarpophalangeal joint hyperextension in association with trapeziometacarpal osteoarthritis. J Hand Surg Eur Vol. 2014;39(3):272–5. PubMed.
8. Gvozdenovic R, Boeckstyns M. Collateral ligament reconstruction of the chronic thumb injury with bio-tenodesis screw fixation. Tech Hand Up Extrem Surg. 2014;18(4):160–4. PubMed.
9. Bezwada HP, Sauer ST, Hankins ST, Webber JB. Long-term results of trapeziometacarpal silicone arthroplasty. J Hand Surg. 2002;27(3):409–17. PubMed.

10. Creighton Jr JJ, Steichen JB, Strickland JW. Long-term evaluation of silastic trapezial arthroplasty in patients with osteoarthritis. J Hand Surg. 1991; 16(3):510–9. PubMed.
11. Lluch A. Is there a role for silicone trapezial replacement in the rheumatoid hand? In: Hayton M, editor. Trail I surgery of the rheumatoid hand and wrist. Amsterdam: Elsevier; 2006. p. 169–77.
12. Chacko AT, Rozental TD. The rheumatoid thumb. Hand Clin. 2008;24(3):307–14, vii. PubMed.
13. Vermeulen GM, Slijper H, Feitz R, Hovius SE, Moojen TM, Selles RW. Surgical management of primary thumb carpometacarpal osteoarthritis: a systematic review. J Hand Surg. 2011;36(1):157–69. PubMed.
14. Giddins G. Thumb arthroplasties. J Hand Surg Eur Vol. 2012;37(7):603–4. PubMed.
15. Fulton DB, Stern PJ. Trapeziometacarpal arthrodesis in primary osteoarthritis: a minimum two-year follow-up study. J Hand Surg. 2001;26(1):109–14. PubMed.
16. Salem H, Davis TR. Six year outcome excision of the trapezium for trapeziometacarpal joint osteoarthritis: is it improved by ligament reconstruction and temporary Kirschner wire insertion? J Hand Surg Eur Vol. 2012;37(3):211–9. PubMed.
17. Li YK, White C, Ignacy TA, Thoma A. Comparison of trapeziectomy and trapeziectomy with ligament reconstruction and tendon interposition: a systematic literature review. Plast Reconstr Surg. 2011;128(1): 199–207. PubMed.
18. Gangopadhyay S, McKenna H, Burke FD, Davis TR. Five- to 18-year follow-up for treatment of trapeziometacarpal osteoarthritis: a prospective comparison of excision, tendon interposition, and ligament reconstruction and tendon interposition. J Hand Surg. 2012;37(3):411–7. PubMed.
19. Belt E, Kaarela K, Lehtinen J, Kautiainen H, Kauppi M, Lehto MU. When does subluxation of the first carpometacarpal joint cause swan-neck deformity of the thumb in rheumatoid arthritis: a 20-year follow-up study. Clin Rheumatol. 1998;17(2):135–8. PubMed.

Case-Based Examples of Management of the Rheumatoid Hand

22

Kevin C. Chung and Alexandra L. Mathews

Introduction

The techniques for performing rheumatoid hand surgery are not particularly complex; however, what to do and when to do them can be challenging. The treating surgeon must determine the most predictable procedure that will yield the best outcomes for patients, understand the patient's needs and expectations, and organize the sequential approach of a number of surgical options by considering the effects that each joint in the wrist and hand have on each other.

The most predictable outcomes for patients are to achieve pain relief and stability of critical joints. Therefore, thumb MCP fusion and wrist fusion procedures are outstanding options for RA patients. Synovitis of the thumb MCP joint causes a weak pinch because the thumb subluxes when the patient attempts to pinch. After thumb MCP fusion, the patient typically has more assurance when gripping as the thumb becomes much more stable. Wrist fusion is a time-honored procedure for the RA hand. Volar subluxation and deviation of the carpus alter the biomechanics of the hand and contribute to deformities of the hand joints owing to the link effect of multiple joints in the hand. For example, collapse of the radial wrist causes radial deviation of the metacarpals and fosters ulnar subluxation of the fingers. Therefore, a stable and aligned wrist through wrist fusion establishes the foundation for the hand, which improves outcomes for future reconstructive procedures. Although wrist arthroplasty is an enticing choice for wrist reconstruction, predictably failure will occur, either fracture around the stem or dislocation. Therefore, patient expectations must be tempered with the elegant wrist arthroplasty procedure. I will perform wrist arthroplasty for patients who have good bone stock, similar to those with osteoarthritis, and can accept the sequela of future implant failure and the need for additional revision wrist surgery.

The distal radioulnar joint is often the first place for discomfort in RA patients. Synovitis in the DRUJ disrupts the ligamentous support of the DRUJ by weakening the TFCC, collateral ligaments, and the ECU subsheath. All of these primary and secondary stabilizers of the wrist are stretched, which cause the misnomer of "dorsal subluxation" of the ulna. In reality, the ulna serves as the central axis of the forearm by articulating with the humerus. The ulna is stable and

K.C. Chung, MD, MS (✉)
Comprehensive Hand Center, Section of Plastic Surgery, Department of Surgery, The University of Michigan Health System, 2130 Taubman Center, SPC 5340, 1500 E. Medical Center Drive, Ann Arbor, MI 48109-5340, USA
e-mail: kecchung@med.umich.edu

A.L. Mathews, BS
Section of Plastic Surgery, Department of Surgery, The University of Michigan Health System, Ann Arbor, MI, USA

K.C. Chung (ed.), *Clinical Management of the Rheumatoid Hand, Wrist, and Elbow*,
DOI 10.1007/978-3-319-26660-2_22

does not sublux, but rather it is the radius that descents to give the relative change in the DRUJ relationship. Although ligament stabilization of the DRUJ is certainly a worthwhile goal in early deformity, most patients presenting with pain at the DRUJ already had arthritic change in the sigmoid notch, which causes intractable pain with forearm pronation and supination. The choices of treatment are rather straightforward. If the radiocarpal joint is already auto-fused or the lunate sits squarely within the lunate fossa, then distal ulna excision will predictably improve pain and restore rotation. On the other hand, if the carpal is deviating off the radius as shown by the lunate migrating off the lunate fossa on the radius, then distal radioulna joint fusion with osteotomy of the ulna proximal to the sigmoid notch provides a platform for the carpus.

As the wrist sets the platform for the hand, the MCP joints of the fingers establish the fulcrum for the fingers. The MCP joints of the fingers require motion and stability. Unfortunately, our current implant designs and surgical procedures cannot achieve these two goals. Silicone implants are rather simplistic designs that provide stability in the constraint joint design at the expense of motion, whereas the non-constraint two-piece implants theoretically give better motion but are prone to instability that leads to rather early recurrent ulnar subluxation of the fingers. For the finger MCP joints, our outcome studies using silicone implants over the past decades have shown remarkably good outcomes in improving function and aesthetic appearance, which patients value. I do not perform two-piece implants for the MCP joints because recurrent deformity is too common.

The fingers are often the anatomic region for reconstruction. I do not perform simultaneous finger MCP joint reconstruction and finger boutonniere/swan neck deformity correction. Finger MCP joint reconstruction requires fastidious postoperative therapy, and the effect of the reconstructed MCP joints on the distal joints are often uncertain. For example, one of the etiologies of finger swan neck deformities is MCP joint subluxation. By correcting the finger MCP joint, it is quite possible that the swan neck deformity may be remedied.

For the RA fingers, the DIP deformity and pain are treated with joint fusion with *K*-wires. The distal joints in the fingers require stability, similar to the MCP joint of the thumb. Therefore, the main quandary is the PIP joint. My concept for the RA PIP joint is whether the joints are flexible or fixed. If the joint is fixed because of articular destruction, then the option is either fusion or arthroplasty. Again, my choice for the PIP arthroplasty is silicone implant. However, if the joint is fixed because of ligament tightness, then the ligaments can be released to achieve a flexible joint that can be reconstructed with soft tissue alignment procedures.

There is a distinct difference in patients' hand function between boutonniere and swan neck deformity. Patients with swan neck deformity cannot flex the PIP joint to curl their fingers around an object. Therefore, their need is mainly flexion that can be achieved with joint ligament releases. However, those with boutonniere deformities have mainly an aesthetic problem because of the flexed PIP joint. If the these joints are treated and render the hand in an extended posture, particularly for the ulnar fingers, the patient may complain of functional problems because now they cannot grip their golf club or grocery bag, even though the fingers may look better. Therefore, I am much more aggressive in treating swan neck deformity than boutonniere. And I spend quite a bit of time gauging the patient's expectations and needs, as well as patient education, to be sure the patient's goals align with the expected outcomes.

The following are illustrative cases to reinforce the concepts articulated above. The key to a successful RA hand surgical treatment is to listen, to think, and to understand the expected outcomes. It is not what one can do, but what one should do and not do to achieve the best outcome for the patient.

Case 1

A 61-year-old female with a 25-year history of rheumatoid arthritis who presented with intractable pain over her right wrist. She wore a splint at all times to stabilize her wrist. The wrist was quite

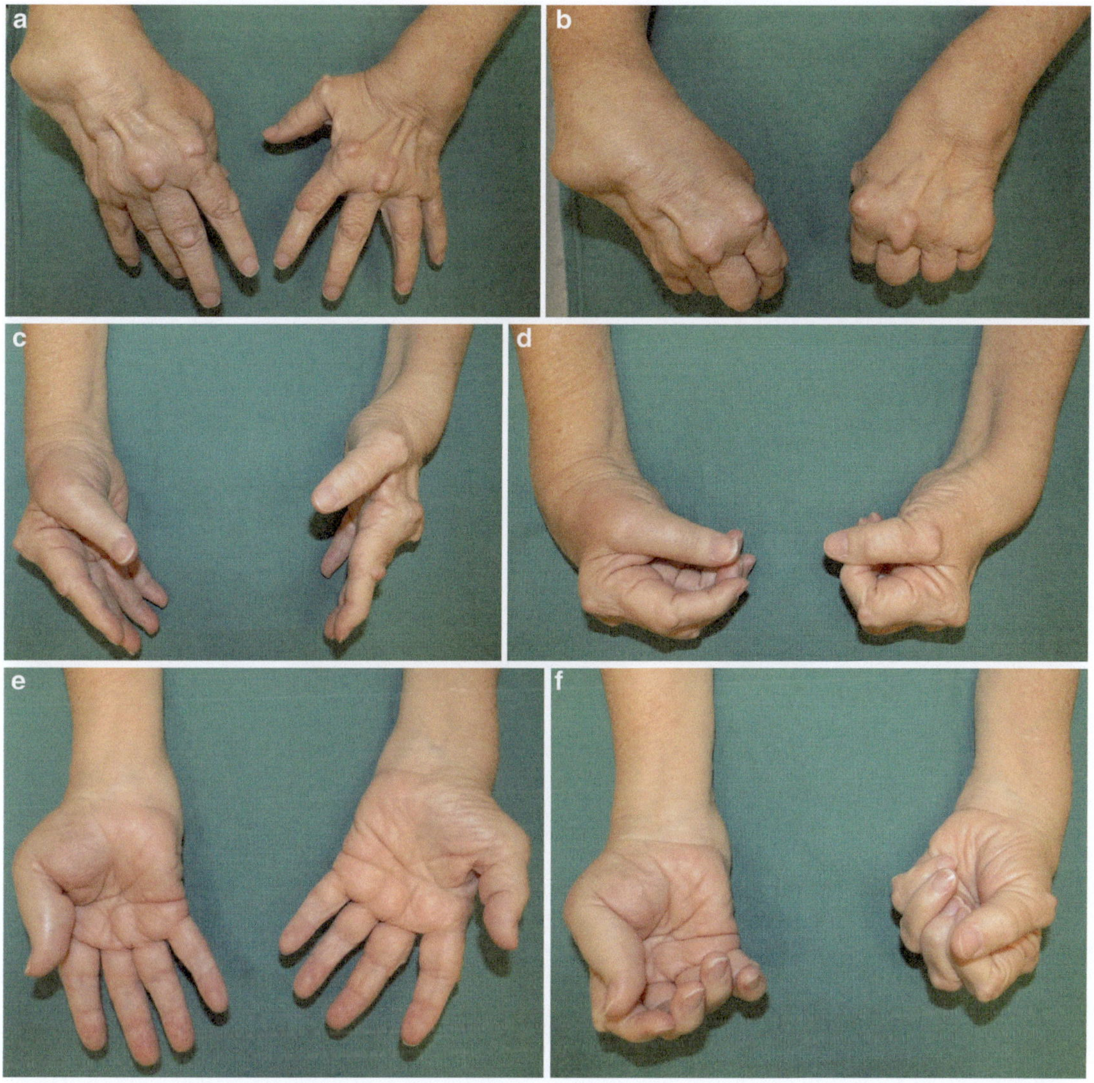

Fig. 22.1 Case #1—Preoperative images of a 61-year-old female with a 25-year history of RA

painful during movement and had no stability. Additional complaints included multiple rheumatoid nodules over the hand and the proximal forearm. Furthermore, she complained of an inability to fully extend the thumb that happened a few years ago when suddenly she lost thumb extension. Physical examination of the right wrist indicated subluxation of the hand and a prominent distal ulna. She also demonstrated loss of thumb extension. Preoperative images are presented in Fig. 22.1.

Discussion

1. Which anatomical parts are responsible for the pain?

Initial X-rays were presented (Fig. 22.2). These X-rays revealed severe erosion and loss of carpal bones in both wrists. There was no stability to the wrist and her pain was caused by subluxation of the wrist and bone-to-bone contact between the distal radius

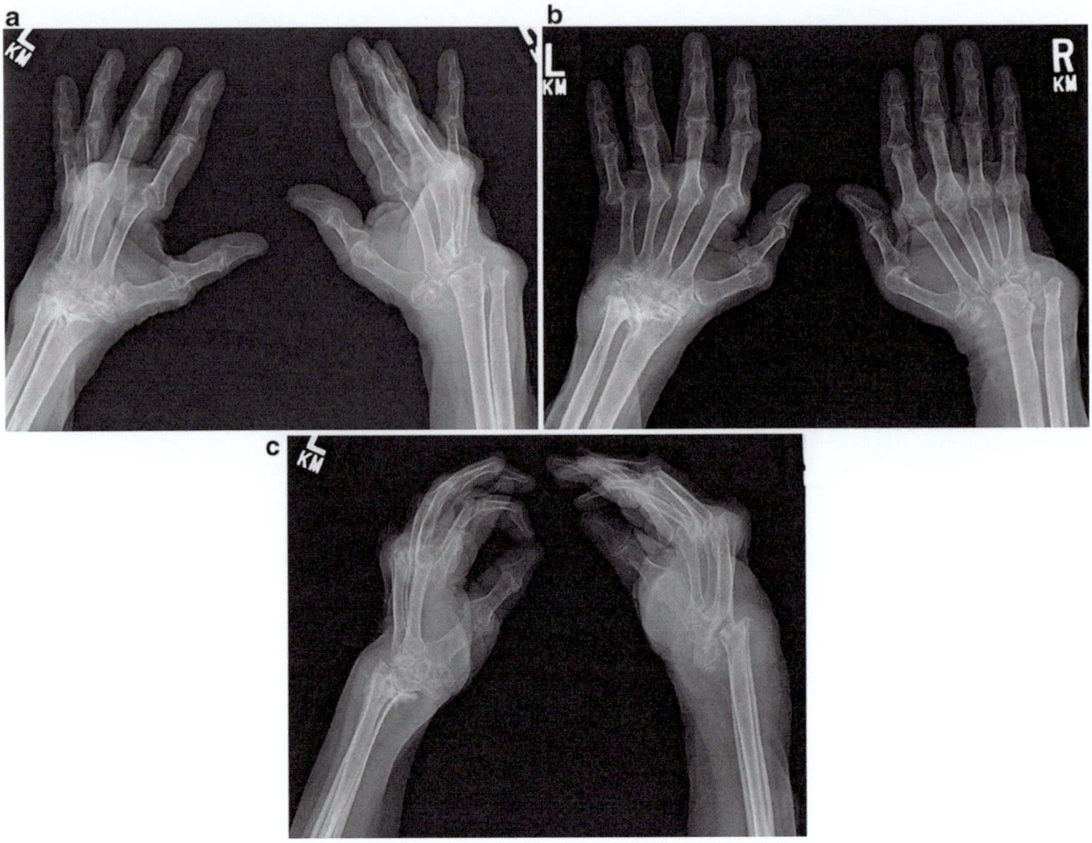

Fig. 22.2 Case #1—Initial X-rays showing severe erosion and loss of the carpal bones in both wrists

and the carpal bones and metacarpal. Furthermore, the X-rays showed classic volar subluxation of the carpus, and erosion of the carpal bones, in particular her dominant right wrist.

2. Is surgery indicated?

   The patient's wrist was unstable and her fingers did not move well. She explained that she would ultimately like to be able to hold something in her right hand independently and oppose her right thumb to her fingers to obtain some degree of function. Our recommended plan to the patient included a right total wrist fusion using a locking 2.4 mm plate. A distal ulna excision would also be performed, and the distal ulna bone would be used for bone grafting material in the wrist fusion. Tenosynovectomy of the right dorsal wrist and extensor tendons and tendon transfers as needed were indicated to restore extension of the digits and the thumb. Possible tendon transfers included FDS of the ring finger to EPL or using the expendable ECRL.

3. Procedure performed

   The ulna head was resected to prevent ulnar impaction of the carpus. We used a low-profile plate to fuse the wrist after decortication of the articular surface and used the ulna head for a bone graft interposing between the radius and carpal bones. The wrist was stabilized using this plate and extensive synovectomy was performed to clean out the entire wrist joint. The tendon transfer was then performed. Figure 22.3 is illustrative, showing the series of procedures. The wrist was short after fusion and all of the tendons were lengthened. We imbricated the tendons to shorten them so that the patient could have sufficient finger exten-

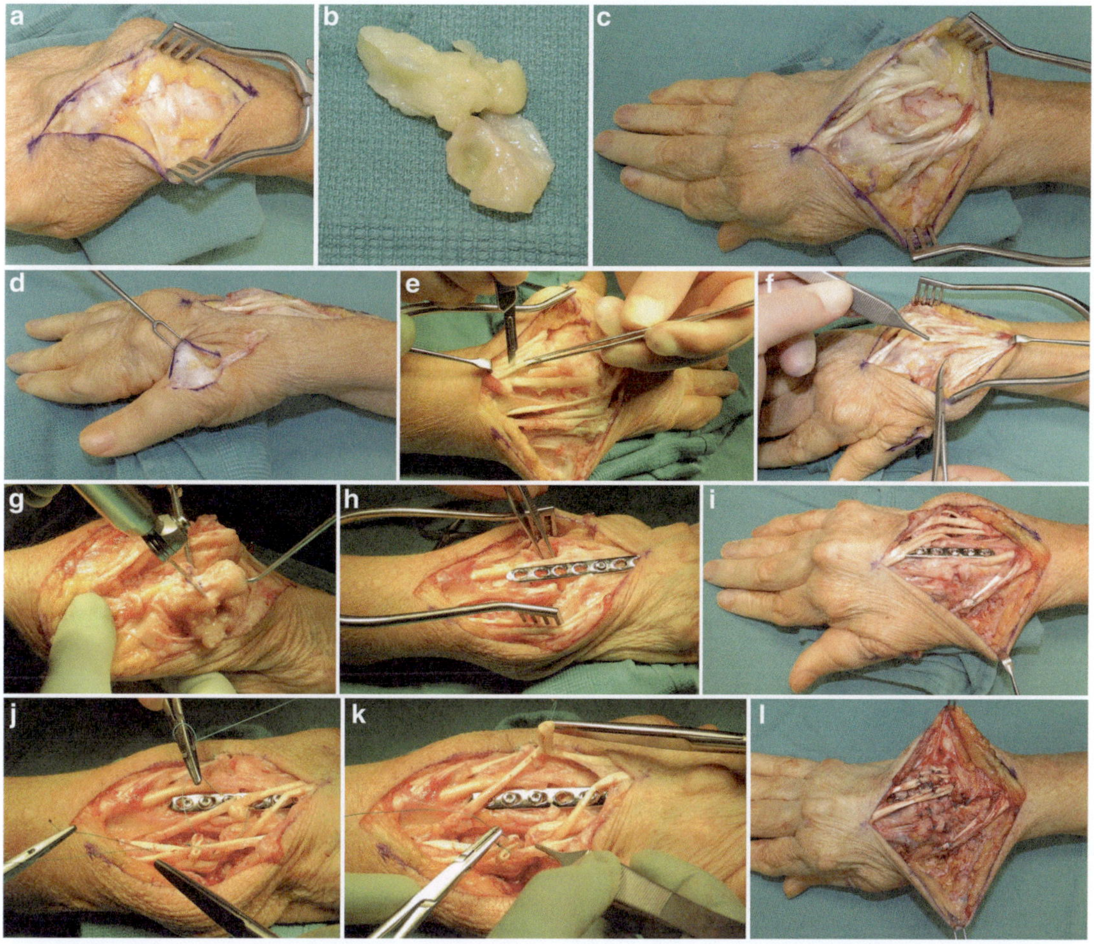

Fig. 22.3 Case #1—Series of procedures including right total wrist fusion using a 2.7 mm Synthes locking plate; extensive synovectomy of the second, third, fourth, fifth, and sixth compartments; shortening of the EDC tendon of the index, middle, ring, and little finger; right distal ulna excision using the ulna bone for bone grafting to the right wrist fusion site, and ECRL turnover tendon flap to EPL tendon for rupture of the EPL tendon

sion. The extensor retinaculum was then repaired by passing half of it under the extensor tendon to protect the extensor tendon from the underlying bone, and the proximal retinaculum was used to close over the extensor mechanism to present a pulley for the extensor tendons. The EPL tendon was reconstructed with an ECRL turnover tendon flap.

4. Postoperative care and outcomes

   Her wrist and fingers were splinted for 4 weeks to allow the tendon junctures to heal, and after 4 weeks, finger range-of-motion exercises were initiated. Several months follow-up showed that she had excellent extension of the fingers with stability of the wrist (Fig. 22.4). Comparing both sides, her finger posture improved greatly and she is functional.

Case 2

A 57-year-old female with a long history of rheumatoid arthritis and multiple hand operations to improve hand dysfunction. The patient had previous implant arthroplasty procedures for the MCP joints in her left hand and some joints in her right hand as well. She was concerned that her left hand was continuing to lose function, especially

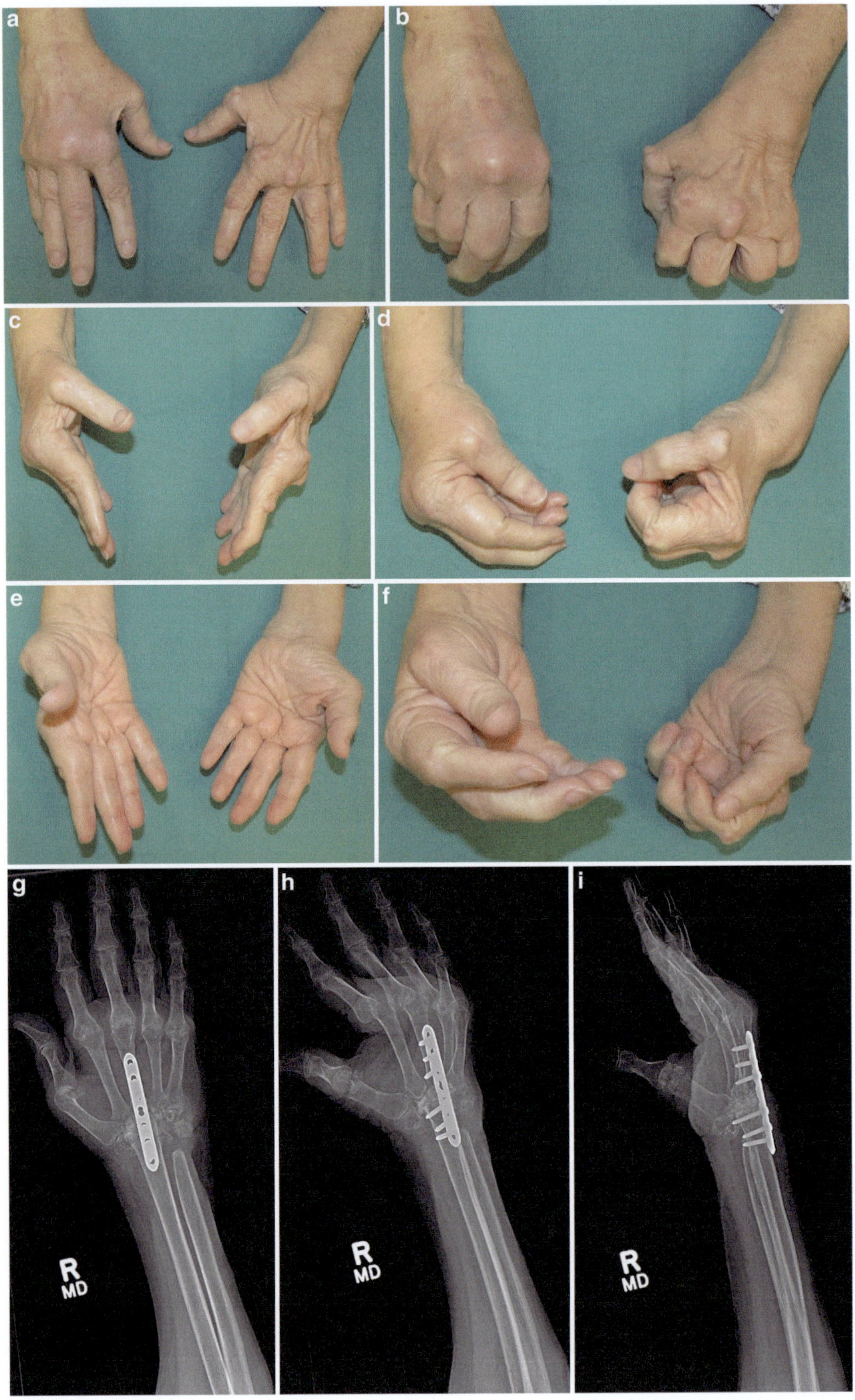

Fig. 22.4 Case #1—Six-month follow-up

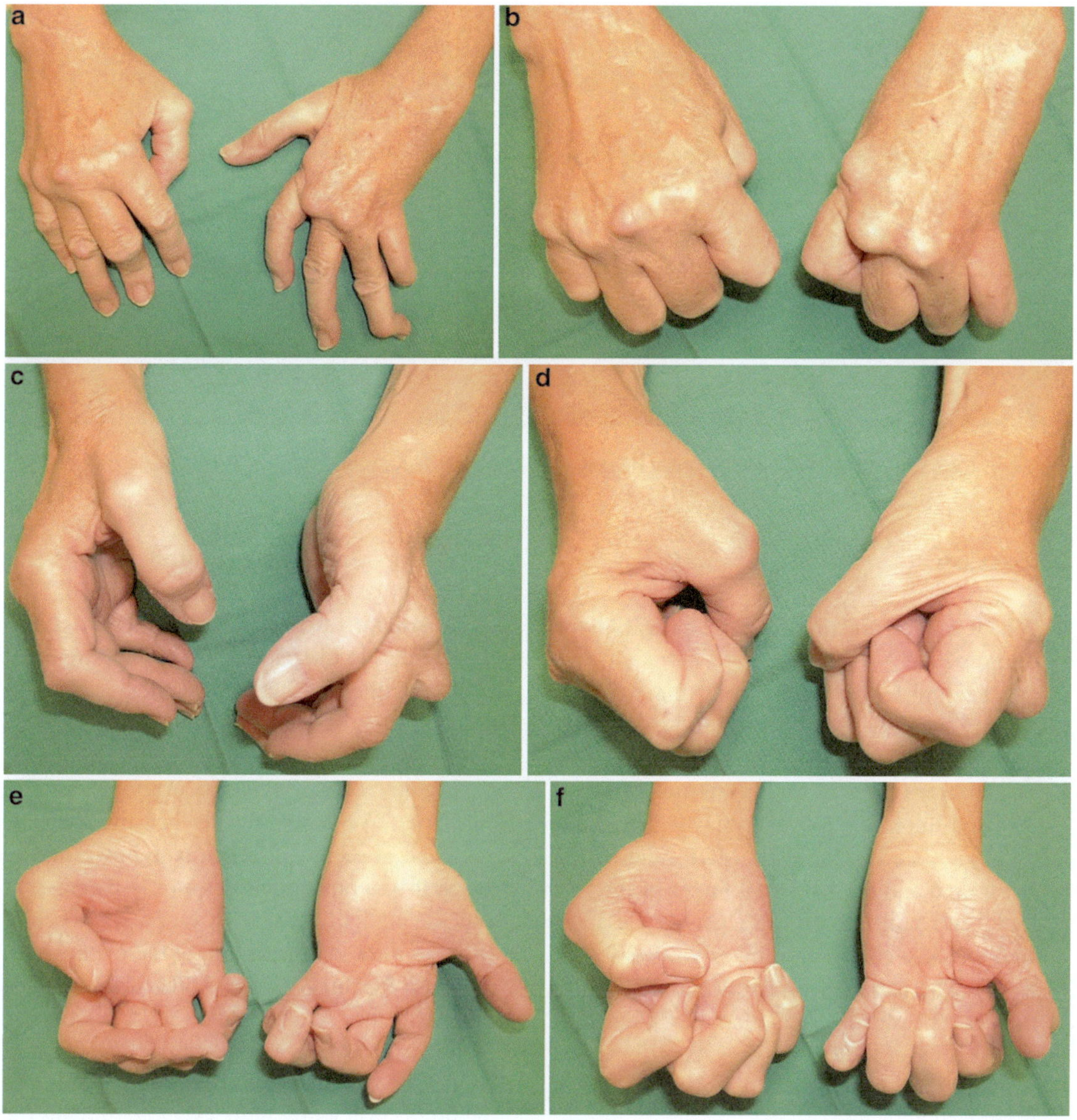

Fig. 22.5 Case #2—Preoperative images of a 57-year-old female with a long history of RA

with keyboarding which was important for her job. Additional complaints were that she could not put a glove on her hand or put her hand in her pocket and had difficulty with buttons and fastening jewelry. She felt it was becoming more and more of a problem. The patient previously consulted with a surgeon from another facility who recommended stabilizing the left wrist prior to addressing the hand. However, the patient explained that she would like to have her hand addressed first. Evaluation of the left hand indicated severe deformity of the fingers with ulnar deviation and subluxation in the MCP joints of the index, middle, ring, and small finger. She had mild wrist instability with synovitis associated with the ulnar head. The patient demonstrated normal function with the left hand as far as flexion and extension of the fingers. The right hand appeared to have difficulties with motion of the fingers, however, was much more functional than the left and had excellent wrist range of motion. Preoperative pictures are presented (Fig. 22.5).

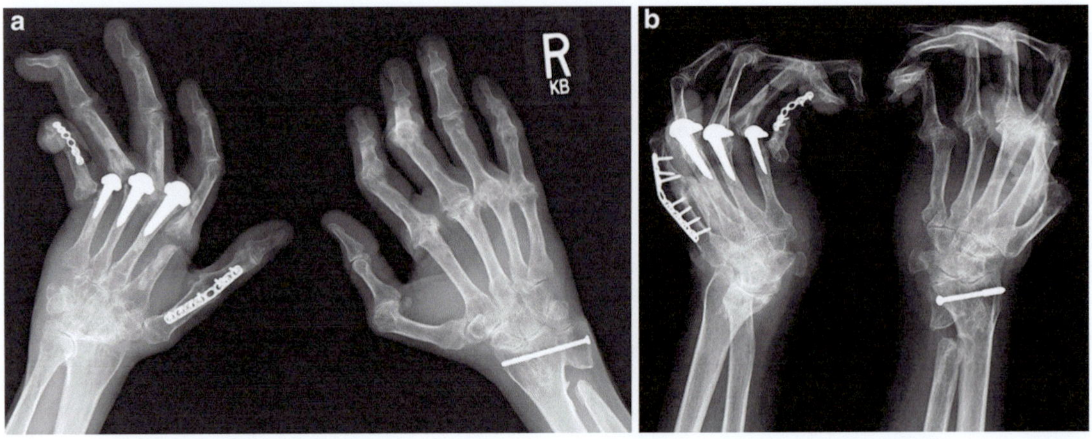

Fig. 22.6 Case #2—Preoperative radiographic images showing severe deformity of the fingers

Discussion

1. Which anatomical parts are responsible for the pain?

   Radiographic examination of the patient's bilateral hands showed dislocation and deviation of implants in the left middle, ring, and small fingers (Fig. 22.6). Furthermore, X-rays revealed implant removal from the left index finger, a plate fusion of the MCP joint of the left thumb and the left small finger of the PIP joint, and multiple arthritic changes associated with the carpus and finger joints on both hands. The patient's severe deformity of the fingers, specifically the ulnar deviation and subluxation of the MCP joints, contributed to her decreased hand function.
2. Is surgery indicated?

   MCP joint arthroplasty is the preferred option for patients demonstrating chronic subluxation of the MCP joints and ulnar deviation of the fingers. Arthrodesis of the MCP joint can be a viable option for treating deformities of the thumb; however, it is rarely performed in the fingers because range of motion is reduced significantly, and patient activity becomes limited [1]. Furthermore, soft tissue reconstruction alone was not indicated in this case owing to the severity of the patient's deformity. The patient was offered implant removal and replacement with silicone implants at the MCP joints of the middle, ring, and small fingers, as well as collateral ligament reconstruction for the left hand. This is a difficult operation with a high risk for failure due to the patient's previous surgeries and significant laxity of her collateral ligaments.
3. Procedure performed

   Figure 22.7a shows the original metallic implants. We attempted to bur the bone at the neck of the metallic implant; however, the cement was embedded within the metacarpal and the implant, making extraction impossible without removing a portion of the metacarpal. Because the fingers were short and dislocated, removing the metacarpals was a reasonable option as it would realign the fingers. The difficulty was that the medullary cavity could not be fitted sufficiently with a sizable implant for silicone arthroplasty; however, this was the only option to realign the fingers. Therefore, the metacarpals were sawed at the midportion of the implant, and the rest of the bone was then burred and the implant was extracted using a vise-grip. All three implants were extracted. The medullary cavity was then approached through the index finger. Although the implants did not fit precisely within the medullary cavity of the respective metacarpals, we were able to place #1 silicone implants into the index and middle fingers, a #3 implant into the ring finger, and a #2 implant into the little finger (Fig. 22.7b).

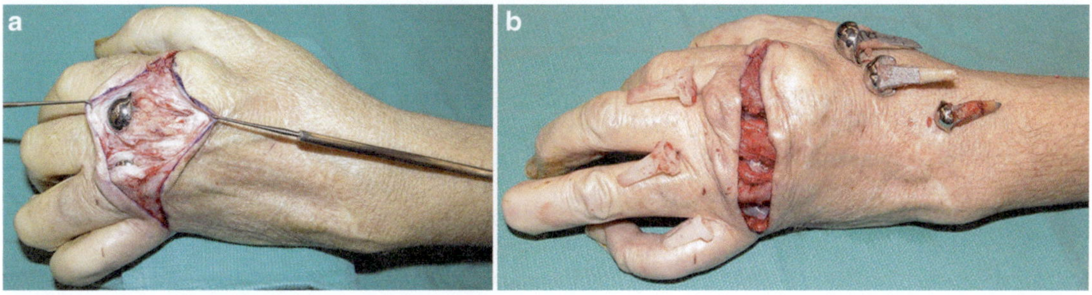

Fig. 22.7 Case #2—Procedures performed: excision of the metacarpal containing the cemented metal implants for the middle finger, ring finger, and little finger of the left hand; silicone arthroplasty of the left index finger, middle finger, ring finger, and little finger using #1 implants for the index and middle finger, #3 implant for the ring finger, and #2 implant for the little finger using silicone implants

4. Postoperative care and outcomes

   The patient's fingers were markedly improved in posture after the operation. She did not follow dynamic splinting protocol because of possible dislocation of the implant. Therefore, the fingers were splinted in a static splint for 4–5 weeks to allow for encapsulation of the implant. The encapsulation process maintained the posture of the implant. The patient was evaluated weekly by a hand therapist, and after 4 weeks of immobilization, she began gentle range-of-motion exercises. Several months after surgery, the patient was able to use her hand more effectively, although the finger posture was not particularly excellent (Fig. 22.8a–f). For the first time, she was able to make a fist because of the relocation of the fingers onto the metacarpals. X-rays revealed persistent subluxation of the small finger MCP joint, which was not a functional problem for her (Fig. 22.8g–i).

Case 3

A 59-year-old female with a known history of rheumatoid arthritis, longstanding. She was referred by her rheumatologist for right hand pain and worsening deformities. The patient complained of difficulty with grasping of the hand and doing things with her hand. Her main problem was not being able to fully extend the middle finger, which was also painful. Physical examination of the patient's right hand revealed ulnar deviation of the index, middle, ring, and small fingers at the MCP joint with subluxation of the joints. Her right thumb also had instability at the MCP joint. Flexion and extension of all the digits remained intact. The patient did have a prominent distal ulna and a tendency to rub over the ulna, but it was painless and she had full supination and pronation of the wrist. Preoperative images are demonstrated in Fig. 22.9.

Discussion

1. Which anatomical parts are responsible for the pain?

   Initial X-rays were presented (Fig. 22.10). These X-rays demonstrated arthritic changes of the wrist, consistent with rheumatoid arthritis and subluxation of the MCP joint, specifically at the index and middle finger. The subluxation at the MCP joint resulted in the patient's inability to fully extend the middle finger, which caused her pain. Arthritis was noted at the thumb as well. The patient's destruction and instability at the thumb greatly limited her hand function, specifically her ability to generate a tip-to-tip pinching motion between her index and middle fingers and the thumb.
2. Is surgery indicated?

   Right MCP joint fusion is indicated to allow the patient to achieve a stable, mobile

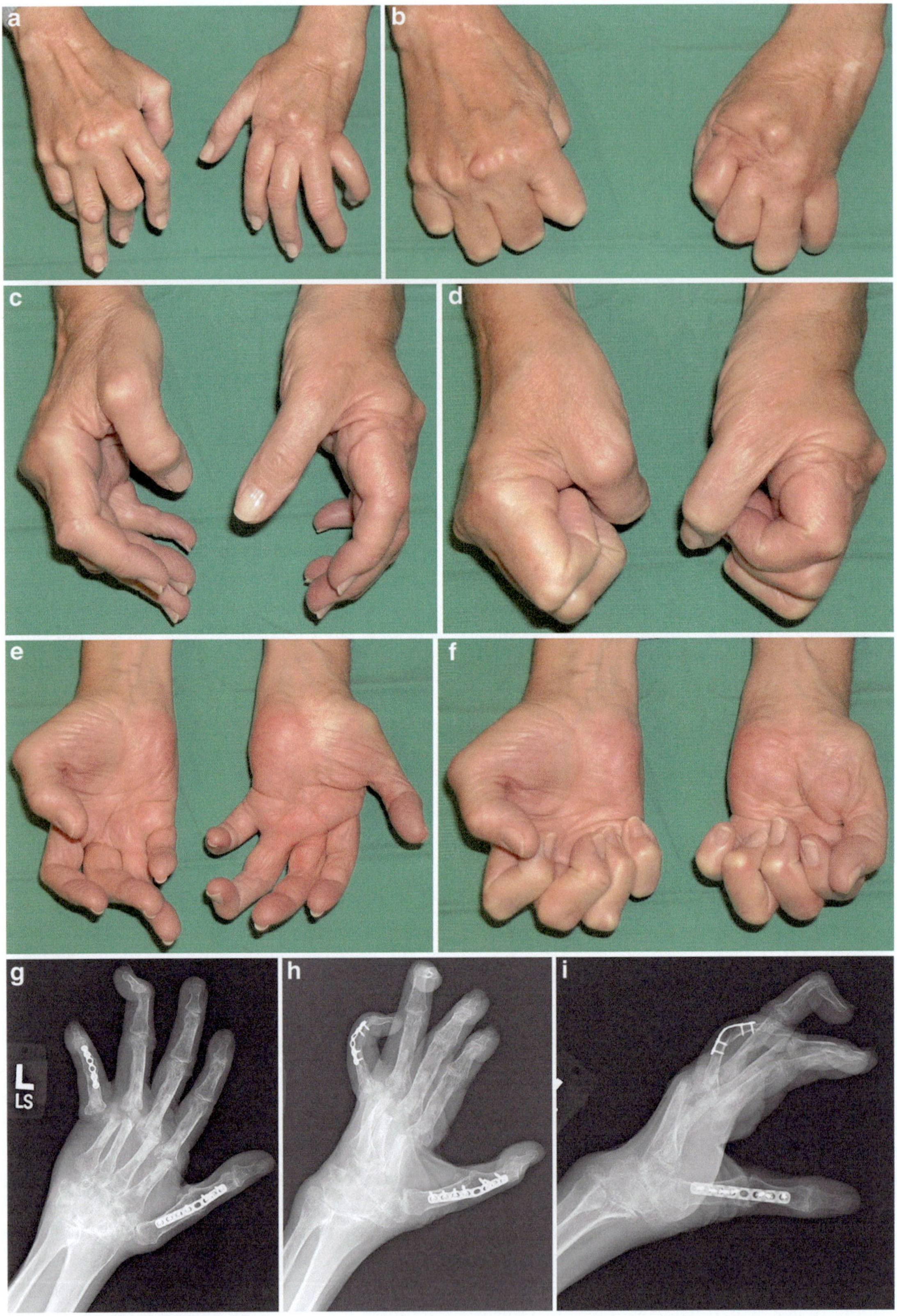

Fig. 22.8 Case #2—Four-month follow-up

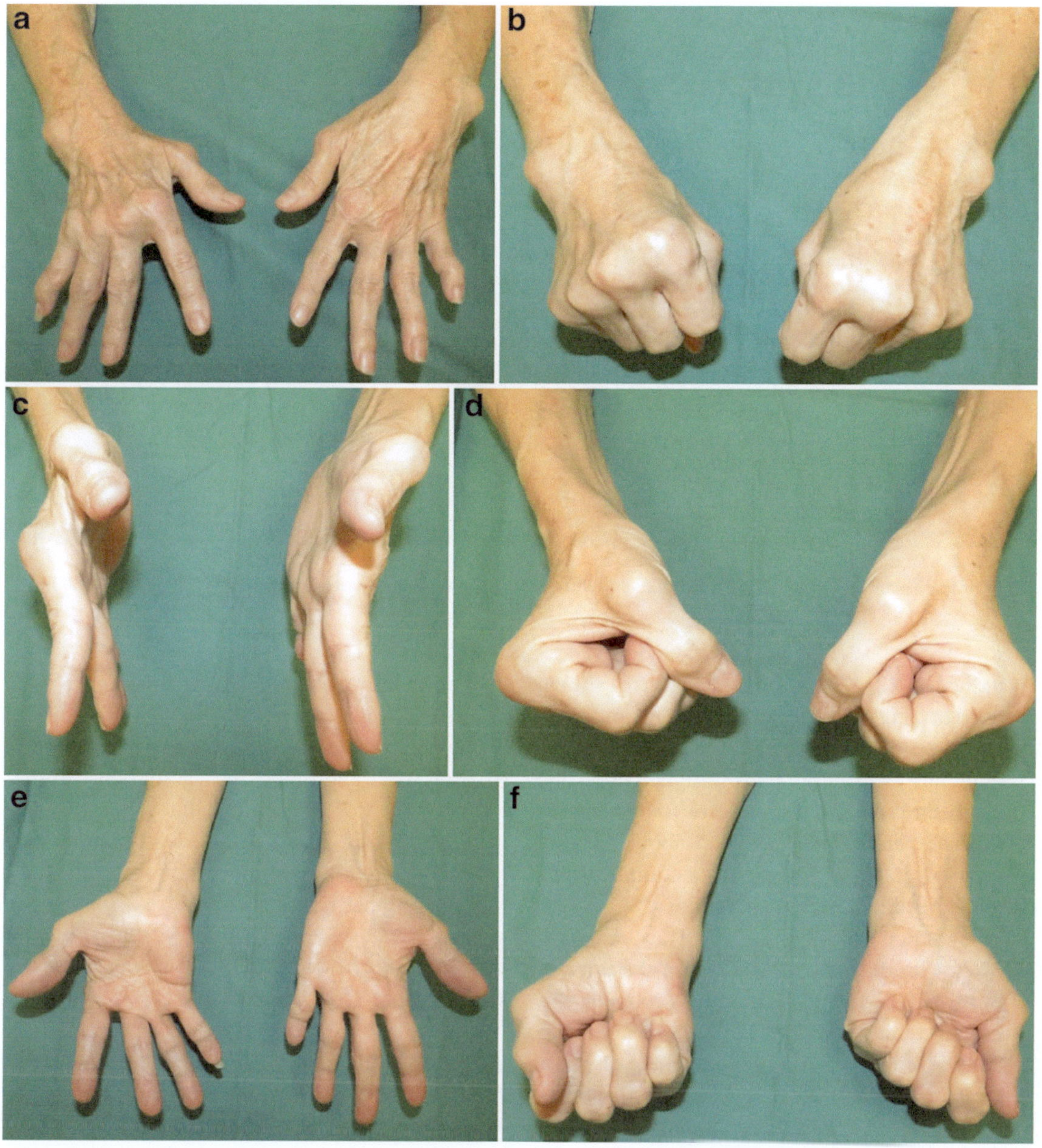

Fig. 22.9 Case #3—Preoperative images of a 59-year-old female with a known history of RA, longstanding

thumb, which will improve grip strength and posture. Furthermore, the patient requested realignment of the fingers, thus, right index, middle, ring, and small finger implant arthroplasty for the MCP joints were recommended. Ulnar drift of the fingers is normally caused by chronic synovitis, which disrupts the ligamentous support of the MCP joint. In early cases, ulnar deviation can be addressed with a cross intrinsic transfer in which the ulnar lateral bands are transferred to either the proximal phalanges or the extensor tendons [1]. For patients demonstrating articular surface damage of the MCP joint or severe volar subluxation, soft tissue reconstruction will not be effective, and MCP joint arthroplasty is

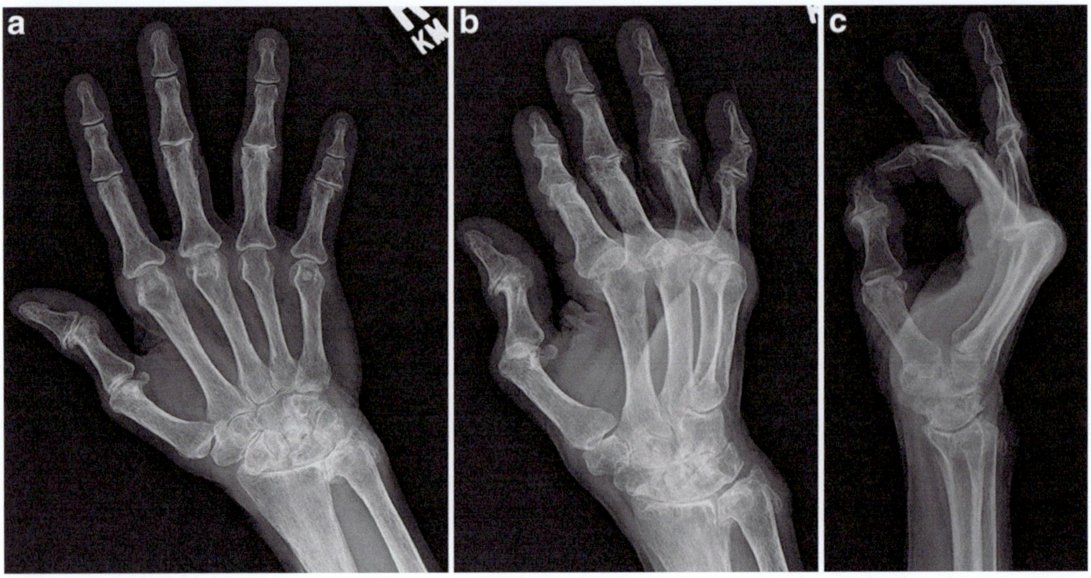

Fig. 22.10 Case #3—Initial X-rays showing subluxation of the index and middle finger MCP joints in the right hand

indicated [2]. Several studies have shown encouraging short-term functional and aesthetic outcomes associated with this procedure; however, a high rate of implant breakage has been reported at long-term follow-up [3–6]. The patient was informed about the surgery expectations and possible complications and agreed to have the procedure.

3. Procedure performed

   A 4 cm incision was made on the dorsum of the MCP joint of the thumb. A rongeur was used to remove the articular surface until cancellous bone was seen. The joint was then compressed, and cross *K*-wires were used to fixate the MCP joint with slight pronation of the tip. A transverse incision was then made over the head of the metacarpals. The radial sagittal bands were incised, and a radical synovectomy was performed. An oscillating saw was used to remove the head of the metacarpals. The medullary cavity was then broached. The #3 implants were placed in the index, middle, and ring fingers, and a #2 implant was placed in the little finger (Fig. 22.11).

4. Postoperative care and outcomes

   The patient was placed in a volar splint with the fingers in a fully extended position. The thumb was splinted for 6–8 weeks until the MCP joint was fused. Once the joint was fused, it was stable enough for strengthening exercises and pinching activities. Three-month follow-up pictures and X-rays are presented in Fig. 22.12. After several months the patient reported improved comfort and function with her right hand.

Case 4

A 63-year-old female with a known history of rheumatoid arthritis presented 6 years after her right hand silicone arthroplasty. The procedure offered excellent results; however, she started to have ulnar subluxation of the fingers which limited her function. She wanted revision of these joints. Preoperative images and X-rays are shown in Fig. 22.13.

Discussion

1. Is surgery indicated?

   Silicone arthroplasty has become the mainstay of MCP joint treatment in rheumatoid

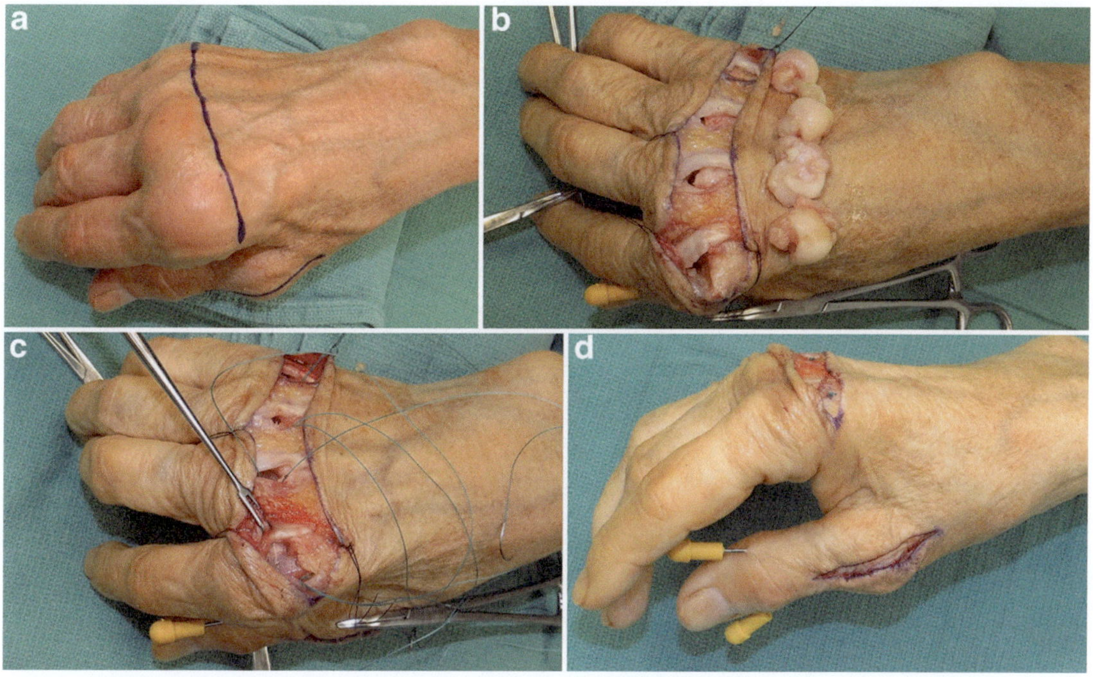

Fig. 22.11 Case #3—Procedures performed: right silicone arthroplasty of the MCP joints of the index, middle, ring, and little fingers and extensor tendons realignment; right thumb MCP joint fusion

patients; however, complications such as implant fracture have been commonly reported [6]. In most cases, implant replacement is not necessary because scar tissue forms around the implants, creating sufficient enough support to maintain hand function [1]. In this case, the patient lost significant hand function owing to the ulnar subluxation of her fingers and requested that the joints be replaced.

2. Procedure performed

   Intraoperative findings indicated that all of the implants were fractured at the stem (Fig. 22.14a). All stems were removed and new implants were then placed; the extensor tendons were all centralized (Fig. 22.14b). The patient's finger posture was much better after the revision arthroplasty.

3. Postoperative care and outcomes

   The patient was placed in a volar splint after the operation and initiated dynamic exercises during the recovery period. Two month follow-up images are demonstrated in Fig. 22.15a–f. Postoperative X-rays show the implant arthroplasty with good position of the implant (Fig. 22.15g–i).

Case 5

A 41-year-old female recently diagnosed with rheumatoid arthritis and was referred for an evaluation of bilateral hand extensor tenosynovitis. The patient complained of bilateral pain with edema on the dorsal aspect of her wrist and hand. The pain had been going on for approximately 8 months but had not been causing the patient significant disability. She was taking a number of rheumatoid medications including Enbrel, methotrexate, and Plaquenil which controlled her rheumatoid arthritis fairly well. The patient denied any weakness, tingling, or numbness in her hands. Focused examination of the patient's left upper extremity revealed an approximately 4 cm × 2 cm cystic mass on the dorsal aspect of her wrist and hand. This mass was soft and mobile and non-tender to palpation. There was no erythema or warmth about the mass, and it felt cystic in nature. Focused examination of the patient's right upper extremity revealed similar findings to her left hand, including an approximately 4 × 3 cystic mass that was without erythema or warmth (Fig. 22.16).

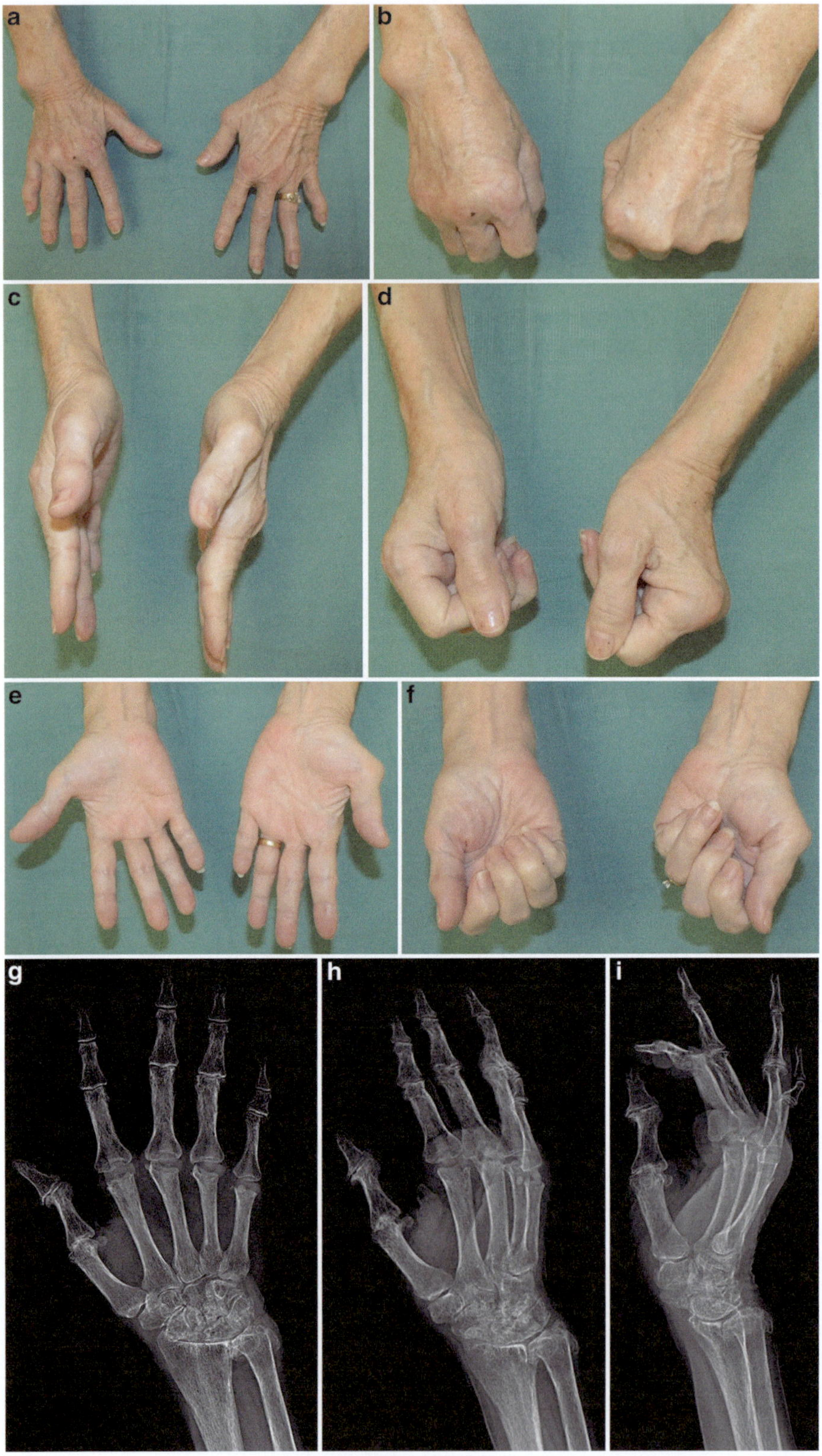

Fig. 22.12 Case #3—Three-month follow-up

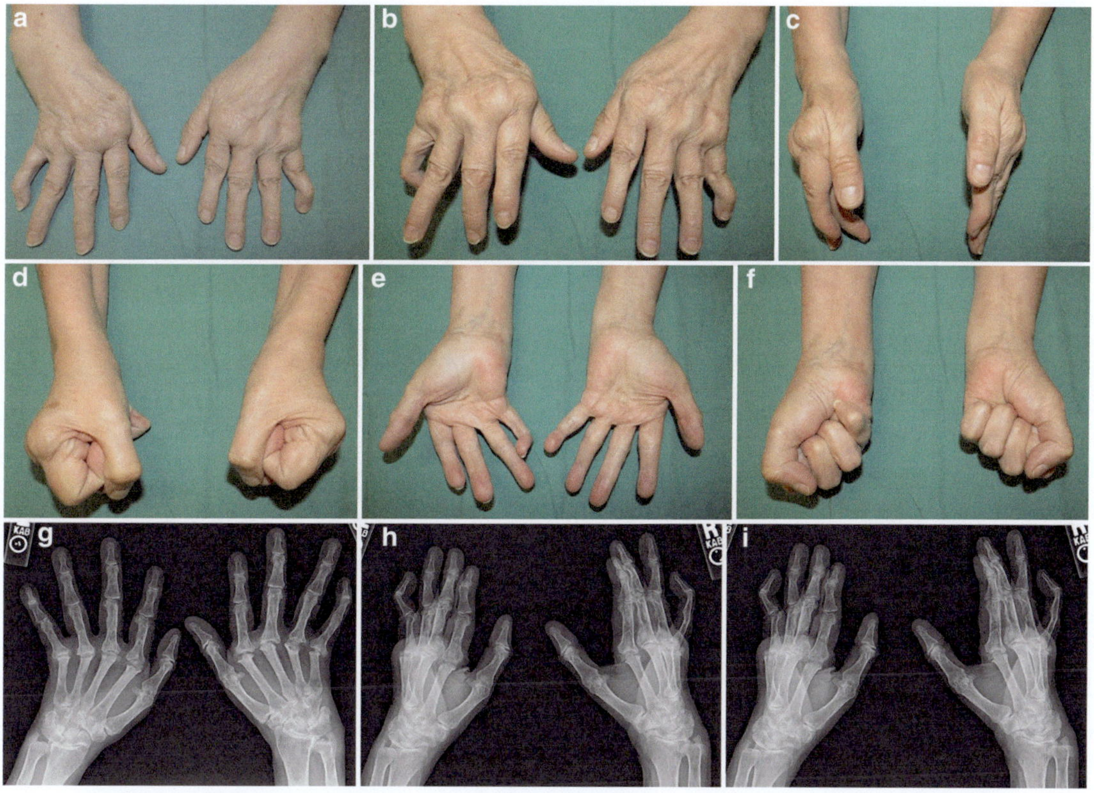

Fig. 22.13 Case #4—Preoperative images and X-rays of a 63-year-old female with a known history of RA and previous silicone arthroplasty

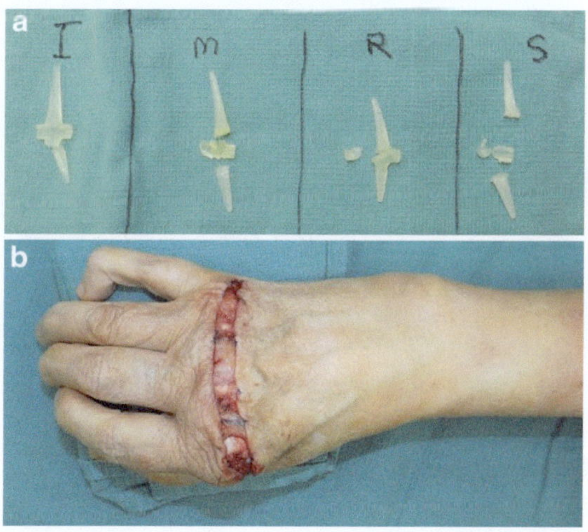

Fig. 22.14 Case #4—Procedure performed: right revision silicone metacarpophalangeal joint arthroplasty for the index, middle, ring, and little fingers

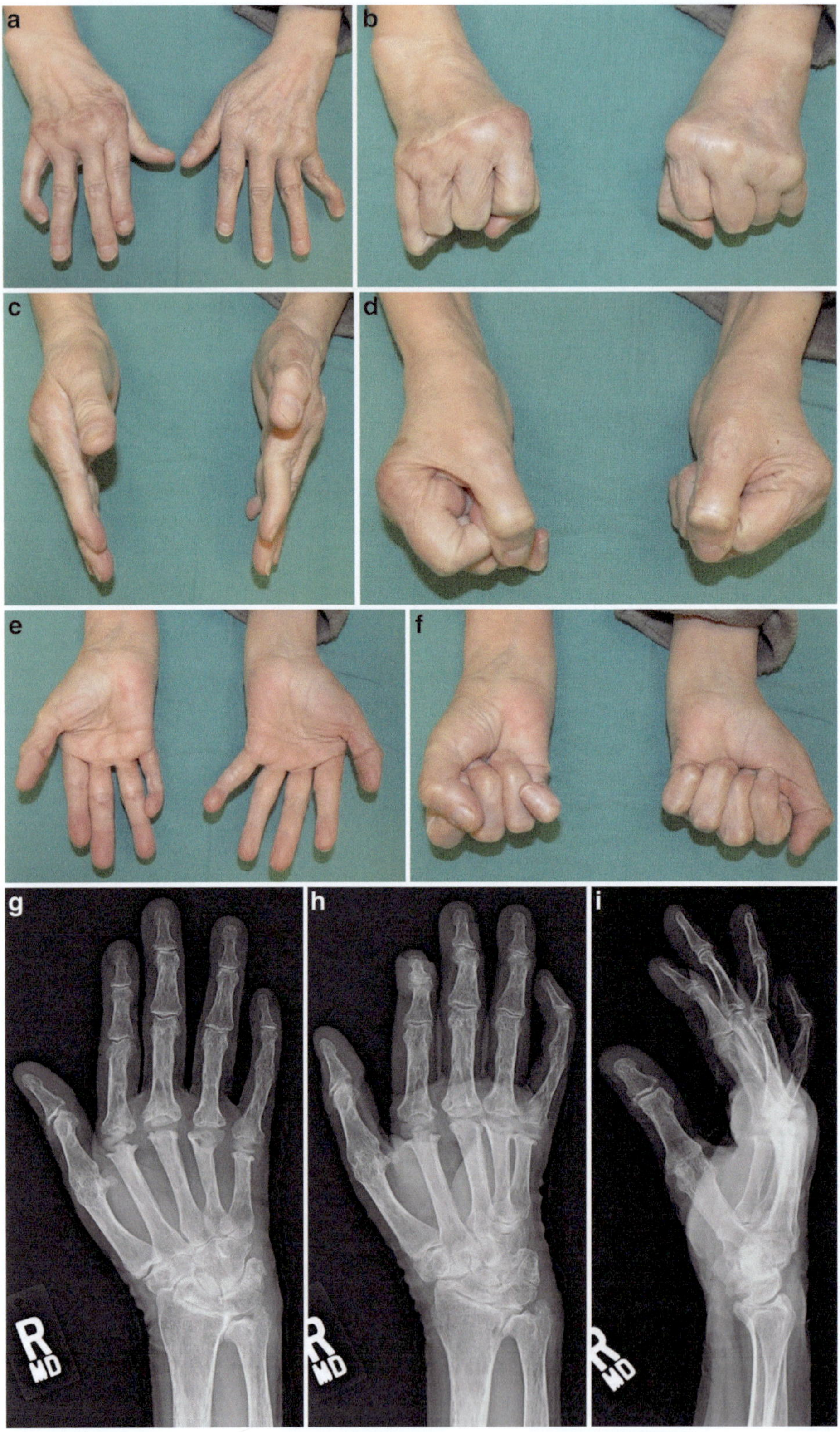

Fig. 22.15 Case #4—Two-month follow-up

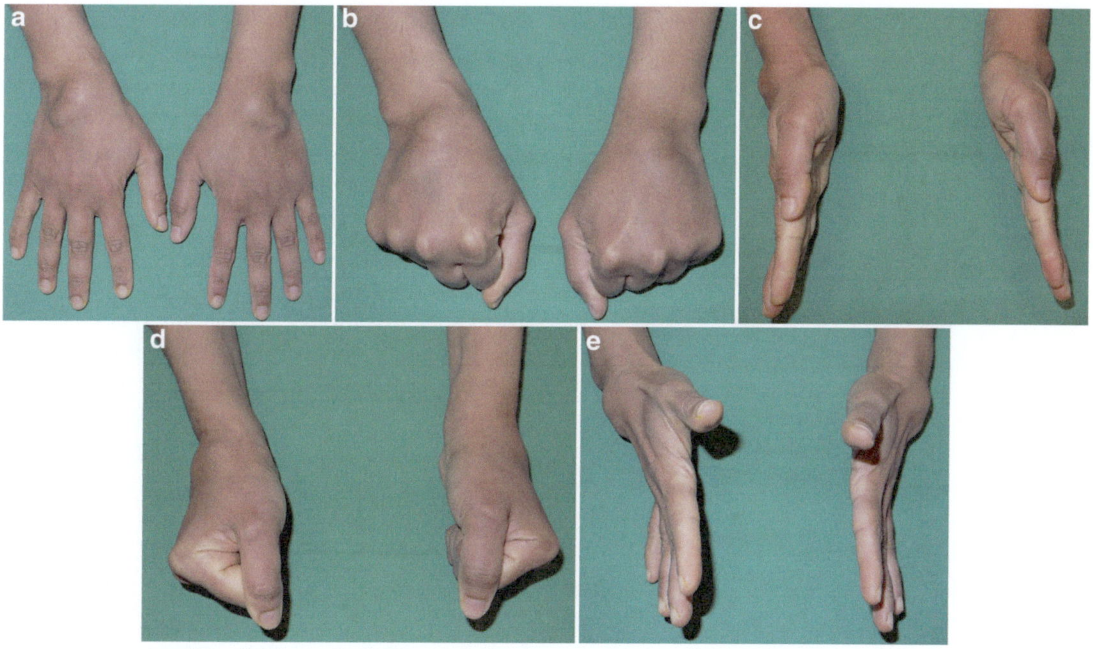

Fig. 22.16 Case #5—Preoperative images showing bilateral hand extensor tenosynovitis of a 41-year-old female recently diagnosed with RA

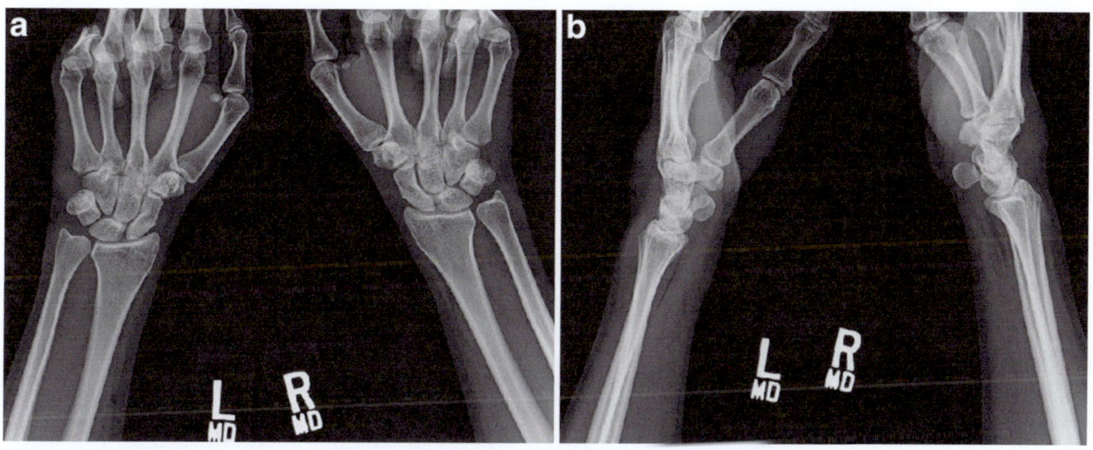

Fig. 22.17 Case #5—Initial X-rays showing edema in both hands but minimal arthritic changes

1. Which anatomical parts are responsible for the pain?

   Initial X-rays revealed minimal arthritic changes in both hands (Fig. 22.17a). Lateral views demonstrated notable edema on the dorsal aspect of the patient's wrist and hand (Fig. 22.17b). The mass over the patient's dorsal wrist was likely caused by extensor tenosynovitis and was responsible for her pain.

2. Is surgery indicated?

   This patient was an excellent candidate for tenosynovectomy because this synovial hypertrophy and inflammation could lead to tendon inflammation and erosion over time. The patient's rheumatologists first attempted to address the inflammation aggressively with medication, but the synovitis persisted for more than a few months. Synovectomy

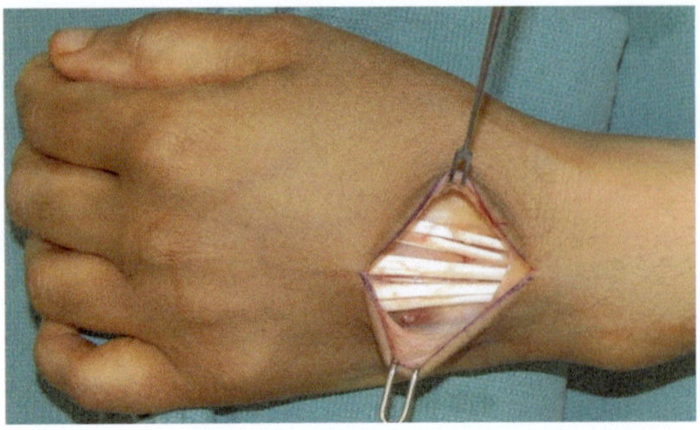

Fig. 22.18 Case #5—Procedure performed: right fourth and fifth compartment synovectomy

was indicated to prevent extensor tendon rupture.

3. Procedure performed

   Radial synovectomy of the fourth dorsal compartment was performed in the left hand. The hypertrophic synovium attached to the extensor tendons was removed successfully, and the extensor tendons had not been frayed (Fig. 22.18). The specimen was sent for a culture and pathology report. The surgical pathology report indicated that the specimen was synovitis with extensive organizing fibrinous exudate.

4. Postoperative care and outcomes

   The patient was told to refrain from aggressive finger range-of-motion exercises immediately after surgery in case of frayed tendons from the synovectomy. The hand and wrist were supported in a volar plaster splint for 2 weeks. Active extension and flexion exercises were introduced after 48 h. The sutures were removed after 2 weeks, and scar massage exercises were initiated. The patient experienced successful results with her left hand; therefore, the same procedure was performed on her right hand. Figure 22.19 shows patient pictures 9 months after surgery.

Case 6

A 29-year-old woman with a history of rheumatoid arthritis and type I diabetes. The patient was referred for evaluation of a right thumb extensor tendon rupture and difficulty extending the small finger. She had started Humira approximately 3 weeks prior to this consultation. On physical examination, the patient's fingers were in good position with no significant ulnar drift (Fig. 22.20). She was able to fully flex all of her fingers into the palm. With extension, she had no extension of the right thumb at the IP joint with evidence of the EPL rupture. The left small finger did extend to neutral; however, she was unable to hyperextend the finger, and the extension seemed to be mediated through the ring finger junctura. On pronation and supination, there was crepitus over her distal ulna bilaterally; her right hand was worse than her left. The DRUJ was stable with stressing.

Discussion

1. Which anatomical parts are responsible for the pain?

   Initial X-rays demonstrate severe degeneration of the carpal bones, distal radius, and ulna bilaterally (Fig. 22.21).Furthermore, the patient experienced limited hand function and pain caused by EPL and small finger extensor tendon ruptures.

2. Is surgery indicated?

   Tendon rupture is a frequent problem for patients with RA and can occur for two reasons. Tendons may become weakened by synovial hypertrophy within the extensor compartment, or tendons can come in contact with bony prominences, such as the eroded distal ulna or the distal pole of the scaphoid, resulting in tendon rupture [1]. The patient presented with a right EPL rupture and small finger extensor tendon rupture that required surgical correction. EIP to EPL tendon transfer is ideal in patients with an EPL rupture. In cases where the little finger extensor tendon is ruptured, the distal end of the intact tendon can be transferred end-to-side to the intact ring finger. The patient also had severe erosion of her right distal ulna. Distal ulna excision was suggested to prevent continued rupture of the remaining tendons.

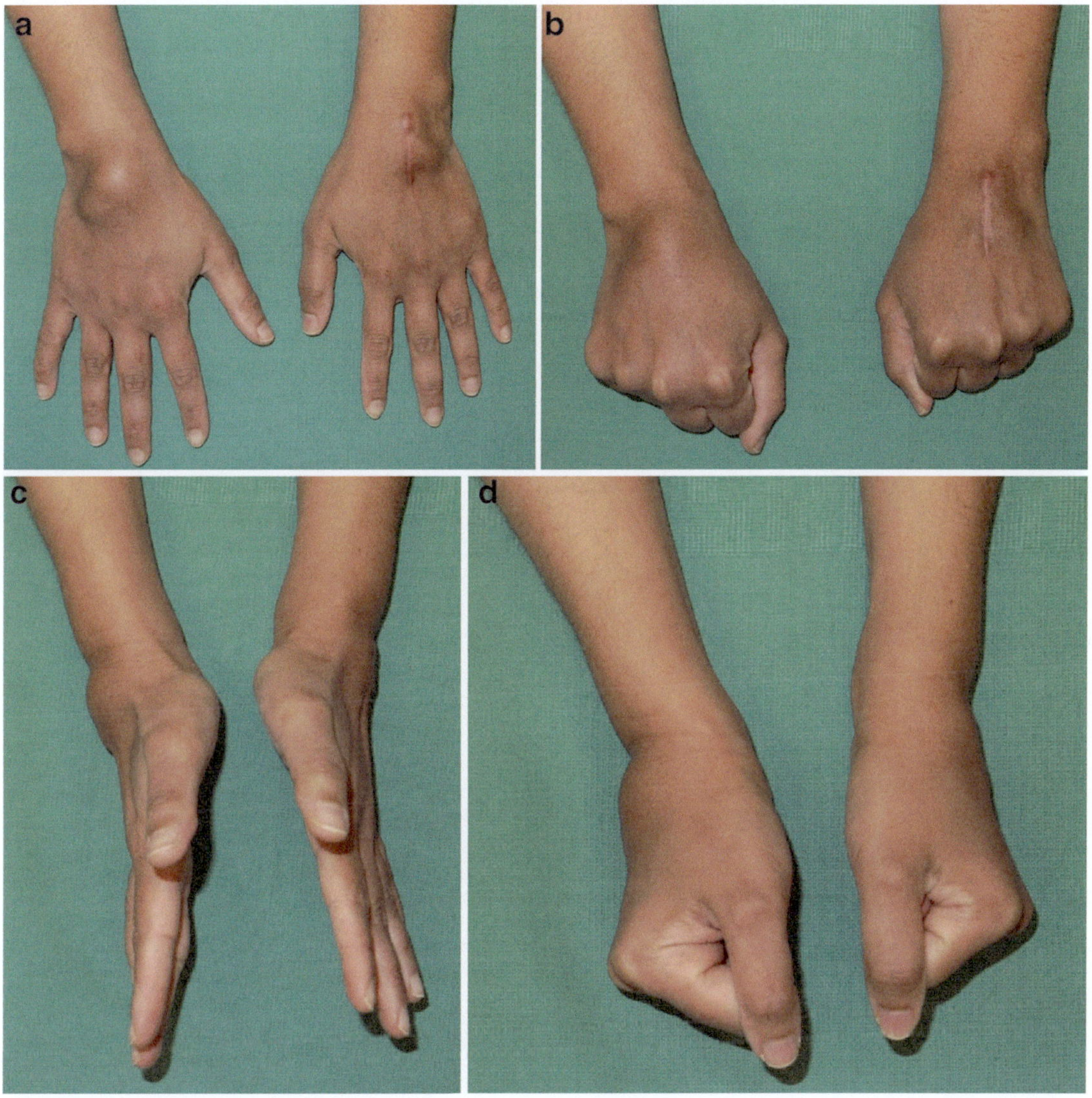

Fig. 22.19 Case #5—Nine-month follow-up

3. Procedure performed

   Intraoperative findings indicated that the little finger extensor tendon was ruptured at the mid-metacarpal. The rupture appeared to be primarily caused by synovitis. The synovitis was removed from the fourth compartment. An end-to-side transfer of the EDC of the little finger to the ring finger was made. The distal ulna was removed proximal to the sigmoid notch, and the dorsal capsule was closed over the distal ulna tightly to prevent recurrent subluxation of the distal ulna. The EIP tendon was harvested at the head of the metacarpal and transferred to the EPL tendon end-to-end. The finger posture appeared to be quite excellent. The extensor retinaculum was then closed. Figure 22.22 is illustrative, showing the steps of the procedure.

4. Postoperative care and outcomes

   The patient was placed in a volar splint with the fingers in a fully extended position. She was splinted in extension for about 3

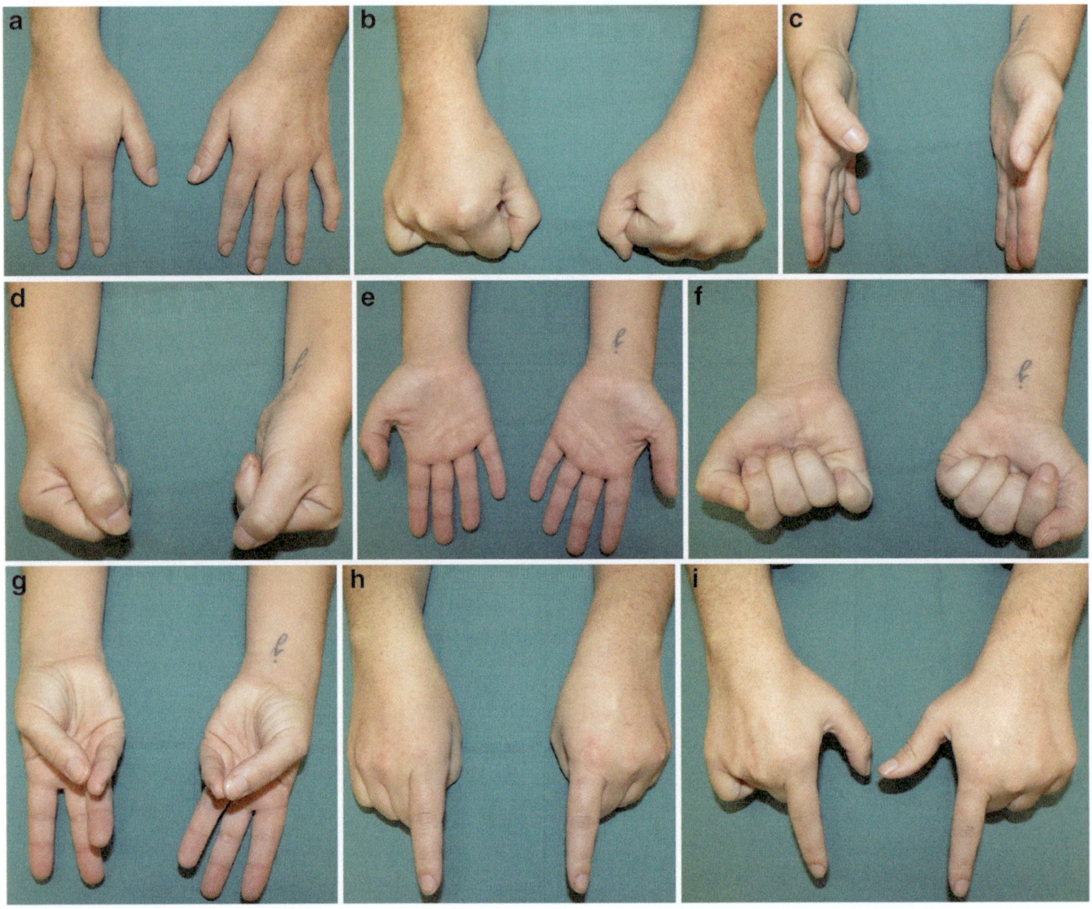

Fig. 22.20 Case # 6—Preoperative images of a 29-year-old woman with RA, presenting with evidence of EPL and small finger extensor tendon ruptures

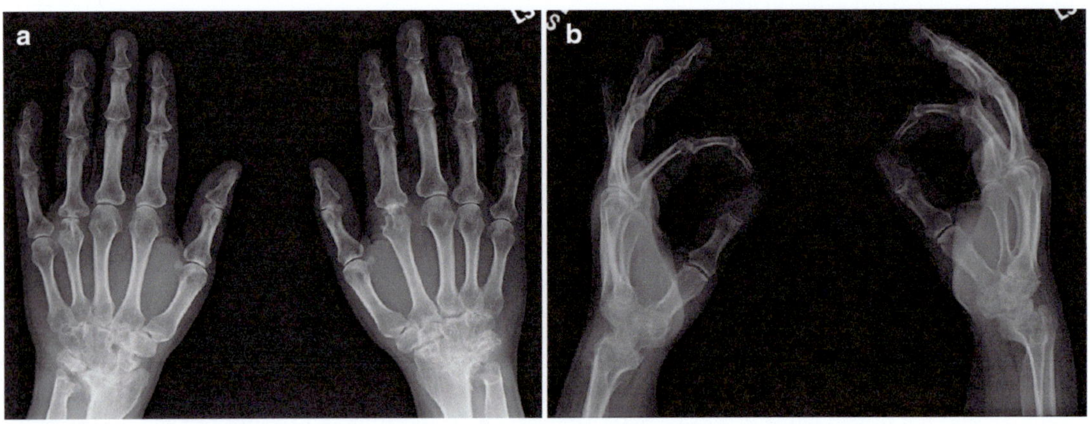

Fig. 22.21 Case #6—Initial X-rays demonstrating severe arthritic changes at the wrist bilaterally

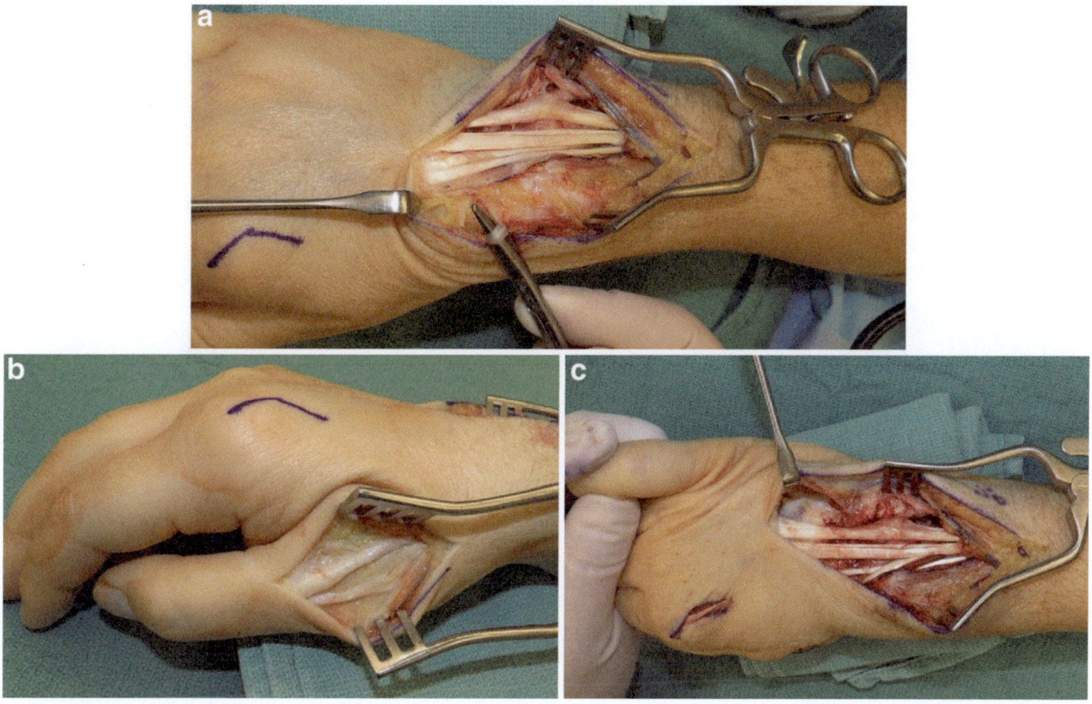

Fig. 22.22 Case #6—Procedures performed: right distal ulna excision, right EDC of the little finger to the ring finger tendon transfer, right EIP to EPL tendon transfer, right fourth dorsal compartment extensive tenosynovectomy

weeks to allow the tendon juncture to heal. After 3 weeks, range-of-motion exercises were initiated. Several months after surgery, the patient demonstrated excellent finger range of motion (Fig. 22.23).

Case 7

A 48-year-old female with a known history of seronegative rheumatoid arthritis and hereditary exostosis who presented with an inability to flex the right thumb. The patient noticed several months ago a difficulty moving her right thumb, particularly at the interphalangeal joint. She admitted that she felt a pop and pain radiating into the volar aspect of her right wrist; however, she did not seek medical attention immediately. She was being treated with Arava therapy and overall was doing well. Focused examination of her bilateral hands and wrists showed her wrist and digital extensors to be intact with some ulnar drift but no subluxation of the extensor tendons off of the metacarpal heads. She had significant swan neck deformities of her index through small finger on both hands, most notably at the index finger; however, she could make a fist relatively easily and did not have any catching due to the swan neck deformity. Her right thumb appeared to be hyperextended at the DIP joint with good EPL function but no function of the FPL tendon (Fig. 22.24).

Discussion

1. Which anatomical parts are responsible for the pain?

   Initial X-rays were presented (Fig. 22.25a–b). These X-rays revealed a very flexed distal pole of the scaphoid which caused an attritional rupture of the right FPL tendon. The FPL tendon rupture resulted in hyperextension

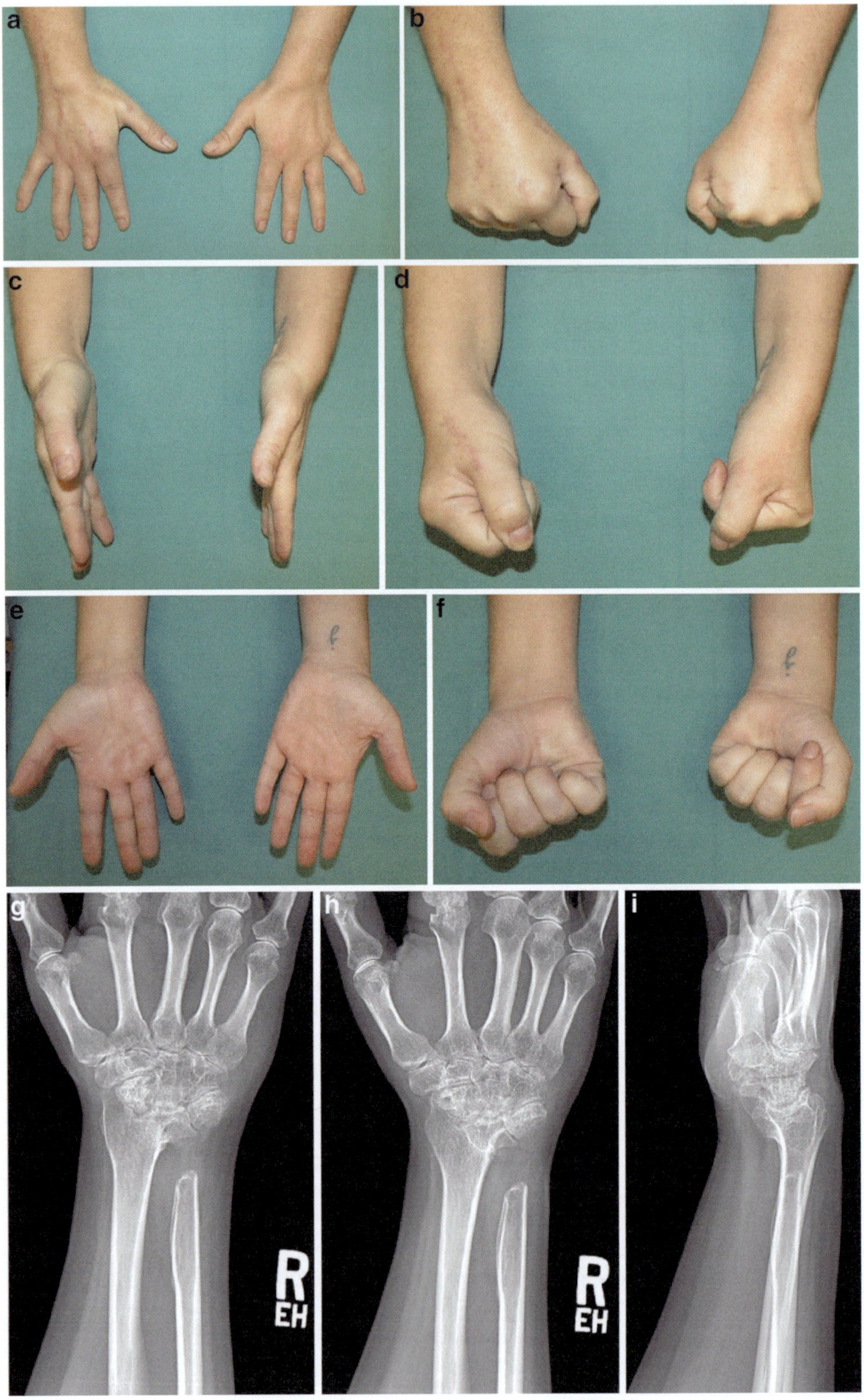

Fig. 22.23 Case #6—Five-month follow-up

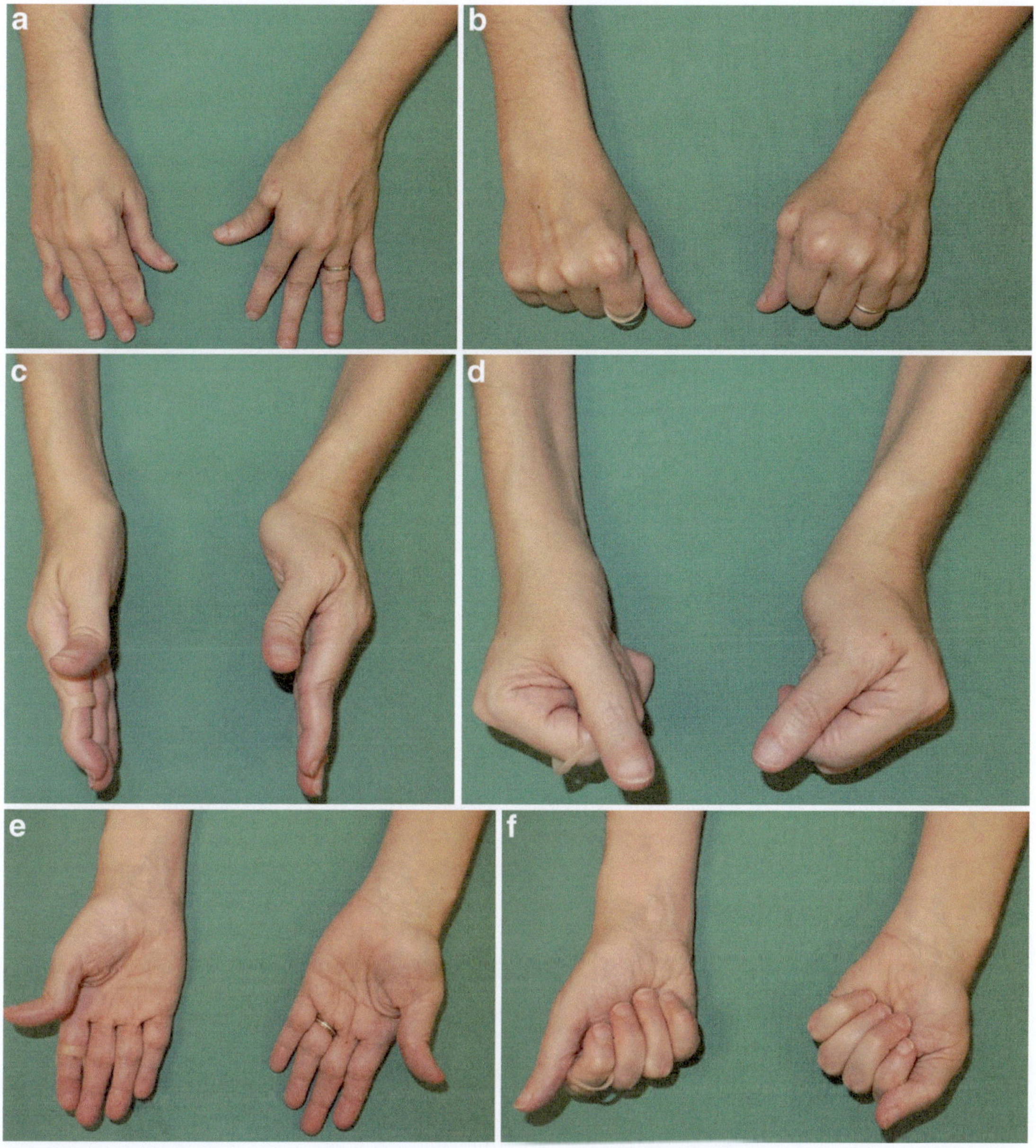

Fig. 22.24 Case #7—Preoperative images of a 48-year-old female with a known history of RA presenting with FPL tendon rupture

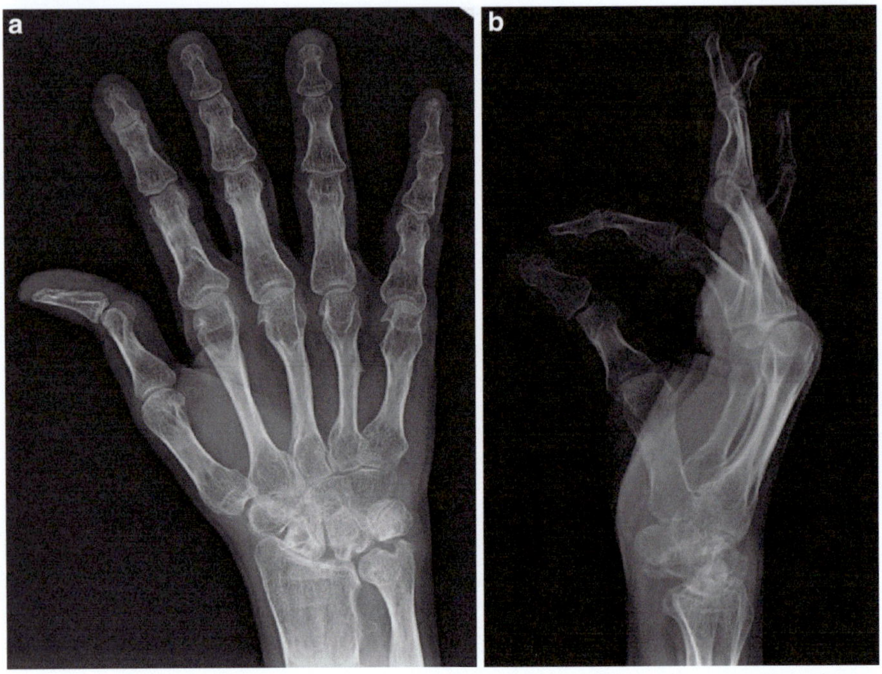

Fig. 22.25 Case #7—Initial X-rays demonstrating a flexed distal pole of the scaphoid in the right hand, which caused an FPL tendon rupture

at the IP joint and caused the patient to experience pain and significant limitations with hand function.

2. Is surgery indicated?

   Surgical intervention is indicated to restore function at the thumb. The FPL tendon can be repaired through a bridging graft from the palmaris longus, or tendon transfer moving the FDS tendon from the right middle finger to the FPL if the excursion of the proximal FPL is minimal from posttraumatic scarring and contracture. There is a risk of repeat rupture; therefore the prominent distal pole of the scaphoid, responsible for the tendon rupture, should be removed and a wrist capsular flap should be used to shield the tendons from the scaphoid.

3. Procedure performed

   Through a carpal tunnel incision, the distal end of the ruptured tendon was found. Proximally, the ruptured tendon was at the level of the wrist (Fig. 22.26a). Therefore, a palmaris longus tendon graft could be used to bridge the defect through the carpal tunnel into the distal FPL tendon at the A1 pulley level (Fig. 22.26b–e). The etiology was quite apparent that the flexed scaphoid caused this attritional rupture of the FPL tendon. The distal pole of the scaphoid which was flexed was partially removed using a rongeur. A capsule closure was then made over the distal pole of the scaphoid to prevent eroding of the bone on the reconstructed tendon.

4. Postoperative care and outcomes

   The patient was placed in a dorsal wrist splint after the operation. She was splinted fulltime for three and a half weeks. Several months after surgery, the tendon graft appeared to be in good position and thumb position was excellent (Fig. 22.27a–f).

Case 8

A 76-year-old male with a known history of rheumatoid arthritis, diagnosed over 35 years ago, presented for evaluation and treatment of his

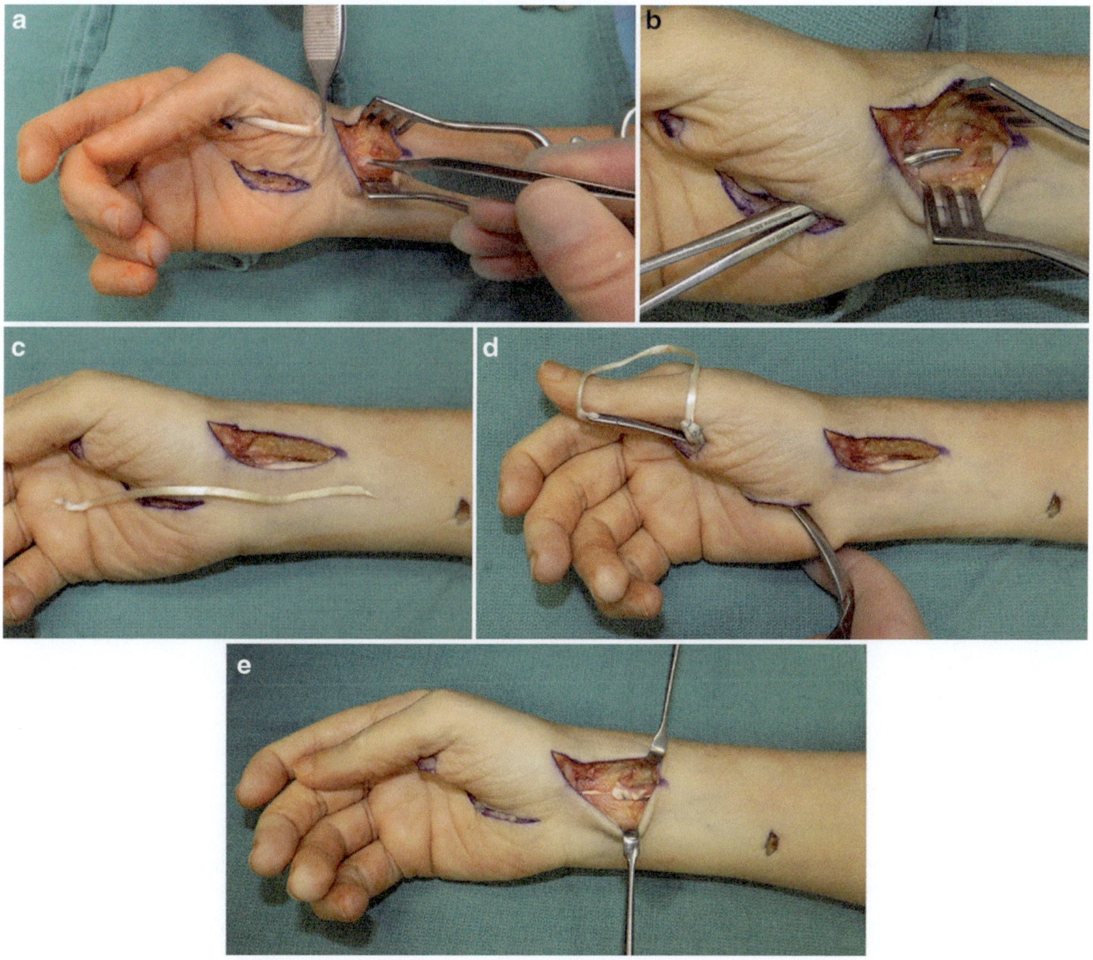

Fig. 22.26 Case #7—Procedures performed: right palmaris longus tendon grafting to the flexor pollicis longus tendon, removal of the flexed distal pole of the scaphoid, wrist capsular closure over the excised scaphoid

right thumb hyperextension deformity at the MCP joint and instability of the CMC joint. He had many hand surgeries in the past, including a right total wrist fusion with proximal row carpectomy and right wrist Darrach procedure. Furthermore, he previously had right index, middle, ring, and small finger silicone implant arthroplasties, left hand cross intrinsic transfer, and left thumb MCP joint fusion. Preoperative pictures are shown in Fig. 22.28a–f.

Discussion

1. Which anatomical parts are responsible for the pain?

   Initial X-rays were presented (Fig. 22.29). These X-rays showed significant arthritic changes of both hands, hardware in place of the left thumb, and left index, middle, ring, and small finger implant arthroplasties. He also had a right wrist proximal row carpectomy, wrist

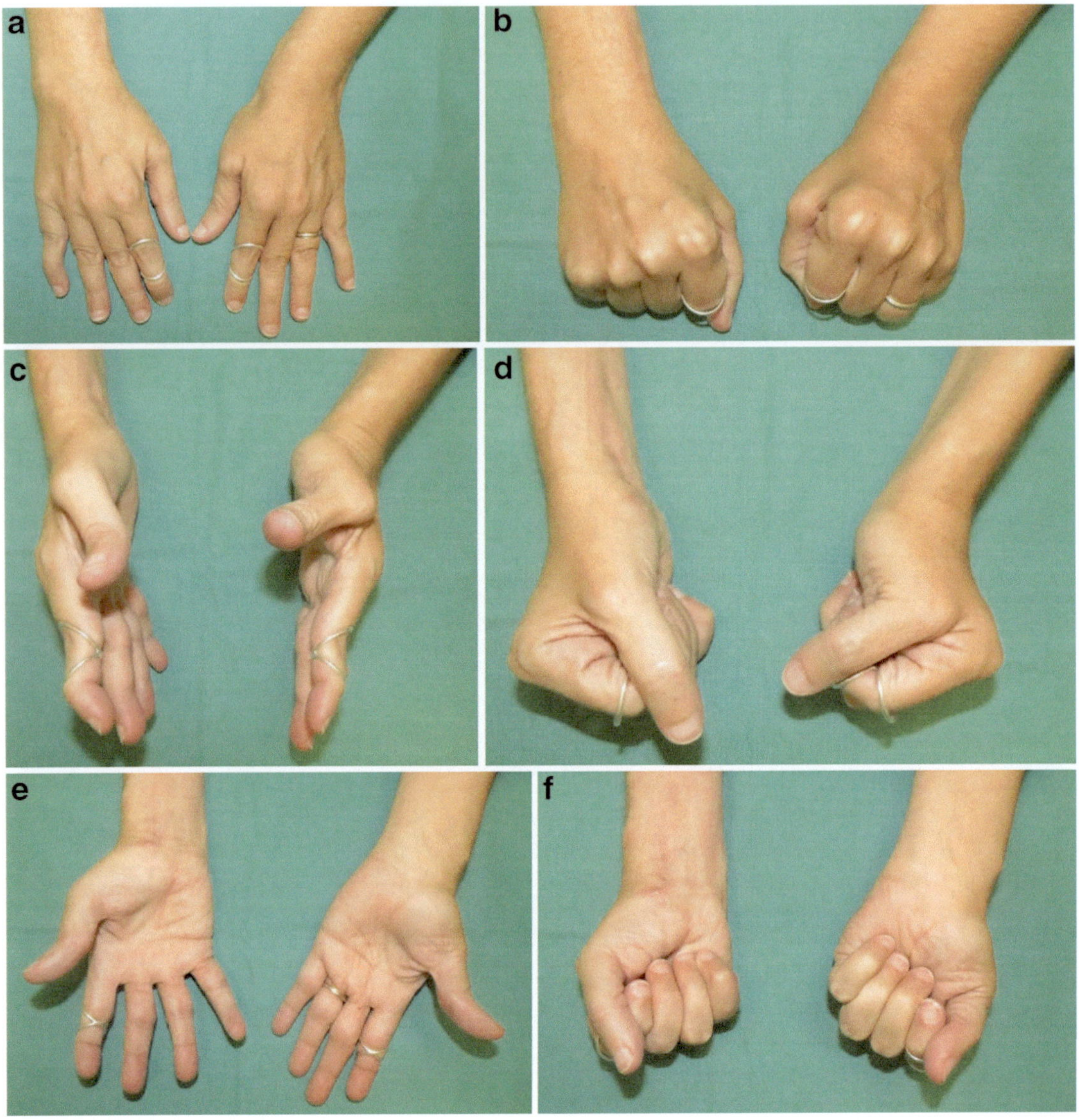

Fig. 22.27 Case #7—Five-month follow-up

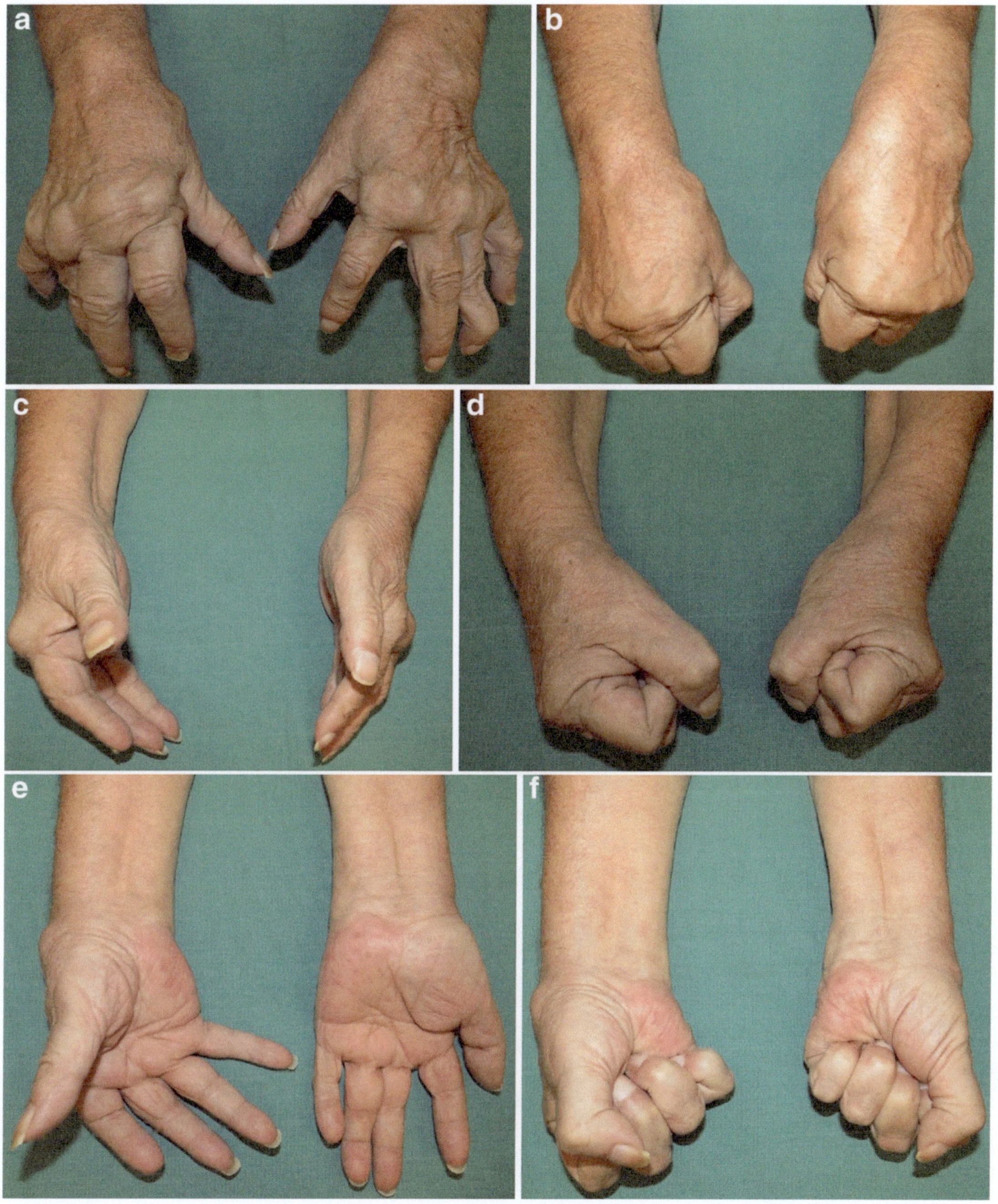

Fig. 22.28 Case #8—Preoperative images of a 76-year-old male with a known history of RA presenting with a right thumb hyperextension deformity at the MCP joint and CMC joint instability

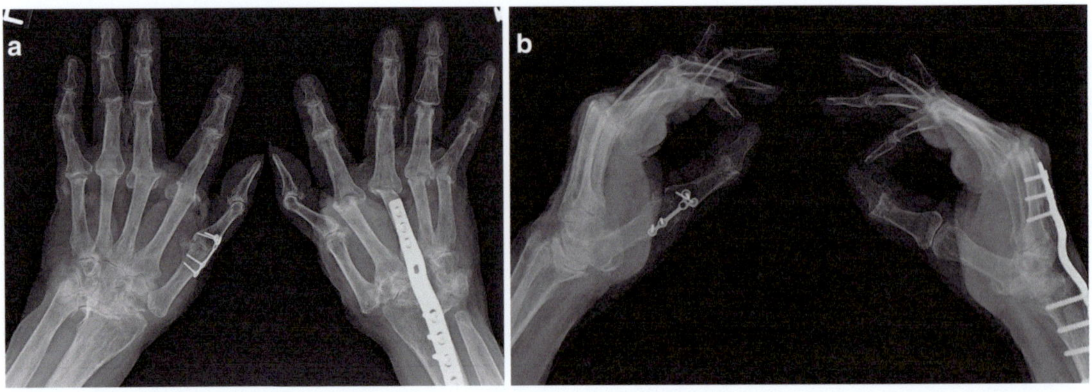

Fig. 22.29 Case #8—Initial X-rays demonstrating severe arthritic changes bilaterally

fusion plate, and distal ulna excision. Physical examination of the patient's bilateral hands indicated multiple arthritic deformities of the MCP joints, hyperextension deformity of the thumb MCP joint, flexion deformity at the DIP joint, and instability at the CMC joint.

2. Is surgery indicated?

   The patient's severe right thumb CMC arthritis with degeneration of the trapezium and subluxation of the thumb CMC joint demands surgical treatment. Surgery can significantly improve the patient's thumb stability and function. We recommended a right thumb MCP joint fusion at 30° of flexion and tendon procedure to stabilize the CMC joint.

3. Procedure performed

   The diseased trapezium was removed, and the thumb CMC joint was stabilized using a slip of the APL tendon (Fig. 22.30a–b). Because the patient had a wrist fusion, the patient's wrist extensors were expendable. Therefore, an extensor carpi radialis brevis tendon graft was harvested, sutured into a cushion, and placed under the thumb CMC joint for stabilization (Fig. 22.30c–d). To prevent hyperextension of the thumb MCP joint, which will destabilize the thumb CMC joint, the thumb MCP joint was fused in neutral position to give the patient a much better posture of the thumb. The patient's thumb was placed in an abducted position to stabilize the thumb CMC joint (Fig. 22.30e).

4. Postoperative care and outcomes

   The pins were in place for 6–8 weeks to allow the fusion to heal at the MCP joint, after which time, range of motion exercises were started for the thumb CMC joint. Several months after surgery, the patient was able to use the thumb moderately well and demonstrated a good return of key activities of daily living with his right thumb. Postoperative pictures and X-rays are shown in Fig. 22.31.

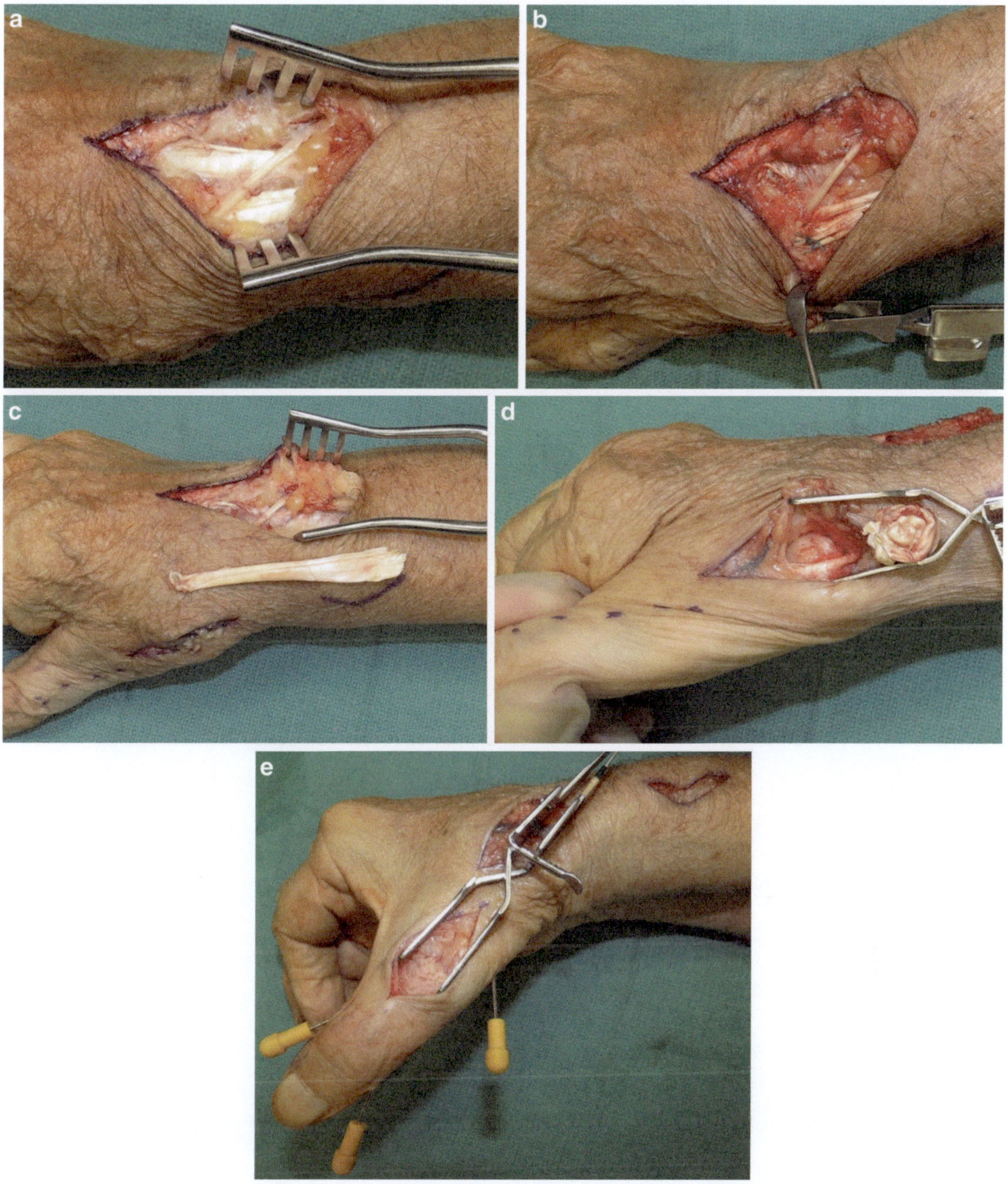

Fig. 22.30 Case #8—Procedures performed: right thumb carpometacarpal joint arthroplasty with abductor pollicis longus tendon stabilization, extensor carpi radialis brevis tendon graft for interpositional arthroplasty at the base of the thumb, right thumb MCP joint fusion with bone grafting

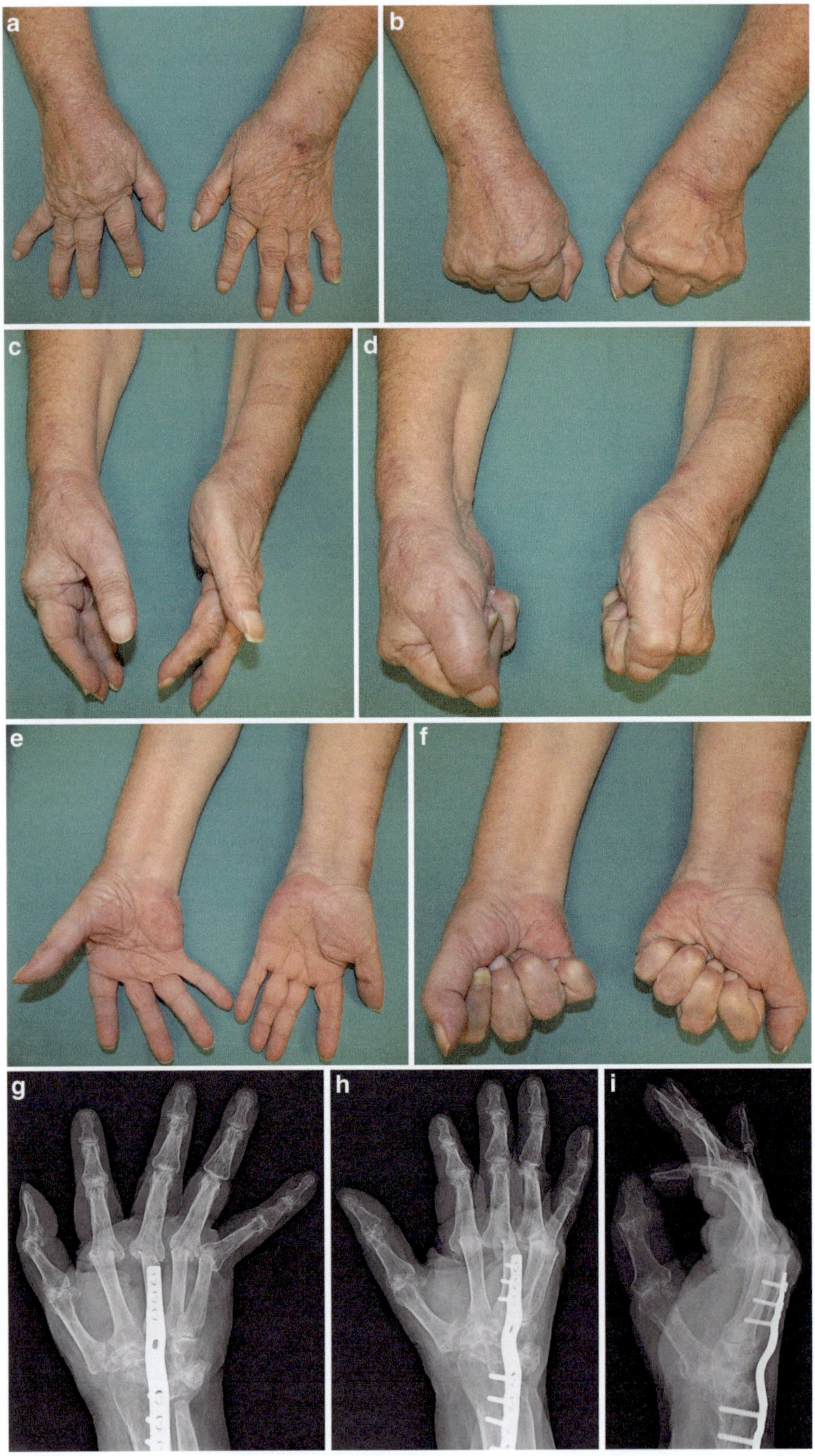

Fig. 22.31 Case #8—Three-month follow-up

References

1. Chung KC, Pushman AG. Current concepts in the management of the rheumatoid hand. J Hand Surg Am. 2011;36(4):736–47.
2. Longo UG, Petrillo S, Denaro V. Current concepts in the management of rheumatoid hand. Int J Rheumatol. 2015;2015:648073.
3. Chung KC, Burns PB, Wilgis EF, Burke FD, Regan M, Kim HM, et al. A multicenter clinical trial in rheumatoid arthritis comparing silicone metacarpophalangeal joint arthroplasty with medical treatment. J Hand Surg Am. 2009;34(5):815–23.
4. Chung KC, Kotsis SV, Wilgis EF, Fox DA, Regan M, Kim HM, et al. Outcomes of silicone arthroplasty for rheumatoid metacarpophalangeal joints stratified by fingers. J Hand Surg Am. 2009;34(9):1647–52.
5. Chung KC, Burns PB, Kim HM, Burke FD, Wilgis EF, Fox DA. Long-term followup for rheumatoid arthritis patients in a multicenter outcomes study of silicone metacarpophalangeal joint arthroplasty. Arthritis Care Res. 2012;64(9):1292–300.
6. Burgess SD, Kono M, Stern PJ. Results of revision metacarpophalangeal joint surgery in rheumatoid patients following previous silicone arthroplasty. J Hand Surg Am. 2007;32(10):1506–12.

Part IV

Rheumatoid Elbow

Soft Tissue Management of Elbow Deformities

23

Takeshi Ogawa and Kevin C. Chung

Introduction

Among patients with rheumatoid arthritis (RA), 25 % have severe disability affecting the elbow and half of those patients report having pain. The majority of RA patients have some symptoms involving the elbow, with only 28 % having no symptoms affecting the elbow [1]. RA of the elbow usually starts with the proliferation of synovium. The disease progression leads to destruction of the articular cartilage and distension of the collateral ligament. In advanced stages, significant destruction and loss of subchondral bone occur, along with loss of normal articular contour. This combination of the loss of bone and soft tissue causes instability and pain [2]. Issues concerning the bone or joint are primarily treated with surgery, including synovectomy and arthroplasty using prostheses. On the other hand, damage to soft tissue, including rheumatoid nodules, bursitis, and skin ulcers, is not treated as easily [1, 2]. Soft tissue defects at the elbow that expose bones, tendons, nerves, and articular surfaces, including prostheses, are all considered failures. These failures, especially in a wide zone injury, can develop edema that cause functional deficit of the elbow resulting from long-term immobilization. The aim of treatment for soft tissue defects is to close the wound, decrease the risk of infection or the edema of tissues, and permit early mobilization and rehabilitation of the elbow. Early reconstruction facilitates maximum functional recovery, and a familiarity with treatment of the soft tissue loss at the elbow is valuable for surgeons.

T. Ogawa, MD, PhD (✉)
Department of Orthopaedic Surgery and Sports Medicine, Tsukuba University Hospital, Mito Clinical Education and Training Center, Mito, Ibaraki, Japan
e-mail: oga-take@pg7.so-net.ne.jp

K.C. Chung, MD, MS
Comprehensive Hand Center, Section of Plastic Surgery, Department of Surgery, The University of Michigan Health System, 2130 Taubman Center, SPC 5340, 1500 E. Medical Center Drive, Ann Arbor, MI 48109-5340, USA
e-mail: kecchung@med.umich.edu

Rheumatoid Nodule

Rheumatoid nodules are classically associated with RA and indicate severe arthritis. Rheumatoid nodules appear in 20–25 % of patients with RA [3, 4]. The most common sites at the elbow are the olecranon and the extensor side of the forearm (Fig. 23.1). Other frequent sites include the dorsum of hand, the knee, the ears, the scapula, and sites that experience repetitive trauma. Rheumatoid nodules present subcutaneously and adhere to deep tissues including the periosteum, tendon sheaths, and bursa. The pathogenesis is not known, but it is thought to occur in the immune complex

K.C. Chung (ed.), *Clinical Management of the Rheumatoid Hand, Wrist, and Elbow*,
DOI 10.1007/978-3-319-26660-2_23

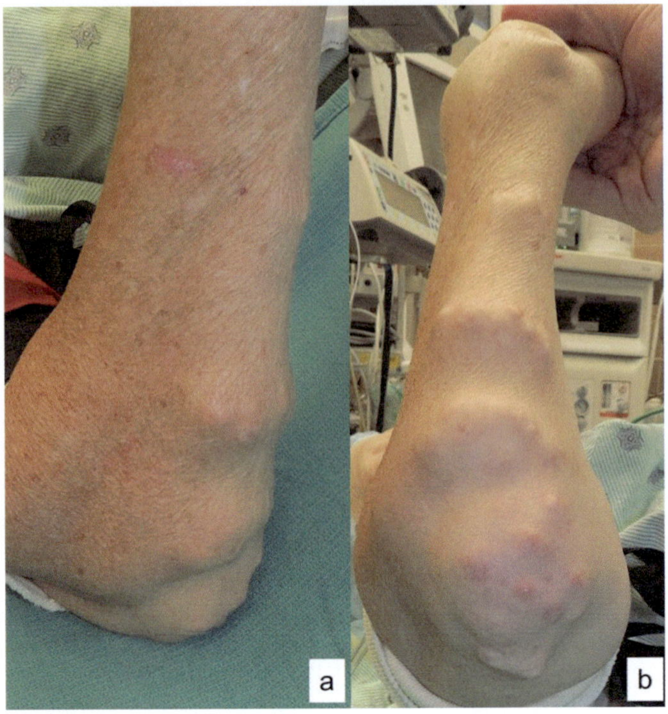

Fig. 23.1 (**a**, **b**) Rheumatoid nodules on the olecranon to the extensor side of the forearm

of small vessels and caused by vascular inflammatory change following tissue necrosis [5]. Necrosis of the subcutaneous nodules causes proteinases and collagenase to be produced by the cellular palisade. Trauma has also been proposed as a mechanism for nodule formation.

Rheumatoid nodules are diagnosed clinically, and care must be taken to ensure the correct diagnosis. Differential diagnoses associated with subcutaneous nodules similar to those found in RA are broad and include rheumatic fever, Jaccoud's arthritis, granuloma annulare, basal cell carcinoma, necrobiosis lipoidica diabeticorum, and infectious disease [5, 6]. Atypical rheumatoid nodules, such as those in uncommon locations, of abnormal color, or those that are accompanied by skin ulcers, should undergo a biopsy. Approximately 5–7 % of patients with systemic lupus erythematosus, another chronic autoimmune disease, develop rheumatoid nodules [7]. In rare instances, rheumatoid nodules occur in the lung, larynx, nasal septum, and heart [8].

The histological features of rheumatoid nodules include a palisaded granulomatous pattern, the deposition of many IgG with central necrosis, and a few depositions of IgA and C3. Vasculitis may be recognized in early stage lesions, and fibrosis in late stage lesions. Similar to rheumatoid nodules, deep granuloma annulare presents with a comparable pattern but generally contains mucin in the center and few palisades. It contains many giant cells and also shows perivascular cuffing of lymphocytes around the new vessels of peripheral lesion [9].

Most rheumatoid nodules are asymptomatic and therefore treated conservatively. Disease-modifying antirheumatic drugs (DMARD) typically inhibit formation of the nodules, with the exception of methotrexate which promotes formation of the nodules [10, 11]. Many surgeons tend to avoid treating nodules with corticosteroid injection because it increases the risk of infection [12]. Ching reported that patients experienced substantial reduction in nodule size after receiving a corticosteroid injection, but no significant decrease in pain, compared with a placebo [13]. There is only one report, which noted four successful cases, for surgical treatment of rheumatoid nodules [14]. We recommend conservative, nonoperative treatment, which should include pain control using nonsteroidal anti-inflammatory drugs (NSAID). However, for patients with rheumatoid nodules that have pain, infection, ulceration, or limited range of motion, operative treatment should be considered. Operative treatment may require coverage with skin flap at the site of the excision because of the possibility of local granular proliferation. Surgery should not be done solely for aesthetic purposes.

Rheumatoid nodulosis is a condition involving subcutaneous nodules that does not develop as typical RA, although it is almost identical to RA in histological features. It is distinguished by having rheumatoid nodules, with no systemic evidence of RA. Ginsberg named the condition rheumatoid nodulosis in 1975 [15]. In 1988, Couret referred to the four criteria for the diagnosis of rheumatoid nodulosis [16]:

1. Multiple subcutaneous rheumatoid nodules identified using biopsy
2. Recurrent joint symptoms with minimal radiological or clinical involvement
3. Benign clinical course
4. No or mild systemic manifestations of rheumatoid arthritis

Methotrexate therapy is known to induce the nodulosis as a benign side effect. Colchicine, D-penicillamine, and hydroxychloroquine are effective treatments [17, 18].

Synovial Cyst

RA is identified as the chronic inflammation of synovial tissues. This synovial tissue inflammation stimulates synovial cyst formation around the joints. The condition may develop owing to several different pathologic mechanisms [19]:

1. Accumulation of fluid in communicating bursae
2. Distention of bursae by fluid originating in the joint
3. Herniation of the joint capsule in response to increased intra-articular pressure

Synovial cysts at the elbow mostly occur posteriorly, and a cyst of the antecubital space is rare. These cysts are similar to the Baker's cyst that occurs in the popliteal space of the knee. Synovial cysts can sometimes rupture, leading to pain and edema from the elbow to forearm. The treatment of synovial cysts is similar to treatment of elbow arthritis, including rest, administration of NSAIDs, and possible corticosteroid injections [20]. Synovial cysts should be addressed before they rupture or become large enough to cause entrapment neuropathy. There are several reports of ulnar nerve and posterior interosseous nerve palsy caused by synovial cysts [21] (see Chap. 6).

Olecranon Bursitis

Olecranon bursitis may occur in RA patients, and because it is typically caused by repetitive trauma, there may not be a large benefit in routine removal of the inflamed bursa. Bursitis can cause the area around the olecranon to become swollen and unsightly, which alone is not reason for removal. However, if the bursa is infected or a skin ulcer forms, removal is justified. Nonetheless, the recurrence rate is high among RA patients. Stewart et al. described the results of open resection of 21 cases of aseptic olecranon bursitis. The success rates of those with RA and those without RA were 40 % and 94 %, respectively [22]. If surgery is justified, olecranon bursa excision is useful to reduce repetitive trauma. The elbow is the primary bearing joint for patients with RA, especially for severe or noncontrolled patients who have functional loss of one or both of their lower extremities. Quayle described 11 cases of olecranon process excision and found no recurrence of bursitis and no loss of triceps function [23]. Based on the above, conservative treatment is recommended. If surgery is necessary, the olecranon process should be excised along with the bursa.

Flap Management of the Wound

Principle

In RA patients, complicated wounds may develop because of vulnerability of the vessels, exposure of the prosthesis, or chronic infection, even without severe trauma. Various factors should be considered when determining the reconstruction method for wounds. First, the defect should be clearly evaluated by focusing on the components that need reconstruction. Before forming a complex restructuring plan, it is important to take into consideration the condition of the wound. The wound should be systematically evaluated on what has been lost and the steps necessary for restoring function and aesthetic. Second, neurovascular assessment should be performed before the reconstruction, and if there is any uncertainty about the blood supply, arteriography should be done. Third, for contaminated wounds, debridement of the contaminated bones and soft tissues should precede reconstruction. Thorough debridement of the wound is the most important step to minimize infection and should be performed promptly. After debridement, various options of reconstruction can be considered. The ultimate selection of flap coverage depends on elements including size, wound complexity, the condition of the donor site, the general condition of the patient, and the final desired outcome of the elbow joint. The reconstruction plan should match not only the needs of the wound but also the needs of the patient. Patients with RA have compromised immune system, which may lead to complications such as wound healing failure and an increased risk of infection.

Timing of Surgery

Surgery should be done as early as possible. The success of the early wound closure is dependent on thorough debridement. Delayed wound closure is indicated only if debridement is deemed inadequate. Wound infection is one factor that delays the surgery; however, early soft tissue coverage reduces edema and pain and controls further infections. This concept applies to emergency cases as well as RA patients. Early closure is specifically required when the prosthesis or other vital structures including bones, joints, or tendons are exposed. Prompt surgery allows rehabilitation to begin sooner and leads to an improved success rate of flap coverage [24, 25].

Algorithm

The reconstruction algorithm for determining elbow coverage is viewed in a "step ladder" fashion, which means choosing a simple procedure before a more complicated option. However, with the development of microsurgery techniques, this "step ladder" is becoming overlooked, and surgical procedures are being chosen first because they provide the best outcome for the patient. The process of choosing a reconstruction technique is now referred to as an "elevator" and is one of the important concepts in wound management (Fig. 23.2) [26]. It starts out with the simple technique of direct closure, followed by skin graft, local flap, and then distant flap. With recently improved microsurgical techniques, it has become possible to choose a suitable strategy depending on the situation of the wound [27]. Moreover, with the advent of the vacuum-assisted closure (VAC) system and the development of the dermal matrices, the treatment options are widespread [28]. The elbow is surrounded by minimal soft tissue covered by thin and mobile skin. For defects of soft tissue around the elbow, a fasciocutaneous flap, frequently from the radial forearm, or a lateral arm flap is indicated. For local situations, brachioradialis (BR) or flexor carpi ulnaris (FCU) muscle flap can be used, with both muscles having minimal loss of function. Latissimus dorsi (LD) is available as a functional muscle transfer to replace the biceps and triceps and preserves the pedicle that reaches to the elbow. It can be used for a wide range of defects that may spread to the forearm and upper arm. In summary, options for elbow wound treatment in RA patients are limited. For large to massive-sized wounds, choices for flap reconstruction include using the anterolateral thigh (ALT) as a free flap and the LD as a distant flap. For the small- to medium-sized wound, options include local random flaps (advancement flap, rotational flap, Z-plasty, and rhomboid flaps) and regional axial flaps (BR, FCU, anconeus, radial forearm, and reverse lateral arm as a muscle or fasciocutaneous flap).

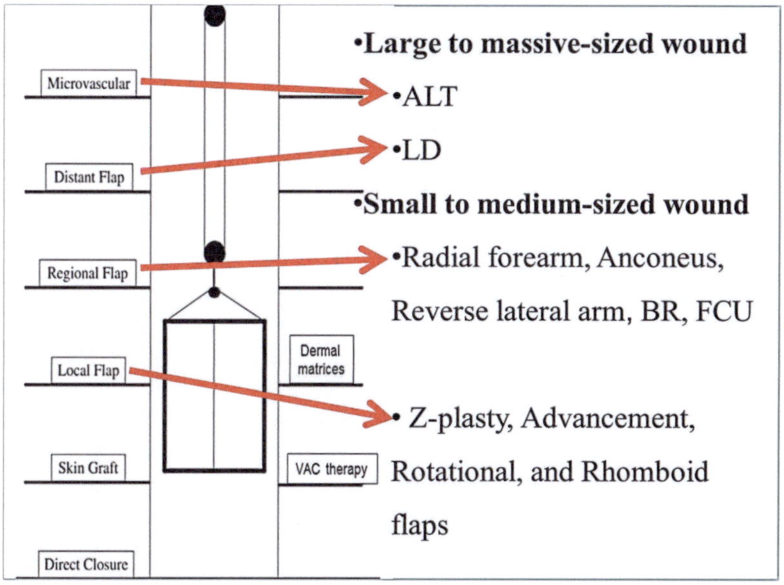

Fig. 23.2 Options for elbow wound treatment in RA patients

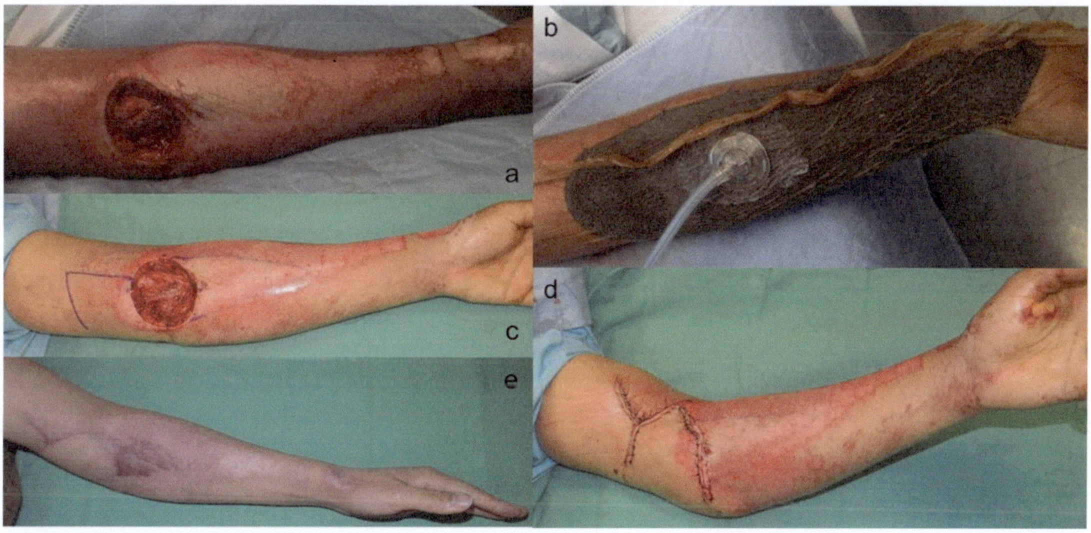

Fig. 23.3 (**a**) Antecubital skin defect measuring 6×7 cm. (**b**) VAC system was performed. (**c**) The wound is shown at 4 days after the injury. (**d**) Rhomboid fasciocutaneous flap. (**e**) Five months after skin closure

Cases of Reconstruction of the Elbow in RA Patients

Postoperative complications after total elbow arthroplasty (TEA) occur frequently and can be attributed to the skin at the tip of the olecranon being thin and mobile. Jeon and colleagues reported that 5.5 % of TEA patients suffered postoperative wound complications such as delayed healing, wound dehiscence, and necrosis [24]. In their report, 33 % (32/97) of patients had RA, and 24 % of RA patients had signs of sepsis. The number of sepsis cases was significantly higher in RA patients than in osteoarthritis (OA) patients. In this paper, the authors noted that a small superficial necrotic area of less than 3 cm in diameter may heal with local wound care, but surgical debridement is generally required for necrosis greater than 3 cm or with full thickness muscle loss (Fig. 23.3). An FCU flap can be used safely after TEA if the feeding artery is not damaged [29]. Jeon and colleagues used a radial forearm flap to cover small and noninfected defects and preferred a pedicled muscle flap for infected wound or to fill a dead space around the elbow. They used an LD flap in four patients and a radial forearm flap in three patients. ALT flap was also used in several cases that involved infection with a soft tissue defect. In a different study, Gill and Morrey reported two cases of muscle flaps (BR and LD) to cover the elbow after debridement for deep infection [25]. Dee performed a radial forearm flap to cover the bare metal of an exposed prosthesis [30].

Small- to Medium-Sized Wounds

Radial Forearm Flap

A skin flap is harvested from the volar aspect of the forearm between the antecubital fossa and the wrist crease. The maximum flap size is 10 × 30 cm, but for elbow coverage, a flap no larger than 8 × 16 cm is generally used. Perforating branches of the radial artery act as the blood supply. The venous drainage of the flap relies on both the deep and superficial system and the cephalic vein. The sensory component of the flap is the medial and lateral antebrachial cutaneous nerves. The Allen test must be done preoperatively. The central axis of the pedicle is designed along the line from the midpoint of the antecubital fossa to the radial border of the wrist. Next, the pivot point is determined, and the distance from the point to the defect is transposed to the donor site. The tendons of the BR and flexor carpi radialis (FCR) must be identified because the radial artery usually lies between the two tendons. Before distal radial artery ligation, it is imperative to confirm flow through the superficial palmar arch to the ulnar artery. The distal radial artery and venous continuity are ligated and divided, and the flap is raised distal to proximal, including the antebrachial fascia, radial vessels, and fasciocutaneous perforators. Care must be taken to preserve the paratenon over the BR and FCR for recovery following the skin graft. The flap is raised and transposed to cover the elbow defect. The donor site is covered with a non-meshed split-thickness skin graft from the anterior thigh. The wrist and fingers are immobilized with a splint for a week to prevent skin graft loss [31, 32].

Reverse Lateral Arm Flap

The blood supply of the reverse lateral arm flap is the posterior radial collateral artery and has collateral flow through the radial recurrent artery in the proximal forearm. The radial recurrent vessels provide inflow to the reverse lateral arm flap, with a lesser contribution from a recurrent branch of the posterior interosseous artery. It can cover up to 8 × 15 cm, although primary skin closure can be difficult if the width exceeds 6 cm. The blood supply is the 3–5 septocutaneous perforator arteries in the lateral intermuscular septum of the upper arm, which are derived from the radial collateral artery. This artery is a branch of the profunda brachii artery and runs between the triceps and brachialis distally along the humerus. The reverse lateral arm flap can be distally extended with blood supply over the lateral epicondyle of the humerus because of anastomoses with recurrent arteries of the periarticular plexus of the elbow joint (Fig. 23.4) [33, 34]. The maximum flap size is 8 cm in width and 20 cm in length. The pedicle length can be up to 11 cm long and 2–2.5 mm in diameter. The operation is done in a supine position, and a tourniquet is not applied because the flap is harvested from the upper arm. It starts on a virtual axis between the deltoid apex and the lateral epicondyle of the humerus. Starting posteriorly, the fascia is dissected from the muscle and elevated toward the intermuscular septum until the blood vessels appear. The same procedure is then done from the anterior side. The average length of the pedicle is 7.8 cm, which is shorter than the radial forearm flap or the ALT. The donor site can usually be closed primarily if the width of the flap is no more than 8 cm. The posterior antebrachial cutaneous nerve often cannot be preserved. Hypoesthesia in the forearm remains in more than 50 % of the patients (Fig. 23.5) [35, 36].

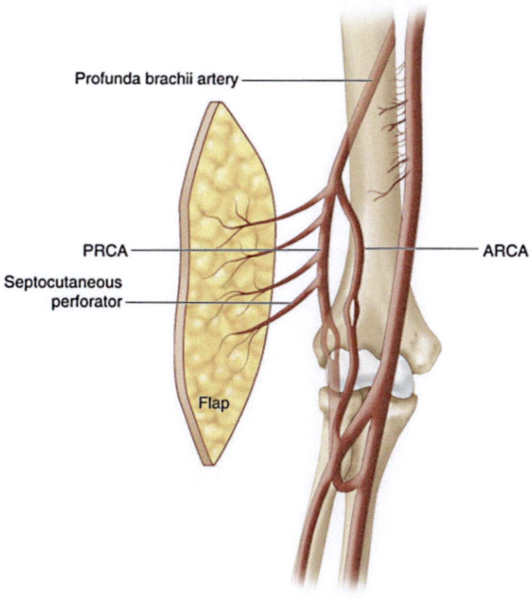

Fig. 23.4 The anatomy of lateral arm flap. *PRCA* posterior radial collateral artery, *ARCA* anterior radial collateral artery [33]. This article was published in Hand and Wrist Surgery, 2nd ed., Teoh L-C, Lateral arm flap for upper limb coverage, 444–450, Copyright Elsevier (2012)

Anconeus Flap

The anconeus muscle is approximately 2.5 cm in width and 7 cm in length. It can cover an area of 5–7 cm^2 and is used for a defect of the lateral radiocapitellar joint, the distal triceps tendon at its insertion, or the olecranon. The anconeus functions as a minor elbow extensor and helps maintain the lateral stability of the elbow [37]. The blood supplies are the recurrent posterior interosseous artery and the medial collateral artery, which is a terminal branch of the profunda brachii and has anastomoses within the muscle belly. The innervation is the radial nerve branch. The subsequent functional deficit is negligible. A split-thickness skin graft is used to cover the muscle. Commonly, the VAC system is used to help the muscle and the skin graft to be adherent to the wound. The elbow must remain immobilized for approximately 2 weeks (Fig. 23.6).

Brachioradialis Flap

The brachioradialis flap is contraindicated in patients who have weak elbow flexion. The BR lies superficially on the radial side of the forearm. It originates from the upper two-thirds of the lateral epicondyle and inserts into the radial styloid. The base of the muscle is 7–8 cm in width and tapers distally, providing approximately 15 cm of muscle. The blood supply arises from the radial artery, the radial recurrent artery, or both. The pedicle is approximately 3 cm in length, with a diameter of 1 mm. The innervation is the radial nerve. The skin incision is along a line from the lateral epicondyle to the radial styloid. Just volar and deep to the BR are the dorsal and lateral antebrachial cutaneous nerve, the superficial radial nerve, and the radial artery. The BR is cut slightly distal to the musculotendinous junction, and the tendon cuff is used for the flap inset. The rotation arc can be increased by safely ligating several perforating branches from the radial artery. It is not necessary to identify the recurrent radial artery or to release the origin of the BR. The subcutaneous tunnel is useful for reaching the defect site; however, that might compress the flap. Therefore, it is recommended to extend the skin incision. The muscle flap is inset and covered with a split-thickness skin graft if necessary (Fig. 23.7) [32].

Flexor Carpi Ulnaris Flap

This flap is a good choice for an antecubital lesion; however, it can also cover a defect of less than 3 cm for an olecranon tip lesion. The muscle belly of the FCU is 5 cm in width by 20 cm in length and extends to the proximal two-thirds of the forearm. The blood supply is the ulnar artery, with a smaller contribution from the posterior ulnar recurrent artery. The pedicle is approximately 2–3 cm in length and 1–2 mm in diameter. The skin incision is at the proximal third of the forearm on a line from the medial epicondyle to

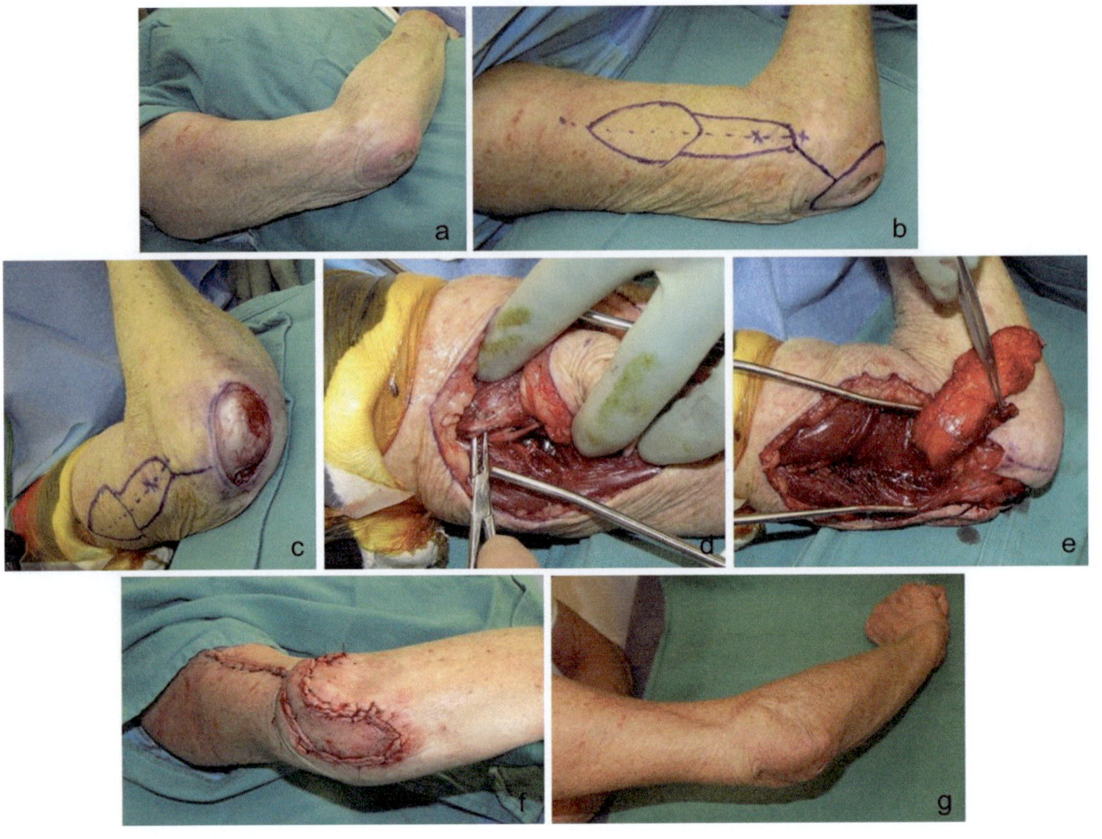

Fig. 23.5 (**a**) Chronic bursitis. (**b**) Flap design. (**c**) After debridement for olecranon bursitis. (**d**) The proximal pedicle is ligated (radial collateral artery). (**e**) The pedicle was dissected distally until it reached the lateral epicondyle. (**f**) The flap was rotated 180° and able to cover the entire elbow wound. (**g**) Four months postoperatively

the pisiform, taking care to preserve the medial antebrachial cutaneous nerve. The FCU muscle is identified and cut at the level of the musculotendinous junction. After identifying a feeding artery, the branches from the ulnar artery can be found in the proximal third of the forearm. The pivot point is approximately 6–8 cm from the elbow flexion crease (Fig. 23.8). Mobilize the FCU only enough to cover the defect, and then use a split-thickness skin graft to cover the exposed muscle belly. The FCU can also be split into its two heads, retaining one for ulnar deviation strength of the wrist [38]. The FCU flap is also used as the musculocutaneous flap. The donor skin lies on the muscle belly of the FCU in proximal third of the forearm. The skin paddle can be harvested with muscle for an area up to 6 by 10 cm.

Large to Massive-Sized Wounds

Latissimus Dorsi Musculocutaneous Flap

The LD muscle originates from the lower six thoracic vertebrae, thoracolumbar fascia, and the iliac crest. The insertion is the biceps groove of the humerus. The dominant vascular pedicle arises from the thoracodorsal artery with segmental perfusion from multiple lumbar perforators. The muscle is innervated by the thoracodorsal nerve, which originates from the posterior cord of the brachial plexus. With dimensions averaging 25–35 cm, this flap is a versatile, reliable, and technically straightforward option for pedicle coverage of the elbow and proximal forearm or

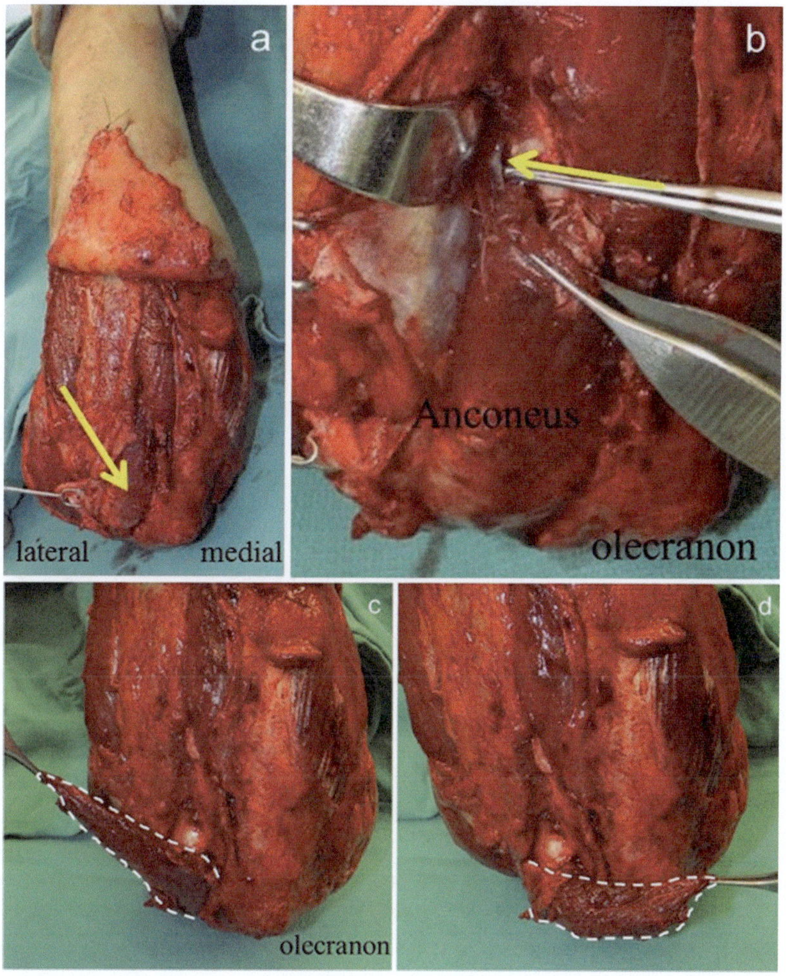

Fig. 23.6 (**a**) Exposure (*arrow*: anconeus). (**b**) The recurrent branch of the posterior interosseous artery. (**c, d**) The mobility of anconeus (*dotted line*: anconeus). Photos courtesy of Dr. Jennifer Waljee

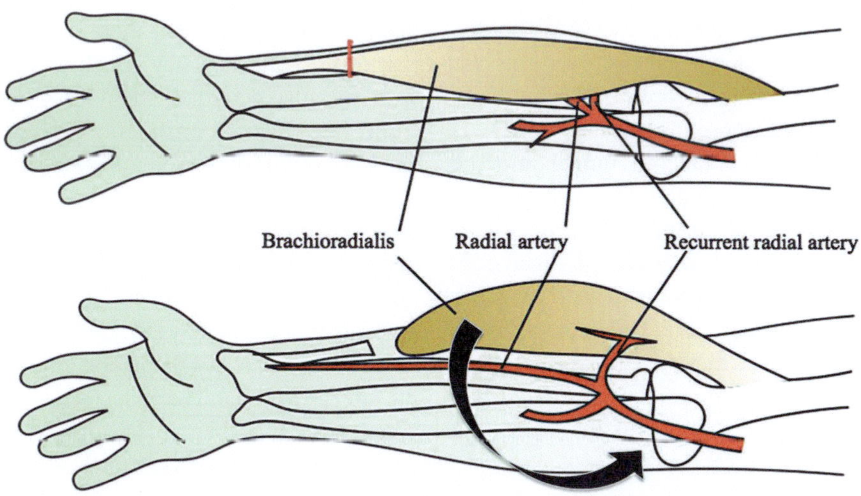

Fig. 23.7 The anatomy of BR and the arteries. After BR was cut, it is rotated to the olecranon

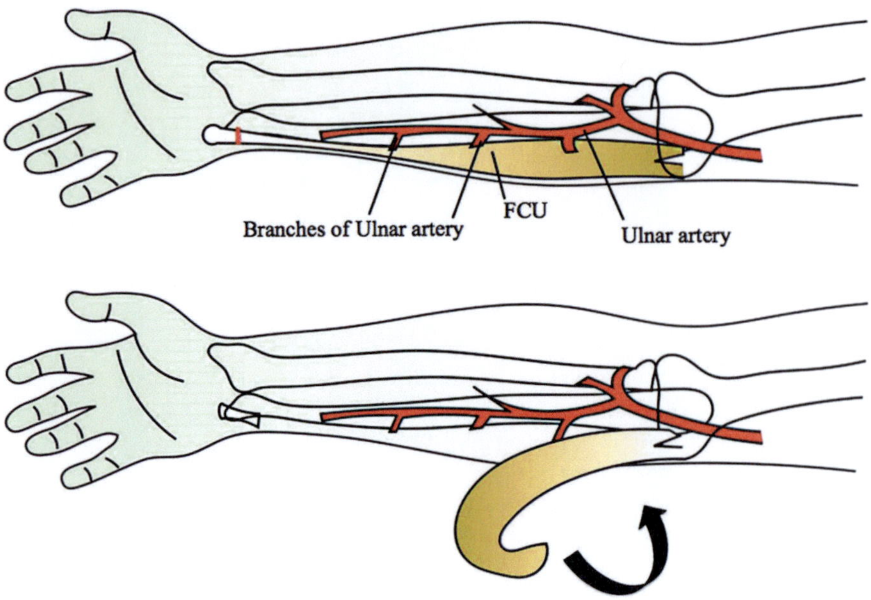

Fig. 23.8 The anatomy of FCU and the arteries. After FCU was cut, it is rotated to the olecranon

free flap coverage of massive forearm defects. The flap may also be used as a functional muscle transfer to restore elbow flexion or extension [24, 32]. The patient is placed in a lateral decubitus position. The incision is drawn several centimeters posterior of the LD and parallel with the anterior border of the LD. Then the dissection is made anteriorly to divide between the serratus anterior and the LD, and thoracodorsal neurovascular bundle is identified and preserved. The dissection is carried distally, the distal origins are cut, and then LD muscle is mobilized proximally and freed from the teres major. The muscle is passed through a subcutaneous tunnel into the arm to the elbow wound site. The technique of rotating the superficial surface to the deep surface of the flap allows more wide and distal coverage and avoids twisting the pedicle. The donor site is closed primarily, and drains need to be inserted for 1–2 weeks to reduce the formation of a seroma. A common complication is distal flap loss. Doppler scanning is useful for evaluating perfusion [39].

Anterolateral Thigh Flap

Considering the vulnerability of the blood vessels, a free flap that includes ALT is not recommended for patients with RA. However, Jensen and Moran reported a good clinical result of an ALT flap case for an RA patient who had an exposed elbow prosthesis [27]. Wang et al. reported on a review of 32 free flaps in patients with collagen vascular disorders and found that there was no increased risk of thrombosis. They concluded that patients with vascular disorders should not be precluded from free flap reconstruction. However, their reconstruction sites were the breast, head, and neck, not the elbow [40]. The potential flaps for reconstruction are cutaneous flap, musculocutaneous flap with tensor fascia lata and vastus lateralis muscle, and sensate flap with the lateral femoral cutaneous nerve. The blood supply is the descending branch of the lateral circumflex femoral artery (LCFA). The innervation is the lateral cutaneous femoral nerve. Perforators connect two veins; however, the perforator is absent in 2 % of people. The perforator of ALT flap is usually located within 3–4 cm of the midpoint of the line between the anterior superior iliac spine and lateral upper border of the patella. The Doppler device is useful for searching the perforator. The incision should be started from medial side. Because the perforator is easily found, the risk of perforator injury is low. If the perforator is absent, the anteromedial thigh flap can be used. The dissection is made from the supra fascia to the deep fascia and continues laterally. The perforator is identified under the deep fascia and is easily found at the medial portion of vastus lateralis muscle. Then the vascular pedicle is released for the bifurcation of LCFA. Thinning should be done before the vascular pedicle is cut. The coverage area extends up to 35 cm × 15 cm. The donor site can be closed primarily if the width of the flap is less than 8 cm. When the flap width is larger than 8 cm, a split-thickness skin graft is needed. The subsequent functional deficit is practically nonexistent [41, 42].

Postoperative Care

Various methods have been used to decrease complications that may occur following flap reconstruction:

1. Avoid applying excessive tensions to the vascular pedicle.
2. Elevate the elbow if possible in order to reduce edema and venous return.
3. Insert closed aspiration drains in both the donor and recipient sites.
4. Administer antibiotics for an appropriate period for chronic infection and exposure of the prosthesis.
5. Use aspirin to inhibit thrombosis and platelet aggregation in the anastomotic site.
6. Regularly monitor the flap for signs of ischemia and compromised venous return. If insufficiency of the artery or vein is confirmed early postoperatively, the pedicle should be explored as soon as possible.
7. Excessive edema may cause decreased blood supply, so release sutures until the edema decreases. If the insufficiency of the vein continues, repair is needed. If that is impossible, consider using leaches.

References

1. Souter WA. Surgery of the rheumatoid elbow. Ann Rheum Dis. 1990;49(Supp 2):871–82.
2. Mansat P. Surgical treatment of the rheumatoid elbow. Joint Bone Spine. 2001;68(3):198–210.
3. Munns JJ, Ruff ME. Rheumatoid nodules. J Hand Surg Am. 2014;39(4):765–7.
4. Gordon A, Stein L. The extra-articular features of rheumatoid arthritis a systematic analysis of 127 cases. Am J Med. 1973;54(4):445–52.
5. Kaye B, Kaye R, Bobrove A. Rheumatoid nodules review of the spectrum of associated conditions and proposal of a new classification, with a report of four seronegative cases. Am J Med. 1983;76(2):279–92.
6. Ruben BS, Connolly MK. Nodules in rheumatoid arthritis. In: Matucci-Cerinic M, Furst D, Fiorentino D, editors. Skin manifestations in rheumatic disease. New York: Springer; 2014. p. 133–8.
7. Hahn BH, Yardley JH, Stevens MB. Rheumatoid nodules in systemic lupus erythematosus. Ann Intern Med. 2014;72:49–58.
8. Khurana R, Berney SM. Clinical aspects of rheumatoid arthritis. Pathophysiology. 2005;12(3):153–65.
9. Ziff M. The rheumatoid nodule. Arthritis Rheum. 1990;33(6):761–7.
10. Verstappen SMM, Jacobs JWG, Bijlsma JWJ, Heurkens AHM, van Booma-Frankfort C, Ter Borg EJ, et al. Five-year follow-up of rheumatoid arthritis patients after early treatment with disease-modifying antirheumatic drugs versus treatment according to the pyramid approach in the first year. Arthritis Rheum. 2003;48(7):1797–807.
11. Kremer JM, Lee JKL. The safety and efficacy of the use of methotrexate in long-term therapy for rheumatoid arthritis. Arthritis Rheum. 1986;29(7):822–31.
12. Rosen A, Weiland AJ. Rheumatoid arthritis. Rheum Dis Clin North Am. 1998;24:101–28.
13. Ching DWT, Petrie JP, Klemp P, Jones JG. Injection therapy of superficial rheumatoid nodules. Rheumatology. 1992;31(11):775–7.
14. Arnold C. The management of rheumatoid nodules. Am J Orthop. 1996;25(10):706–8.

15. Ginsberg MH, Genant HK, Yu TF, Mccarty DJ. An unusual variant of rheumatoid disease. Arthritis Rheum. 1975;18(1):49–58.
16. Couret M, Combe B, Chuong VT, Leroux JL, Blotman F, Sany J. Rheumatoid nodulosis: report of two new cases and discussion of diagnostic criteria. J Rheumatol. 1988;15(9):1427–30.
17. Patatanian E, Dennis F. A review of methotrexate-induced accelerated nodulosis. Pharmacotherapy. 2002;22(9):1157–62.
18. Agarwal V, Aggarwal A, Misra R. Methotrexate induced accelerated nodulosis. J Assoc Physicians India. 2004;52:538–40.
19. Ishikawa H, Hirota K. Posterior interosseous nerve syndrome associated with rheumatoid synovial cysts of the elbow joint. Clin Orthop Relat Res. 1988; 254:134–9.
20. Millender L, Nalebuff E, Holdsworth D. Posterior interosseous-nerve secondary to rheumatoid syndrome synovitis. J Bone Joint Surg Am. 1973;55(4): 753–7.
21. Keret D, Porter K. Synovial cyst and ulnar nerve entrapment. A case report. Clin Orthop Relat Res. 1984;188:213–6.
22. Stewart NJ, Manzanares J, Morrey B. Surgical treatment olecranon bursitis. J Shoulder Elbow Surg. 1997;6:49–54.
23. Quayle J, Robinson M. A useful procedure in the treatment of chronic olecranon bursitis. Injury. 1978;9(4):299–302.
24. Jeon I-H, Morrey BF, Anakwenze OA, Tran NV. Incidence and implications of early postoperative wound complications after total elbow arthroplasty. J Shoulder Elbow Surg. 2011;20(6):857–65.
25. Gill DRJ, Morrey BF. The Coonrad-Morrey total elbow arthroplasty in patients who have rheumatoid arthritis. J Bone Jt Surg Am. 1998;80(9):1327–35.
26. Janis JE, Kwon RK, Attinger CE. The new reconstructive ladder: modifications to the traditional model. Plast Reconstr Surg. 2011;127 Suppl 1:205S–12.
27. Jensen M, Moran SL. Soft tissue coverage of the elbow: a reconstructive algorithm. Orthop Clin North Am. 2008;39(2):251–64.
28. Leininger BE, Rasmussen TE, Smith DL, Jenkins DH, Coppola C. Experience with wound VAC and delayed primary closure of contaminated soft tissue injuries in Iraq. J Trauma. 2006;61(5):1207–11.
29. Okamoto S, Tada K, Ai H, Tsuchiya H. Flexor carpi ulnaris muscle flap for soft tissue reconstruction after total elbow arthroplasty. Case Rep Surg. 2014; 2014:1–3.
30. Dee R. Total replacement arthroplasty of the elbow for rheumatoid arthritis. J Bone Joint Surg Br. 1972;54(1):88–95.
31. Jones NF, Jarrahy R, Kaufman MR. Pedicled and free radial forearm flaps for reconstruction of the elbow, wrist, and hand. Plast Reconstr Surg. 2008;121(3): 887–98.
32. Stevanovic M, Sharpe F. Soft-tissue coverage of the elbow. Plast Reconstr Surg. 2013;132(3):387e–402.
33. Teoh L-C. Lateral arm flap for upper limb coverage. In: Chung KC, editor. Operative techniques: hand and wrist surgery. 2nd ed. p. 444–50.
34. Maruyama Y, Takeuchi S. The radial recurrent fasciocutaneous flap: reverse upper arm flap. Br J Plast Surg. 1986;39(4):458–61.
35. Stevanovic M, Sharpe F, Schnall S, Angeles L, Itamura JM. Latissimus dorsi pedicle flap for coverage defects about the elbow of soft tissue. J Shoulder Elbow Surg. 1999;8(6):634–43.
36. Wang TY, Serletti JM, Kolasinski S, Low DW, Kovach SJ, Wu LC. A review of 32 free flaps in patients with collagen vascular disorders. Plast Reconstr Surg. 2012;129(3):421e–7.
37. Kimura N, Saito M, Sumiya Y, Itoh N. Reconstruction of hand skin defects by microdissected mini anterolateral thigh perforator flaps. J Plast Reconstr Aesthet Surg. 2008;61(9):1073–7.
38. Wang HT, Fletcher JW, Erdmann D, Levin LS. Use of the anterolateral thigh free flap for upper-extremity reconstruction. J Hand Surg Am. 2005;30(4):859–64.
39. Graham B, Adkins P, Scheker L. Complications and morbidity of the donor and recipient sites in 123 lateral arm flaps. J Hand Surg Br. 1992;17(2):189–92.
40. Adkinson JM, Chung KC. Flap reconstruction of the elbow and forearm: a case-based approach. Hand Clin. 2014;30(2):153–63.
41. Schmidt C, Kohut G, Greenberg J, Kann S, Idler R, Kiefhaber T. The anconeus muscle flap: its anatomy and clinical application. J Hand Surg Am. 1999;24(2): 359–69.
42. Wysocki RW, Gray RL, Fernandez JJ, Cohen MS. Posterior elbow coverage using whole and split flexor carpi ulnaris flaps: a cadaveric study. J Hand Surg Am. 2008;33(10):1807–12.

24 Arthroplasty Procedures for the Rheumatoid Elbow

Michael C. Glanzmann
and Hans-Kaspar Schwyzer

Introduction

Rheumatoid arthritis (RA) is characterized by polyarticular involvement, which typically manifests between the third and fifth decade of life. Almost two out of three patients suffering from RA have elbow problems. Data from our own patient experience showed that 53 % of rheumatoid patients developed elbow symptoms within the first 10 years after confirmation of the diagnosis [1]. Cases of isolated affected elbow are rare in RA. Pain is the main symptom for the affected elbow. Loss of extension as well as limitation of supination may be seen as an early sign of the disease, but a flexion deficit is rare. In contrast, juvenile RA is associated with an early loss of motion and ankylosis is more common, which makes treatment difficult. At the level of the elbow joint, progression of the disease is usually slow. In late-stage RA, bilateral elbow involvement is common. Radiographic findings usually correlate with clinical presentation for the rheumatoid elbow, in contrast to other joints such as the wrist and shoulder in which despite severe radiographic degenerative changes, patients may have reasonable function. Radiologic staging of the disease is based on the well-established classification of Larsen, Dale, and Eek (LDE, Fig. 24.1). Initially, osseous erosion is usually observed at the capitellum followed by the lateral epicondyle and olecranon [2]. A positive fat pad sign may be present in the case of exuberant joint effusion and distension of the fibrous capsule. Concomitant radiographic changes include bone demineralization and subchondral radiolucency. The inflammatory disease alters bony and ligamentous stabilizers leading to joint instability. Consequently, valgus deformity may occur. In the case of annular ligament destruction, volar subluxation of the radial head is typical. Approximately one out of five patients with rheumatoid elbow pathology may present with pressure neuropathies around the elbow. The primary goals of treatment are pain relief and restoration of joint function.

In the last decade, the introductions of effective pharmaceutical agents, namely, tumor necrosis factor (TNF) inhibitors, have contributed to reducing the signs and symptoms of the disease as well as slowing or halting radiographic damage. Pain remains the dominant complaint of RA patients, which may require surgical options if inflammation and swelling cannot be controlled by modern pharmacotherapy.

M.C. Glanzmann, MD (✉) • H.-K. Schwyzer, MD
Orthopaedics Upper Extremities, Schulthess Clinic
Zurich, Lengghalde 2, Zurich 8008, Switzerland
e-mail: michael.glanzmann@kws.ch

K.C. Chung (ed.), *Clinical Management of the Rheumatoid Hand, Wrist, and Elbow*,
DOI 10.1007/978-3-319-26660-2_24

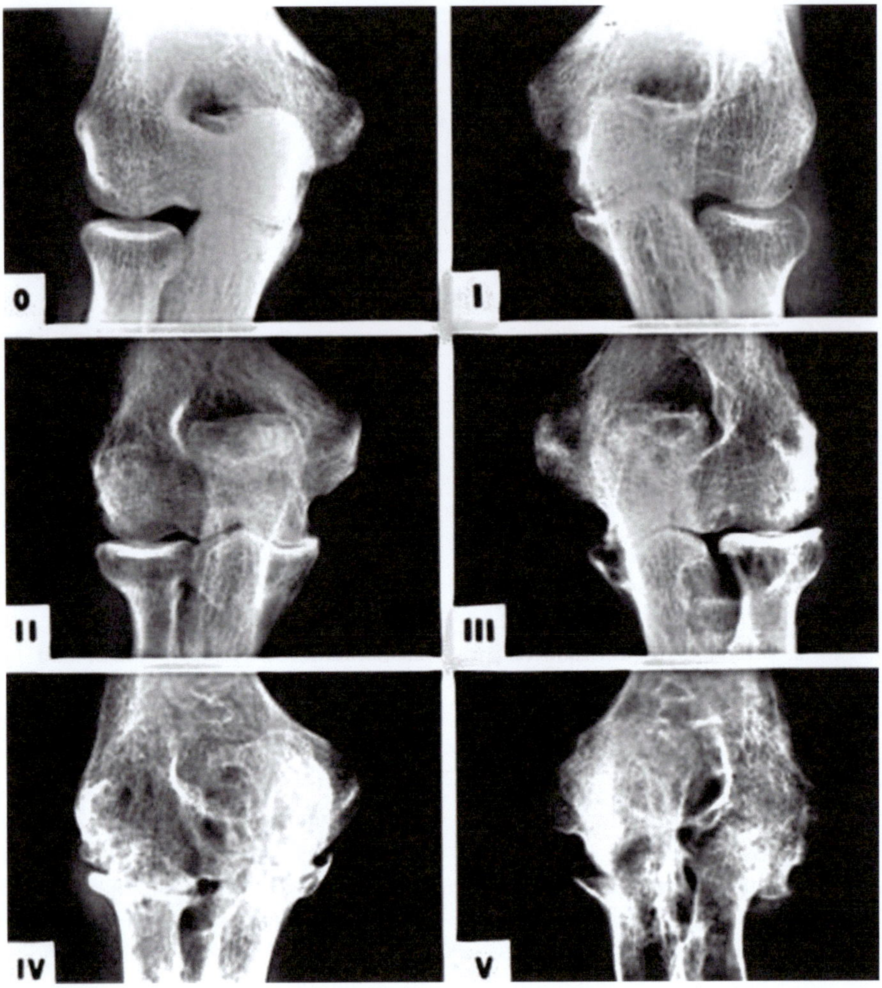

Fig. 24.1 Radiologic staging according to the Larsen–Dale–Eck classification

Surgical Options and Decision Making

Synovectomy

Removal of the inflamed synovial tissue from the affected joint by joint synovectomy and tenosynovectomy was an effective and common procedure for treating rheumatoid patients. Following the introduction of novel disease modifying antirheumatic drugs, the number of these procedures has dropped dramatically in our clinic. However, synovectomy is still a valuable option for patients with resistant synovitis unresponsive to pharmaceutical treatment and without articular surface destruction. By removing the inflamed synovium, antigen load within the joint is substantially reduced. In a study following 54 patients (70 rheumatoid elbow joints) after synovectomy, marked pain relief was documented in 40 % of the patients after a mean follow-up time of 7.5 years. Moderate improvement was still present in 38.5 % of all individuals [3]. Early synovectomy consistently offers a more favorable outcome compared to late-stage intervention [4]. Based on our experience, synovectomy at a late stage of RA is only justified to remove mechanical obstacles such as loose bodies. Arthroscopy offers the advantages of a minimally invasive technique as well as complete removal of the inflamed tissue. In general, it is considered as a valuable tool to postpone prosthetic procedures as long as the articular surface shows no major erosion. In a Scandinavian study, the reoperation rate following synovectomy of the rheumatoid elbow was 23 % within an average follow-up period of 5.2 years [5]. Synovectomy may be combined with radial head resection in cases of severe impairment of pronation and supination. In a cohort of age-matched patients, 45 cases of synovectomy and radial head excision were compared with the same number of cases who underwent total elbow joint replacement [6]. Both interventions appeared to be equally effective in restoration of range of motion and function, but the rate of complications was greater in the endoprosthetic group. Previous synovectomy does not have an effect on future attempts of elbow arthroplasty. In the case of apparent joint instability, synovectomy or radial head resection is contraindicated.

Resection Arthroplasty

In order to restore motion of ankylotic joints, Ollier described a resection arthroplasty as early as 1878. Due to his pioneer role in the surgical field of the locomotor apparatus, he is also named "the father of bone and joint surgery." During his time, Ollier felt that joint excision should be considered as a "last resort" procedure. Resection arthroplasty concurrently involves two competing states of instability and mobility, and the correct amount of bone to be removed is critical. Today, resection arthroplasty still plays a role in elbow revision surgery when periprosthetic joint infection is present or bone stock does not allow for implantation of an elbow prosthesis. Our experience shows that despite the imperfection of resection arthroplasty, it is not uncommon to still observe major clinical improvement in the overall status of the elbow. For the patient, a custom-made, light orthosis provides sufficient stability for daily activities and facilitates their ability to tolerate an otherwise flail elbow.

Total Elbow Replacement

Progression of elbow joint erosion in RA is usually slow. Owing to the natural course of the disease, regular radiographic surveillance of the patient is crucial. Severe bone loss may substantially impair reconstructive interventions. In the case of progressive articular surface destruction, pain and loss of function may become insufficiently handled with nonoperative means, and more aggressive options will need to be discussed with the patient. Despite the successful introduction of pharmaceutical agents, RA is still the most common diagnosis leading to the implantation of a total joint prosthesis. RA characteristically impairs the stability of the elbow. Therefore, total elbow replacement must be performed with an implant that provides some degree of stability within its design. Three elbow arthroplasty designs have these unique features:

1. *Constrained implants* have been abandoned due to the associated unacceptable high rates of loosening. This design allowed for motion in only one plane and led to high shear stresses at the bone–implant interface.
2. *Semiconstrained implants* provide an important amount of stability. A so-called floppy hinge allows between 8 and 10° of freedom in varus, valgus, and axial rotation. This feature significantly reduces the stress on the bone–cement interface that permits absorption of the forces through the surrounding soft tissues. Semiconstrained implants such as the Coonrad Morrey (Fig. 24.2) or GSB III prostheses have been used for more than three decades with only minor design modifications. The former prosthesis was adapted in terms of the central locking pin as well as the surface structure.
3. *Non-constrained implants* do not provide a mechanical link between the humeral and ulnar part. Approximately 25 % of rheumatoid elbows present with at least moderate instability, and as a result, these implants should not be used for RA patients. Under conditions

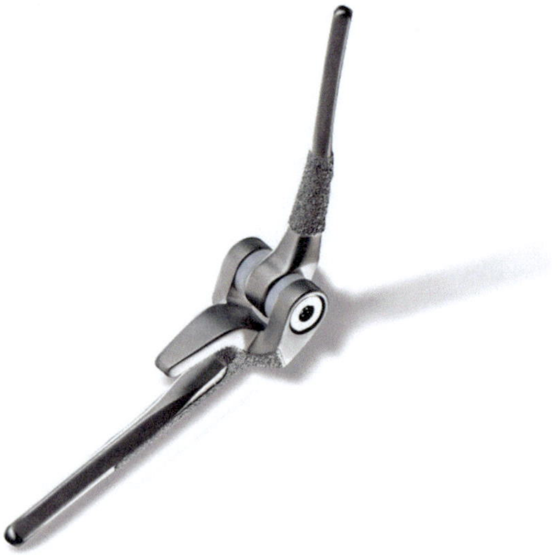

Fig. 24.2 The Coonrad–Morrey total elbow arthroplasty represents a semiconstrained implant allowing for 8–10° of freedom in varus, valgus, and axial rotation. The design has proven successful clinical results over the last three decades (with permission of Zimmer, Winterthur, Switzerland)

other than those associated with RA, this design may offer better preservation of elbow kinematics and bone stock.

Convertible implants have been designed in recent years and allow implantation of a hemiarthroplasty with the option of conversion to a conventional total joint replacement as required. In our clinic, these designs play no role in the surgical treatment of rheumatoid patients.

Fixation of the elbow prosthesis is generally achieved by cementing both humeral and ulnar components. Specific features of the implant such as a humeral flange provide additional rotational stability. In the case of a previously implanted shoulder arthroplasty, interference between the humeral stems can occur and must be taken into account when choosing the size of an elbow prosthesis, particularly the length of its humeral stem.

Indications for total elbow replacement in RA include symptomatic joint destruction (>grade III according to the LDE classification) and instability and/or loss of range of motion (<100°). In addition, total elbow replacement may be a valid option for acute rheumatoid elbow fractures with advanced degenerative changes.

In the presence of an acute or chronic infection, muscular paresis, critical skin conditions, or a lack of patient compliance, total elbow replacement is contraindicated. Planning of the intervention requires utmost diligence. Disease-modifying antirheumatic TNF-alpha blockers must be stopped in advance according to their half-life period, generally between 4 and 8 weeks prior to the surgery. Only after the wound has healed may TNF-alpha blockers be readministered. A multidisciplinary approach involving the surgeon, rheumatologist, and physical therapist is particularly important in managing rheumatoid patients prior to and after a surgical intervention. Frequently used agents such as methotrexate, sulfasalazine, and leflunomide may be continued perioperatively. Furthermore, detailed patient information is essential prior to the intervention. Patients must be aware that in the postoperative period, the physical capacity of the elbow will remain limited and weight placed on the operated arm must not exceed 5 kg.

Surgical Approaches

Whenever possible, a posterior approach preserving the extensor apparatus is performed. This allows for faster and less restricted rehabilitation and avoids extensor mechanism deficiency. Several surgical alternatives have been described to gain sufficient access while preserving the triceps. The entire triceps can be elevated and reflected either from the medial to the lateral side or vice versa from the lateral to the medial side as published by Bryan and Morrey [7]. After a straight posterior skin incision avoiding the tip of the olecranon, two skin flaps are raised and the ulnar nerve is identified. Transposition of the nerve is dependent on the surgeon's preference. Proximally the medial part of the triceps is developed, while at the distal end preparation follows the interval between the flexor carpi ulnaris and anconeus. Even for rheumatoid elbows, release of the medial and lateral collateral ligaments may be required to gain sufficient access to the joint. Furthermore, release of contracted flexor pronator and common extensor muscles allows for rebalancing of the soft tissues and should avoid later prosthesis malpositioning. Elevation of the triceps from the proximal ulna may incorporate a sliver of bone to enhance later healing. In this case, reattachment of the extensor apparatus is best performed through bone tunnels. If more exposure is needed, a triceps-reflecting anconeus pedicle (TRAP) approach offers a more extensile option to expose the elbow joint [8]; O'Driscoll described this approach for distal humerus fractures and nonunions with the advantage of avoiding an olecranon osteotomy. To develop the anconeus pedicle, the interval between the anconeus muscle and extensor carpi ulnaris is incised. The anconeus is dissected subperiosteally off the ulna and reflected with the entire triceps. On the medial side, the TRAP approach is similar to the Bryan–Morrey approach. Based on our practice, this approach is mainly used for revision cases.

Long-Term Outcome

Recent registry studies revealed similar survival rates associated with total elbow replacements. The overall survival rate for primary TEA in a Danish study of 324 prostheses was 90 % at 5 years and 81 % at 10 years [9]. Furthermore, the relative risk for revision was increased when a non-linked design was implanted [9]. These results are slightly inferior when compared to those associated with total shoulder arthroplasty. Current data show a revision-free survivorship of 96.1 % and 92.9 % at 5 and 10 years, respectively, for total shoulder replacement in rheumatoid patients. Within our institution, the survival rates of rheumatoid patients following implantation of a GSB III elbow prosthesis are 85 % at 10 years and 69 % at 20 years [10]. The risk of revision in rheumatoid patients is generally lower compared to post-traumatic conditions. Plaschke et al. (2013) found a 1.8-times increased relative risk for revision in post-traumatic elbow arthroplasties. In terms of recovery of function, both rheumatoid and post-traumatic elbow joints benefit from total elbow replacement. Pain-free and normal quality of life is restored in both groups, but functional deficits are reported to be larger in the rheumatoid group [11].

Complications

Gschwend and co-workers reported a high complication rate of 43 % after TEA. According to Cook et al., total elbow replacement in rheumatoid patients is not generally associated with an increased risk of perioperative complications compared to nonrheumatoid patients [12].

Intraoperative fractures rarely occur during TEA. Nevertheless, inflammatory erosion may weaken the osseous stability. Resection of the humeral trochlea and rasping of the canal must be performed meticulously to prevent a fracture of the condyles. Even for preparation of the ulna, similar technical diligence is also required. Excessive resection of the olecranon will compromise reattachment of the extensor apparatus. Perforation of the humeral or ulnar cortices must be avoided during reaming of the canals. Extrusion of bone cement may cause thermal injuries at a later stage of the procedure.

Wound healing following TEA is a sensitive issue and is even more critical for rheumatoid elbows because soft tissue protection around this joint is minimal. Postoperative bracing in extension may reduce tension on the skin flaps. Active range of motion exercises may be started early, but forced extension must be avoided for 6–8 weeks after surgery to allow healing of the extensor apparatus.

Infections occur more frequently following elbow arthroplasty compared to replacement surgery of other joints. Rheumatoid patients are particularly at risk when undergoing concomitant immunosuppressive treatment. The deep infection rate is approximately 3–17 % with both *Staphylococcus aureus* and *epidermidis* being the pathogens. Management of periprosthetic infection is dependent on the time after the last surgical intervention, the duration of symptoms, microbial results, and the degree of the damaged infected tissue. Repetitive debridement with implant retention is often the first line of defense. If septic loosening is present, exchange of the prosthesis becomes necessary. The authors' surgical preference involves a two-stage exchange with a prosthesis-free interval and antibiotic treatment spanning several months before reimplantation of the prosthesis [13]. According to published data from the Mayo Clinic, 5 % of all patients undergoing primary TEA will sustain a *periprosthetic fracture* in the future. The reasons for this "difficult-to-treat" complication are manifold, in which the main risk factors of poor bone quality and osteoporosis particularly affect the rheumatoid patient. Aseptic loosening, noncompliance of the weight restriction for the elbow (5 kg), or previous surgeries are further risk factors for periprosthetic elbow fractures. Nonoperative treatment of a periprosthetic elbow fracture is associated with a high risk of fibrous nonunion. If the stability of the implant is compromised, its exchange in combination with the use of a long-stem design is often mandatory. Especially for rheumatoid patients, the surgeon must consider the possibility of interference with a shoulder implant when planning a revision. Severe loss of bone stock often calls for bone grafting using allograft struts. In the case of intact implant stability, a humeral shaft fracture may be treated with immobilization.

Rheumatoid patients undergoing TEA are specifically vulnerable to *triceps insufficiency* owing to poor bone and tendon quality in the area of the olecranon. From the basic concept of "staying out of trouble is easier than getting out of trouble," surgical techniques involving elbow exposures have evolved. Approaches used for rheumatoid patients must prevent triceps splitting and should try to reflect the entire extensor apparatus either to the medial or lateral side. Despite preservation and meticulous reattachment of the triceps, some degree of weakness of the extensor mechanism is a common outcome following TEA.

Exposure of the *ulnar nerve* is a standard part of every elbow joint replacement surgery. Depending on the surgeon's preference, the ulnar nerve can be transposed anteriorly. Ulnar neuropathies are not uncommon in the early postoperative phase, but spontaneous resolution of the symptoms can be expected as long as traction and thermal injuries are avoided during the procedure. For revision cases that require strut allografts, a more extensile approach is needed that can compromise the radial nerve. For enhanced protection in such cases, we recommend the dissection of the radial nerve during its course below the lateral head of the triceps.

Revision of Total Elbow Arthroplasty

Several studies have demonstrated a decreasing trend in the number of orthopedic surgical procedures undertaken for the treatment of lower and upper limbs affected by RA. Although the prevalence of RA and the demographic characteristics have remained significantly unchanged throughout the last two decades, modern therapeutic drug regimens are largely responsible for this trend. At the authors' institution, these trends are also clearly visible: in 1985, 12 primary TEAs were implanted and two revisions of a TEA were performed. In 2012, this number decreased to seven primary implantations, whereas the number of revisions increased to 16. Another interesting finding is a diverging trend between shoulder and elbow replacements. In 1985, the relation between total elbow arthroplasty (TEA) and total shoulder arthroplasty was 12:14, whereas these numbers shifted to 7:216 for primary arthroplasty surgery and 16:26 for revision arthroplasty interventions by 2012. At the level of the elbow, RA is still the main indication for placing an elbow prosthesis, yet rheumatoid shoulder patients are a rare group in patient cohorts receiving a TSA.

Revision of a failed elbow arthroplasty demonstrates common crucial points. Frequently, bone stock has to be augmented following aseptic loosening or in case of a two-stage revision after a periprosthetic infection. Strut allografts may be used in combination with cerclage wires or plates. Invagination of a strut allograft is another technique available to support the intramedullary canal of the ulna.

Clinical Case 1

Eight years after implantation of a TEA, a 60-year-old female patient experienced a superficial skin lesion at the operated elbow. Oral antibiotics were prescribed by the general practitioner. Symptoms were progressive and due to persistent signs of local infection, the patient was referred to the orthopedic center. Radiographic assessment indicated intact implant stability but laboratory tests and outcome of the arthrocentesis

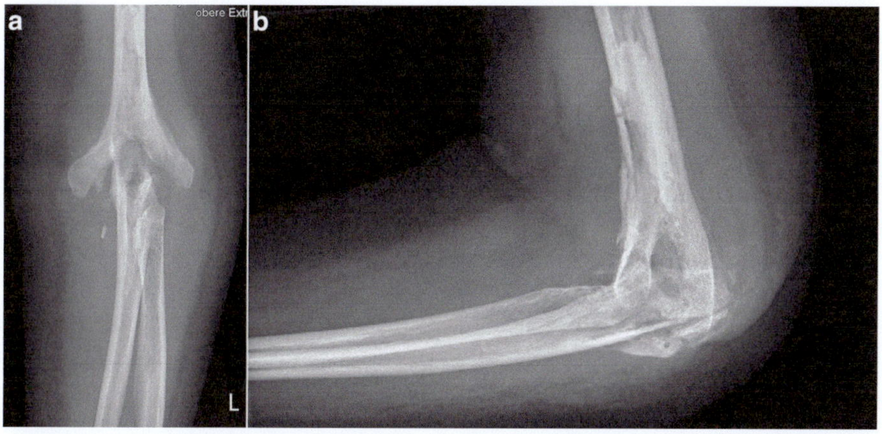

Fig. 24.3 (**a**, **b**) Anteroposterior and lateral radiograph of the left elbow after the first stage of the revision showing remnants of cement in the humeral intramedullary canal after explantation of an infected TEA. The condyles remained intact but moderate bone loss was noted due to the infection and perioperative trauma

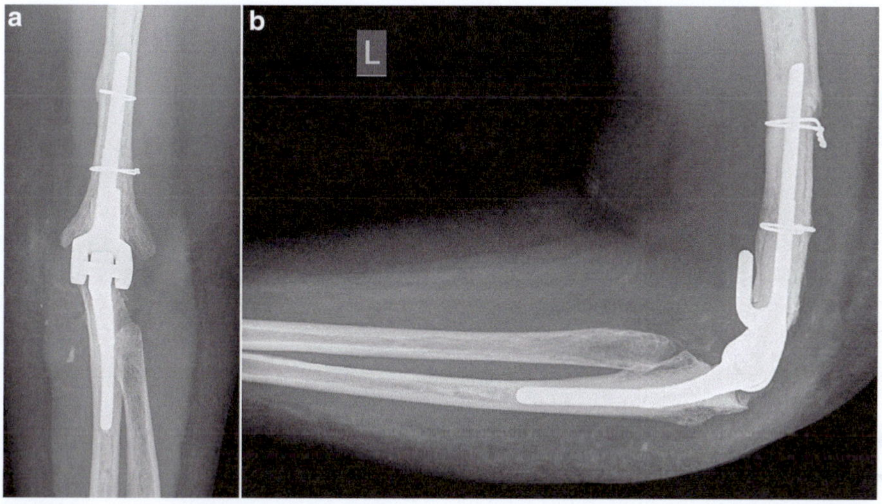

Fig. 24.4 (**a**, **b**) Radiographs after the second stage of revision demonstrate the cemented semiconstrained TEA (Coonrad–Morrey) in situ. In order to completely remove the cement remnants, fenestration of the distal humerus was performed with two cerclage wires

showed clear signs of a bacterial infection. After interdisciplinary discussion of the case, a two-stage revision was performed. The explanted prosthesis was sonicated and a total of eight bone and soft tissue samples were obtained for cultivation. All microbiological tests were positive for *Staphylococcus aureus* (Fig. 24.3). After a 2-week intravenous antibiotic treatment regime, an oral course of the antimicrobial therapy was undertaken for a further 6 weeks. Reimplantation was performed following an antibiotic free interval of 3 weeks. During the revision surgery, a prophylactic antibiotic regimen was carried out until all samples obtained during reimplantation were reported negative. Despite the infection and prior removal of a cemented implant, bone stock was still favorable and allowed for implantation of the same type of implant (i.e., Coonrad–Morrey; Zimmer, Winterthur, Switzerland; Fig. 24.4).

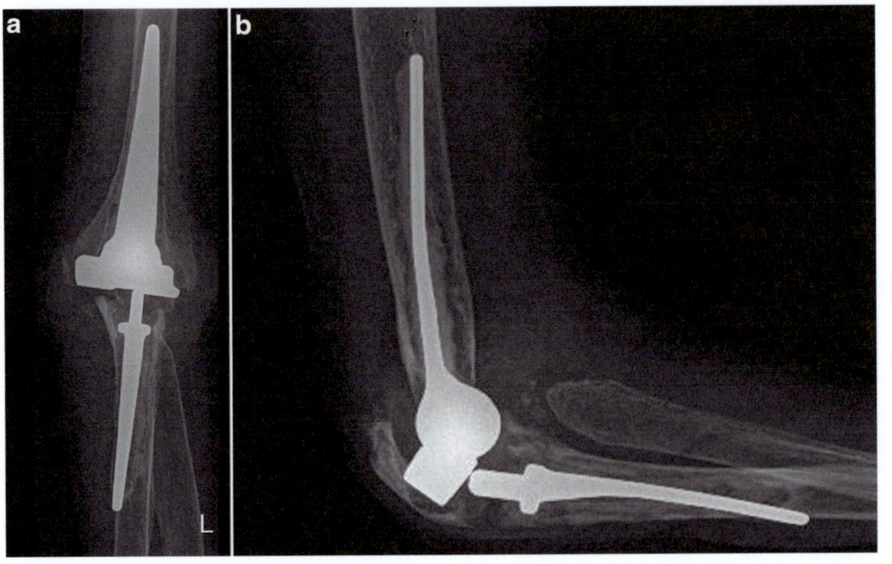

Fig. 24.5 (**a**, **b**) Eleven years post-TEA, the radiographs show decoupling of the two components and perforation of the ulnar stem through the posterior cortex. Furthermore, there is discontinuity of the extensor apparatus due to an olecranon fracture. Marked signs of loosening can be identified at the bone–cement interface on both the humeral and ulnar side

Clinical Case 2

A 72-year-old female rheumatoid patient presented with ongoing elbow pain and major functional deficits of her dominant left arm. A cemented semiconstrained TEA (GSB III, Zimmer, Winterthur, Switzerland) had been implanted 11 years ago. Radiographic work-up demonstrated a combination of several complications: aseptic loosening of the humeral and ulnar component, distal perforation of the ulnar stem, decoupling of the components, and an olecranon fracture (Fig. 24.5). Signs of infection were absent. A one-stage revision was performed using a long-stem prosthesis with a different design offering fixed coupling (Coonrad–Morrey). In addition, a strut allograft was invaginated into the proximal ulna to support bony stability. Using a plate, the extensor apparatus including the fractured tip of the olecranon was reattached to the ulna. Interference with the proximal and distal implants of the adjacent shoulder and wrist joint could be avoided (Figs. 24.6, 24.7, 24.8, and 24.9).

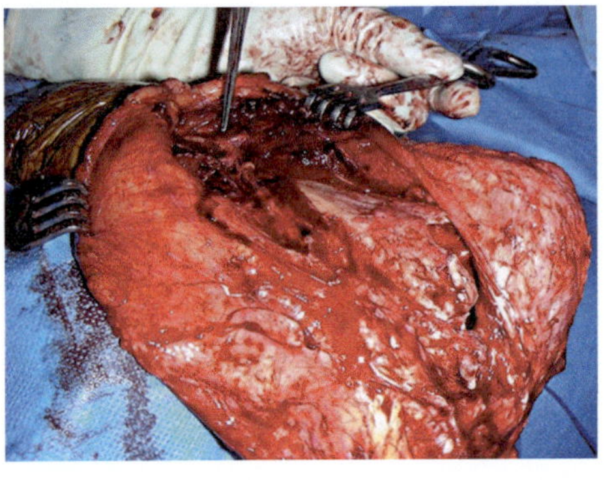

Fig. 24.6 Intraoperative situs of a hanging left elbow with the patient in a lateral decubitus position: an extensile approach was used for improved visualization. The pincers mark the radial nerve, which has been dissected under the lateral head of the triceps. In order to avoid weakening of the extensor mechanism, the triceps was elevated and reflected in toto

Conclusion

The number of TEAs in rheumatoid patients is decreasing owing to the efficacy of modern drug therapies. Nevertheless, TEA is a powerful tool to treat advanced joint degeneration and instability.

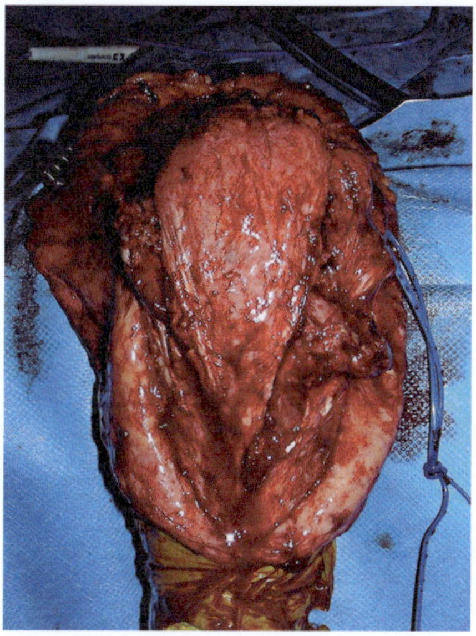

Fig. 24.7 Upon completion of the revision, the extensor apparatus is put back in its original position and secured with transosseous sutures. The ulnar nerve was not transposed based on the authors' discretion

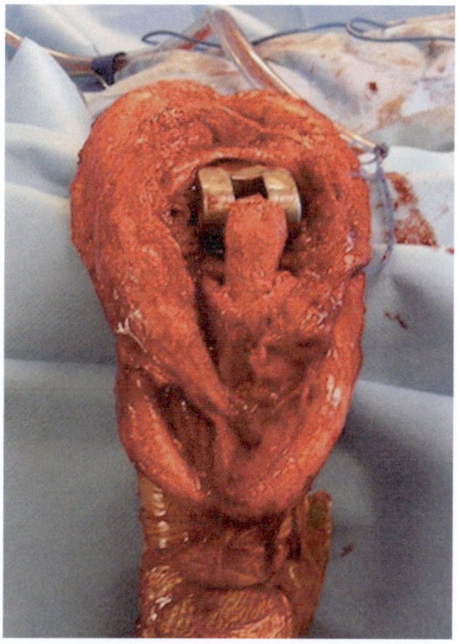

Fig. 24.8 Intraoperative photograph of the final assembled prosthesis and the strut allograft, which was introduced into the ulnar shaft

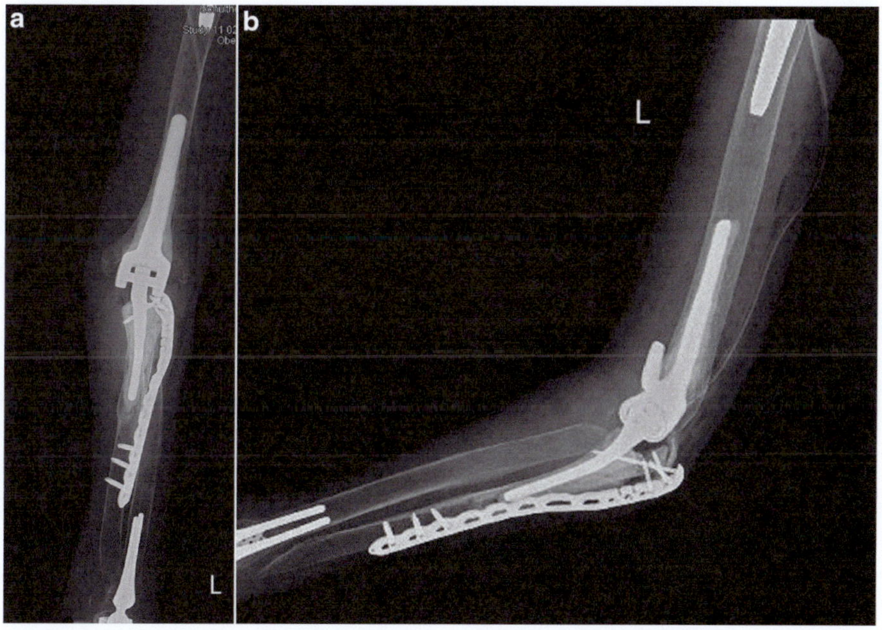

Fig. 24.9 (**a**, **b**) Radiographs after the one-stage revision show the new cemented semiconstrained implant in place. Augmentation of the proximal ulna was achieved with a strut allograft invaginated into the intramedullary canal. The olecranon fracture was reduced with a locking compression plate. Interference with the neighboring arthroplasties of the shoulder and wrist joints was avoided

The potential risks are high and must be minimized by every means: careful preoperative planning together with the treating rheumatologist is imperative and improved surgical techniques should help to avoid extensor mechanism insufficiencies. Once a TEA has been implanted, lifelong meticulous skin care and compliance in terms of weight restrictions are mandatory to optimally protect the prosthesis from infection and aseptic loosening. In the case of a periprosthetic infection, implant stability and the duration of symptoms are the guiding signs for further treatment. If symptoms are acute and implant stability is intact, irrigation and debridement with retention of the implant are the first line of defense. In the case of septic loosening, a two-stage revision is recommended. For recurrent infections, a resection arthroplasty might offer less risk with comparable pain reduction in contrast to additional reimplantations, which the authors only consider with great caution.

References

1. Gschwend N. Die operative Behandlung der chronischen Polyarthritis. Thieme. 1977;47–68.
2. Lehtinen JT, Kaarela K, Ikavalko M, et al. Incidence of elbow involvement in rheumatoid arthritis. A 15 year endpoint study. J Rheumatol. 2001;28(1): 70–4.
3. Vahvanen V, Eskola A, Peltonen J. Results of elbow synovectomy in rheumatoid arthritis. Arch Orthop Trauma Surg. 1991;110(3):151–4.
4. Tanaka N, Sakahashi H, Hirose K, Ishima T, Ishii S. Arthroscopic and open synovectomy of the elbow in rheumatoid arthritis. J Bone Joint Surg Am. 2006;88(3):521–5.
5. Maenpaa HM, Kuusela PP, Kaarela K, Kautiainen HJ, Lehtinen JT, Belt EA. Reoperation rate after elbow synovectomy in rheumatoid arthritis. J Shoulder Elbow Surg. 2003;12(5):480–3.
6. Woods DA, Williams JR, Gendi NS, Mowat AG, Burge PD, Carr AJ. Surgery for rheumatoid arthritis of the elbow: a comparison of radial-head excision and synovectomy with total elbow replacement. J Shoulder Elbow Surg. 1999;8(4):291–5.
7. Bryan RS, Morrey BF. Extensive posterior exposure of the elbow. A triceps-sparing approach. Clin Orthop Relat Res. 1982;166:188–92.
8. O'Driscoll SW. The triceps-reflecting anconeus pedicle (TRAP) approach for distal humeral fractures and nonunions. Orthop Clin North Am. 2000;31(1): 91–101.
9. Plaschke HC, Thillemann T, Belling-Sorensen AK, Olsen B. Revision total elbow arthroplasty with the linked Coonrad-Morrey total elbow arthroplasty: a retrospective study of twenty procedures. Int Orthop. 2013;37(5):853–8.
10. Schoni M, Drerup S, Angst F, Kyburz D, Simmen BR, Goldhahn J. Long-term survival of GSB III elbow prostheses and risk factors for revisions. Arch Orthop Trauma Surg. 2013;133(10):1415–24.
11. Angst F, Goldhahn J, John M, Herren DB, Simmen BR. Comparison of rheumatic and post-traumatic elbow joints after total elbow arthroplasty. Comprehensive and specific evaluation of clinical picture, function, and quality of life. Orthopade. 2005;34(8): 794, 6–800.
12. Cook C, Hawkins R, Aldridge 3rd JM, Tolan S, Krupp R, Bolognesi M. Comparison of perioperative complications in patients with and without rheumatoid arthritis who receive total elbow replacement. J Shoulder Elbow Surg. 2009;18(1):21–6.
13. Spormann C, Achermann Y, Simmen BR, et al. Treatment strategies for periprosthetic infections after primary elbow arthroplasty. J Shoulder Elbow Surg. 2012;21(8):992–1000.

Case-Based Examples of Management of Rheumatoid Elbow

25

Massimo Ceruso, Prospero Bigazzi, and Sandra Pfanner

Case-Based Examples of Management of Rheumatoid Elbow

The algorithm of treatment of the rheumatoid elbow is derived from the understanding of the developmental aspects of the disease [1, 2]. Similarly to what has been clearly outlined for the wrist [3], three evolving patterns may be described for the rheumatoid elbow: the lytic, the degenerative type, and the ankylotic. Accordingly, the therapeutic choices vary in line with the stage of the disease [4, 5] and its evolution trend [6]. There is, however, a substantial difference in dealing with the surgical options for the wrist or the elbow, because joint fusion is an absolute contraindication for the elbow as this represents an unsuitable functional limitation for the patient.

In planning the surgical treatment of a rheumatoid elbow, one should also take into account the condition of the ipsilateral DRUJ, given the strict biomechanical link between the proximal radioulnar joint (PRUJ) and distal radioulnar joint (DRUJ) in forearm pronosupination [7]. Further issues to be considered are the potential coexisting involvement of the radiocarpal joint and hand, the rotator cuff, and shoulder joint, as well as the multi-articular pattern of the disease. The patient's functional needs and expectations should also be discussed, and they should concur to the tailoring of the surgical program and rehabilitation.

A classification of the different modalities of the rheumatoid elbow involvement should be able to support the therapeutic indication. The bone stock quality and the tendency to bone resorption, cyst formation, and progressive instability versus ankylosis [8–10] should be clearly appraised. In this regard, the Larson's staging, even if handy to be used, should only be considered as a radiographic definition of the current state of the affected joint and may not have sufficient clinical relevance.

Our algorithm of treatment is based on classifying five different conditions:

1. Synovitis, antalgic ROM reduction; normal appearing joint.
2. Synovitis, minor ROM reduction; loss of joint space, maintenance/minimal alteration of the subchondral architecture:
   a. Uniform
   b. Prevailing involvement of the radial compartment

M. Ceruso, MD (✉) • P. Bigazzi, MD, PhD
S. Pfanner, MD
Orthopaedics, Division of Hand Surgery and Microsurgery, Azienda Ospedaliero-Universitaria Careggi, Firenze, CTO largo P.Palagi 1, Florence 50139, Italy
e-mail: cerusom@tin.it

K.C. Chung (ed.), *Clinical Management of the Rheumatoid Hand, Wrist, and Elbow*,
DOI 10.1007/978-3-319-26660-2_25

3. Joint stable, ROM reduction, marked joint space narrowing, cyst formation
4. Instability; gross deformity ("wet type")
5. Ankylosis

Treatment options can be referred to each stage or pattern as follows:

1. Synovitis, antalgic ROM reduction; normal appearing joint:
   i. Synovectomy (either arthroscopic or open)
2. Synovitis, minor ROM reduction; loss of joint space, maintenance/minimal alteration of the subchondral architecture:
   a. Uniform:
      i. Synovectomy
   b. Prevailing involvement of the radial compartment:
      i. Synovectomy + radial head resection (stable joint)
      ii. Synovectomy + lateral elbow implant (unstable joint, capitulum humeri involved)
      iii. Synovectomy + anconeus muscle arthroplasty (JIA)
3. Joint stable, ROM reduction, marked joint space narrowing, cyst formation
   i. Late synovectomy
   ii. Resurfacing TEA (stable joint—well preserved capsuloligamentous structures)
   iii. Semi-constrained TEA (tendency to instability)
4. Instability gross deformity ("wet type")
   i. Semi-constrained TEA
5. Ankylosis
   i. Semi-constrained TEA
   ii. Interposition arthroplasty (JIA)

Case Examples

Case 1 (Elbow Late Synovectomy)

A 48-year-old patient affected by rheumatoid arthritis since the age of 25. The onset of the disease was synovitis of the left wrist. She has multiple joint involvement including the contralateral wrist, the right elbow, the left knee, bilateral ankle, forefoot, and cervical spine. In her 30s she underwent an open synovectomy of both wrists, Darrach procedure on the left wrist, and a hemiresection of the ulnar head on the right. In 2004 she underwent right ankle synovectomy and left subtalar fusion. She is under medication with a weekly administration of etanercept—50 mg, since 9 years.

Two years ago she was referred to us because of increasing pain and functional impairment of her right elbow. Her joint was stable with an antalgic ROM limitation. X-ray showed joint space narrowing and cyst formation (Fig. 25.1). After discussing with her the available treatment options, and taking into consideration her age, activity and preferences, an open "late" synovectomy of the right elbow was performed (Fig. 25.2) [11, 12]. A posterior triceps sparing approach was used in order not to interfere with a possible future revision to a total elbow arthroplasty. To date she has good pain control and she has regained a complete elbow ROM (Figs. 25.3 and 25.4). She was recently scheduled for a left wrist arthrodesis.

Case 2 (Bilateral Total Elbow Implant)

Long-standing systemic RA. The patient had been first diagnosed at the age of 52. At the age of 66, he was referred to us with a bilateral painful elbow. Radiographs showed marked bilateral joint space narrowing and articular erosions (Figs. 25.5 and 25.6). Medical treatment had been hydroxychloroquine for the first 10 years; it had later been changed to methotrexate and steroids.

In 1998 he underwent a semi-constrained total left elbow arthroplasty (Coonrad–Morrey implant); 2 years after, he had a contralateral right elbow TEA.

The right ulnar component had to be revised after 3 years for aseptic loosening due to the anterior impingement of the humeral component flange with the coronoid (Figs. 25.7 and 25.8). He is now pain-free with a good functional long-term result (Fig. 25.9. Left TEA FU, 16 years; right elbow FU, 14 years).

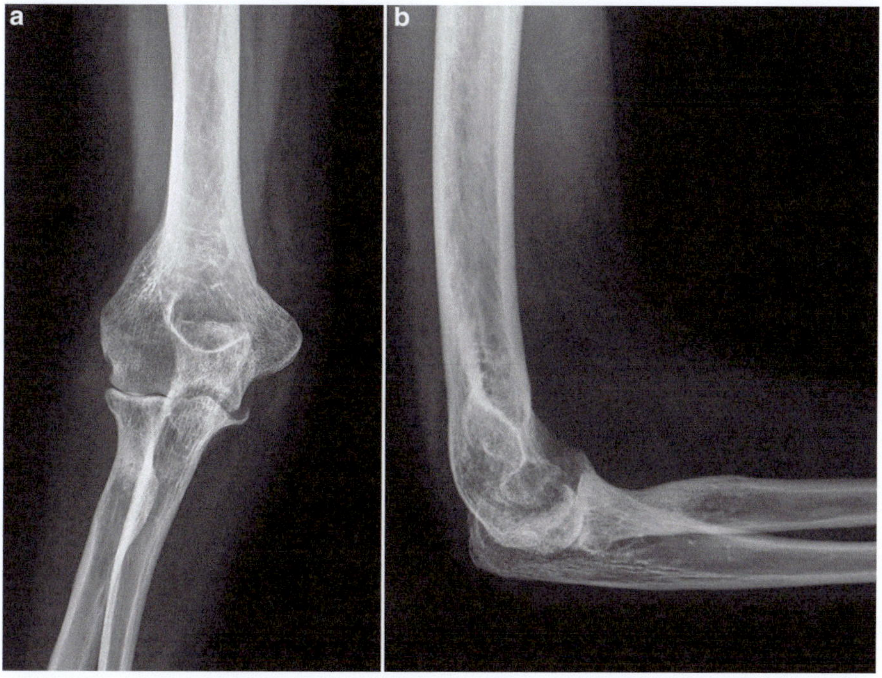

Fig. 25.1 (**a**, **b**) Elbow late synovectomy: preoperative X-rays. Note joint space narrowing and cyst formation, no major bone deformity

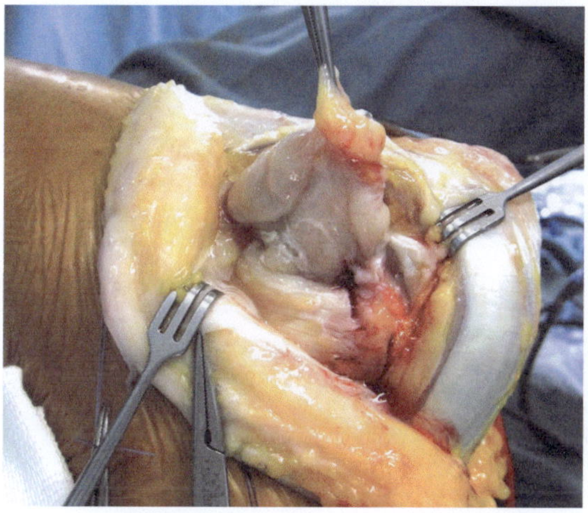

Fig. 25.2 Elbow late synovectomy: posterior triceps sparing approach

Case 3 (Homolateral TEA and TWA)

Juvenile idiopathic arthritis. The patient was referred to us at the age of 37. She had a multi-articular involvement, with the upper limb joints prevailing. In 2003 she had a total left wrist fusion together with EIP to EPL tendon transfer as EPL tendon rupture had occurred some months before. Eight months later she underwent a total right elbow arthroplasty (Figs. 25.10 and 25.11—Coonrad–Morrey implant). In 2005 the evolution of her right wrist arthropathy led us to consider a new surgical treatment. Given the pre-existing homolateral elbow implant, the contralateral wrist arthrodesis, and the age and work requirements of the patient, we discussed with her the pros and cons of a total wrist arthroplasty versus a bilateral wrist fusion. A total wrist implant was then chosen (Fig. 25.12).

In 2010 a CMC arthroplasty of the basal joint of her left thumb was also performed; a pyrocarbon spacer was implanted and a MP thumb fusion was associated (Fig. 25.13).

Two years ago the humeral component of the right elbow implant had to be revised for aseptic loosening due to the polyethylene wear debris (Fig. 25.14).

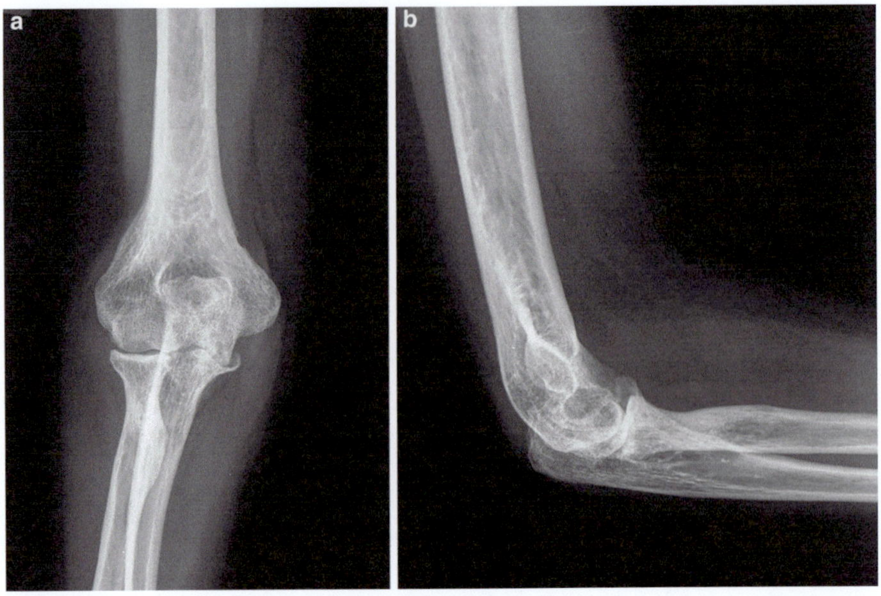

Fig. 25.3 (**a**, **b**) Elbow late synovectomy: X-rays at 2-year follow-up

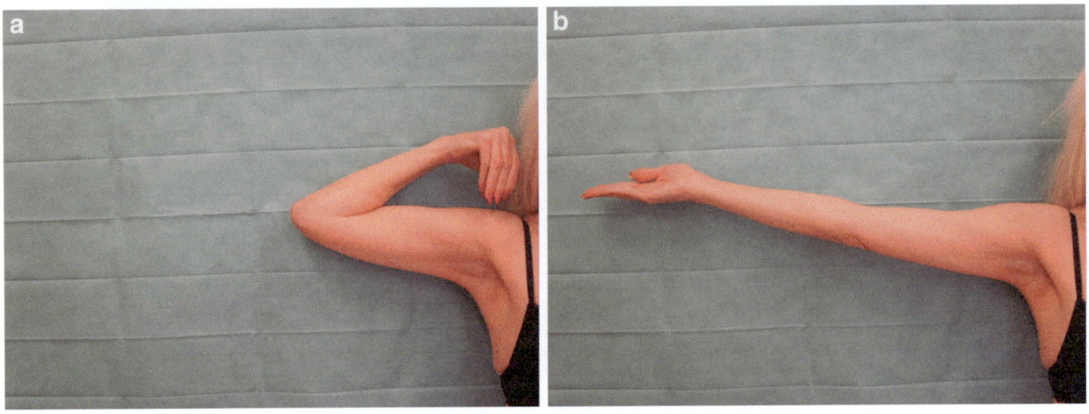

Fig. 25.4 (**a**, **b**) Elbow late synovectomy: ROM at 2-year follow-up

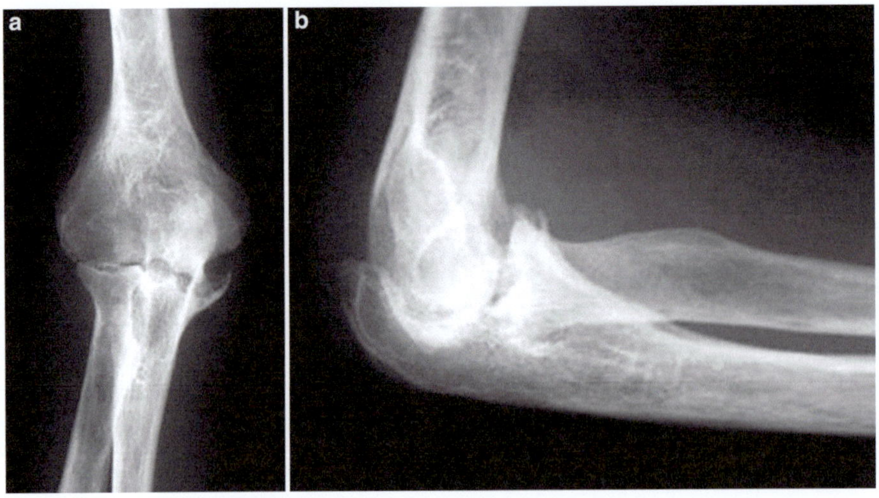

Fig. 25.5 (**a**, **b**) Bilateral TEA: right elbow preoperative X-rays

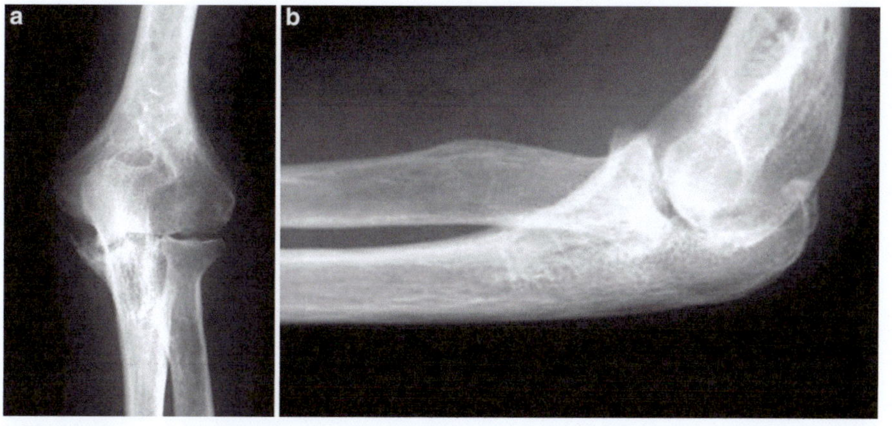

Fig. 25.6 (**a**, **b**) Bilateral TEA: left elbow preoperative X-rays

Fig. 25.7 (**a**, **b**) Bilateral TEA: right elbow X-rays at 14-year follow-up

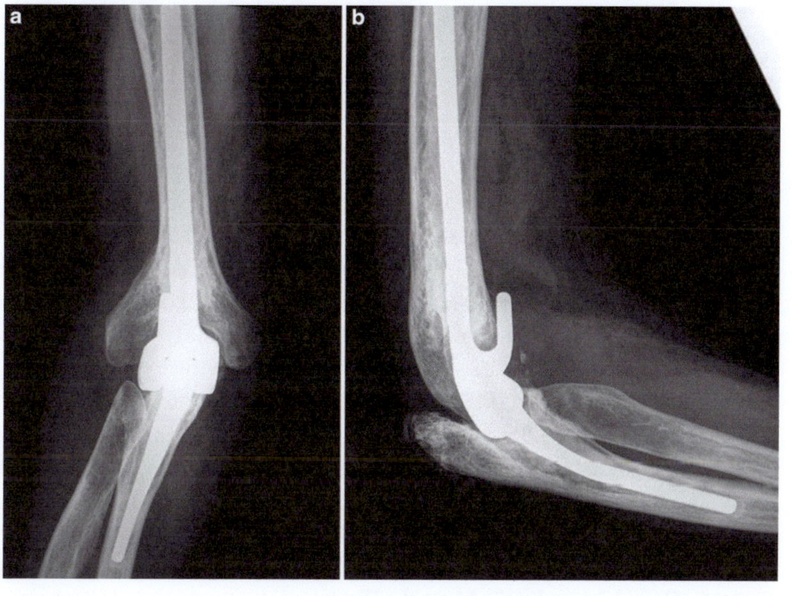

Case 4 (Total Semi-constrained Discovery Implant)

Psoriatic oligoarthritis. Pain and swelling at the right elbow started at the age of 35. Since then, the right elbow condition remained the patient's major complaint because of the synovitis and painful joint instability that prevented him from doing his job. Despite biologic medication (methotrexate and adalimumab), his articular conditions continued to get worse. Daily activities and bed rest were also impaired. At the age of 54 he had an Achilles tendon rupture, treated with a percutaneous suture and complicated by

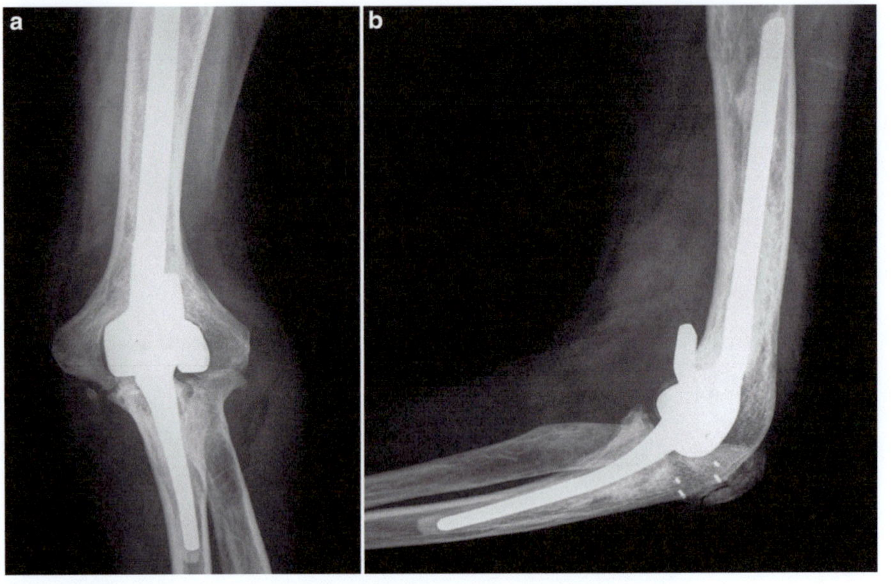

Fig. 25.8 (**a**, **b**) Bilateral TEA: left elbow X-rays at 16-year follow-up

thrombosis of the superficial femoral vein. At the age of 55 X-rays show gross deformity, malalignment and major erosion of the elbow joint (Fig. 25.15). A semi-constrained TEA (Discovery Elbow System) was implanted [13]. At 2-year follow-up he has a stable, painless joint and a subtotal functional ROM (flexion–extension: 10°–130°) (Fig. 25.16). He was able to resume his previous activity as a clay and bronze sculptor. He wears an elbow brace for his heavier activities.

Case 5 (Brachioradialis Muscle Flap to Repair Dorsal Skin Dehiscence after TEA)

Polyarticular RA. Onset of the disease at the age of 20. The patient had undergone multiple total joint arthroplasties (bilateral elbow, bilateral knee and left hip).

She responded poorly to biologic therapy, and she needed high doses of corticosteroids and NSAIDs (nonsteroidal anti-inflammatory drugs). In 2004 she was operated on the right elbow (stage 4) with a semi-constrained Coonrad–Morrey total elbow implant. Six months later she fell on her contralateral elbow and caused a fracture at the distal third of the humerus. Taking account of the severe pre-existing arthritic condition of the joint and the distal site of the fracture, we chose to treat both lesions with a total joint replacement. Two months after surgery, she developed a dystrophic skin lesion over the olecranon that eventually evolved into a pressure ulcer exposing the bone (Fig. 25.17). A brachioradialis muscle rotation flap was then performed (Fig. 25.18) [14] to reconstruct the posterior soft tissue coverage and padding of the elbow with a good long-term follow-up (Fig. 25.19).

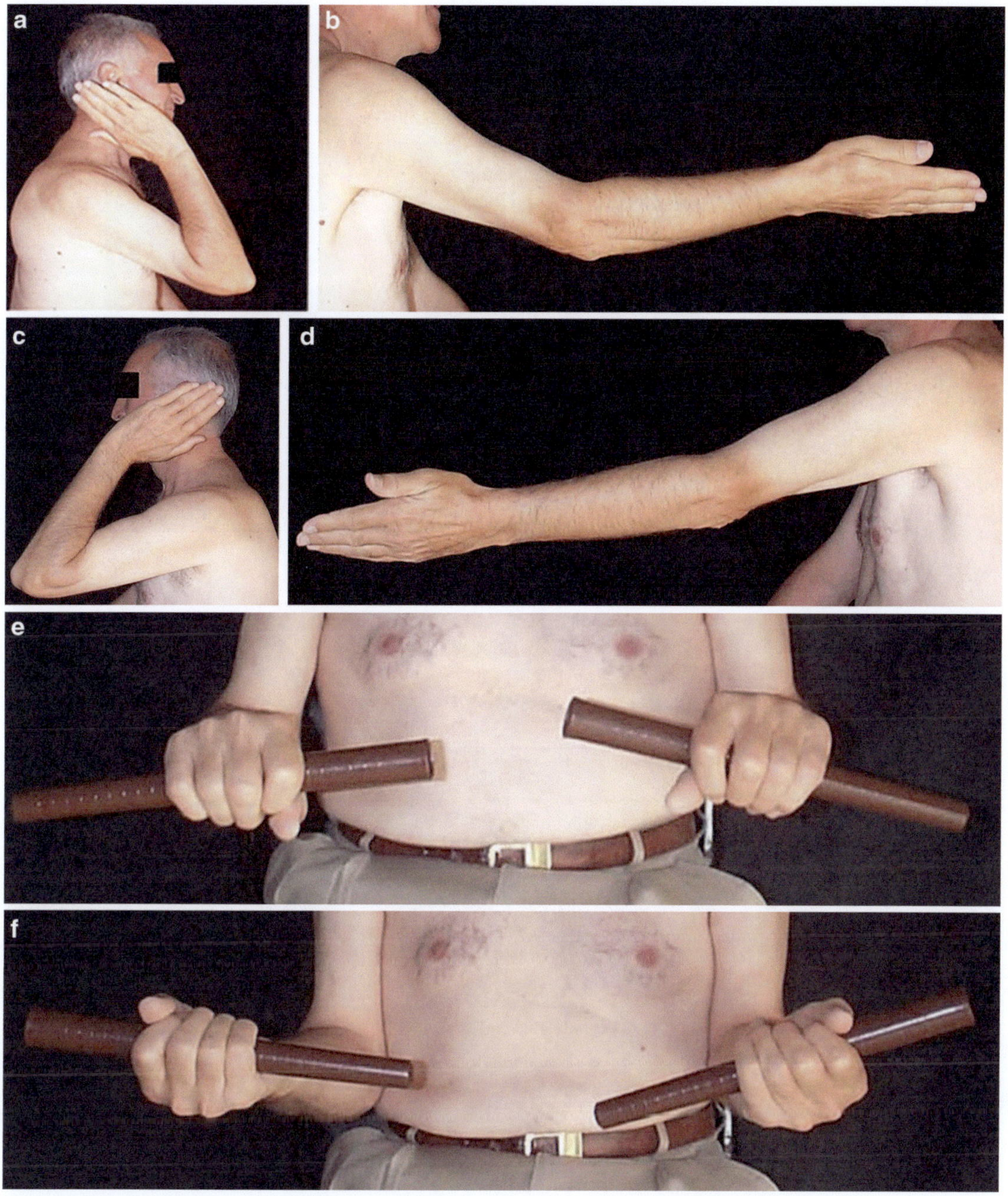

Fig. 25.9 (**a**, **b**): Bilateral TEA: right elbow flexion–extension at 14-year follow-up. (**c**, **d**) Bilateral TEA: left elbow flexion–extension at 16-year follow-up. (**e**, **f**) Bilateral TEA: bilateral pronation–supination

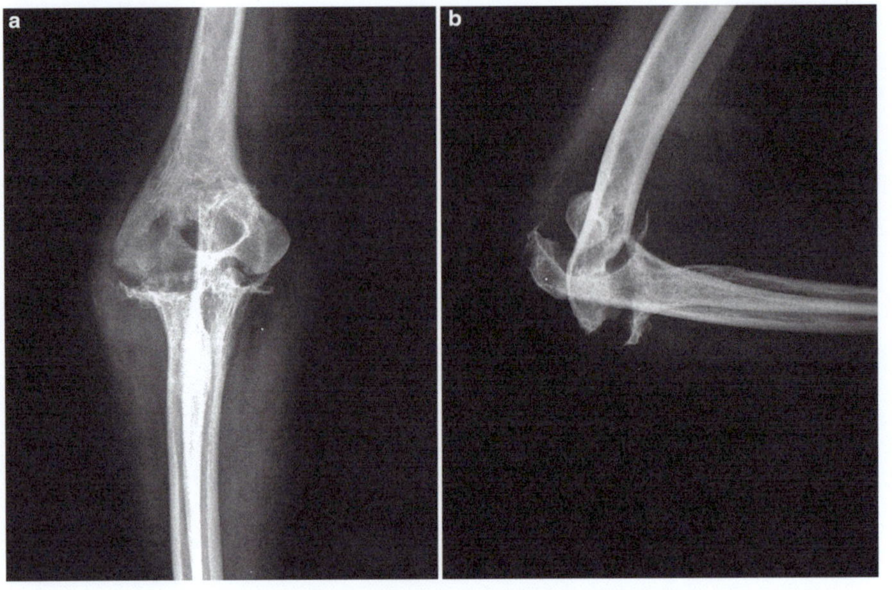

Fig. 25.10 (**a**, **b**) Homolateral TEA and TWA. Right elbow preoperative X-rays

Fig. 25.11 (**a**, **b**) Homolateral TEA and TWA. Right Coonrad–Morrey TEA. X-rays at 9-year follow-up

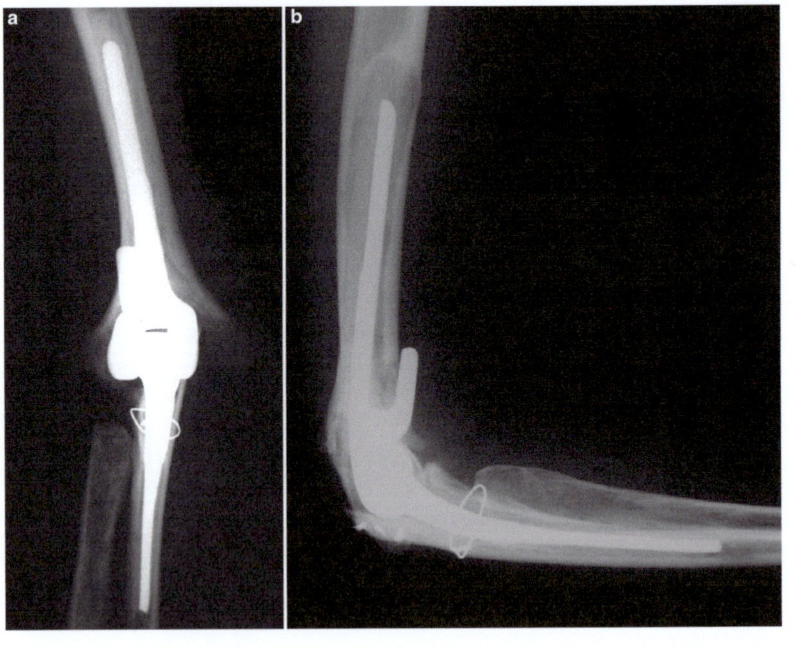

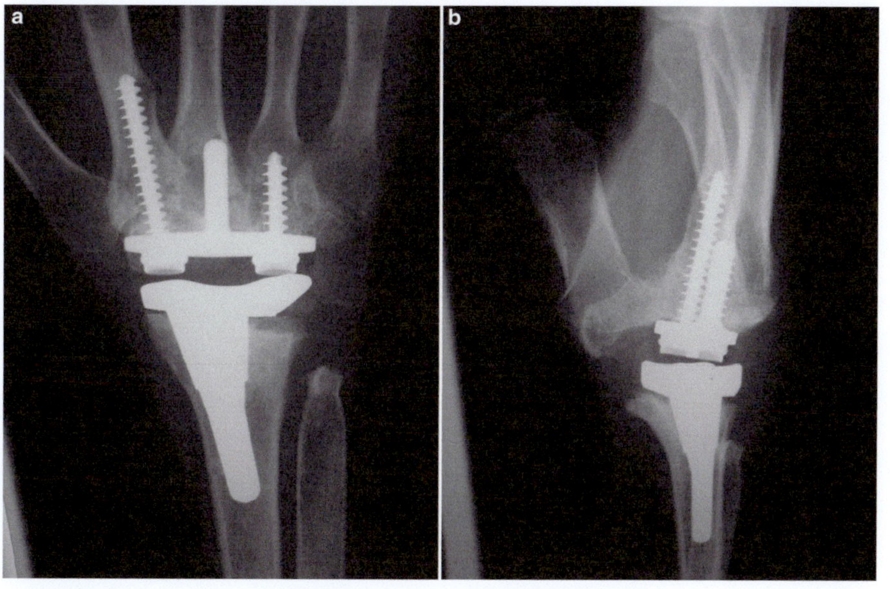

Fig. 25.12 (**a**, **b**) Homolateral TEA and TWA. Right wrist implant at 9-year follow-up

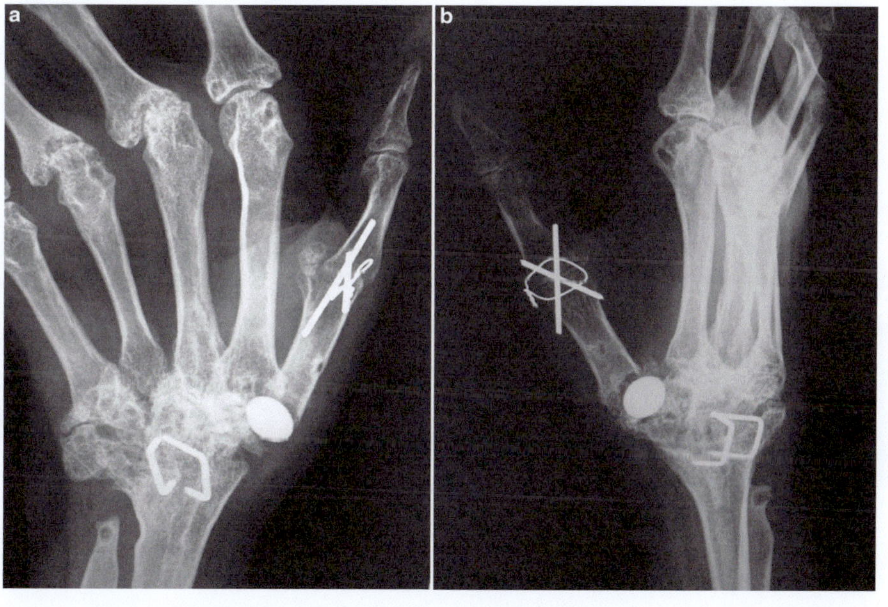

Fig. 25.13 (**a**, **b**) Homolateral TEA and TWA. Left wrist fusion associated to pyrocarbon CMC spacer and MP thumb fusion

Fig. 25.14 Homolateral TEA and TWA. Humeral component revision for aseptic loosening

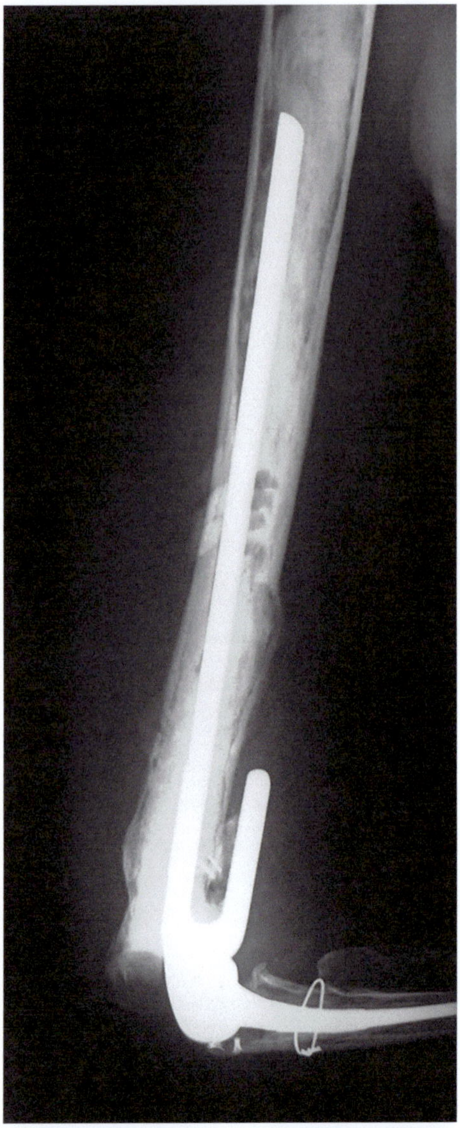

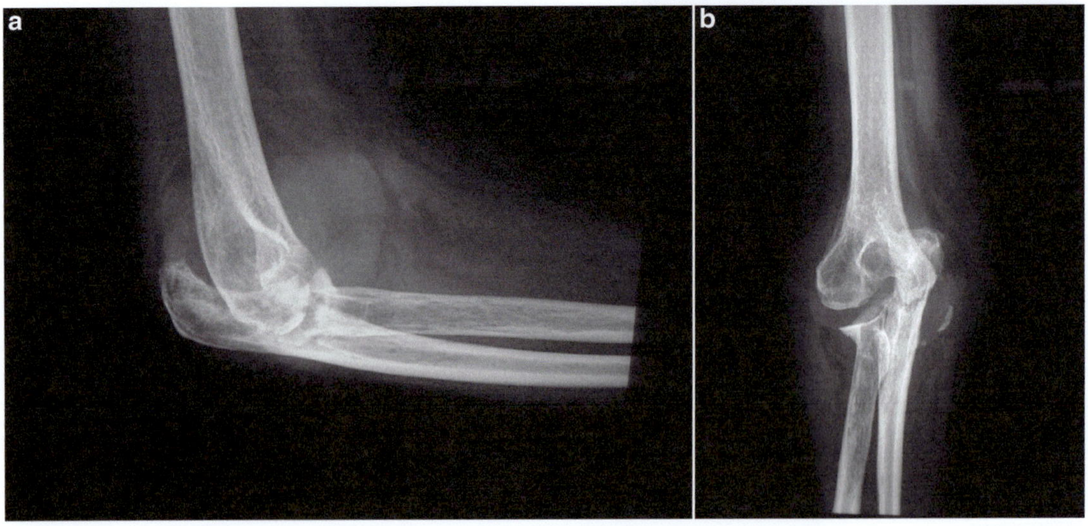

Fig. 25.15 (**a**, **b**) TEA in psoriatic oligoarthritis. Right elbow preoperative X-rays

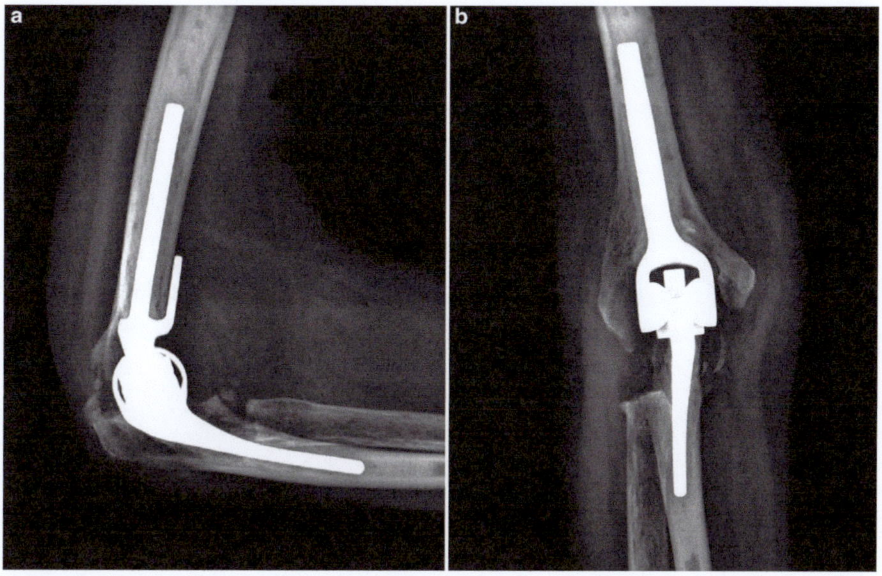

Fig. 25.16 (**a**, **b**) TEA in psoriatic oligoarthritis. Total semi-constrained discovery implant at 2-year follow-up

Fig. 25.17 Polyarticular RA. Dorsal skin dehiscence following left TEA

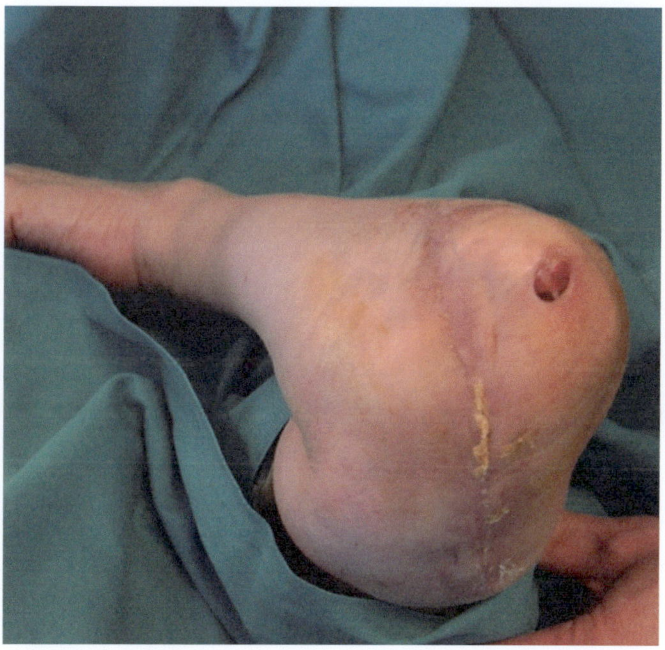

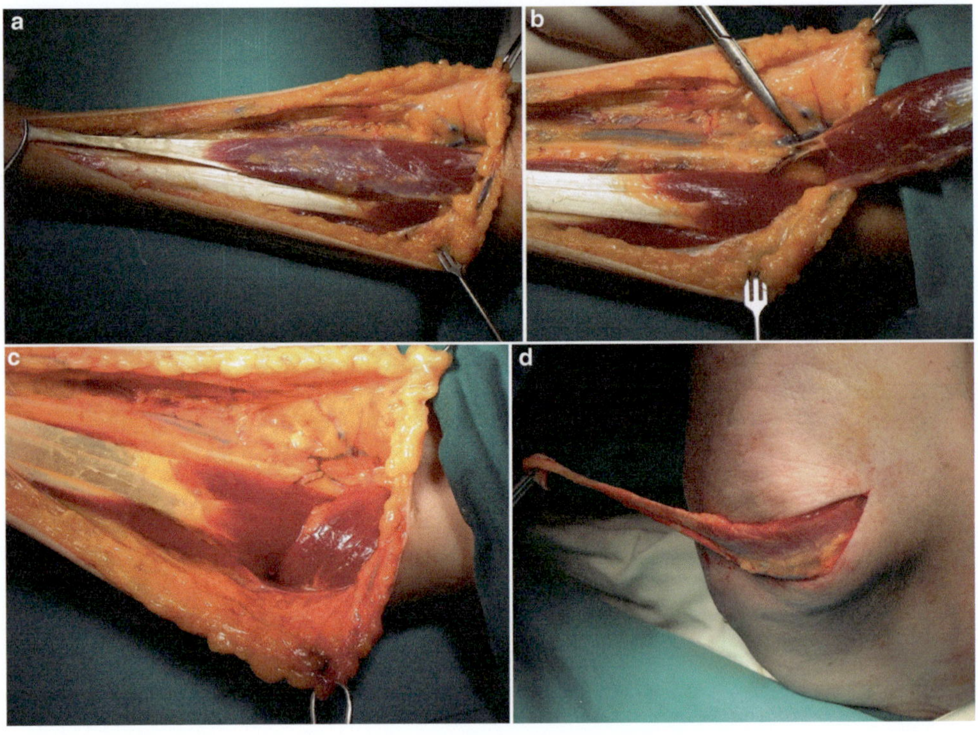

Fig. 25.18 Dorsal skin dehiscence: pedicled brachioradialis muscle flap. (**a**) The BR muscle is isolated, (**b**) the proximal vascular pedicle is identified, and (**c**, **d**) rotation of the flap and coverage of the olecranon exposure

Fig. 25.19 BR flap. Clinical control at 7-year follow-up

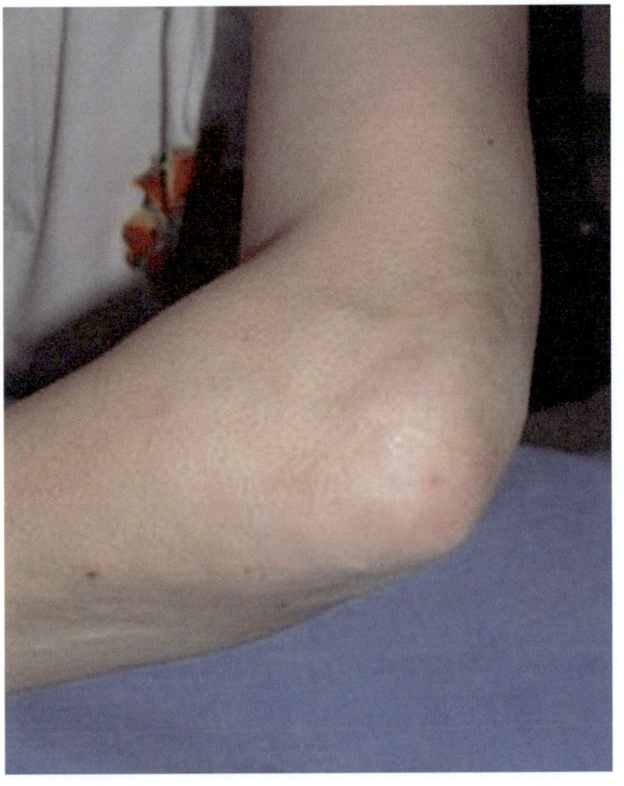

References

1. Studer A, Athwal GS. Rheumatoid arthritis of the elbow. Hand Clin. 2011;27(2):139–50.
2. Kapetanovic MC, Lindqvist E, Saxne T, et al. Orthopaedic surgery in patients with rheumatoid arthritis over 20 years: prevalence and predictive factors of large joint replacement. Ann Rheum Dis. 2008;67:1412–8.
3. Flury MP, Herren DB, Simmen BR. Rheumatoid arthritis of the wrist. Classification related to the natural course. Clin Orthop Relat Res. 1999;366:72–7.
4. Dyer GS, Blazar PE. Rheumatoid elbow. Hand Clin. 2011;27(1):43–8.
5. Bernardino S. Total elbow arthroplasty: history, current concepts and future. Clin Rheumatol. 2010;29:1217–21.
6. Kaneko A, et al. Development and validation of a new radiographic scoring system to evaluate bone and cartilage destruction and healing of large joints with rheumatoid arthritis: Arashi (Assessment of rheumatoid arthritis by scoring of large joint destruction and healing in radiographic imaging) study. Mod Rheumatol. 2013;23(6):1053–62.
7. Soubeyrand M, Wassermann V, Hirsch C, Oberlin C, Gagey O, Dumontier C. The middle radioulnar joint and triarticular forearm complex. J Hand Surg Eur Vol. 2011;36(6):447–54.
8. Baghdadi YM, et al. The outcome of total elbow arthroplasty in juvenile idiopathic arthritis (juvenile rheumatoid arthritis) patients. J Shoulder Elbow Surg. 2014;23(9):1374–80.
9. Peden JP, Morrey BF. Total elbow replacement for the management of the ankylosed or fused elbow. J Bone Joint Surg Br. 2008;90:1198–204.
10. Celli A, Morrey BF. Total elbow arthroplasty in patients forty years of age or less. J Bone Joint Surg Am. 2009;91:1414–8.
11. Ishii K, Inaba Y, Mochida Y, Saito T. Good long-term outcome of synovectomy in advanced stages of the rheumatoid elbow 64 elbows followed for 10–23 years. Acta Orthop. 2012;83(4):374–8.
12. Fuerst MB, Fink B, Rüther W. Survival analysis and long-term results of elbow synovectomy in rheumatoid arthritis. J Rheumatol. 2006;33:892–6.
13. Hastings H, Lee DH, Pietrzak WS. A prospective multicenter clinical study of the discovery elbow. J Shoulder Elbow Surg. 2014;23:95–107.
14. Rohrich RJ, Ingram Jr AE. Brachioradialis muscle flap: clinical anatomy and use in soft-tissue reconstruction of the elbow. Ann Plast Surg. 1995;35(1):70–6.

Index

K.C. Chung (ed.), *Clinical Management of the Rheumatoid Hand, Wrist, and Elbow*,
DOI 10.1007/978-3-319-26660-2

T

U

V

W

X

Z

MIX
Papier aus verantwortungsvollen Quellen
Paper from responsible sources
FSC® C105338

If you have any concerns about our products,
you can contact us on
ProductSafety@springernature.com

In case Publisher is established outside the EU,
the EU authorized representative is:
Springer Nature Customer Service Center GmbH
Europaplatz 3, 69115 Heidelberg, Germany

Printed by Libri Plureos GmbH
in Hamburg, Germany